Management of CANCER
IN THE OLDER PATIENT

Management of
CANCER
IN THE OLDER PATIENT

Arash Naeim, MD PhD
Director of Geriatric Oncology
Director of the Hematology-Oncology Fellowship Program
Divisions of Hematology-Oncology and Geriatric Medicine
Associate Professor, David Geffen School of Medicine
University of California Los Angeles
Los Angeles, California

David B. Reuben, MD
Director, Multicampus Program in Geriatric Medicine and Gerontology
Chief, Division of Geriatrics
Archstone Professor of Medicine
David Geffen School of Medicine
University of California Los Angeles
Los Angeles, California

Patricia A. Ganz, MD
Professor, David Geffen School of Medicine
School of Public Health
University of California Los Angeles
Director, Division of Cancer Prevention and Control Research
Jonsson Comprehensive Cancer Center
Los Angeles, California

ELSEVIER
SAUNDERS

1600 John F. Kennedy Blvd.
Ste 1800
Philadelphia, PA 19103-2899

MANAGEMENT OF CANCER IN THE OLDER PATIENT   ISBN: 978-1-4377-1398-5

Library of Congress Cataloging-in-Publication Data

Management of cancer in the older patient / [edited by] Arash Naeim, David B. Reuben,
Patricia A. Ganz.
   p. ; cm.
 Includes bibliographical references and index.
 ISBN 978-1-4377-1398-5 (hardback : alk. paper) 1. Geriatric oncology. I. Naeim, Arash.
II. Reuben, David B. III. Ganz, Patricia.
 [DNLM: 1. Neoplasms—therapy. 2. Aged. QZ 266]
 RC281.A34M36 2012
 618.97′6994—dc23

                                               2011016975

Acquisitions Editor: Kate Dimock
Developmental Editor: Kate Crowley
Publishing Services Manager: Hemamalini Rajendrababu
Senior Project Manager: Srikumar Narayanan
Designer: Ellen Zanolle

Printed in China
Last digit is the print number: 9 8 7 6 5 4 3 2 1

To Arya and Shayan for their inspiration. My hope is that I can be nearly as good a father to you as my dad is to me.

To all those older individuals with cancer who have taught me that life is richer when living with dignity, quality, and passion.

Arash Naeim

For all my older patients, friends, and family members who have fought their battles with cancer.

David Reuben

Thanks to my family for the love and support and especially to my parents and my husband's parents who have taught us so much about aging and its impact on health and quality of life.

Patricia Ganz

CONTRIBUTORS

Sunil Amalraj, MD
Geriatric-Oncology Fellow
Divisions of Hematology and
  Geriatric Medicine
David Geffen School of Medicine
University of California Los Angeles
Los Angeles, California

Lodovico Balducci, MD
Professor of Oncologic Sciences
University of South Florida College
  of Medicine
Medical Director of Affiliates and
  Referring Physician Relations
Program Leader of Senior Adult
  Oncology
Moffitt Cancer Center
Tampa, Florida

Daniel Becker, MD
General Medicine, Geriatrics and
  Palliative Care
University of Virginia Health System
Charlottesville, Virginia

Susan Charette, MD
Assistant Professor of Medicine,
  Geriatrics
Department of Medicine
University of California Los Angeles
Los Angeles, California

Octavio Choi, MD, PhD
Department of Psychiatry
Department of Medicine
University of California Los Angeles
Los Angeles, California

Kerri M. Clough-Gorr, DSc, MPH
National Institute for Cancer
  Epidemiology and Registration
  (NICER) Institute of Social and
  Preventive Medicine (ISPM)
University of Zürich
Zürich, Switzerland
Institute of Social and Preventive
  Medicine (ISPM)
University of Bern
Bern, Switzerland
Section of Geriatrics
Boston University Medical Center
Boston, Massachusetts

Melissa Cohen, MD
Geriatric-Oncology Fellow
Divisions of Hematology and
  Geriatric Medicine
David Geffen School of Medicine
University of California Los Angeles
Los Angeles, California

Jennifer M. Croswell, MD, MPH
Acting Director
Office of Medical Applications of
  Research
National Institutes of Health
Bethesda, Maryland

Lucia Loredana Dattoma, MD
Geriatric Medicine
Ronald Reagan UCLA Medical
  Center
Santa Monica UCLA Medical
  Center and Orthopaedic Hospital
Stewart and Lynda Resnick
  Neuropsychiatric Hospital
University of California Los Angeles
Los Angeles, California

James W. Davis Jr., MD
Clinical Professor
Division of Geriatrics
University of California Los Angeles
Los Angeles, California

Roxana S. Dronca, MD
Assistant Professor of Oncology
Instructor in Medicine
Department of Oncology
Mayo Clinic
Rochester, Minnesota

Amy A. Edgington, RN, NP-BC
Division of Cancer Prevention and
  Control Research
Jonsson Comprehensive Cancer
  Center
David Geffen School of Medicine
School of Public Health
University of California Los Angeles
Los Angeles, California

William B. Ershler, MD
Deputy Clinical Director
Intramural Research Program
National Institute on Aging
National Institutes of Health
Bethesda, Maryland

Randall Espinoza, MD, MPH
Professor
Department of Psychiatry and
  Biobehavioral Sciences
David Geffen School of Medicine
University of California Los Angeles
Director
Geriatric Psychiatry Fellowship
  Training Program
Medical Director
ECT Program
Associate Director
Center on Aging
University of California Los Angeles
Los Angeles, California

**Betty Ferrell, PhD, MA, FAAN,
  FPCN**
Professor and Research Scientist
Nursing Research and Education
Department of Population Sciences
City of Hope Comprehensive
  Cancer Center
Duarte, California

Bruce Ferrell, MD
Professor of Medicine/Geriatric
  Medicine
David Geffen School of Medicine
University of California Los Angeles
Los Angeles, California

Patricia A. Ganz, MD
Professor
David Geffen School of Medicine
School of Public Health
University of California Los Angeles
Director, Division of Cancer
  Prevention and Control Research
Jonsson Comprehensive Cancer
  Center
Los Angeles, California

Barbara A. Given, PhD, RN, FAAN
University Distinguished Professor
Associate Dean of Research and Doctoral Program
College of Nursing
Michigan State University
East Lansing, Michigan

Charles W. Given, PhD
Professor
Department of Family Medicine
College of Human Medicine
Michigan State University
East Lansing, Michigan

Erin E. Hahn, MPH
Division of Cancer Prevention and Control Research
Jonsson Comprehensive Cancer Center
David Geffen School of Medicine
School of Public Health
University of California Los Angeles
Los Angeles, California

David M. Heimann, MD
Assistant Professor of Surgery
Mt. Sinai School of Medicine
Surgical Oncologist
Queens Cancer Center
Jamaica, New York

Dawn L. Hershman, MD, MS
Assistant Professor of Medicine and Epidemiology
Co-Director
Breast Cancer Program
Herbert Irving Comprehensive Cancer Center
Department of Medicine
Columbia University
New York, New York

Arti Hurria, MD
Associate Professor
Department of Medical Oncology and Experimental
    Therapeutics and Cancer Control and Population
    Sciences Program
Director
Cancer and Aging Research Program
City of Hope Comprehensive Cancer Center
Duarte, California

William Irvin Jr., MD
Assistant Professor of Medicine
University of North Carolina at Chapel Hill Division of
    Hematology/Oncology
Lineberger Comprehensive Cancer Center
Chapel Hill, North Carolina

Michael R. Irwin, MD
Norman Cousins Professor of Psychiatry and
    Biobehavioral Sciences
David Geffen School of Medicine
Professor of Psychology
College of Letters and Sciences
Director
Cousins Center for Psychoneuroimmunology
Semel Institute for Neuroscience
University of California Los Angeles
Los Angeles, California

Pattie Jakel, RN, MN, AOCN
Clinical Nurse Specialist
Clinical Research Center
University of California Los Angeles
Los Angeles, California

Bindu Kanapuru, MD
Clinical Research Fellow
Clinical Research Branch
National Institute on Aging
National Institutes of Health
Baltimore, Maryland

M. Margaret Kemeny, MD, FACS
Professor of Surgery
Mt. Sinai School of Medicine
Director
Queens Cancer Center
Jamaica, New York

Barnett S. Kramer, MD, MPH
Editor-in-Chief
Journal of the National Cancer Institute
Data Query (PDQ) Screening and Prevention Editorial
    Board
Rockville, Maryland
Associate Director for Disease Prevention
Office of Disease Prevention
National Institutes of Health
Bethesda, Maryland

Stuart M. Lichtman, MD
Attending Physician
Clinical Geriatrics Program
Memorial Sloan-Kettering Cancer Center
New York, New York

Charles Loprinzi, MD
Regis Professor of Breast Cancer Research
Division of Medical Oncology
Mayo Clinic
Rochester, Minnesota

Jeffrey Mariano, MD
Assistant Clinical Professor of Medicine/Geriatric
    Medicine
David Geffen School of Medicine
University of California Los Angeles
Los Angeles, California

Susan McCloskey, MD
Department of Radiation Oncology
Ronald Reagan UCLA Medical Center
Santa Monica UCLA Medical Center and Orthopaedic
    Hospital
University of California Los Angeles
Los Angeles, California

Joseph Albert Melocoton, RN, MSN, OCN
Oncology Nurse Practitioner
Wilshire Oncology Medical Group, Inc.
Pasadena, California

Lillian C. Min, MD
Assistant Professor
Department of Internal Medicine
University of Michigan
Ann Arbor, Michigan

Hyman B. Muss, MD
Professor of Medicine
University of North Carolina at Chapel Hill
Director of Geriatric Oncology
Lineberger Comprehensive Cancer Center
Chapel Hill, North Carolina

Arash Naeim, MD PhD
Director of Geriatric Oncology
Director of the Hematology-Oncology Fellowship Program
Divisions of Hematology-Oncology and Geriatric
    Medicine
Associate Professor
David Geffen School of Medicine
University of California Los Angeles
Los Angeles, California

Sumanta Kumar Pal, MD
Assistant Professor
Division of Genitourinary Malignancies
Department of Medical Oncology and Experimental
    Therapeutics
City of Hope Comprehensive Cancer Center
Duarte, California

Janet Pregler, MD
Professor of Clinical Medicine
Director
Iris Cantor–UCLA Women's Health Center
David Geffen School of Medicine
University of California Los Angeles
Los Angeles, California

Scott D. Ramsey, MD, PhD
Associate Professor of Medicine and Health Services
Associate Member
Cancer Prevention Research Program
Fred Hutchinson Cancer Research Center
Division of General Internal Medicine
University of Washington
Seattle, Washington

David B. Reuben, MD
Director
Multicampus Program in Geriatric Medicine and
    Gerontology
Chief
Division of Geriatrics
Archstone Professor of Medicine
David Geffen School of Medicine
University of California Los Angeles
Los Angeles, California

Lisa M. Schwartz, MD
Medical Director
Integrative Medicine
Roy and Patricia Disney Family Cancer Center
Providence Saint Joseph Medical Center
Burbank, California

John F. Scoggins, PhD, MS
Senior Research Fellow
Fred Hutchinson Cancer Research Center
University of Washington
Seattle, Washington

Mary E. Sehl, MD, PhD
Physician
Divisions of Geriatrics and Hematology-Oncology
David Geffen School of Medicine
University of California Los Angeles
Los Angeles, California

Veena Shankaran, MD
Assistant Professor
Medical Oncology
Assistant Member
Clinical Research Division
Fred Hutchinson Cancer Research Center
University of Washington
Seattle, Washington

Paula Sherwood, PhD, RN, CNRN
Associate Professor
University of Pittsburgh School of Nursing
Pittsburgh, Pennsylvania

Rebecca A. Silliman, MD, PhD
Professor
Department of Medicine
Department of Epidemiology
Boston University School of Medicine
Boston, Massachusetts

Michael L. Steinberg, MD
Professor and Chair
Department of Radiation Oncology
David Geffen School of Medicine
University of California Los Angeles
Los Angeles, California

Virginia Sun, RN, PhD
Assistant Research Professor
Division of Nursing Research and Education
Department of Cancer Control and Population Sciences
City of Hope
Duarte, California

Tiffany A. Traina, MD
Assistant Attending Physician
Breast Cancer Medicine Service
Memorial Sloan-Kettering Cancer Center
New York, New York

Anne Walling, MD
Ronald Reagan UCLA Medical Center
Santa Monica UCLA Medical Center and Orthopaedic
    Hospital
University of California Los Angeles
Los Angeles, California

Peter Ward, MD
Geriatric-Oncology Fellow
Divisions of Hematology and Geriatric Medicine
David Geffen School of Medicine
University of California Los Angeles
Los Angeles, California

Neil S. Wenger, MD, MPH
Professor of Medicine
Director
UCLA Health System Ethics Center
Chair
Ethics Committee
Ronald Reagan UCLA Medical Center
Santa Monica UCLA Medical Center and Orthopaedic
    Hospital
University of California Los Angeles
Los Angeles, California

Elizabeth Whiteman, MD
Department of Geriatric Medicine
University of California Los Angeles
Los Angeles, California

Jeffrey Wu, MD
Division of Radiation Oncology
David Geffen School of Medicine
University of California Los Angeles
Los Angeles, California

Jerome W. Yates, MD, MPH
Senior Vice President
Population Sciences and Health Services Research
Roswell Park Cancer Institute
Professor of Medicine
State University of New York at Buffalo
Buffalo, New York

Marjorie G. Zauderer, MD
Hematology-Oncology Fellow
Department of Medicine
Memorial Sloan-Kettering Cancer Center
New York, New York

The population is aging. It is estimated that 1 in 5 individuals will be older than 65 years by the year 2030. The risk of cancer increases with age, with persons older than age 75 having the highest risk. Individuals older than age 65 also account for greater than two thirds of all cancer deaths. The demand for cancer care will steadily grow, but workforce projections for the next decade demonstrate that the supply of oncologists will not meet this demand. Therefore it is critically important for primary care providers (general practitioners, family practitioners, internists, and nurse practitioners) to become more familiar with the *Management of Cancer in the Older Patient*.

A frequent comment among general oncologists is that they mostly see older individuals, a viewpoint supported by the epidemiologic data. It is important to note that most of the evidence supporting treatment recommendations in oncology is derived from clinical trials where older individuals were significantly underrepresented. Moreover, those older individuals who did participate in clinical trials usually represented a healthy cohort with minimal competing comorbid conditions and little impairment in physical functioning. As a result, it is often hard to know how to generalize the evidence base to everyday practice or apply it to the average older patient with cancer.

Older individuals tend to be a more heterogeneous population. Although only 1 in 10 individuals has a functional impairment between the ages of 65 and 74, this number increases to almost half for patients over the age of 85. Similarly, as individuals age, the number of other co-existing conditions (comorbidity) increases as well, with individuals over the age of 75 having, on average, 5 other health conditions. Age, functional status, and comorbidity alter the lens through which providers view the older patient with cancer. These perceptions affect their approach to screening and prevention, diagnosis, treatment, supportive care, and survivorship care. In these areas, the role of the primary care provider extends beyond just screening, diagnosis, and referral to also include comanagement, aftercare, and long-term surveillance.

In parallel to the clinical practice of cancer care, the field of oncology is quickly being transformed. There is a large growth of research in molecular and cell biology, as well as immunology. Over the last decade, numerous new targeted therapies have received approval from the Food and Drug Administration. These newer therapies often have a more pronounced therapeutic effect but have different side effect profiles than traditional chemotherapy. There is an increasing trend toward personalizing or individualizing treatment based on the underlying biology of the individual and/or the tumor. In older patients with cancer, it will be important to combine these advances with the recognition that host factors that are markers for frailty also need to be factored into the process of individualizing care. The drug advances in cancer care are also associated with the high cost of treatment, which, when combined with increasingly large numbers of elderly patients, will put a strain on the resources allocated to health care.

The *Management of Cancer in the Older Patient* examines the key issues that a primary care provider would encounter in providing and supporting the care of an older patient. The book is divided into six sections. Section I, Screening/Prevention, examines key guidelines for screening and discusses populations for which screening may be underutilized or overutilized. Section II, Diagnosis/Assessment, examines diagnostic workup, assessment (geriatric assessment, functional assessment, and comorbidity), as well as the value of a second opinion. Section III, Treatment, examines modalities of treatment (surgery, radiation, and chemotherapy) with special chapters on novel and targeted therapies, clinical trials in the elderly, and shared treatment decision making. Section IV is focused entirely on supportive care with special chapters on insomnia and complementary and alternative care. Section V focuses on rehabilitation, surveillance, and survivorship. Section VI, the last section, examines important issues including home care, caregiver burden, communication, end of life and hospice, ethical issues, and economic issues important to managing the older cancer patient.

Most of the chapters in *Management of Cancer in the Older Patient* are case based with the use of summary and key tables to help synthesize the information. Whenever possible, we have included a suggested reading list that may be valuable to the reader. The goal of this book is to take a multidisciplinary approach to traditional topics such as prevention, screening, diagnosis, treatment, and survivorship while applying a geriatric lens to these issues, focusing on functioning, assessment, frailty, quality of care, quality of life, caregivers, and cost. Our hope is that this book makes a very practical contribution to improve the decision-making process of primary care providers, who often serve as the central resource or "quarterback" in the care of older complex patients. The editors are excited to contribute to a field that will be increasingly important as the number of older Americans with cancer rises dramatically in the coming decades.

ACKNOWLEDGMENTS

There are many people who contributed to this book project. First, I would like to thank my father who is a great role model and shared his experiences associated with the several books he has published to date.

This book would not exist without the tremendous efforts of the Elsevier publishing and editorial team. Mara Conner went out of her way to help me find the right home for this book and connecting me to Druanne Martin, who was the force to get this book proposed and approved at Elsevier. Along the way this book was shepherded by many individuals including Dolores Meloni and Taylor Ball. The team that did the heavy lifting in the end to put this book together at Elsevier included Srikumar Narayan (Senior Project Manager),

Kate Crowley (Editorial Assistant), and Kate Dimock (Senior Acquisitions Editor). I would also like to thank the individuals at Elsevier who worked behind the scenes to make this book possible, including Patricia Tannian, Ellen Zanolle, Lesley Frazier, Cara Jespersen, Hemamalini Rajendrababu, and Claire Kramer. I really appreciate the help of all the staff and team at Elsevier.

I would like to thank my own assistant, Chelsea Starkweather, who spent countless hours reading through the chapters of this book and providing editorial suggestions.

Lastly, I would like to thank my co-editors, who placed their faith and time in this project.

Arash Naeim

CONTENTS

Screening/Prevention

SECTION

Screening/Prevention

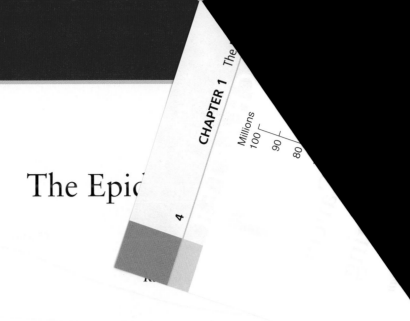

The Epid

Aging, a highly individualized process, is known to be related to changes in the physical, cognitive, emotional, social, and economic status of older adults. Increasing age is primarily associated with negative changes in these areas (e.g., increased comorbidity, decreased function, limited social support). These age-associated changes may occur singly or in combination, with broad variation among older adults. Moreover, they often result in considerable consequences not just for aging individuals themselves but simultaneously for health care systems, families, and caregivers.

A common late-life experience is a cancer diagnosis. According to the National Cancer Institute (NCI), aging is the most important risk factor for cancer, with most cancers occurring in persons aged 65 years and older. Over the last several decades, cancer trends have been changing contemporaneously with our knowledge of aging. Because of the increased heterogeneity of older populations, treating older cancer patients seldom means treating only the cancer. Furthermore, with improved screening and treatments, larger numbers of older cancer patients are experiencing longer-term survival. Unfortunately, even though older adults make up the largest segment of the cancer population, they are often undertreated and are seldom included in clinical trials. Few clinical trials are even designed to identify optimal treatments for them.

The combined effects of cancer and aging are of concern because of graying populations worldwide (a larger proportion aging in industrialized countries; greater numbers aging in developing countries). Although we cannot truly anticipate the changes that rapid population aging will bring, we can attempt to understand the epidemiological patterns of aging and cancer, where they intersect, and their potential implications. Such understanding will provide a frame of reference to address age-related disparities in research, education, and treatment in the older adult cancer population. Because of growing numbers alone, it is certain that management of cancer in older adults will continue to be a complex, resource-intensive, and increasingly common problem.

What follows herein is an overview of top... ing to the epidemiology of cancer and aging. in cancer incidence and mortality are examined, and the specific characteristics and unique issues related to older cancer patients are described. Special attention is provided to the survivorship experience of older cancer patients, along with a summary of the challenges associated with studying them.

INCIDENCE AND MORTALITY: THEN AND NOW

There have been remarkable changes in the United States population over the last century. One hallmark of these changes is the expansion of the older (65 years and older) population (Figure 1-1).[1] U.S. Census Bureau estimates show that the percentage of Americans 65 years and older has more than tripled (from 4.1% in 1900 to 12.8% in 2008). The older population itself is getting older; in 1940, 4.1% of the older population was 85 years or older (the "oldest old"), whereas in 2008, 14.7% was in this group. This trend toward greater longevity is reflected by tremendous growth in the centenarian population (approximately 120% from 1990 to 2008) and the current life expectancy estimates of older adults (Figure 1-2).[5,7] After the middle of the twentieth century, life expectancy at age 65 years increased moderately (5 years for men, 8 years for women) relative to life expectancy gains at birth. In recent years (1990 to 2005), the gap in life expectancy between older white and black people has been stable and narrower than at birth (difference at age 65 years approximately 2 years for men and 1 year for women).[8]

These aging trends will hasten with the senescence of the Baby Boom generation, but, on the basis of previous life expectancies, not necessarily uniformly across sex and race/ethnicity. The number of older Americans is expected to more than double by 2050 (increasing from 39 million in 2008 to 89 million) with substantial growth in older minority segments (Figure 1-3) and increasingly in female "oldest-olds."[2] The U.S. Census

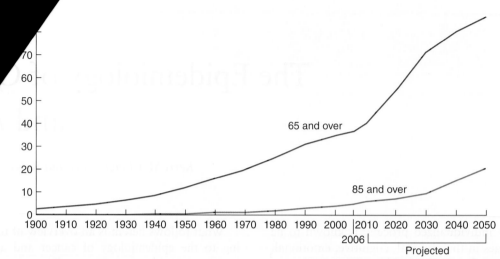

FIGURE 1-1 Number of people age 65 and older in the United States, by age group, selected years 1900-2006 and projected 2010-2050. *(Adapted from U.S. Department of Health and Human Services: A Profile of Older Americans: 2008. Washington, DC: Administration on Aging, 2008.)*

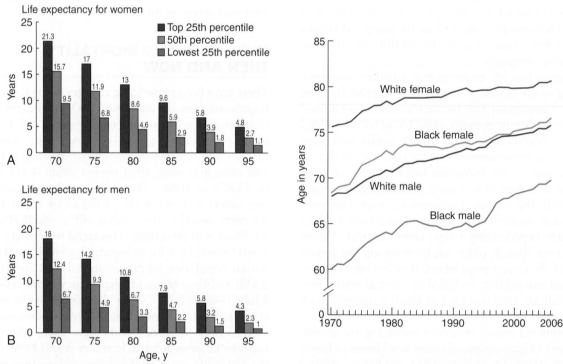

FIGURE 1-2 Life expectancy of older adults in the United States **A,** Upper, middle, and lower quartiles of life expectancy by sex at selected ages. *(Adapted from Walter LC, Covinsky KE. Cancer screening in elderly patients: a framework for individualized decision making. JAMA 2001;285:2750-6.)* **B,** Life expectancy for women and men by race 1970-2006. *(Adapted from Heron et al. Deaths: final data for 2006. National Vital Statistics Reports; Vol 57, No 14. Hyattsville, MD: National Center for Health Statistics; 2009.)*

Bureau also projects by 2050 a nearly 225% increase in persons aged 100 years and older (from 2008) and that, for the first time in United States history, the population older than 65 years will outnumber the population younger than 15 years. Figure 1-4 shows the overall projected age shift in the U.S. population pyramid from 2000 to 2050.[2]

As older Americans live longer than ever before, the inevitable shift in the population age structure foreshadows many challenges. Importantly, whether or

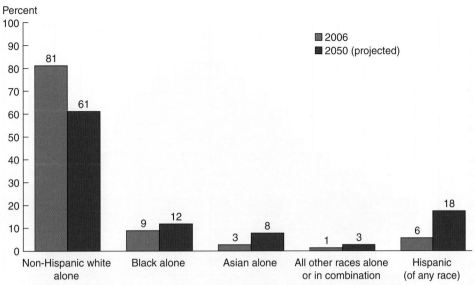

FIGURE 1-3 United States population age 65 and older by race and Hispanic origin, selected years 2006 and projected 2050. *(Adapted from U.S. Department of Health and Human Services: A Profile of Older Americans: 2008. Washington, DC: Administration on Aging, 2008.)*

not years added later in life are healthy, enjoyable, and productive depends in large part on prevention and control of potentially debilitating and sometimes fatal chronic diseases such as cancer. Figure 1-5 shows that cancer is the fourth most common chronic disease and the second leading cause of death in older adults in the United States.[1] Cancer is a disease that disproportionately affects older adults. Over the past decades, cancer incidence and mortality trends in the oldest population showed a greater burden than for those in the so-called young-old (65 to 74 years) and younger populations (Figure 1-6).[3]

The increased risk of cancer in older adults is proposed to be related to two main age-linked processes. Because cancer is a multistep process, over the course of longer lives there is both increased opportunity for DNA damage and longer exposure to potential carcinogens. Older adults, therefore, may have greater potential for accrued molecular damage coexisting with age-related decreased cellular repair activity leading to malignancies. This is supported by the epidemiological evidence, which consistently shows at least twofold or higher all-cause cancer mortality and incidence rates in older adults since SEER reporting began in 1975. From 2002 to 2006, the median age at diagnosis for cancer of all sites was 66 years.[9] However, looking at more finely stratified older age groups during the same period, approximately 24.9% of all cancers were diagnosed between 65 and 74 years, 22.2% between 75 and 84 years, and 7.6% at 85 years of age and older. These patterns hold across most primary cancer types. Within the older age groups, controversies exist over evidence pointing to a potential drop of cancer incidence and mortality in the oldest-old group. These data raise unresolved questions as to whether the effect is real and, if so, whether it is due to selective survival, an interaction with late-life biology, or both.

Trends in recent years in the older U.S. population show decreases in age-adjusted all-cause cancer mortality and incidence (–1.1 and –1.2 annual percent change 1997 to 2006, respectively).[3,6] However, trends and risks vary considerably by primary cancer site and sex (Figure 1-7 and Table 1-1).[6,10] In people 65 years of age and older, lung cancer incidence and mortality increased for women and decreased for men. Nonetheless, it was the second leading cancer site and the most fatal cancer (approximately 30% of all cancer deaths) in both women and men. The second- and third-ranked fatal cancers were breast and colorectal cancers in women and colorectal and prostate cancers in men. All showed varied but decreased mortality and incidence over time. The risk of colorectal cancer rose precipitously with age, with 91% of cases diagnosed in individuals aged 50 years of age and older, with moderate decreases in mortality and incidence (–2.9 and –3.0 annual percent change 1997 to 2006, respectively).[6,9,10]

There are also considerable differences in cancer burden and survival across race and ethnic populations (Figures 1-8 and 1-9).[4,6] All-cause cancer incidence and mortality rates have been higher, and relative survival rates lower, for African-Americans in comparison to whites. Hispanic, Asian, Pacific Islander, American Indian, and Alaska Native persons generally have lower incidence rates than whites, except for several specific cancers (e.g., stomach, liver, cervix, kidney, and gallbladder). This general pattern of lower incidence among racial and ethnic minorities has been attributed to younger age structures. However, cancer disparities in incidence, mortality, and late-stage presentation also exist within these groups by geography, national origin, economic status, and other factors. By 2050 and beyond, these disparities are expected to transition into the older age groups as demographic changes (i.e., growth in older

Text continued on p. 10

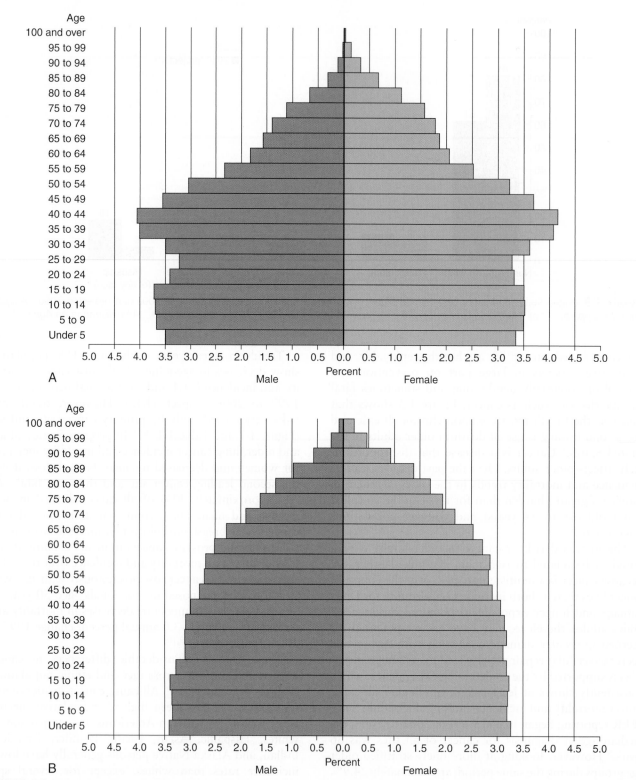

FIGURE 1-4 Population pyramids of the United States (*left*) 2000 and (*right*) projected 2050. *(Adapted from U.S. Census Bureau: Projections of the Population by Age and Sex for the United States: 2010 to 2050 (NP2008-T12). Washington, DC: Population Division, U.S. Census Bureau; 2008.)*

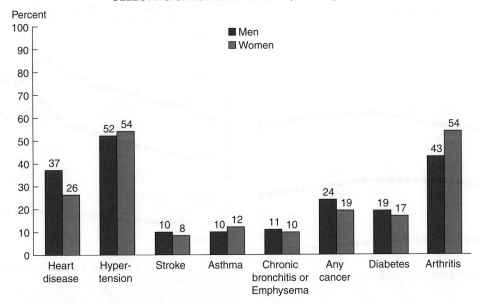

PERCENTAGE OF PEOPLE AGE 65 AND OVER WHO REPORTED HAVING
SELECTING CHRONIC CONDITIONS, BY SEX, 2005–2006

Note: Data are based on a 2-year average from 2005–2006.
Reference population: These data refer to the civilian noninstitutionalized population.
A   Source: Centers for Disease Control and Prevention, National Center for Health Statistics, National Health Interview Survey.

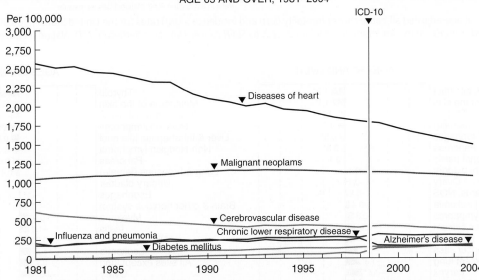

DEATH RATES FOR SELECTED LEADING CAUSES OF DEATH AMONG PEOPLE
AGE 65 AND OVER, 1981–2004

Note: Death rates for 1981–1998 are based on the 9th revision of the *International Classification of Diseases* (ICD-9). Starting in
1999, death rates are based on ICD-10 and trends in death rates for some causes may be affected by this change.[11] For the period
1981–1998, causes were coded using ICD-9 codes that are most nearly comparable with the 113 cause list for the ICD-10 and may
differ from previously published estimates. Rates are age adjusted using the 2000 standard population.
Reference population: These data refer to the resident population.
B   Source: Centers for Disease Control and Prevention, National Center for Health Statistics, National Vital Statistics System.

FIGURE 1-5 Incidence and mortality of chronic conditions in the population aged 65 and older in the United States. **A,** Percentage of population 65 years and older, by chronic condition and sex, 2005-2006. **B,** Mortality rates in population 65 years and older, by leading causes of death, 1981-2004. *(Adapted from U.S. Department of Health and Human Services: A Profile of Older Americans: 2008. Washington, DC: Administration on Aging, 2008.)*

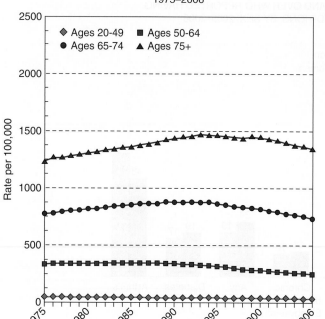

AGE-ADJUSTED U.S. MORTALITY RATES BY AGE AT
DIAGNOSIS/DEATH ALL SITES, ALL RACES, BOTH SEXES
1975–2006

Ages 20-49 Ages 50-64
Ages 65-74 Ages 75+

Rate per 100,000

Year of death

A

Cancer sites include invasive cases only unless otherwise noted.
Mortality source: US Mortality Files, National Center for Health Statistics, CDC.
Rates are per 100,000 and are age-adjusted to the 2000 US Std Population (19 age groups -
Census P25-1130). Regression lines are calculated using the Joinpoint Regression Program
Version 3.3.2, June 2008, National Cancer Institute.

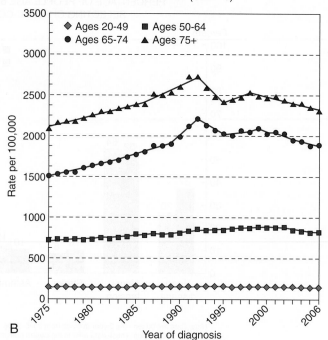

AGE-ADJUSTED SEER INCIDENCE RATES BY AGE AT
DIAGNOSIS/DEATH ALL SITES, ALL RACES, BOTH SEXES
1975–2006 (SEER 9)

Ages 20-49 Ages 50-64
Ages 65-74 Ages 75+

Rate per 100,000

Year of diagnosis

B

Cancer sites include invasive cases only unless otherwise noted.
Incidence source: SEER 9 areas (San Francisco, Connecticut, Detroit, Hawaii, Iowa, New
Mexico, Seattle, Utah and Atlanta).
Rates are per 100,000 and are age-adjusted to the 2000 US Std Population (19 age groups -
Census P25-1130). Regression lines are calculated using the Joinpoint Regression Program
Version 3.3.2, June 2008, National Cancer Institute.

FIGURE 1-6 Trends of age-adjusted all-cause cancer mortality (*left*) and incidence (*right*) rates for the United States population, by age group, 1975-2006. (*Adapted from FastStats: An interactive tool for access to SEER cancer statistics. Bethesda, MD, National Cancer Institute, 2009.*)

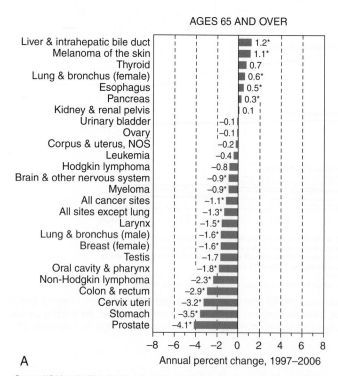

AGES 65 AND OVER

	Annual percent change, 1997–2006
Liver & intrahepatic bile duct	1.2*
Melanoma of the skin	1.1*
Thyroid	0.7
Lung & bronchus (female)	0.6*
Esophagus	0.5*
Pancreas	0.3*
Kidney & renal pelvis	0.1
Urinary bladder	−0.1
Ovary	−0.1
Corpus & uterus, NOS	−0.2
Leukemia	−0.4
Hodgkin lymphoma	−0.8
Brain & other nervous system	−0.9*
Myeloma	−0.9*
All cancer sites	−1.1*
All sites except lung	−1.3*
Larynx	−1.5*
Lung & bronchus (male)	−1.6*
Breast (female)	−1.6*
Testis	−1.7
Oral cavity & pharynx	−1.8*
Non-Hodgkin lymphoma	−2.3*
Colon & rectum	−2.9*
Cervix uteri	−3.2*
Stomach	−3.5*
Prostate	−4.1*

A

Source: US Mortality Files, National Center for Health Statistics, Centers for Disease Control
and Prevention. For sex-specific cancer sites, the population was limited to the population of
the appropriate sex.
* Underlying rates are per 100,000 and age-adjusted to the 2000 US Std Population (19 age
groups - Census P25-1103). The Annual Percent Change is significantly different from zero
(p<.05).

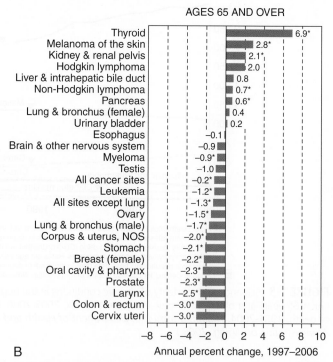

AGES 65 AND OVER

	Annual percent change, 1997–2006
Thyroid	6.9*
Melanoma of the skin	2.8*
Kidney & renal pelvis	2.1*
Hodgkin lymphoma	2.0
Liver & intrahepatic bile duct	0.8
Non-Hodgkin lymphoma	0.7*
Pancreas	0.6*
Lung & bronchus (female)	0.4
Urinary bladder	0.2
Esophagus	−0.1
Brain & other nervous system	−0.9
Myeloma	−0.9*
Testis	−1.0
All cancer sites	−0.2*
Leukemia	−1.2*
All sites except lung	−1.3*
Ovary	−1.5*
Lung & bronchus (male)	−1.7*
Corpus & uterus, NOS	−2.0*
Stomach	−2.1*
Breast (female)	−2.2*
Oral cavity & pharynx	−2.3*
Prostate	−2.3*
Larynx	−2.5*
Colon & rectum	−3.0*
Cervix uteri	−3.0*

B

Source: US Mortality Files, National Center for Health Statistics, Centers for Disease Control
and Prevention. For sex-specific cancer sites, the population was limited to the population of
the appropriate sex.
* Underlying rates are per 100,000 and age-adjusted to the 2000 US Std Population (19 age
groups - Census P25-1103). The Annual Percent Change is significantly different from zero
(p<.05).

FIGURE 1-7 Change in trends of age-adjusted all-cause cancer mortality (*left*) and incidence (*right*) rates for the population aged 65 and older in the United States, by primary cancer site, 1997-2006. (*Adapted from SEER Cancer Statistics Review, 1975-2006. Bethesda, MD, National Cancer Institute, 2009.*)

| TABLE 1-1 | Probability of Developing Cancer for Selected Age Groups in the United States,* by Sex, 2003 to 2005 |

Cancer Site	Sex	Birth to 39 Years (Percentage)	40 to 59 Years (Percentage)	60 to 69 Years (Percentage)	70 Years and Older (Percentage)	Birth to Death (Percentage)
All sites†	Male	1.42 (1 in 70)	8.44 (1 in 12)	15.71 (1 in 6)	37.74 (1 in 3)	43.89 (1 in 2)
	Female	2.07 (1 in 48)	8.97 (1 in 11)	10.23 (1 in 10)	26.17 (1 in 4)	37.35 (1 in 3)
Urinary bladder‡	Male	0.02 (1 in 4448)	0.41 (1 in 246)	0.96 (1 in 104)	3.57 (1 in 28)	3.74 (1 in 27)
	Female	0.01 (1 in 10,185)	0.12 (1 in 810)	0.26 (1 in 378)	1.01 (1 in 99)	1.18 (1 in 84)
Breast	Female	0.48 (1 in 208)	3.79 (1 in 26)	3.41 (1 in 29)	6.44 (1 in 16)	12.03 (1 in 8)
Colon and rectum	Male	0.08 (1 in 1296)	0.92 (1 in 109)	1.55 (1 in 65)	4.63 (1 in 22)	5.51 (1 in 18)
	Female	0.07 (1 in 1343)	0.72 (1 in 138)	1.10 (1 in 91)	4.16 (1 in 24)	5.10 (1 in 20)
Leukemia	Male	0.16 (1 in 611)	0.22 (1 in 463)	0.35 (1 in 289)	1.17 (1 in 85)	1.50 (1 in 67)
	Female	0.12 (1 in 835)	0.14 (1 in 693)	0.20 (1 in 496)	0.77 (1 in 130)	1.07 (1 in 94)
Lung and bronchus	Male	0.03 (1 in 3398)	0.99 (1 in 101)	2.43 (1 in 41)	6.70 (1 in 18)	7.78 (1 in 13)
	Female	0.03 (1 in 2997)	0.81 (1 in 124)	1.78 (1 in 56)	4.70 (1 in 21)	6.22 (1 in 16)
Melanoma§	Male	0.16 (1 in 645)	0.64 (1 in 157)	0.70 (1 in 143)	1.67 (1 in 60)	2.56 (1 in 39)
	Female	0.27 (1 in 370)	0.53 (1 in 189)	0.35 (1 in 282)	0.76 (1 in 131)	1.73 (1 in 58)
Non-Hodgkin lymphoma	Male	0.13 (1 in 763)	0.45 (1 in 225)	0.58 (1 in 171)	1.66 (1 in 60)	2.23 (1 in 45)
	Female	0.08 (1 in 1191)	0.32 (1 in 316)	0.45 (1 in 223)	1.36 (1 in 73)	1.90 (1 in 53)
Prostate	Male	0.01 (1 in 10,002)	2.43 (1 in 41)	6.42 (1 in 16)	12.49 (1 in 8)	15.78 (1 in 6)
Uterine cervix	Female	0.15 (1 in 651)	0.27 (1 in 368)	0.13 (1 in 761)	0.19 (1 in 530)	0.69 (1 in 145)
Uterine corpus	Female	0.07 (1 in 1499)	0.72 (1 in 140)	0.81 (1 in 123)	1.22 (1 in 82)	2.48 (1 in 40)

Adapted from Jemal et al. Cancer statistics, 2009. CA Cancer J Clin 2009;59:225-49.
*For people free of cancer at beginning of age interval.
†All sites exclude basal and squamous cell skin cancers and in situ cancers except urinary bladder.
‡Includes invasive and in situ cancer cases.
§Statistics for whites only.

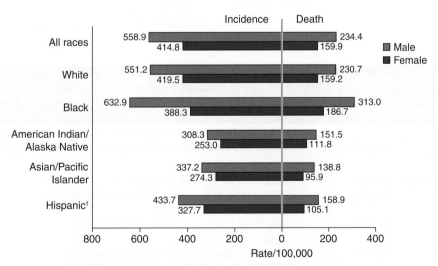

FIGURE 1-8 All-cause age-adjusted cancer incidence and mortality rates in the general United States, by sex, race, and ethnicity, 2001-2005. *(Adapted from Centers for Disease Control and Prevention: Health Disparities in Cancer. Atlanta, GA, National Center for Chronic Disease Prevention and Health Promotion, Division of Cancer Prevention and Control, 2008.)*

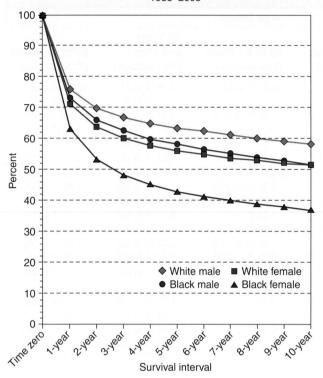

RELATIVE SURVIVAL RATES BY SURVIVAL TIME
BY RACE AND SEX ALL SITES, AGES 65+,
1988–2005

Cancer sites include invasive cases only unless otherwise noted.
Survival source: SEER 9 areas (San Francisco, Connecticut, Detroit, Hawaii, Iowa, New Mexico, Seattle, Utah, and Atlanta).
Survival rates are relative rates expressed as percents. The annual survival estimates are calculated using monthly intervals.

FIGURE 1-9 Relative all-cancer-site survival rates by survival time, race, and sex in the population age 65 and older in the United States, 1988-2005. *(Adapted from SEER Cancer Statistics Review, 1975-2006. Bethesda, MD: National Cancer Institute; 2009.)*

and minority populations) intersect to drive increases in cancer incidence.

CHARACTERISTICS OF OLDER PATIENTS WITH CANCER

As has been noted, age is the single most important risk factor for the development of cancer; yet, many risk factors that affect the general population are also contributors to cancer risk in older adults. These same risk factors are often associated not only with cancer, but also with common diseases and disabilities of aging (e.g., chronic diseases such as heart disease or hypertension, limitations in physical function). In turn, these risk factors and associated conditions can greatly affect treatment decision making, responses to treatment, and outcomes. Some risk factors such as smoking, diet, and physical exercise are modifiable, whereas others such as family history and race are not (for example, genetic factors are estimated to account for up to 10% of prostate, breast, and colorectal cancers).[11-13] The World Health Organization estimates that more than 30% of cancer deaths in the general population can be prevented by modifying risk factors (Table 1-2).[14] The effect of these factors may be magnified in older adults because of their association not just with cancer but with other common causes of morbidity and death as well. What follows is an examination of some common modifiable risk factors and their impact in relation to cancers and treatment-related issues in older adults. Genetic risk factors are not addressed because of their tendency to be less age-specific, nor are environmental risk factors addressed because of their overall variability in older adults.

TABLE 1-2	Number of Attributable Deaths and Population Attributable Fractions (PAF) Estimating Individual and Joint Contributions of Selected Modifiable Risk Factors by Cancer Site, Worldwide and in High-Income Countries		
	Total Deaths	PAF (%) and Number of Attributable Cancer Deaths (Thousands) for Individual Risk Factors	PAF Due to Joint Hazards of Risk Factors
Worldwide			
Mouth and oropharynx cancers	311 633	Alcohol use (16%; 51), smoking (42%; 131)	52%
Esophageal cancer	437 511	Alcohol use (26%, 116), smoking (42%; 184), low fruit and vegetable intake (18%; 80)	62%
Stomach cancer	841 693	Smoking (13%; 111), low fruit and vegetable intake (18%; 147)	28%
Colon and rectum cancers	613 740	Overweight and obesity (11%; 69), physical inactivity (15%; 90), low fruit and vegetable intake (2%; 12)	13%
Liver cancer	606 441	Smoking (14%; 85), alcohol use (25%; 150), contaminated injections in health-care settings (18%; 111)	47%
Pancreatic cancer	226 981	Smoking (22%, 50)	22%
Trachea, bronchus, and lung cancers	1 226 574	Smoking (70%; 856), low fruit and vegetable intake (11%; 135), indoor smoke from household use of solid fuels (1%; 16), urban air pollution (5%; 64)	74%
Breast cancer	472 424	Alcohol use (5%; 26), overweight and obesity (9%; 43), physical inactivity (10%; 45)	21%
Cervix uteri cancer	234 728	Smoking (2%; 6), unsafe sex (100%; 235)	100%

TABLE 1-2	Number of Attributable Deaths and Population Attributable Fractions (PAF) Estimating Individual and Joint Contributions of Selected Modifiable Risk Factors by Cancer Site, Worldwide and in High-Income Countries—cont'd		
	Total Deaths	**PAF (%) and Number of Attributable Cancer Deaths (Thousands) for Individual Risk Factors**	**PAF Due to Joint Hazards of Risk Factors**
Corpus uteri cancer	70 881	Overweight and obesity (40%; 28)	40%
Bladder cancer	175 318	Smoking (28%; 48)	28%
Leukemia	263 169	Smoking (9%; 23)	9%
Selected other cancers	145 802	Alcohol use (6%; 8)	6%
All other cancers	1 391 507	None of selected risk factors	0%
All cancers	7 018 402	Alcohol use (5%; 351), smoking (21%; 1493), low fruit and vegetable intake (5%; 374), indoor smoke from household use of solid fuels (0·5%; 16), urban air pollution (1%; 64), overweight and obesity (2%; 139), physical inactivity (2%; 135), contaminated injections in health-care settings (2%; 111), unsafe sex (3%; 235)	35%
High-Income Countries			
Mouth and oropharynx cancers	40 559	Alcohol use (33%; 14), smoking (71%; 29)	80%
Esophageal cancer	57 752	Alcohol use (41%; 24), smoking (71%; 41), low fruit and vegetable intake (12%; 7)	85%
Stomach cancer	146 267	Smoking (25%; 36), low fruit and vegetable intake (12%; 17)	34%
Colon and rectum cancers	256 791	Overweight and obesity (14%; 37), physical inactivity (14%; 36), low fruit and vegetable intake (1%; 3)	15%
Liver cancer	102 033	Smoking (29%; 29), alcohol use (32%; 33), contaminated injections in health-care settings (3%; 3)	52%
Pancreatic cancer	110 154	Smoking (30%; 33)	30%
Trachea, bronchus, and lung cancers	455 636	Smoking (86%; 391), low fruit and vegetable intake (8%; 36), indoor smoke from household use of solid fuels (0%), urban air pollution (3%; 12)	87%
Breast cancer	155 230	Alcohol use (9%; 14), overweight and obesity (13%; 20), physical inactivity (9%; 15)	27%
Cervix uteri cancer	16 663	Smoking (11%; 2), unsafe sex (100%; 17)	100%
Corpus uteri cancer	26 955	Overweight and obesity (43%; 12)	43%
Bladder cancer	58 636	Smoking (41%; 24)	41%
Leukemia	73 110	Smoking (17%; 12)	17%
Selected other cancers	57 095	Alcohol use (8%; 5)	8%
All other cancers	509 507	None of selected risk factors	0%
All cancers	2 066 388	Alcohol use (4%; 88), smoking (29%; 596), low fruit and vegetable intake (3%; 64), indoor smoke from household use of solid fuels (0%; 0), urban air pollution (1%; 12), overweight and obesity (3%; 69), physical inactivity (2%; 51), contaminated injections in health-care settings (0·5%; 3), unsafe sex (1%; 17)	37%

From Danaei G, Vander Hoorn S, Lopez AD et al. Causes of cancer in the world: comparative risk assessment of nine behavioural and environmental risk factors. Lancet 2005;366:1784-93.
PAF, Population Attributable Fraction

Smoking is considered the leading cause of preventable death in the United States, accounting for nearly one of five deaths each year.[15,16] Regardless of age, smoking is by far the most important risk factor for the development of lung cancer (about 90% of lung cancer deaths in men and 80% in women are due to smoking).[9] The longer one smokes, and the greater amount smoked daily, the more lung cancer risk increases. Thus, older smokers are at particularly high risk, as evidenced by their having the highest probabilities of having lung cancer overall (Table 1-1). According to the U.S. Surgeon General, smoking is also associated with an increased risk of at least 14 other types of cancer (nasopharynx, nasal cavity and paranasal sinuses, lip, oral cavity, pharynx, larynx, esophagus, pancreas, uterine cervix, kidney, bladder, stomach, and acute myeloid leukemia).[16] Although the U.S. Surgeon General does not currently recognize smoking as a risk factor for colorectal cancer, there is evidence that it is.[17-20] The increased colorectal cancer risk among smokers is hypothesized to be due to cancer-causing substances in tobacco and/or the relation between smoking and alcohol use (colorectal cancer has been linked to alcohol use). Smoking is also known to be a major cause of other chronic conditions commonly affecting older adults, such as heart disease, cerebrovascular disease, and chronic lower respiratory disease (Figure 1-5), all of which can greatly complicate cancer treatment options and tolerance. Although older adults have the lowest current smoker rates (under 10%), older former smokers may represent considerable past exposures.[21] With the actual number of older adults increasing and the higher smoking rates in minorities, interactions of smoking-related health problems in the older population will continue to be of serious concern.

Obesity is a growing epidemic in the United States and is not limited to younger populations. The Centers for Disease Control (CDC) estimates that nearly 30% of the 65-and-older population is obese, with even higher rates in minority populations. There are many negative health outcomes associated with obesity. It is associated with excess mortality, as well as with increased risk of heart disease, diabetes, osteoarthritis, cancer, and disability.[22-29] In the case of cancer, studies have estimated that obesity may contribute to up to 6% of U.S. incident cancer cases.[30, 31] It has been linked to cancers of the colon, breast (postmenopausal), endometrium, kidney, esophagus, gallbladder, ovaries, and pancreas.[22] Furthermore, obesity has been associated with a worse prognosis for certain cancers (e.g., breast, colon, lymphoma, and prostate) and a greater risk for disease recurrence.[22,32,33] Unfavorable survival rates in obese cancer patients may be related to the higher likelihood of associated comorbid conditions or unfavorable tumor characteristics.[34] Detection of breast tumors is more difficult in obese than in lean women and may explain findings that higher body mass is associated with advanced stage breast cancer and, in turn, poorer prognosis.[35] In addition, studies demonstrating systematic underdosing of chemotherapy in overweight and obese breast cancer patients suggest another potential factor in poorer survival rates.[34,36-38] The unique challenges and increased complications associated with older obese cancer patients directly influence planning, delivery, and tolerance of cancer treatments. Current demographics predict a rise in the risk of morbidity and death from obesity-related cancers common in older adults, resulting from the burgeoning numbers of older Americans (especially minorities), the increasing prevalence of obesity, and persistent racial differences in obesity.

Diet and physical activity are two other important modifiable risk factors for common cancers in older adults.[14] As with smoking and obesity, diet and physical activity are closely related to some cancers (e.g., prostate, colorectal, breast) and to other diseases and conditions of aging. For instance, eating well and exercising may reduce the risk not only of cancer but also of heart disease, stroke, type 2 diabetes, bone loss, and anemia. Diet and exercise are, obviously, also related to obesity and being overweight, as discussed previously. Importantly,

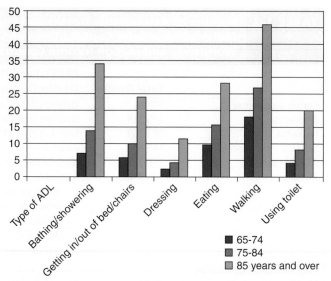

FIGURE 1-10 Percent of community-dwelling older adults reporting a limitation in activities of daily living, by age, 2006. *(Adapted from U.S. Department of Health and Human Services: A Profile of Older Americans: 2008. Washington, DC: Administration on Aging, 2008.)*

this constellation of health-related factors may play a key role in cancer treatment decision making and tolerance. Unfortunately, physical activity may be less modifiable in older adults than in younger populations because a sedentary lifestyle in older adults may not actually be a choice but a consequence of coexisting functional limitations. Figure 1-10 shows how age is associated with a decreased ability to accomplish daily activities in community-dwelling older adults.[1] Older minorities, especially African-Americans and Hispanics, have an even greater number of functional disabilities than their white counterparts.[39,40] In general, older adults who are functionally dependent have a lower life expectancy and stress tolerance, including tolerance for the stress of cancer treatment.[41] Difficulty shopping, preparing meals, or eating can greatly affect the diet of older adults, for whom nutrition is a health concern that directly affects cancer treatments and tolerance. Even though regular physical activity, maintenance of a healthy body weight, and a healthy diet are widely considered to reduce cancer risk, the lifestyle changes required to achieve them may not be feasible in older adults.

The issues surrounding modifiable risk factors previously outlined are by no means the only matters of concern in the treatment of older cancer patients. Studies show documented undertreatment of older cancer patients across cancer types. Common reported reasons for undertreatment are the high prevalence of comorbidities, lower life expectancies, limited data on treatment efficacy from clinical trials, and increased adverse effects of treatment.[42] Paradoxically, undertreatment persists even though studies have shown that older adults are prepared to receive cancer treatments just as readily as younger patients and most appear to benefit from treatment to a similar extent as younger patients.[43-48] Likewise, treatments such as surgery and adjuvant therapy are well tolerated, effectively decrease relapse, and improve survival in many older cancer patients.[42,49-59] Defining treatment strategies specific to older adults is hampered by limited age-specific evidence and the fact that treating older adults for cancer seldom means treating their cancer alone. Chronological age is a poor indicator of future life expectancy, functional reserve, or the risk of treatment complications.[60,61] Because aging is so highly individualized, recent guidelines suggest that clinical decision making for cancer treatments based on geriatric assessment is most likely to result in positive outcomes in older cancer patients.[52,60,62] The key to managing older cancer patients is the ability to accurately assess whether the expected benefits of treatment will outweigh the risks.[63] In fact, once they are adequately evaluated, fewer older patients should have to be excluded from treatment because of reduced tolerance.[64] To date, the lack of systematic comprehensive evaluation and age-specific evidence restricts treatment-modification decision making to factors such as chronological age and slows the development of interventions to optimize cancer treatment in older adults. Our expanding knowledge and understanding of the aging process will eventually allow us to accurately identify older cancer patients who will benefit from prevention and treatment options and distinguish them from those who are not candidates for treatments with curative intent. Future research will provide a more robust foundation for targeting treatments to older cancer patients for the purpose of maximizing clinical benefit and cost-effectiveness, as well as eliminating undertreatment.

UNIQUE ISSUES OF CANCER AND AGING

The prospect of a longer life span is generally considered desirable, as long as one is healthy. With longer life, though, the biological changes, diseases, and conditions known to be associated with aging become precipitously more prevalent. Older adults face many more health care concerns than do younger adults. In 2006, only 39% of community-dwelling older adults in the United States assessed their health as excellent or very good, compared with 65% of persons younger than 65 years, and most older Americans reported having at least one chronic condition.[21] African-American and Hispanic Medicare beneficiaries are both more likely than whites to have serious health problems and long-term care needs.[39] As previously discussed, cancer incidence and mortality trends in the older population differ from those in the younger population and also by race (e.g., consistently higher rates in persons 65 years and older and certain types of cancer consistently higher in minority groups, such as prostate cancer in African-Americans).[6] This may be due to the influence of age on cancer biology, prolonged exposures, systemic effects of aging, or quality of care. In addition, older adults with cancer and their families often have different needs than younger adults. For example, they may not always have access to transportation, social support, or the financial resources required to successfully undergo cancer treatments. The nexus of cancer and aging presents some unique issues for older cancer patients and their caregivers (familial and professional) alike.

There is evidence indicating that cancers may behave differently depending on the age of the patient.[62,65,66] It is hypothesized that, basically, two types of mechanisms are involved: (1) changes in the intrinsic biology of the tumor cells and (2) changes in the ability of an older host to sustain and stimulate tumor growth. The biology of aging and its interactions with cancer are not completely understood and are further complicated by their heterogeneity across cancer type. Table 1-3 shows how the biology of certain tumors changes with increasing age, and Table 1-4 lists some of the biological interactions of cancer and aging.[67, 68] With increased age, some cancers become more aggressive (e.g., leukemias, lymphomas, ovarian), and others become more indolent (e.g., breast, lung). As an example, in the case of breast cancer, age-specific incidence profiles differ between

TABLE 1-3	Age-Related Changes in Tumor Biology by Selected Cancer Type and Hypothesized Mechanism	
Neoplasm	**Change with Increasing Age**	**Possible Mechanism**
Acute myeloid leukemia	Resistance to chemotherapy	Tumor cells show increased expression of the multidrug resistance protein (MDR1) and unfavorable cytogenetic changes
Non-Hodgkin lymphoma	Reduced response to chemotherapy Reduced duration of response and survival	Stromal cells show increased concentration of interleukin-6 in the circulation, stimulating lymphocyte proliferation; Immune senescence and increased growth rate of highly immunogenic tumors is also evident
Breast cancer	More indolent	Tumors show higher concentrations of well-differentiated hormone-receptor–rich neoplastic cells and decreased tumor growth fraction; Stromal cells exhibit endocrine senescence; Immune system senescence
Non-small cell lung cancer	More indolent	Development of cancer in elderly ex-smokers
Ovarian cancer	Decreased response to chemotherapy and reduced survival	Unknown

From Balducci L, Aapro M. Epidemiology of cancer and aging. Cancer Treat Res 2005;124:1-15.

TABLE 1-4	**Biological Interactions of Cancer and Aging**

Molecular Changes of Aging That Could Favor Carcinogenesis

- Accumulation of DNA adducts, DNA hypermethylation, and point mutations, which prime the cells to "late-stage" carcinogens
- Higher concentration of cells in advanced carcinogenesis; therefore more likely to be hit "at random" by environmental carcinogens
- The exposure of tissues from young and old rodents to the same dose of carcinogen results in higher numbers of tumors in the older tissues.

Molecular Changes of Aging That Could Inhibit Carcinogenesis

- Progressive telomere shortening, leading to senescence
- Activation of genes that oppose cell replication, such as the gene encoding ARF, the cyclin-dependent kinase inhibitor

Cellular Changes of Aging That Could Favor the Development of Cancer

- Premature senescence of fibroblasts associated with production of tumor growth factors and metalloproteinases that favor metastatic spread
- Premature senescence associated with loss of apoptosis and development of immortal cells. A possible mechanism to explain some slow-growing malignancies in older individuals, such as follicular lymphomas.

Physiological Changes of Aging That Could Influence Tumor Growth

- Endocrine senescence might cause slower growth of endocrine-dependent tumors (such as breast, prostate and endometrial cancer).
- Immune senescence might favor the growth of highly immunogenic tumors, such as large cell lymphomas, renal cell carcinomas, and aggressive sarcomas. Alternatively, the growth of less immunogenic tumors might be slowed in older patients, owing to a reduced immune cell infiltrate and decreased inflammatory cytokine expression.
- Premature senescence of stromal cells associated with increased production of growth factors and metalloproteinases
- Increased concentration of catabolic cytokines in the circulation, which might lead to muscle loss and oppose the growth of highly proliferative tissues and neoplasias

From Balducci L, Aapro M. Epidemiology of cancer and aging. Cancer Treat Res 2005;124:1-15.

early- and late-onset breast cancers.[69] Early-onset breast cancers are thought to be primarily due to inherited or early-life cellular damage of immature breast tissue, whereas late-onset breast cancers are considered to be due to extended exposures and age-related cellular damages. Clinical observations and biomarker studies indicate that late-onset breast cancers grow more slowly and are biologically less aggressive than early-onset breast cancers, even when hormone and growth factor receptor expression are taken into account.[70] In general, some cancers in older adults have a worse prognosis than in younger adults (e.g., non-Hodgkin lymphoma), whereas others have an improved prognosis (e.g., breast, lung); this may be confounded by the fact that older adults tend to be diagnosed at more advanced stages than do young persons.[67,71] Age-related physiological changes due to both genetic (e.g., organ and systems functional reserve) and environmental influences (e.g., disease, physical and emotional stresses, lifestyle, and carcinogenic exposures) involve a progressive loss of the body's ability to cope with stress.[72,73] Age-related physiological changes may be particularly relevant to cancer biology and treatment. They may affect the growth rate of the tumor, the pharmacokinetics of drugs, and the risk of drug-related toxicity.[73] There is little doubt the mechanisms and pathways of cancer and aging are interrelated.[68] Their interactions can have an impact on cancer risk, tumor activity, and older patients' responses to treatment.[73-75] Moreover, evidence must be cautiously interpreted and translated because our ability to understand the effects of underlying aging biology may be obscured by age discrepancies between study populations and general cancer populations.[70] This may be particularly problematic for older cancer patients, for whom treatment complications can have a serious ripple health effect.

As previously described, the diseases most commonly associated with aging (Figure 1-5) are chronic, are usually progressive in nature, often negatively affect physical health, and are related to modifiable cancer risk factors, as well as to outcomes (e.g., functional reserve, morbidity, mortality). Because age is considered the most important risk factor for cancer and is associated with increasing comorbidity, coexisting diseases are of substantial concern in older cancer patients. Indeed, cancer patients 70 years and older have, on average, three comorbidities.[76,77] The consequences of coexisting illnesses are related to pathophysiology, prognosis, diagnosis, treatment, and etiology and may have broad-ranging serious implications in the lives of older adults, especially for those with cancer.[78] Table 1-5 shows the biomedical framework for interactions of comorbidities as outlined in the report of the National Institute on Aging Task Force on Comorbidity.[78] The framework highlights the substantial potential for synergism between concomitant diseases. It emphasizes that health issues related to cancer and its treatment should not be considered in isolation but in relation to other prevalent diseases. There is evidence suggesting that a primary cancer diagnosis interacts with comorbidity, that survival is inversely related to the number of comorbidities, and that death more commonly results from comorbidity, rather than from cancer, with advancing age.[79-85] However, cause of death varies according to the aggressiveness of the cancer (i.e., cancer-specific cause of death for aggressive cancers and comorbidity-related cause of death for less aggressive cancers). It is difficult to fully isolate the individual contributions of comorbidity, functional status, and treatment modification to prognosis.[76,81,85] Interactions of comorbidity and cancer may also result in more severe

TABLE 1-5	Biomedical Framework for Interaction of Comorbidity

Pathophysiology and Prognosis

1. One condition worsens another (faster progression, poorer outcomes, more disabling).
2. One condition increases risk for another.
3. Combination of two conditions has synergistic effects on other poor outcomes.

Diagnosis

4. One condition creates problems for diagnosing or assessing another.

Treatment

5. A treatment for one condition worsens or causes another condition.
6. Response to a treatment for one condition is affected by another condition.
7. The combination of treatments for more than one condition creates new problems.

Etiology

8. Two or more conditions combined occur more frequently than expected (common cause?).

From Yancik et al. Report of the national institute on aging task force on comorbidity. J Gerontol A Biol Sci Med Sci 2007;62:275-80.

morbidity, disability, or both, with subsequently higher levels of dependence on family, friends, and local services. Some of the latter issues in relation to survivorship will be addressed later in the chapter.

Because each person ages at a different rate and with actual age being a poor mirror of physiological age (an estimation of age based on how a person functions), the evaluation of function and coexisting illnesses is essential, especially when evaluating older adults for cancer treatment. The specific issues of cancer and aging beg important and unique questions that should be considered whenever managing older adults with cancer: Will the patient die of or with cancer? Will the cancer compromise the function and the quality of life of the patient? Will the patient be able to tolerate complications of treatment?[71,74] Unlike younger patients, the main determinants of outcomes (including survival) in older cancer patients are not age or tumor characteristics alone but also comorbidities and functional reserve.

SURVIVORSHIP OF OLDER CANCER PATIENTS

With improvements in cancer screening and treatment over the past several decades, the risk of death from cancer following diagnosis has steadily decreased. This has resulted in the number of cancer survivors in the United States increasing to nearly 11.4 million, most (60%) of whom are 65 years of age and older.[86] An important aspect of cancer survivorship is that cancer survivors of all ages are at greater risk for recurrence and for developing multiple primary malignancies (MPMs). In fact, one of the

most serious events experienced by cancer survivors is the diagnosis of a new cancer. The National Cancer Institute estimates that the risk of developing a second primary or multiple primaries varies from 1% to 16%, depending on the primary cancer site, and this risk is increasing.[87-89] As with first primary cancers, the incidence of multiple primaries increases with age, and nearly 7% of older cancer survivors are affected[90-93]; yet, in this largest group of cancer survivors (65 years and older), multiple primary malignancies and their consequences remain understudied. Multiple primary cancers in older survivors may reflect late sequelae of treatment, as well as the effects of aging, lifestyle factors, environmental exposures, host factors, and combinations of influences, including gene-environment and gene-gene interactions.[94-96]

Breast cancer survivors represent one of the largest groups of survivors with multiple primary malignancies, the most common site being contralateral breast cancers, followed by prostate and colorectal cancers.[90,97] This ranking may reflect both the high incidence and survival rates for the first primary cancer but not necessarily greater risks for a subsequent cancer. Cross-sectional studies of MPM suggest that their prevalence peaks in the seventh or eighth decade; longitudinal studies indicate that the incidence of MPM increases with survival after the diagnosis and treatment of the first malignancy.[93] Despite documented disparities in cancer treatment and survival related to age, race/ethnicity, residence, and socioeconomic status, the impact of these characteristics on MPM risk has not been well studied.[98-106] Radiation therapy has been linked to excess risk for contralateral breast cancer, lung cancer, soft tissue sarcoma, and esophageal cancer.[91,107-113] Excess endometrial cancer is considered to be related to previous tamoxifen therapy.[114,115] An increased risk of leukemia after a primary cancer has been associated with both chemotherapy and radiation therapy.[97,116-119] The few studies that have examined nontreatment and multiple primaries that are not cancer-site specific are inconsistent.[120-123] The American Cancer Society recommends primary prevention (i.e., tobacco avoidance and cessation, healthy diet, weight control, physical activity) as the main strategy to reduce the burden of multiple primary cancers related to lifestyle factors.[97]

CHALLENGES OF EPIDEMIOLOGICAL STUDY OF OLDER PATIENTS WITH CANCER

Older adults remain understudied in general, and this is particularly true in cancer research.[39,124] Unfortunately, the lack of participation of older adults in research studies reduces opportunities for discoveries that may be particularly relevant to their care.[125] There are many challenges in the study of older adults that are unique and must be considered to ensure validity and reliability of the evidence. Some of these challenges are reviewed, and their consequences for research and for the care of older adults with cancer are considered.

Although most new cancer cases occur in older adults and it is accepted that well-conducted randomized controlled trials (RCTs) provide the highest level of evidence to guide clinical management, relatively few older cancer patients participate in RCTs of new cancer treatments. Conducting RCTs in vulnerable patient populations is challenging, and oncology treatment trials have documented low participation rates among older adults.[39,71] Barriers to participation and retention include study design; physician, patient, and logistic issues (e.g., availability of caregivers, travel constraints); and financial costs.[125] By design, RCTs enroll participants with similar characteristics to ensure results of the trial are due to the intervention and not to other factors. Eligibility criteria are implemented to achieve accurate and meaningful results. Age-based criteria, common in cancer trials, are a means to exclude the inherent variability of older cancer patients and to minimize the risk of other comorbidities worsening by study participation. Notably, evidence is accumulating that persons older than 65 years who are reasonably fit tolerate aggressive chemotherapy treatments as well as younger persons.[125,126] According to these studies, age alone should not be a barrier to participation in clinical trials of new cancer treatments.[124,125] However, the heterogeneity of older cancer patients necessitates large samples or increased duration of observation to achieve adequate study power. Nevertheless, RCTs of older cancer patients are feasible.

Longitudinal studies—of any design—can play a major role in understanding the natural history, the analysis of change of disease, and the impact of treatment on older patients.[127] However, the validity and integrity of studies in which data are collected from participants over time can be severely compromised by attrition.[128,129] Longitudinal studies of older adults are particularly challenging to conduct because of age, disease, and functional status of the study population. Older, sicker, more disabled persons are less likely to enroll in studies, and these characteristics similarly affect the likelihood of continued study participation.[130,131] Common reasons for loss to follow-up in longitudinal studies of older adults include illness, being hospitalized, and moving to nursing homes. In most studies of older adults, dropouts differ from completers in demographic characteristics, physical and mental health indices, and extent of social support.[132-135] These realities are magnified in the setting of a cancer diagnosis, and the attrition of respondents can create methodological challenges (e.g., bias in data analysis) and must be seriously considered in study design.[136-138] On the other hand, outcome-based retrospective cohort and case-control studies evaluating the effectiveness of cancer-related care can be alternatives to RCTs. Retrospective studies circumvent the challenges of enrollment, retention, and attrition, as well as the high costs of prospective studies, with the use of existing data sources. However, if not properly designed, they can be more prone to confounding and bias.

Translation of evidence to evidence-based practice requires a specific and adequate knowledge base. Because older patients and minorities continue to be underrepresented in studies, there is limited evidence about the efficacy and tolerability of standard treatments in these patients. In the not so distant future, the older populations in the U.S. will more than double, with sizeable increases in the minority segments. It is estimated that by 2030, a 67% increase in cancer incidence for older adults will occur, accompanied by a 99% increase in minorities compared with 31% in whites.[139] It is essential to expand and accelerate our production of cancer-related evidence in this growing and changing population, regardless of study design. The current lack of efficacy data restricts the basis of treatment choice and modifications, and has retarded the development of interventions to optimize cancer treatment in older adults.

Summary

The aging of the U.S. population and the consequence of increased cancer incidence with longer life spans require physicians to develop a better understanding of the epidemiology of cancer, aging, and their intersection. Today, a person 65 years old can expect to live an average of 18.5 additional years, and a person 85 years old, 6.4 more years. These represent a considerable number of years at the end of the life course, which has become progressively more entwined with cancer. Thus, the treatment of older adults with cancer should be focused on maintaining or strengthening the quality of those years.

As has been discussed in this chapter, aging and cancer share pathways and interact to form a complex setting, full of challenges for identifying risk and devising optimal care for older cancer patients. The consequences of cancer and its treatment have a greater impact in older patients, particularly because of the interaction of cancer treatment effects, comorbidities, and age-related disabilities. Comorbidity is of particular concern in older cancer patients because of its prevalence and because it may be affected by cancer and, in turn, affect cancer and its treatment. Although primary prevention through lifestyle changes is promoted as the primary means to reduce cancer burden, some of these changes cannot be achieved in older adults. A greater understanding of cancer and aging will provide valuable opportunities to devise treatment strategies that maximize survival, minimize morbidity, and maintain quality of life in older cancer patients. Development and cogent use of cancer treatments in the complex setting of the older cancer patient require an understanding of the epidemiology of cancer and aging.

See expertconsult.com for a complete list of references and web resources for this chapter

SUGGESTED READINGS

1. *A Profile of Older Americans: 2008*, Washington, DC, 2008, Administration on Aging U.S. Department of Health and Human Services.
2. Balducci L, Aapro M: Epidemiology of cancer and aging, *Cancer Treat Res* 124:1–15, 2005.
3. Balducci L, Beghe C: Cancer and age in the USA, *Crit Rev Oncol Hematol* 37:137–145, 2001.
4. Balducci L, Ershler WB: Cancer and ageing: a nexus at several levels, *Nat Rev Cancer* 5:655–662, 2005.
5. Danaei G, Vander Hoorn S, Lopez AD, et al: Causes of cancer in the world: comparative risk assessment of nine behavioural and environmental risk factors, *Lancet* 366:1784–1793, 2005.
6. Ershler WB: Cancer: a disease of the elderly, *J Support Oncol* 1:5–10, 2003.
7. Extermann M: Interaction between comorbidity and cancer, *Cancer Control* 14:13–22, 2007.
8. From Cancer Patient to Cancer Survivor: *Lost in Transition*, Washington, D.C, 2007, Institute of Medicine and National Research Council of the National Academies.
9. National Center for Health Statistics: *Health, United States, 2008 With Chartbook*, Hyattsville, MD, 2009, National Center for Health Statistics.
10. Irminger-Finger I: Science of cancer and aging, *J Clin Oncol* 25:1844–1851, 2007.
11. Jemal A, Siegel R, Ward E, et al: Cancer statistics, 2009, *CA Cancer J Clin* 59:225–249, 2009.
12. *SEER Cancer Statistics Review, 1975-2006*, Bethesda, MD, 2009, National Cancer Institute.
13. Smith BD, Smith GL, Hurria A, et al: Future of cancer incidence in the United States: burdens upon an aging, changing nation, *J Clin Oncol* 27:2758–2765, 2009.
14. Travis LB: The epidemiology of second primary cancers, *Cancer Epidemiol Biomarkers Prev* 15:2020–2026, 2006.
15. Yancik R, Ershler W, Satariano W, et al: Report of the National Institute on Aging task force on comorbidity, *J Gerontol A Biol Sci Med Sci* 62:275–280, 2007.

SUGGESTED READINGS

Cancer Screening and Prevention in the Older Patient

Jennifer M. Croswell and Barnett S. Kramer

CASE 2-1 **CASE DESCRIPTION**

A husband and wife, aged 76 and 77, respectively, are new patients to a medical practice. The wife mentions that along with having seen multiple direct-to-consumer promotions emphasizing the importance of "healthy living" and the role of early detection in cancer, they recently watched a close friend die of prostate cancer. The wife mentions that she has had "about seven or eight mammograms" in her life, starting when she was 44 years old, but her last test was several years ago, and she is now very worried that she has not been sufficiently proactive about her health. She has come to schedule a mammogram. She would also like to get a prescription for raloxifene, after seeing an advertisement about its bone and breast health benefits in *Ladies Home Journal*. She states that her husband has "never liked going to the doctor," and has never previously had a serum prostate-specific antigen (PSA) test, but she has decided, on the basis of their friend's experience, to "put her foot down." She also would like to schedule both of them for colonoscopies. Both are now retired; the husband was a construction worker, and the wife, an elementary school teacher. The husband states that except for an incarcerated hernia requiring surgical intervention and a traumatic crush injury to his left shoulder caused by an on-the-job accident, he has no significant medical history. Her medical history is significant for mild hypertension, controlled with the use of a thiazide.

Public health messaging about the power of prevention and early detection has been both pervasive and persuasive. However, given its intuitive, "common sense" appeal, it is also frequently presented in an overly simplistic manner that belies the true complexity of decision making in this field, particularly in the elderly. Benefits may be overstated, and potential harms unrecognized or unconsidered. This chapter is intended to provide a review of the general principles of cancer screening and prevention, as well as a focus on the specific issues unique to older adults; these concepts should facilitate informed, individualized discussions with patients.

First and foremost, it is essential to realize that screening and prevention are fundamentally different activities from treatment of established disease. In the case of treatment, the baseline status of the population is one of symptomatic illness; individuals are actively seeking relief from a specific problem. Screening and prevention, however, deal with a population not overtly affected by the condition of interest and in whom the vast majority will never go on to acquire the disease. It is difficult to make an essentially healthy person better off than he or she already is; as such, the level of acceptable harm due to screening and prevention is lower than for a treatment scenario. The concept of *primum non nocere* is of particular relevance in the arena of prevention and screening, where the potential for the balance of benefits and harms to tip in the wrong direction rests at a different baseline than with treatment.

ANALYTIC FRAMEWORK: REJECTING INTUITIVE THINKING IN SCREENING AND PREVENTION

One of the most efficient tools developed to help clinicians and researchers sort through the salient elements related to the utility of a screening or prevention intervention is the analytic framework. Figure 2-1 depicts sample analytic frameworks (adapted from the U.S. Preventive Services Task Force) for prevention and screening activities, respectively.[1]

The analytic framework demands that attention be paid to (1) the population under consideration for the intervention (different groups might benefit more or less from a given screening or intervention practice, and proof of efficacy in one group does not automatically equate to utility for all populations); (2) the specifics of the intervention in question; (3) potential harms generated by the application of screening test or preventive agent; (4) potential harms generated by diagnostic follow-up or treatment of a disease; and (5) the precise nature of the potential beneficial outcomes of the intervention. The framework makes a point of explicitly delineating the difference between an intermediate outcome and a true health outcome. This is a useful reminder in screening and prevention efforts because a change in a laboratory value or radiographic examination does not necessarily equate to a decrease in deaths or a clinically meaningful

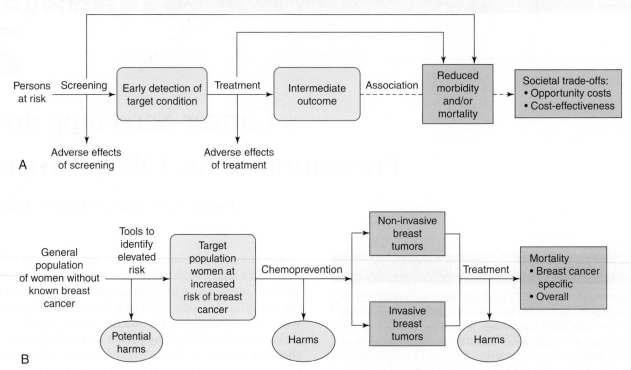

FIGURE 2-1 Sample analytic frameworks developed by the U.S. Preventive Services Task Force for both screening and preventive interventions. The analytic framework is a useful tool when evaluating the overall net benefit to harm ratio of an intervention, because it makes explicit each of the necessary links of the chain of evidence proving an intervention's efficacy, and also demands careful consideration of potential harms. **A,** Screening Analytic Framework. **B,** Prevention Analytic Framework. *(From Harris RP, Helfand M, Woolf SH, et al. Current methods of the US Preventive Services Task Force: a review of the process. Am J Prev Med 20(3 Suppl):21-35, 2001. Used with permission.)*

reduction in morbidity for the patient. Although intermediate outcomes are quicker and easier to obtain in studies of screening and prevention interventions because they occur with far greater frequency in an asymptomatic population than "hard" outcomes such as death, it is frequently difficult if not impossible to project with confidence how well they truly predict for endpoints with more clinical impact.

The framework's careful elucidation of the possible burdens associated with a given screening or prevention behavior is also of great importance: because these practices generally appear essentially innocuous (e.g., a blood draw, an x-ray, or ingestion of a substance already found in other foods) in an asymptomatic population, any associated potential harms are frequently overlooked or discounted. As the framework shows diagrammatically, any benefit of screening or prevention is linked to resulting therapy, so both the benefits and harms of therapy must be considered. Even if an intervention has been demonstrated to reduce disease-specific mortality in some individuals, the practice could still potentially be of net harm to a population, depending on the frequency and severity of associated complications that its use generates.

Finally, the framework is also useful in that it rejects mental shortcuts and a reliance on personal experience, opinion, or assumptions in favor of a series of defined links in a chain of evidence to prove the final net utility of an intervention. This is absolutely critical in the realm of prevention and screening activities because there are

strong obfuscating biases operating that can mislead even the most astute clinician, if he or she relies on experience, personal observation, or logical deduction to evaluate the worth of these practices.

BIASES IN SCREENING AND PREVENTION STUDIES

The first of these biases is known as the *healthy volunteer effect*. This bias occurs because there are fundamental differences between people who are interested in and choose to participate in screening and prevention activities, and those who do not. Persons who participate in early detection or preventive efforts are often more attuned to health messages (e.g., exercise more, smoke less), come from higher educational and socioeconomic strata, are more likely to be compliant with medical advice, and have a generally superior baseline health status, as compared with those who are not interested in such activities. The healthy volunteer effect has been documented in a range of screening and prevention studies: for example, in the Prostate, Lung, Colorectal, and Ovarian (PLCO) Cancer screening trial, investigators found that participants in both the screening and control arms consistently showed lower-than-expected mortality rates (when compared with the general population) for cardiovascular, respiratory, and digestive diseases, diabetes, and all cancers other than those screened for in the study. Even injuries and poisonings occurred about half

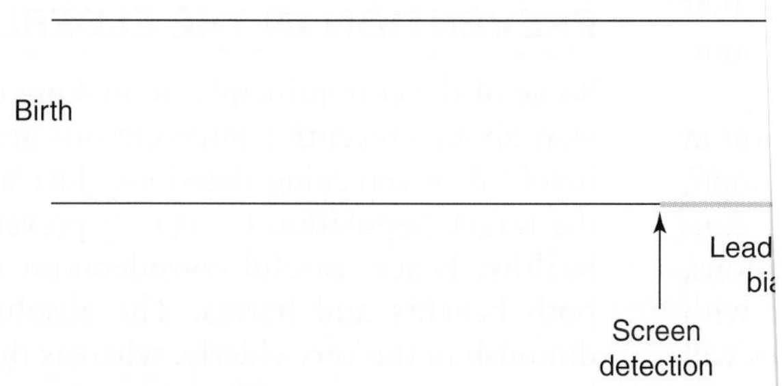

Birth

Lead[...]
bi[...]

Screen
detection

FIGURE 2-2 Lead-time bias. Early detection will advance the date of cancer diagn[...] case, although the individual lives longer with the diagnosis of cancer, there is no [...]

as frequently as would be expected. An intervention's apparent success may be entirely attributable to other confounding characteristics that track with the desire to be screened or engage in preventive activities.

A second confounding factor related to screening is known as *lead-time bias*. Any early detection tool will advance the date of diagnosis forward in time from that of symptomatic presentation. However, it does not automatically follow that a person will live longer as a result of this activity. Figure 2-2 depicts this concept. In this case, it can be seen that although early detection, by definition, shifts the date of diagnosis to an earlier point of time and, as a result, lengthens the period of life during which the person is known to have disease, it has no impact on the time of death. She simply spends more of her life as a cancer patient.

Lead-time bias explains why survival is a particularly misleading endpoint in screening trials, as opposed to disease-specific mortality. To demonstrate this conceptually, take as a hypothetical example a disease that kills 100% of people 4 years after the onset of physical symptoms. The 5-year survival rate is therefore 0%. A new screening test is developed that can diagnose the disease 5 years before symptom onset. The 5-year survival for screen-detected disease therefore rises to 100%, even though nothing has been done in this scenario that will affect the outcome of the disease. Mortality rates are not subject to lead-time bias because they deal with an entirely different denominator: whereas 5-year survival is the number of individuals with the disease alive after 5 years divided by the number of individuals diagnosed with the disease, mortality is the number of individuals who have died from the disease divided by the total population at risk for the disease.

This highlights an important difference between trials of screening and prevention: the usual endpoint used to evaluate efficacy. In the case of cancer screening, as noted previously, the primary endpoint should be *cause-specific mortality*. However, in prevention trials, the primary endpoint is generally cumulative cancer *incidence*. The ultimate goal of primary disease prevention is to decrease mortality. Practically speaking, however, few

if any [...]
enough [...]
tality. In fact, none of the chemoprevention trials that are discussed in this chapter have shown an improvement in cause-specific or overall mortality. In the case of the elderly, a reduction in cancer incidence may never translate into improved cancer mortality because of limited life expectancy. However, the diagnosis of cancer is important in and of itself as a health outcome because it has such a major impact on overall health and because treatments triggered by the diagnosis can be so morbid, particularly in the elderly.

Length-biased sampling is a third form of bias inherent in screening programs. Early detection tools are more effective at identifying slower-growing, less lethal lesions than rapidly progressing ones. This occurs because although every tumor has a given window of time between the threshold of detectability and the appearance of symptoms (the target period of early detection efforts), less aggressive cancers will have a longer preclinical period of growth than more rapidly fatal cancers. As such, a screening tool applied at set intervals has a greater likelihood of detecting these slowly progressive, more favorable lesions than those tumors that quickly advance to a symptomatic state. This does not automatically mean that early detection has had a beneficial impact on the course of the disease; screening programs may simply "stack the deck" with more indolent lesions.

The most extreme form of length-biased sampling is a highly counterintuitive concept termed *overdiagnosis*. Overdiagnosis occurs when a cancer is detected that would never have gone on to cause problems for the individual. This can occur for two reasons: (1) despite its histological appearance, the lesion is essentially indolent and has no malignant potential or (2) the lesion is so slow growing that the individual would die of another competing cause of death before the cancer would have ever become a health concern. This second mechanism is particularly of concern in older persons; cancer is largely a disease of aging and, even in those who coincidentally have slow-growing cancers, competing causes of death can account for a large proportion of deaths.

Overdiagnosed individuals cannot, [...] from the treatment(s) received, [...] all of the potential morbiditie[...] may accompany the therap[...] mary of these important[...] The potential bene[...] mortality (overall [...] clinically impo[...] cer. As effecti[...] because a[...] age, it [...] be a[...]

by definition, benefit
... ut they are exposed to
... s and even mortality that
... y. Table 2-1 provides a sum-
... biases.

... its of screening are a reduction in
... or disease-specific), or, at minimum,
... tant morbidity associated with the can-
... ve screening is applied to older populations,
... l causes of death become more common with
... becomes less likely that overall mortality rates will
... ffected and more probable that only disease-specific
... ortality will change.

TABLE 2-1	Key Clinical Pearls
Important biases in cancer screening	**Healthy volunteer bias:** There are fundamental differences between people who choose to participate in screening and those who do not; persons that participate may tend to be more attuned to health messages, come from higher educational and socioeconomic strata, and have a generally superior baseline health status **Lead-time bias:** The interval between diagnosis at the asymptomatic stage (by screening) and by symptoms; by advancing the date of diagnosis, screening adds apparent survival time compared with symptomatic detection, but this may not translate into a longer life span **Length-biased sampling:** Screening tools disproportionately detect slower-growing, more latent cancers compared with symptomatic detection **Overdiagnosis:** A situation where, despite its pathological appearance, a cancer either has no malignant potential or will not affect remaining life span as the person will die of another cause first
Important considerations for screening and prevention in the older patient	**Limited life expectancy and presence of comorbidities:** Can increase probability of overdiagnosis and overtreatment, as absolute potential for benefit of screening and prevention decreases with age Increasing likelihood of harm from preventive agents, treatments: Older populations may not be as resilient to the toxic effects of chemopreventive agents or the stresses of surgical interventions **Limitations of most screening and prevention efficacy trials in the older population:** Most trials have excluded older patients, meaning that evidence of benefit is extrapolated/assumed to be true in this group

COMMONALITIES BETWEEN CANCER SCREENING AND PREVENTION IN THE ELDERLY

Some of the core principles in making the personal decision about preventive interventions are similar to those involved in screening decisions. Just as with screening, the target population for cancer prevention is generally healthy; hence, careful consideration must be given to both benefits and harms. The absolute benefits often diminish in the very elderly, whereas the absolute rate of harms may increase. The harms associated with screening and related diagnostic follow-up and treatment often increase with age. For example, advancing age has an adverse effect on postoperative mortality for a range of surgical procedures and associated complication rates. In the case of cancer prevention, strategies frequently involve pharmacologic interventions, which may have unfavorable toxicity profiles in the elderly compared to the young. These considerations may even reverse the benefit-harm balance of screening tests or preventive interventions in the elderly.

Just as with screening, powerful biases can confound the interpretation of prevention studies, leading to overestimation of benefits. "Healthy volunteer" bias is particularly important in prevention studies because adherence to (and interest in) preventive interventions is often associated with underlying robust health and favorable outcomes independent of the actual effect of the intervention. Healthy volunteer bias in clinical screening and prevention trials may therefore make accurate generalization of both benefits and harms to the very elderly difficult.

UNIQUE ASPECTS IN JUDGING BENEFITS AND HARMS OF CANCER PREVENTION IN THE ELDERLY

There are also important differences between screening and primary prevention interventions in the elderly. As previously discussed, limited life expectancy may amplify overdiagnosis in screening because even progressive tumors may not grow quickly enough to cause medical problems before the individual dies of competing causes. Delay in time to benefit can also represent an important difference between screening and prevention strategies. "Lead time" before a cancer screening test confers benefit may be on the order of 3 to 15 years. However, the delay in benefits from certain preventive interventions could, in some cases, be far longer if the intervention acts at early stages of carcinogenesis and may be even more likely than screening interventions to fall beyond the remaining life expectancy of an elderly person considering, for example, difficult changes in lifestyle. In contrast, risk for lung cancer begins to drop within a few years after quitting smoking, so tobacco cessation programs are likely to produce benefits even in the elderly.

With some exceptions, such as episodic single cervical cancer or colon cancer screening tests to detect and remove preneoplastic lesions, preventive interventions are usually long term and require prolonged effort. This is particularly true of dietary change and exercise but also applies to the need to take pharmacologic agents for years. These long-term interventions can be especially challenging in a cognitively impaired person or in someone with the physical limitations of advancing age that limit exercise. This stands in contrast to screening interventions, which are repeating but episodic in nature, and although they may cause distress in a cognitively impaired person (who might not understand what is being done), are usually brief, time-limited encounters.

Case Study: Screening Interventions

The Husband: Prostate Cancer Screening. Although this female patient firmly believes in the power of PSA screening to avert prostate cancer death in her husband, experts strongly disagree over the utility of this modality. Despite explosive uptake of this technology in the United States, for many years only observational studies existed to guide practitioners' judgement, and such studies are particularly prone to the biases previously mentioned. In 2009, the publication of two randomized controlled trials shed new light onto the issue. The first trial was the Prostate, Lung, Colorectal, and Ovarian (PLCO) cancer screening trial. It assigned approximately 77,000 men, aged 55 to 74 years, at 10 U.S. study sites to receive annual PSA testing for 6 years or to usual care. After 7 to 10 years of follow-up, no statistically significant difference in prostate cancer mortality rates was observed, with a trend toward *increased* death in the screened group (rate ratio 1.13; 95% CI, 0.75-1.7). Between 40% and 50% of participants in the control group did receive PSA screening at least once outside the confines of the trial, which may have had an impact on the observed effect size, although any potential benefit would remain small.[2]

The second trial, the European Randomized Study of Screening for Prostate Cancer (ERSPC), was a multinational study that randomized approximately 162,000 men between ages 50 and 74 years (with a predefined "core" group of 55 to 69 years) to receive PSA testing (at varying intervals, and with digital rectal examination and transrectal ultrasound, depending on screening center, or no screening). There was about a 20% relative reduction in the risk of prostate cancer death in the "core" screening group after a median follow-up of 9 years. Of note, no statistically significant difference in prostate cancer mortality was observed in the overall study population, and, again, there was a trend toward *increased* mortality in the oldest enrolled subgroup (70 to 74 years) (rate ratio 1.26, 95% CI, 0.80-1.99). The trial also raised considerable concerns about resulting overdiagnosis; it found that 48 cases of prostate cancer needed to be treated to avert one death from the disease.[3]

Neither of these trials provides direct evidence concerning the efficacy of PSA screening for men—such as this patient—who are 75 years and older. Additionally, because most men 75 years and older have a reduced life expectancy, few would be expected to live long enough to experience a mortality benefit from screening. There is also evidence to suggest that any net benefit of treatment with radical prostatectomy for diagnosed prostate cancer may be largely limited to men younger than 65 years.

As stated previously, potential harms must always be weighed against likelihood of benefit when deciding the worth of a clinical intervention. In the case of PSA testing, important possible harms to the individual besides the documented potential for overdiagnosis and overtreatment of latent disease include false-positive results and resulting unnecessary diagnostic procedures (including repeat biopsies). Analysis of the PLCO trial has shown that the cumulative probability for a man to receive at least one false-positive PSA test is 13%, and the probability of undergoing resulting invasive testing is 6%, after four rounds of testing.[4] False-positive tests have been shown to have an impact on men's mental health. Multiple studies have shown that men with false-positive PSA screening test results are more likely to worry about prostate cancer, have an inaccurately elevated perceived risk for the disease, and have sexual function issues compared with those with normal results. These psychological findings have been documented to persist for at least 1 year after the false-positive test, despite diagnostic resolution of the issue (a normal biopsy).

Finally, potential harms associated with therapy for the disease must also be factored into the overall risk-benefit profile of a screening test because the test can confer no benefit without resulting treatment. In the case of prostate cancer, the harms of treatment can be considerable. A study of quality of life among survivors of localized prostate cancer after treatment with radical prostatectomy, brachytherapy, or external-beam radiotherapy found that at 1 year after treatment, depending on choice of therapy, 54% to 75% could not maintain erections for intercourse, 3% to 14% experienced bowel urgency described as "a moderate or big problem," and 6% to 16% had urinary incontinence at least once a day.[5] Multiple studies have also shown that the postoperative mortality from radical prostatectomy increases with age; as noted previously, this may occur in the context of absence of potential for benefit from the therapy.

This careful review of the uncertainty of benefits, along with the potential harms of screening and therapy, convinces this patient and his wife that he should forgo PSA screening.

The Wife: Breast Cancer Screening. The wife remains concerned that she has not been getting regular mammograms. There have been a number of randomized controlled trials of mammography performed; however, most of these trials are older (approximately 30 years) (which could reduce the true importance of screening relative to treatment, as new therapies have emerged over time) and have important methodological limitations. Several meta-analyses of these trials have estimated an approximate 15% relative reduction in breast cancer deaths after 10 to 14 years of regular mammography screening in women aged 39 to 74 years.[6] However, age is a critical factor affecting the magnitude of risk reduction. The most recent systematic review performed for the U.S. Preventive Services Task Force found that for women ages 50 to 59, the relative risk was 0.86 (95% CrI [credible interval], 0.75-0.99); for women 60 to 69, 0.68 (95% CrI, 0.54-0.87); and for women 70 to 74, there was a (not statistically significant) trend towards *increased* breast-cancer mortality with screening (RR, 1.12, 95%; CrI, 0.73-1.72).[7] Importantly, of all of the studies, only the Swedish Two-County trials included women between the ages of 70 and 74 years, and no trial has directly evaluated the efficacy of mammography in women aged 75 years and older.

As with prostate cancer screening, potential harms of mammography screening include the risk of overdiagnosis and overtreatment, adverse effects of treatment, and false-positive results, with resulting psychological effects and unnecessary diagnostic procedures. The potential for radiation-induced breast carcinogenesis has also been cited as a concern, although younger populations (e.g., 40 to 49 years) would be at greatest risk for this outcome. Rates of overdiagnosis associated with the use of screening mammography have been estimated at 10% to 30% of all breast cancers diagnosed.[8] Another way of framing these findings is that for every 2000 women screened regularly for 10 years, 10 women will be treated unnecessarily and 1 death from breast cancer will be averted (the latter after a delay of about 5 to 10 years). Importantly, because overall mortality rates (competing causes of death) rise with increasing age, the probability of overdiagnosis and overtreatment in women 70 years and older is likely higher than for other age groups.

False-positive test results are common with screening mammography. One analysis found that after 10 years of regular screening, nearly 50% of women would have at least one false-positive test, and 20% a resulting biopsy.[9] However, the frequency of false-positive results is thought to decrease with increasing age. Screening also may increase the overall frequency of mastectomies. A pooled analysis of randomized trials found that the relative risk of mastectomy after mammography compared with no screening was 1.35 (95% CI, 1.26-1.44).[8]

Psychological distress associated with false-positive mammography screening has been documented as well. A systematic review of the long-term effects of false-positive mammograms found that, compared with women who had received normal results, women with false-positive test results used mental health care professionals more frequently and had higher levels of anxiety, apprehension, and intrusive thoughts specific to breast cancer.[10] False-negative tests (that is false reassurance

that the woman does not have breast cancer) can also be of concern; mammography is estimated to miss 1 breast cancer per 1000 women screened per screening round.[7]

After a careful discussion regarding the unavailability of high-quality evidence about the efficacy of mammography for women in this patient's age range, along with a review of the important potential associated harms—particularly overdiagnosis and overtreatment—the wife decides that she would like to take some time to further consider the information before deciding on whether to be screened for breast cancer.

> The wife is also interested in pursuing colonoscopy screening for colorectal cancer for both herself and her husband. She notes that neither has previously received a colonoscopy, although her gynecologist had occasionally performed an in-office guaiac smear; the results of these have always been negative. Her physician points out to her that in-office guaiac smears are not considered an acceptable form of colorectal cancer screening, having never been tested in prospective studies.

Husband and Wife: Colorectal Cancer Screening. Until recently, only the home based fecal occult blood test (FOBT) had randomized, controlled evidence available to demonstrate reductions in colorectal cancer deaths. Several trials of FOBT have consistently shown relative reductions in colorectal cancer mortality of between 15% and 33%, depending on whether the test was administered annually or biennially; this translates into an absolute risk reduction of about one to five deaths per 1000 participants.[11] Of note, most trials only included individuals up to 74 years of age; a single study provides evidence for up to 80 years. Newer fecal immunochemical tests have demonstrated improved sensitivity and specificity compared with guaiac-based tests and have been recommended for use by the U.S. Preventive Services Task Force (Table 2-2).

Flexible sigmoidoscopy (which can evaluate the left side of the colon up to the splenic flexure) is another screening option for the couple to consider. A recently published randomized, controlled trial of one-time flexible sigmoidoscopy versus usual care in 170,000 men and women ages 55 to 64 years demonstrated a statistically significant 30% relative reduction in colorectal cancer mortality.[12] Although colonoscopy has the least evidence available to directly demonstrate its efficacy in reducing colorectal cancer mortality, because the procedure is integral to diagnostic follow-up and polyp removal for the other screening options (and, as such, is a necessary step in colorectal cancer screening programs), this has been thought to represent sufficient indirect evidence of efficacy to support its use as a stand-alone screening option. Colonoscopy generally allows for visualization of the entire colon (to the cecum). On the other hand,

TABLE 2-2	Age-Specific Recommendations for Screening and Prevention from the U.S. Preventive Services Task Force*	
Intervention	**Modality**	**Recommendation**
Prostate cancer screening	PSA	Men, <75 years: the current evidence is insufficient to assess the balance of benefits and harms ("I") Men, 75+ years: Recommends against screening ("D")
Breast cancer screening	Mammography	Women, 50-74 years: Recommends biennial screening ("B") Women, 75+ years: The current evidence is insufficient to assess the balance of benefits and harms ("I")
Colorectal cancer screening	Fecal occult blood testing, annually Flexible sigmoidoscopy, every 5 years Colonoscopy, every 10 years CT colonography Fecal DNA testing	Men and women, 50-75 years: Recommends screening ("A") Men and women, 76-85 years: Recommends against routine screening; there may be considerations that support screening in an individual patient ("C") Men and women, 86+ years: Recommends against screening ("D") The current evidence is insufficient to assess the balance of benefits and harms ("I")
Breast cancer chemoprevention	Tamoxifen Raloxifene	Women, any age, low to average risk for breast cancer: Recommends against routine use ("D") Women, any age, high risk: Recommends clinicians discuss chemoprevention ("B")
Colorectal cancer prevention	Aspirin/NSAIDs	Men and women, all ages: Recommends against routine use ("D")
Cancer chemoprevention, general	Vitamins A,C, E Multivitamins with folic acid Antioxidants	Men and women, any age: The evidence is insufficient to recommend for or against use ("I")

*For more detailed information regarding these recommendations, go to: http://www.ahrq.gov/clinic/uspstf/uspstopics.htm

two recent epidemiologic studies have suggested that the benefits of colonoscopy may be restricted to the left side of the colon. Other screening options under development include computed tomography (CT) colonography and fecal DNA testing; however, evidence regarding the effectiveness of these modalities is still being acquired.

Harms associated with screening vary by the modality used. FOBT in and of itself appears to have the lowest risk of associated adverse events, although its associated false-positive rate (2% to 10%, depending on whether rehydration is used) is of concern because each positive test leads to further evaluation with colonoscopy, which has higher rates of complications.[11] In the most recent systematic evidence review performed in support of the U.S. Preventive Services Task Force, flexible sigmoidoscopy was found to have a rate of serious complications of about 3.4 per 10,000 procedures (including perforation, major bleeding, diverticulitis, and cardiovascular events requiring hospitalization, as well as death). Colonoscopy appeared to have the highest rate of associated serious complications, at 25 per 10,000 procedures. Perforations alone accounted for about 4 per 10,000 procedures.[13]

Although the relative frequencies of harm by age have not been well studied, at least two trials have shown increased risks of perforation with colonoscopy in older adults (older than 60 years). A modeling study performed by two groups from the Cancer Intervention and Surveillance Modeling Network (CISNET) found that although colorectal adenoma incidence does increase with advancing age, for individuals between the ages of 75 and 85,

any gains in life-years acquired through screening were small in comparison to the risks of associated complications. Furthermore, as was true for prostate and breast cancer, the increasing frequency of important comorbidities and competing causes of death in this population reduces the likelihood that any benefits of screening (which may take up to a decade or more to appear) will be actualized.

After reviewing the limitations of the evidence for persons aged 75 and older, and after careful discussion of the variable risks associated with each of the colorectal cancer screening strategies, the husband decides he is not interested in pursuing any type of screening. The wife decides that she is uncomfortable with pursuing colonoscopy as a primary screening test, given the review of potential harms, but, as she feels she is in essentially good health, she is interested in at-home FOBT testing.

Case Study: Prevention Interventions

The Husband: Prostate Cancer Prevention

The husband has chosen not to receive prostate cancer screening. However, his friend informed him that a drug that is used to treat benign prostatic hyperplasia (BPH) and baldness has been shown to decrease the risk of developing prostate cancer and that the side effects are relatively mild. This appeals to him, and he wants to know whether he should take it for cancer prevention.

Although not approved by the Food and Drug Administration (FDA) for prostate cancer prevention, a large randomized placebo controlled trial of the 5-alpha reductase inhibitor finasteride (the Prostate Cancer Prevention Trial [PCPT]) does provide good evidence that finasteride at a dose of 5 mg orally per day decreases the risk of prostate cancer.[14] In the trial, 18,882 men aged 55 and older were randomly assigned to take finasteride or placebo for up to 7 years. Over the 7-year period, the rates of prostate cancer diagnosis were 18% and 24% in the finasteride and placebo arms, respectively, for a relative reduction of 25%. Because the study design mandated an end-of-study prostate biopsy in all men who had not previously been biopsied, the high rates of cancer in each study were due to both clinically relevant cancers and those that would not have been detected had it not been for per-protocol biopsy. A subsequent systematic review of the use of 5-alpha reductase inhibitors for prostate cancer prevention estimated the number needed to treat (NNT) to prevent one diagnosis of prostate cancer after about 7 years of finasteride use was about 71.[15]

Side effects of finasteride were modest and included a decrease in volume of ejaculate, a small decrease in libido, and slight increases in erectile dysfunction and gynecomastia. The effects on sexual function were generally reversible. On the plus side, problems associated with urinary obstruction (including urinary urgency, frequency, and retention) were lower in the finasteride arm compared with placebo.

However, the initial report of the PCPT showed a potentially worrisome increase in diagnoses of high-grade (Gleason score 7-10) tumors associated with finasteride (6% compared with 5%). Even though the number of deaths from prostate cancer was the same in each arm, the fear was that the increase in high-grade tumors might ultimately translate into a higher risk of death from prostate cancer. Subsequent analyses have provided evidence that the increase in high grade tumors in men taking finasteride is likely to be spurious because finasteride decreases the size of the prostate gland, leading to an increase in sensitivity of PSA in the detection of high grade tumors.[15] As part of the study design, all men were being routinely screened annually with PSA and digital rectal examinations.

The routine screening of all men in the PCPT brings up a key issue in counseling this patient. Because of the study design, the impact of finasteride on prostate cancer risk is only known in men who are being regularly screened for prostate cancer. PSA testing is known to increase the risk of being diagnosed with prostate cancer by about 100%. Many of these screen-detected cancers are indolent and would never have come to attention had it not been for screening. Therefore finasteride does not bring the risk of being diagnosed with prostate cancer down to the level of risk in a man who is not being screened at all. It is also not known how effective finasteride is in preventing cancers not detected by screening.

Because this man declined prostate cancer screening, finasteride may be of little or no benefit.[15]

Given this caveat, he asks whether a specific diet, dietary supplements, or vitamins are known to prevent prostate cancer. Unfortunately, there are no known dietary interventions known to decrease prostate cancer risk. In a randomized trial, selenium and vitamin E did not decrease prostate cancer risk.[16] Evidence regarding most other nutrients and supplements is inconsistent, and there are no randomized trials to inform decisions.

The wife has heard about the use of the selective estrogen receptor modulators (SERMs) tamoxifen and raloxifene to lower breast cancer risk and would like to know if she should take one. As in the case of counseling on prostate cancer chemoprevention, treatment decisions are complex and must be individualized. The risk-benefit ratio changes with age and also depends on the underlying absolute risk for breast cancer. As in the case of prostate cancer chemoprevention, there is evidence from randomized controlled trials to help guide the decision.

The Wife: Breast Cancer Prevention. In the Breast Cancer Prevention Trial (BCPT), 13,388 women at increased risk of breast cancer were randomly assigned to take tamoxifen (20 mg per day for up to 5 years) or a placebo.[17] In the subsequent Study of Tamoxifen and Raloxifene (STAR), 19,747 women were randomly assigned to take tamoxifen (20 mg per day) or raloxifene (60 mg per day), a SERM that is FDA-approved for the management of osteoporosis of menopause.[18] Both trials required an estimated 5-year absolute breast cancer risk of at least 1.66%, calculated by a validated statistical model (the "Gail model"; see http://www.cancer.gov/bcrisktool/). The model was based on several risk factors: age, race/ethnicity, family history, age at menarche, age at first live birth of a child, and prior biopsy history. Because the average 5-year risk of breast cancer for an American woman is about 1.66% once she reaches the age of 60 years, this patient may meet the criterion for a discussion about chemoprevention with a SERM. However, since 1.66% is the *average* risk for a 60-year-old woman, many elderly women have a risk level lower than this threshold, and the Gail model estimate should be obtained on the basis of the specific additional risk factors of this patient.

In the BCPT, tamoxifen reduced the relative risk of both invasive and noninvasive breast tumors by about 40% after 7 years of follow-up compared with placebo. The number of women at elevated risk of breast cancer needed to treat to avert an invasive breast cancer was about 60 to 65 and about 175 to avert a noninvasive tumor. The preventive effects were limited to estrogen receptor (ER)–positive tumors. Several other randomized trials (the International Breast Intervention Study;

the Royal Marsden Tamoxifen Trial; and the Italian Randomized Tamoxifen Prevention Trial) have demonstrated similar results for invasive cancer.

Tamoxifen has been shown to cause a number of life-threatening side effects, and several of these increase with age. These include endometrial cancer, stroke, and thromboembolic events (e.g., pulmonary embolism). It is therefore important that elderly women explicitly discuss the possible life-threatening toxicities in considering the use of tamoxifen. Tables have been published that show estimates of the benefits and harms of tamoxifen according to a woman's baseline risk of breast cancer, her age, and the presence of a uterus. Those tables show, for example, that women over age 70 who have a uterus do not generally have a favorable benefit-risk balance unless their estimated 5-year risk of breast cancer is at least 6.5%.

Raloxifene, another SERM, has been shown to decrease the risk of invasive breast cancer in placebo-controlled trials for prevention of osteoporotic fractures and cardiovascular events in postmenopausal women at elevated risk for these outcomes. Unlike tamoxifen, raloxifene does not appear to increase the risk of endometrial cancer in women with a uterus. Because of these observations, raloxifene was directly compared with tamoxifen in the previously mentioned STAR trial. The effects of raloxifene on the risk of invasive cancers observed in the STAR trial were similar to tamoxifen and restricted to ER-positive tumors. However, unlike tamoxifen, raloxifene appeared to have little or no preventive effect on noninvasive tumors.

The toxicity profiles between the two drugs differ in important ways. Raloxifene has a lower incidence of thromboembolic events and tends toward fewer endometrial cancers in women with uteri. Taking all of this evidence into account, it is likely that raloxifene would have a more favorable benefit-risk profile in this patient, if she has a high enough risk of developing breast cancer and wishes to use a chemopreventive agent.

This patient is also curious about other potential breast cancer prevention options. Although prophylactic mastectomy has been shown to be associated with a reduced risk of breast cancer in women with highly penetrant predisposing inherited mutations in genes such as BRCA1 and BRCA2, it is reserved for women at extremely high risk, and thus is not a consideration for this 76-year-old woman with no prior history of cancer. Finally, no lifestyle or dietary changes and no vitamins or dietary supplements have been proven to decrease the risk of breast cancer (and certainly not in the very elderly). It is true, however, that the well-established risk of breast cancer associated with combined postmenopausal hormone therapy with estrogen plus progestin decreases rapidly if the hormones are stopped. Therefore this would be a serious consideration if the patient had been taking hormone therapy.

The third area of particular interest to this couple is colorectal cancer prevention. The hormone therapy component of the randomized Women's Health Initiative (WHI) provided evidence that postmenopausal hormone therapy with combined estrogen plus progestin, but not estrogen alone, lowers the risk of colorectal cancer.[19] This protective effect is supported by observational evidence. However, the WHI combined hormone therapy study was halted because of a net unfavorable balance in health outcomes. Therefore, hormone therapy should not be considered a standard option for colorectal cancer prevention in this female patient.

Husband and Wife: Colorectal Cancer Prevention. On the basis of the fact that colorectal cancers overexpress cyclooxygenase-2 (COX-2) and observational evidence that use of the COX-2 inhibitors such as celecoxib and rofecoxib are associated with a lower risk of colorectal cancer, there was strong interest several years ago in the use of COX-2 inhibitors for cancer prevention. However, several randomized trials were launched and then stopped because of an increased risk of several life-threatening toxicities, including myocardial infarction, stroke, and heart failure. Such adverse outcomes would be particularly important in the elderly, who are at increasing risk for them by virtue of their age.

Aspirin, a nonspecific anti-inflammatory drug, is also of interest, and it is often used in low doses (e.g., one "baby aspirin" of about 81 mg per day) to prevent myocardial infarction in men at elevated risk and stroke in women at elevated risk. However, the doses tested for colorectal cancer have generally been far higher than those used to prevent cardiovascular disease. Randomized trials, supported by observational evidence, suggest that taking at least 300 mg of aspirin per day for at least 5 years can prevent colorectal cancer after a latency period of 10 years or more.[20] However, it is likely that the bleeding risks combined with the long latency before the onset of benefit in this elderly couple would weigh strongly against the use of aspirin in the doses needed to prevent colorectal cancer.

Lifestyle changes such as exercise, increased dietary fiber, lower meat intake, high fruit and vegetable intake, or use of vitamins, minerals, or dietary supplements have been of interest for many years for colorectal cancer prevention. Most of the interest arose from retrospective case-control studies. However, prospective cohort studies that are less subject to recall biases are far less supportive of these associations. There may be reasons to recommend dietary and lifestyle changes for prevention of other chronic diseases, but the evidence is too weak and inconsistent to suggest that the changes will lead to reduction in risk of colorectal cancer.

Finally, polyp removal as a result of colorectal cancer screening is a form of primary cancer prevention. Screening has been covered earlier in this chapter.

CONCLUSION

Discussions about cancer screening and prevention are particularly complex in the elderly (Table 2-3). If the adage that it is very difficult to make a healthy person better off than he already is applies to cancer screening and prevention in general, it is of particular relevance to the elderly. Harms of screening and prevention often occur relatively quickly, and benefits, if any, are often delayed by years or decades. Moreover, what evidence that exists to inform personal decision making is often either observational in nature (and therefore subject to strong study biases) or particularly sparse in the elderly; most randomized trials in healthy volunteers attract a relatively young population. Therefore extrapolations of

TABLE 2-3	Controversial Issues
Need for randomized trials in screening and prevention	Because the outcome of interest (death from cancer or cancer incidence) in a healthy population is relatively rare, randomized trials of screening and prevention must often be large, and may require many years of follow-up along with considerable resources. However, because of fundamental biases inherent in observational studies of screening and prevention trials (see Table 2-1), RCTs are the only method by which one can definitely evaluate the efficacy of a given preventive agent or early detection method.
Overdiagnosis	Although counterintuitive, the concept of overdiagnosis itself is now accepted as a harm of screening for most if not all cancers, including prostate, breast, and colorectal. For a given cancer, estimates regarding the magnitude of overdiagnosis (as a proportion of all detected disease) remain areas of debate.
Universal upper age boundaries for screening and preventive interventions	Some guidelines organizations (including the USPSTF) have begun to establish lower and upper age boundaries for screening practices, on the basis of clinical trial evidence and modeling approaches. This has arisen out of the recognition that different age subpopulations are likely to experience different balances of net benefits and harms. However, as individuals may vary in terms of associated comorbidities and life expectancies, not all groups agree with this approach.

existing evidence to the elderly can be difficult. Some of the tools provided in this chapter can facilitate the discussion with patients, but individualization will always play an important role. Across-the-board recommendations in the elderly are usually overly simplistic.

SUMMARY

Prevention and early detection interventions hold immense intuitive appeal; however, public health messages around these issues have often understated the true complexity of decision making in this field. This is particularly true regarding the unique considerations in screening and prevention for older populations. This chapter begins with a review of general principles of cancer screening and prevention. It introduces the analytic framework, a tool to assist researchers and clinicians in basing decisions about the utility of a given preventive or early detection intervention on an explicit chain of evidence that highlights the net balance of benefits and harms for a given population, rather than a reliance on assumptions or simple intuitive reasoning. Major biases associated with screening and prevention studies (particularly observational studies), including the healthy volunteer effect, lead-time bias, length-biased sampling, and the concept of overdiagnosis, are discussed. Important similarities and key conceptual differences between screening and prevention trials and activities are highlighted.

A critical discussion of the specific considerations for screening and prevention activities in older adults in the areas of prostate, breast, and colorectal cancer follows. Unique factors to bear in mind for older populations include (1) a paucity of direct evidence supporting the use of screening and prevention interventions in this subgroup (as most older adults have been excluded from efficacy trials); (2) the impact that limited life expectancy and the presence of comorbid conditions can have on the probability of overdiagnosis and overtreatment; (3) the differential effect that toxicities of chemopreventive agents or treatments may have on older populations; and (4) the fact that the overall potential for benefit from screening or preventive actions will generally decline with age. The concepts presented in this chapter should help to facilitate informed, individualized discussions with patients.

 See expertconsult.com for a complete list of references and web resources for this chapter

SECTION II

Diagnosis/Assessment

Approach to Cancer Diagnosis: Use of Radiology, Pathology, and Tumor Markers

Sunil Amalraj and Arash Naeim

In 1947, the American Cancer Society began a public education campaign about the signs and symptoms of cancer, describing them as "Cancer's Danger Signals," ranging from "unusual bleeding or discharge" to "nagging cough or hoarseness." This approach has evolved over the decades, with the improvement in diagnostic techniques that has made it possible to rapidly diagnose cancer in patients with minimal symptoms or none at all. The primary care physician and geriatrician are on the front lines of diagnosing cancer, especially in its earliest and most treatable stages.[1]

The number of individuals older than 65 years in the United States is expected to more than double over the next 30 years, with the largest increase occurring in the subsegment of individuals aged 75 to 84. More than 60% of new cancers and 70% of cancer deaths occur in people older than 65 years.[2] The primary care physician or geriatrician must not only manage the chronic comorbid medical conditions of older patients, but also display vigilance in the medical examination of this high-cancer-risk population. The evaluation can often be complex, involving multiple imaging modalities, specialized blood tests, and biopsy procedures, and has the potential to be an emotionally distressing experience for the patient. When cancer is suspected in an older patient, a logical and targeted plan of medical tests must be constructed that takes into consideration the impact on the patient's current performance status, his or her goals of care, and the associated financial costs.

Cancer is one of the most common diseases that drastically diminish quality of life and life expectancy. According to the American Cancer Society, over 1.4 million new cancer diagnoses will be made in the United States in 2009. This number does not include basal and squamous cell skin cancers or in situ carcinoma (except bladder). Cancer is the second most common cause of death next to heart disease and accounts for nearly one of every four deaths. The most common sites of new cancer cases for men are prostate (25%), lung/bronchus (15%), and colorectal (10%). For women, they are breast (27%), lung/bronchus (14%), and colorectal (10%). The leading cause of cancer deaths for both men and women was lung cancer, which accounted for 30% of male cancer deaths and 26% of female cancer deaths.[3] Aging and cancer are complex processes that are regulated by multiple factors. Extensive research into the molecular mechanisms of both aging and cancer has demonstrated the convergence of many common biological pathways. The most critical of these pathways are those activated by DNA damage, inflammation, depletion of stem cells, and oxidative stress.[4-7] Hence, cancer can be truly thought of as a disease of aging. The National Cancer Institute, Surveillance Epidemiology and End Results program has found, from data collected between 2003 and 2007, that the median age for cancer diagnosis for prostate is 67 years; for breast, 61 years; for colon/rectum, 70 years; for lung, 71 years; and for leukemia, 66 years. Furthermore, 68.4% of lung cancer diagnoses and 63.4% of colorectal cancer diagnoses were made in patients older than 65 years.[8]

MAJOR IMAGING MODALITIES IN CANCER DIAGNOSIS

Cancer imaging studies have a fundamental role in the diagnosis and management of many types of cancers. Computed tomography (CT), magnetic resonance imaging (MRI), and ultrasound are widely used to help distinguish between malignant and benign lesions, to accurately stage a newly diagnosed cancer, and to provide objective information on tumor size that can be used to determine the response to treatment. Specialized plain film x-ray imaging such as mammography has been established as an important screening method and posttreatment surveillance program for breast cancer.[9] The recent improvements in functional imaging, such as PET-CT scanning, have made it possible to obtain important additional information for treatment decisions.

A.J. is a 78-year-old widowed man with a past medical history of coronary artery disease, hypertension, and glaucoma who presents to his geriatrician with 4 months of epigastric abdominal pain that radiates to the back, along with episodes of nausea. He also reports an 8-pound weight loss over the past 2 months. On physical examination, he has no signs of ascites or gastrointestinal obstruction. Laboratory studies disclosed the following values: hemoglobin, 10.5 g/dL; white blood cell count, 10,500/µL; platelet count, 330,000/µL; total bilirubin, 2.50 mg/dL; direct bilirubin, 1.50 mg/dL; aspartate aminotransferase, 109 U/L; alanine aminotransferase, 115 U/L; alkaline phosphatase, 467 U/L; lactate dehydrogenase, 503 U/L; and CA 19-9, 82 U/mL. The patient's geriatrician orders an upper endoscopy, which is within normal limits.

Continued

Plain X-rays

Traditional plain film x-rays are widely used for the detection of lung cancers and bone cancers. This form of imaging provides high resolution, but with only limited contrast if there are no calcifications located in the tumor. Chest x-ray screening has not been demonstrated to be effective at reducing mortality from lung cancer. A solitary pulmonary nodule 8 mm or larger in diameter requires further evaluation, including repeat chest x-ray, computed tomography, and possibly biopsy.[10] The skeletal survey, which includes plain x-ray films of the skull, axial skeleton, pelvis, and bilateral extremities, has a key role in the evaluation of patients suspected of having osseous involvement from multiple myeloma.[11]

Mammography

Mammography is the main imaging modality used for the early detection of breast cancer. Mammographic screening programs have been shown to save lives when compared with unscreened populations. Mammography has an overall sensitivity of less than 50%, and efforts are underway to improve its effectiveness as a screening tool.[12] Most mammography performed today is based on newer digital imaging systems. A recently completed trial involving over 50,000 women (Digital Mammographic Imaging Screening Trial) found comparable efficacy compared to plain x-ray mammography. Digital mammography is superior for woman with radiodense breasts and those younger than age 50. The sensitivity for digital mammograms is 41%, with 98% specificity and a positive predictive value of 12%.[13] A newer mammographic imaging technique, tomosynthesis, which generates a number of "slices" of the breast for analysis, has shown encouraging results.[14]

Ultrasound

Ultrasound produces high-resolution images from high-frequency sound waves, and its use has many applications in cancer diagnosis. This form of imaging avoids ionizing agents and contrast agents. It is very effective in distinguishing solid from cystic masses, and is an important tool for evaluating breast abnormalities. It is also helpful in locating and evaluating palpable lesions that are not visible with mammography. MRI with ultrasound can also provide accurate imaging guidance for biopsy procedures and information regarding blood flow intensity and direction in affected vascular structures. Ultrasound images are most widely used for the detection of gynecological, liver, and neck malignancies.[15] Endoscopic ultrasound (EUS), also known as echoendoscopy, combines the techniques of endoscopy with ultrasound imaging technologies and is useful for the diagnosis of esophageal cancer, pancreatic cancer, and rectal cancer.[16] High-intensity focused ultrasound has been utilized as a therapeutic option for ablation of localized breast and prostate cancer.

Computed Tomography

CT scans today have a central role in the diagnosis, staging, and surveillance of cancer because of their ability to offer cross-sectional imaging. This technology has rapidly evolved, with increasing simultaneous imaging slices up to 256, and rotational speeds that allow a whole body scan with a single breath hold. Additional advancements have led to three-dimensional reconstruction and angiography. While CT scans can demonstrate detailed measurements of tumor size and location, intravenous and oral contrast must be used in a coordinated function to obtain optimal images. Some major disadvantages of CT include total radiation dose, renal toxicity and allergic reactions to intravenous contrast, and high financial cost.[17] Triphasic CT scanning (arterial phase, portal venous phase, venous phase after a delay) of a suspicious liver lesion greater than 2 cm and demonstrating classic arterial enhancement is sufficient for making the diagnosis of hepatocellular carcinoma.[18] There has been increasing concern about the carcinogenic potential of multiple diagnostic CT scans. Results from epidemiological studies of medical diagnostic radiation exposure have found that cancer risk from all forms of ionizing radiation is cumulative. The only consistently established link involves exposure to medical radiation during pregnancy and the subsequent risk of pediatric cancer in these children.[19] Thus for the geriatric patient, the risk to the individual patient is minimal, and the benefit/risk balance favors the older patient. The current research evaluating the cancer risk of CT scans when used for symptomatic screening has yet to establish any evidence-based guidelines.

Magnetic Resonance Imaging

MRI scanning offers another form of anatomic imaging without ionizing radiation, and provides superior soft tissue contrast and spatial resolution. MRI is the imaging

Date: 31/03/2015 09:33

Transfer to Hold in Bell Library,
New Cross Hospital (NEW)

Pitt, Sheila

- 0063193
-
- 8, Park Meadow Avenue
  Bilston
  => WV14 6HA
- sheila.pitt106@btinternet.com

ITEM ON HOLD

Management of cancer in the
older patient

Naeim, A

- UH00001915
- QZ 266
-

Notes:

modality of choice for primary and metastatic tumors of the brain and spinal cord, as well as for musculoskeletal tumors. It also plays an important role in the detection of breast cancer in women with dense breast tissue, and in the diagnosis of soft tissue sarcoma and hepatocellular carcinoma. Today's MRI machines, at a strength of 1.5 to 3 Tesla units (T), are capable of rapid-pulse sequences and gating of images, allowing the visualization of blood with the use of contrast materials such as gadolinium. As the speed of MRI image acquisition improves and better contrast enhancement is developed, the applications for cancer imaging will only increase.[20] Absolute contraindications for MRI scanning that are especially common in the elderly include cardiac pacemakers, ocular metal, and significantly reduced creatinine clearance. Nephrogenic systemic fibrosis (NSF) has recently been linked to gadolinium-based contrast agents (GBCA). The practitioner should avoid use of these agents in patients whose glomerular filtration rate is less than 30 mL/min/1.73 m^2 unless the diagnostic information is essential and cannot be obtained with noncontrast MRI or other imaging modalities.[21] The technique of diffusion MRI images, used widely for strokes, has showed promise in measuring the response to treatment of brain tumors. This imaging method, which can distinguish between dead and living brain tumor cells, allows assessment of the cancer for therapeutic effectiveness without relying on measurable changes in tumor size.[22]

Nuclear Medicine

Radionuclide bone scans are commonly used to detect bone metastases from such primary malignancies as breast and prostate cancers. The most commonly used isotope for single-photon imaging is technetium-99m, which can be used to image bone (bone scan with ^{99m}Tc-diphosphonate) or thyroid (technetium pertechnetate). In multiple myeloma, the radionuclide bone scan may be falsely negative because of purely osteolytic lesions.[23] Neuroendocrine tumors of the gastrointestinal tract are often located using radiolabeled somatostatin analogues. Metaiodobenzylguanidine (MIBG), which is structurally similar to noradrenaline, can be radiolabeled with radioiodine (^{123}I) and has a sensitivity of approximately 90% for the detection of pheochromocytoma.[24]

The detection of sentinel nodes has an important role in breast cancer and melanoma. Lymphoscintigraphy involves injection of a radiopharmaceutical such as ^{99m}Tc-labeled colloid particles and use of a handheld gamma probe to localize a focus of increased radioactivity. This technique is highly effective in detecting involved local regional lymph nodes.[25] Therapeutic isotope applications include iodine-131 for the treatment of thyroid cancer, and a CD20 monoclonal antibody linked to the radioactive isotope yttrium-90 (Zevalin) used in refractory B-cell non-Hodgkin lymphoma.[26]

TABLE 3-1	Diagnostic Performance of PET-CT and CT with Contrast[33-40]		
Tumor	**CT (Contrast) Staging Accuracy**	**PET-CT Staging Accuracy**	**PET-CT Staging Sensitivity/ Specificity**
Lymphoma	67%	93%	93/100
Lung Cancer/ Solitary Lung Nodule	85%	93%	96/88
Head and Neck Cancer	74%	94%	98/92
Colorectal Cancer	65%	89%	86/67
Thyroid Cancer	75%	93%	95/91
Breast Cancer	77%	86%	84/88
Melanoma	86.3%	98.4%	94.9/100

Positron Emission Tomography

Positron emission tomography (PET) allows functional imaging by using intravenous radiolabeled metabolic tracers such as 18-fluorodeoxyglucose (FDG). PET imaging is most sensitive in fast-growing tumors with strong metabolic activity such as head and neck and colon cancers, melanoma, and aggressive lymphoma. When PET scan is performed with concurrent CT scanning, functional and anatomic information can be obtained rapidly, allowing for more accurate decision making.[27] Initial evaluation of both Hodgkin and non-Hodgkin lymphoma is increasingly performed with PET-CT scanning because of its increased sensitivity, with the ability to detect 20% more malignant lesions, including bone marrow and splenic involvement.[28] It also has an important role in determining whether complete response has been achieved for those lymphomas that were PET-avid at the time of diagnosis.[29] There is also substantial evidence that PET-CT is superior to CT alone for colon cancer patients in recurrent cancer is suspected after previous surgical resection.[30] An increasing amount of research supports the use of PET-CT in determining the need to pursue invasive testing for a solitary pulmonary nodule suspected of cancer. In a recent retrospective meta-analysis, PET-CT showed a sensitivity of approximately 96% and a specificity of approximately 80% for detecting cancer in solitary pulmonary nodules (predominantly ≥1 cm in diameter).[31-32] (Table 3.1).

CANCER PATHOLOGY

The treatment of cancer is almost always based on analysis of tissue pathology. With the exception of hepatocellular carcinoma and emergent situations such as acute leukemia with leukostasis, the first step after detection

---

CASE 3-1 **CONTINUED**

CT scan of the abdomen with/without intravenous contrast showed dilatation of the gallbladder and the intrahepatic and extrahepatic biliary tree, with a 5 cm mass in the head of the pancreas. A histological diagnosis of adenocarcinoma of the pancreas was made by CT-guided fine needle aspiration (FNA) biopsy.

Pancreatic cancer is the fourth most common cause of cancer-related death for men in the United States. Its peak incidence occurs in the seventh and eight decades of life. When the index of suspicion for pancreatic cancer is high, CT scan should be performed with the "pancreas protocol" (triphasic cross-sectional imaging and thin slices). Endoscopic ultrasound (EUS) is frequently used to further evaluate pancreatic masses and determine the degree of periampullary invasion. Endoscopic ultrasound also provides useful staging information such as the assessment of vascular invasion.[16] Reviews of surgical studies have found that curative pancreaticoduodenectomy (Whipple procedure) can be performed safely in selected patients younger than 80, with morbidity rates, mortality rates, and cost analysis similar to those achieved with younger patients.[41]

CASE 3-3

P.M. is a 72-year-old married woman, with a past medical history of insulin-dependent diabetes mellitus, hypertension, gout, and nephrolithiasis, who presents to her geriatrician for further evaluation after a routine complete blood count (CBC) found a significant white blood cell count: leukocytes 35,000/μL with 88% lymphocytes. The hemoglobin level is 12.5 g/dL, and the platelet count is 320,000/μL. She is feeling well and denies weight loss, night sweats, fatigue, shortness of breath, skin changes, or recent infection. Her physical examination is positive for mild splenomegaly (spleen palpable 2 to 3 cm below the costal margin), but is otherwise unremarkable. She has no clinical evidence of lymphadenopathy, or of abnormal bruises.

---

of a possible malignancy is coordinating a procedure to obtain a tissue sample for initial confirmation of the diagnosis and future treatment planning. This involves close cooperation between the primary care provider and the radiology or surgical consultant to pursue the lowest-risk approach for the older patient, who often comes with several comorbidities. The pathology report always includes such information as tumor size, histological classification, tumor grade, and pathologic staging. These anatomic features are augmented by immunohistochemical, cytogenetic, and molecular biologic testing, as indicated, to allow detailed tumor classification and to guide the best therapeutic treatment plan.[42]

CASE 3-2

K.T. is an 80-year-old married woman, with a past medical history of insulin-dependent diabetes mellitus, chronic renal insufficiency, and atrial fibrillation, who presents to her geriatrician for further evaluation after noticing persistent right cervical adenopathy, which is painless. She reports increased fatigue and a low grade fever. Her hemoglobin level is 11.5 g/μL, with a white blood cell count of 6,500/μL, and a platelet count of 330,000/μL. The serum lactate dehydrogenase level is 720 U/L. Renal and liver function are normal. Her physical examination is unremarkable and her weight has been stable.

Fine Needle Aspiration/Image Guided Biopsy

The technique of fine needle aspiration (FNA), which utilizes a fine-gauge needle to obtain a sample of cells from a suspicious mass, has been a cornerstone of diagnosis for many cancers, such as carcinoma of the thyroid. It

is cost-effective, poses minimal risk for complications, and avoids the need for general anesthesia. These factors make FNA especially appropriate for use with older patients. Although accuracy rates range from 90% to 95%, FNA is limited to cancer diagnoses that are dependent on cell features rather than tumor architectural patterns, which require larger tissue samples. Thus, FNA is insufficient in making a diagnosis of lymphoma or testicular cancer. Percutaneous image-guided biopsies are the most common way of making a tissue diagnosis of cancer today. Real-time imagery provided by ultrasound, CT scan, and MRI has advanced the biopsy procedure, allowing for acquisition of larger samples of suspicious tissue. Hence, they usually result in adequate tissue to complete immunohistochemical staining, flow cytometry testing, cytogenetic evaluation, and molecular studies.[43] Image-guided biopsy is most often performed under local anesthesia, and has a relatively low complication rate when performed by an experienced radiologist. A recent retrospective analysis performed at the Mayo Clinic found image-guided biopsy in elderly patients did not carry a greater risk of any major complication as compared with younger patients.[44]

Immunohistochemistry

Light microscopy utilizing conventional hematoxylin-eosin (HE) staining is central to determining the gross structure of the tumor, such as distinguishing between adenocarcinoma and neuroendocrine solid tumors and evaluating important parameters such as the nuclear/cytoplasmic ratio of lymphoma tumor cells. Immunohistochemical staining (IHC) is a technique for identifying and classifying malignant cells by means of antigen-antibody interactions used in conjunction with standard light microscopy. IHC is widely used to analyze the distribution and localization of biomarkers and differentially expressed proteins in tumor biopsy samples. The site of antibody binding can be identified either by direct labeling of the antibody, or by a secondary labeling method.[45] Its most common use is in immunoperoxidase staining, wherein an antibody is conjugated to the enzyme peroxidase, producing a colored chemical reaction. Although not always able to provide a specific diagnosis, these stains can often aid in the differential diagnosis of carcinomas, lymphomas, melanoma, and certain sarcomas when used in conjunction with routine histological examination.[46] Immunofluorescence is an antigen-antibody reaction in which the antibodies are tagged with a fluorescent dye such as such as fluorescein or rhodamine, and the antigen-antibody complex is visualized using an ultraviolet (fluorescent) microscope. Specific cytokeratin proteins that are components of the cytoskeleton of epithelial cells found on certain cancer cells are often identified this way and play an important role in diagnosis. One example of this is discriminating between the diagnosis of primary lung acinar adenocarcinoma and lung metastasis of colorectal cancer. Positive staining of CK7 was observed in most of the primary lung adenocarcinoma samples and positive staining of CK20 was observed in most lung metastases of colorectal cancer.[47]

Flow Cytometry, Cytogenetics, Molecular Testing, and Cancer Diagnosis

Flow cytometry is a method of measuring the number of cells in a sample, and certain characteristics of cells, such as size, shape, and the presence of tumor markers on the cell surface. The cells are stained with a light-sensitive dye, placed in a fluid, and passed in a stream before a laser or other type of light. The measurements are based on how the light-sensitive dye reacts to the light. Among the most common clinical uses of flow cytometry in cancer diagnosis is the classification of chronic lymphoproliferative disorders and acute hematological malignancies.[48] Acute and chronic leukemia display characteristic patterns of surface antigen expression (CD antigens), which facilitate their identification and proper classification and hence play an important role in instituting proper treatment plans. For example, flow cytometry plays a decisive role in distinguishing acute promyelocytic leukemia (APL) from other forms of acute myeloid leukemia (AML), and therefore is critical to determining the initial treatment.[49] Cytogenetic testing involves examining the chromosomes in a cell to detect any abnormality characteristic of a malignancy, such as translocation, inversion, deletion, or duplication. The development of a newer cytogenetic process called fluorescence in situ hybridization (FISH) has expanded molecular diagnostic capabilities. FISH uses special fluorescent dyes to recognize specific chromosome changes in certain types of cancer. The DNA from a biopsy sample is combined with a fluorescently-labeled probe, such as the one for HER-2/neu-positive breast cancer, that is visible under fluorescent microscopy.[50-51] Another DNA analysis technique, called polymerase chain reaction

TABLE 3-2	Recurrent Molecular Abnormalities Associated with Myeloproliferative Neoplasms	
Genetic Abnormality	**Disease**	**Frequency**
BCR-ABL	Chronic myelogenous leukemia	≈99%
JAK2V617F	Polycythemia vera	>95%
	Essential thrombocytosis	≈60%
	Primary myelofibrosis	≈60%
JAK2 exon 12	Polycythemia vera	≈2%
PDGFRA	Myeloid neoplasm +eosinophilia	Undetermined
	Mast cell disease	
PDGFRB	Myeloid neoplasm +eosinophilia	Undetermined
KIT (D816V)	Mast cell disease	Undetermined

From Vannucchi AM, Guglielmelli P, Tefferi A. Advances in understanding and management of myeloproliferative neoplasms. CA Cancer J Clin 2009;59(3):171-91.

(PCR), which makes possible the rapid amplification of DNA, is used to detect the bcr-abl oncogene in blood or bone marrow when the myeloproliferative neoplasm (MPN) chronic myeloid leukemia (CML) is suspected.[52] (Tables 3.2 and 3.3).

CASE 3-2	CONTINUED

The patient was referred to a head and neck surgeon who performs fine needle aspiration (FNA). Cytology studies demonstrate small cleaved lymphocytes and flow cytometry shows a CD5-negative, CD10-positive, CD20-positive monoclonal population suspicious for non-Hodgkin lymphoma (NHL). However, FNA is not adequate to make a diagnosis of lymphoma. The presence of a monoclonal cell population with a CD10-positive immunophenotype is highly suggestive of follicular lymphoma, but an accurate diagnosis cannot be made without lymph node architecture. Furthermore, FNA cannot determine the histological grade of the follicular lymphoma, which strongly influences treatment choice. NHL is the ninth leading cause of cancer deaths among men and the sixth among women.[55] The incidence of NHL has increased significantly in the past three decades, especially in patients in the sixth and seventh decade of life.[56]

Clinical Applications for Biomarkers in Cancer

Since the discovery of the first tumor markers over a century ago (Bence-Jones proteins), numerous molecules have been identified as being associated with various cancers. Tumor markers are biochemical substances produced by malignant cells or by other cells of the body in response to cancer or certain noncancerous conditions. They can be found in the blood, in the urine, in

TABLE 3-3	Immunophenotype for Selected Cancers[54]	
Disorder	Positive	Negative
Large B-cell lymphoma	CD19, CD20, CD22, CD79a,	CD2, CD3, CD5, CD7
Follicular small cleaved cell lymphoma	CD10, CD19, CD20, CD21, CD22, CD24,	CD2, CD3, CD4, CD5, CD7, CD8, CD11c, CD23, CD25, CD43
Mantle cell lymphoma	CD5, CD19, CD20, CD22, CD24, CD43,	CD11c, CD23, CD5/CD19 or CD5/CD20
Hairy cell leukemia	CD11c, CD19, CD20, CD22, CD25, CD79a, CD103	CD2, CD3, CD4, CD5, CD7, CD8, CD10, CD23
Acute promyelocytic leukemia, M3	CD13, CD15, CD33	CD2, CD3, CD5, CD7, CD11b, CD14, CD41, CD42, CD61, CD71
Acute mega-karyoblastic leukemia, M7	CD33, CD41, CD42, CD61	CD2, CD3, CD5, CD7, CD11b, CD13, CD14, CD15, CD71
ALL (T-cell precursor)	CD3, CD7	CD10, CD19, CD20, CD22
ALL (pre-B)	CD10, CD19, CD22, CD79a	CD3, CD4, CD5, CD7, CD8
Sézary syndrome (mycosis fungoides)	CD2, CD3, CD4, CD5	CD1, CD7, CD8, CD10, CD11c, CD16, CD19, CD20, CD22, CD25, CD56, CD57

From Nguyen AN, Milam JD, Johnson KA, Banez EI. A relational database for diagnosis of hematopoietic neoplasms using immunophenotyping by flow cytometry. Am J Clin Pathol, 2000. 113(1): p. 95-106.

CASE 3-3   CONTINUED

A CT scan of the chest, abdomen, and pelvis shows bilateral 1.5 cm axillary lymphadenopathy. A review of the peripheral blood smear shows small, mature-appearing lymphocytes with dense nuclei and a small amount of cytoplasm. Flow cytometry of the peripheral blood reveals a clonal B-cell population that is CD5-positive, CD19-positive, CD23-positive, and, CD10-negative. Cytogenetic studies are remarkable for 13q- and 12q- chromosomal abnormalities. Based on the CBC, flow cytometry, and cytogenetics, early-stage chronic lymphocytic leukemia (CLL) is diagnosed. A bone marrow biopsy is not required. Chronic lymphocytic leukemia is one of the most common hematological malignancies in the United States, with an incidence of 3.5 per 100,000. The median age at diagnosis is 70 years for men and 74 years for women.[57]

the tumor tissue, or in other tissues. Tumor markers can be broadly classified into tumor-specific antigens and tumor-associated markers. The vast majority of tumor markers are tumor-associated antigens that can also be found in normal tissue.[58]

There are few specific situations where tumor markers play an important role in the screening and initial diagnosis of a malignancy; however, in clinical practice, tumor markers are most frequently used in evaluating the progression of disease status after the initial therapy and in monitoring the effectiveness of treatment. Tumor marker use in the United States is influenced by the requirement for their approval by regulatory agencies such as the U.S. Food and Drug Administration (FDA), which affects eventual reimbursement from insurance companies. Recommendations for the use of tumor markers are published by the American Society for Clinical Oncology and the National Comprehensive Cancer Network Practice Guidelines in Oncology.[59]

CASE 3-4

J.B. is a 70-year-old married man, with a past medical history of rheumatoid arthritis, hypertension, and hepatitis B with compensated cirrhosis, who presents to his primary care physician for further evaluation of an elevated serum alkaline phosphatase at 655 U/L. He underwent ultrasonography and was found to have a 4.8 cm hypoechoic tumor in the right lobe of the liver. Serum total bilirubin, alanine aminotransferase, aspartate aminotransferase, and gamma-glutamyl transpeptidase levels were within normal limits, as were coagulation studies. The serum α-fetoprotein concentration was elevated, at 800 ng/mL (normal <20 ng/mL). Serum carcinoembryonic antigen (CEA), and carbohydrate antigen (CA) 19-9 levels were normal. Computed tomography of the liver displayed a tumor in the right lobe, 5.8 cm in diameter, showing a broad zone of peripheral enhancement after administration of intravenous contrast material, and a central low-density area in the arterial-dominant phase. The border of the lesion was irregular and indistinct, and the radiodensity of the tumor was lower than that of the surrounding liver parenchyma.

SCREENING AND EARLY DETECTION

Screening refers to evaluating an asymptomatic patient for the purpose of early detection of cancer. Clinical sensitivity and specificity, in addition to the prevalence of the cancer in the population, will determine the positive predictive value of the screening marker, Although tumor markers were originally developed for identifying a malignancy in a patient without have any focal physical complaints, the only serum tumor marker that is part of any screening program today is prostate-specific antigen (PSA). Other identified tumor markers lack sufficient sensitivity and specificity for widespread use in screening.[60]

The American Cancer Society (ACS) and the American Urological Association recommend PSA and digital rectal examination annually, beginning at age 50, for men who have a life expectancy of at least 10 years. The U.S. Preventive Services Task Force (USPSTF) and American Academy of Family Physicians do not recommend routine prostate cancer screening with PSA, based on insufficient evidence that early detection by PSA improves health outcomes. Furthermore, PSA is organ-specific but not prostate cancer-specific. Elevated PSA levels (>4 ng/mL) can be found in men with benign prostatic hyperplasia (BPH) and prostatitis. Also, a normal PSA level does not exclude a diagnosis of prostate cancer.[61] Age-specific reference ranges for PSA have been developed (0 to 2.5 ng/mL, 3.5 ng/mL, 4.5 ng/mL, and 6.5 ng/mL for age ranges 40 to 49, 50 to 59, 60 to 69, and 70 to 79 years, respectively) in an attempt to produce increased sensitivity of the test in younger men, so that localized tumors can be detected earlier, when surgical cure is still possible, and improved specificity of the test in older men, who are more likely to have benign elevations in PSA. PSA velocity and analysis of free and complexed PSA levels offer methods of improving PSA specificity. At least three PSA measurements 12 to 18 months apart are needed to accurately calculate PSA velocity. A PSA velocity rate (rate of change) greater than 0.75 ng/mL per year is highly suggestive of cancer. Patients with prostate cancer have a lower percentage of free PSA (free PSA/total PSA) compared with men with benign disease.[62–63]

Tumor Markers in Cancer Diagnosis

Hepatocellular carcinoma is the fifth most common cancer in the world, and the third most important cause of cancer mortality. Prognosis for this disease is poor, since hepatocellular carcinoma (HCC) is usually diagnosed at an advanced stage. Alpha-fetoprotein (AFP) is effective as a tool for confirming a diagnosis of HCC in high-incidence populations such as patients with hepatitis and cirrhosis. An elevation in AFP above 20 ng/mL has been shown to have a sensitivity of between 60% and 90% and a corresponding specificity of 70% to 80% for HCC. An AFP level over 200 ng/mL or the presence of classical arterial enhancement on triphasic CT or MRI is considered to be diagnostic of HCC when a liver mass is greater than 2 cm in size.[64-65]

AFP and β-human chorionic gonadotropin (hCG) have an important role in the classification of germ cell tumors. Usual reference values for AFP are 10-15 mg/L, and for hCG 0-5 IU/L in evaluation for testicular cancer. In seminoma (one form of testicular cancer), AFP is not elevated, but hCG is present in 10% to 30% of cases. Either hCG or AFP or both are produced by 60% to 90% of nonseminomatous germ cell testicular tumors at the time of diagnosis. Both hCG or AFP are elevated in embryonal carcinoma (hCG > 65%; AFP >70%) and AFP is elevated in yolk sac tumors. Also, hCG is elevated in choriocarcinomas and hence useful in diagnosing gestational trophoblastic tumors.[66]

The tumor marker CA-125, developed for epithelial ovarian cancer, is useful in distinguishing benign from malignant disease in postmenopausal women who present with ovarian masses and elevated concentrations of CA-125. One study found a CA-125 greater than 95 U/mL has a positive predictive value of 95% in a postmenopausal woman with a pelvic mass.[67-68] A two-stage strategy in which ultrasonography is performed only if CA-125 concentrations are elevated has shown promise in detecting ovarian cancer. In a study of 4000 women, the specificity of CA-125 plus ultrasound was 99.9% compared with 98.3% for CA-125 alone.[69]

Neuroendocrine tumors constitute a heterogeneous group of rare cancers that originate from endocrine glands in various tissues such as the pituitary, parathyroid, and adrenal glands; the pancreas; and the respiratory tract.[70] Tumor markers often play an important role in the detection of these tumors. For example, the diagnosis of pheochromocytoma usually is established by finding an increase in the urinary excretion of catecholamines or catecholamine metabolites such as vanillylmandelic acid (VMA) and homovanillic acid (HVA).[71] The urinary serotonin metabolite 5-hydroxyindoleacetic acid (5-HIAA) is the primary test for determining the overproduction of serotonin that is characteristic of carcinoid tumors.[72]

CASE 3-4 **CONTINUED**

Elevation of the tumor marker α-fetoprotein (AFP) to 800 ng/mL, in the presence of a liver lesion greater than 2 cm in diameter, is sufficient for the diagnosis of hepatocellular carcinoma (HCC). The presence of classical arterial enhancement on triphasic CT further confirms this diagnosis. Tissue biopsy is not required to confirm the diagnosis in this case.[64] The median age at diagnosis for HCC is 64, with 48% of cases occurring in people older than 65 years. The overall 5-year survival for the period 1999 to 2006 was 13.8%.[3] Treatment options for this patient include liver transplantation, surgical resection, ablation (radiofrequency, cryoablation, microwave) and chemoembolization. Short- and long-term results for liver transplantation in patients older than 65 have found outcomes to be comparable to those younger than 65, if older candidates are carefully selected.[73] (Table 3.4).

Summary

Men in the United States have a one in two lifetime risk of developing cancer and women have a one in three lifetime risk of developing cancer. During the last 3 decades there has been steady improvement in the relative 5-year survival rate for all cancers, with a 50% survival from 1975-1977 improving to a 66% survival from 1996-2004.[3] There has also been an increase in the incidence of certain cancers, such as breast cancer (4.3%) and prostate cancer (7.6 %), since 1975.[8] The factors behind these two trends include advances in treatment, the aging population, and significant improvements in our ability to detect cancer at a less advanced stage. As a result of increasing life expectancy, the incidence of cancer is elevenfold higher in persons older than 65 years compared to those younger than 65.[76] The development of imaging

TABLE 3-4	Malignancies Associated with Elevated Tumor Marker Levels						
Tumor Marker	Primary Tumor	Diagnosis	Screening	Normal Value	Benign disease unlikely	Benign conditions
PSA	Prostate cancer	Adenocarcinoma of unknown primary	Yes	<4 ng/mL	>10 ng/mL	Prostatitis, BPH
CA=125	Ovarian cancer	Pelvic mass in postmeno-pausal women	No	<35 units/mL	>200 units/mL	Menstruation, pregnancy, fibroids, ovarian cysts
AFP	Hepatocellular cancer	Liver mass and cirhosis	No	<5.4 ng/mL	>500 ng/mL	Cirrhosis, hepatitis, pregnancy
β-hCG	Germ cell tumor	Adenocarcinoma of unknown primary	No	<5 mIU/mL	>30m mIU/mL	Hypogonadal states, marijuana use
CA 19-9	Pancreatic cancer	Selected pancreatic masses	No	<37 units/mL	>1000 units/mL	Pancreatitis, biliary diease, cirrhosis
CEA	Colorectal cancer	No	No	<2.5 ng/mL <5.0 ng/mL	>10 ng/mL	Cigarette smoking, pan-creatitis, peptic ulcer disease, cirrhosis
CA 27.29	Breast cancer	No	No	<38 units/mL	>100 units/mL	Breast, liver, kidney disor-ders, ovarian cysts

From Perkins GL, Slater ED, Sanders GK, Prichard JG. Serum tumor markers. Am Fam Physician, 2003. 68(6): p. 1075-82; and Manne U, Srivastava RG, Srivastava S. Recent advances in biomarkers for cancer diagnosis and treatment; Drug Discov Today 2005;10(14):965-76.

modalities such as PET-CT, biomarker assays, histological staining techniques, and molecular testing has made possible the earlier diagnosis and treatment of many solid tumors and hematological malignancies.

A multidisciplinary health care team should be involved with planning from the earliest stage of the cancer evaluation, but a single physician should assume the lead role in communicating with the patient. The primary care physician or geriatrician is often in the best position to assess the severity of the patient's comorbid conditions and understand the patient's goals of care. A geriatric oncology tumor board format adapted from those frequently used in medical oncology for specific cancer types and involving the primary care physician could be an effective tool to develop a personalized diagnostic plan for each older patient. The decision to utilize all the medical technology available to prove the final diagnosis of a suspected cancer must be balanced with an individualized assessment of the patient's capacity to tolerate the toxicity of the likely treatment options. Diagnostic decision making in modern oncology continues to strive to integrate the application of technological advances and patient autonomy with the best understanding of the probability of enhancing patient quality of life when cure is not possible.

See expertconsult.com for a complete list of references and web resources for this chapter

SUGGESTED READINGS

1. American Cancer Society: *Cancer Facts & Figures 2009*, Atlanta, 2009, American Cancer Society.
2. Altekruse SF, Kosary CL, Krapcho M, et al, editors: *SEER Cancer Statistics Review, 1975-2007*, Bethesda, MD, National Cancer Institute. http://seer.cancer.gov/csr/1975_2007/, based on November 2009 SEER data submission, posted to the SEER web site, 2010.
3. Jemal A, Siegel R, Ward E, et al: Cancer statistics, *CA Cancer J Clin* 58(2):71–96, 2008.
4. Czernin J, Allen-Auerbach M, Schelbert HR: Improvements in cancer staging with PET/CT: literature-based evidence as of September 2006, *J Nucl Med* 48(Suppl 1):78S–88S, 2007.
5. Miles KA: Functional computed tomography in oncology, *Eur J Cancer* 38(16):2079–2084, 2002.
6. Rosai J: Standardized reporting of surgical pathology diagnoses for the major tumor types. A proposal. The Department of Pathology, Memorial Sloan-Kettering Cancer Center, *Am J Clin Pathol* 100(3):240–255, 1993.
7. Wick MR, Ritter JH, Swanson PE: The impact of diagnostic immunohistochemistry on patient outcomes, *Clin Lab Med* 19(4):797–814, 1999:vi.
8. Nguyen AN, Milam JD, Johnson KA, Banez EI: A relational database for diagnosis of hematopoietic neoplasms using immunophenotyping by flow cytometry, *Am J Clin Pathol* 113(1):95–106, 2000.
9. Varella-Garcia M: Molecular cytogenetics in solid tumors: laboratorial tool for diagnosis, prognosis, and therapy, *Oncologist* 8(1):45–58, 2003.
10. Vannucchi AM, Guglielmelli P, Tefferi A: Advances in understanding and management of myeloproliferative neoplasms, *CA Cancer J Clin* 59(3):171–191, 2009.
11. Perkins GL, Slater ED, Sanders GK: Prichard JG Serum tumor markers, *Am Fam Physician* 68(6):1075–1082, 2003.
12. Manne U, Srivastava RG, Srivastava S: Recent advances in biomarkers for cancer diagnosis and treatment, *Drug Discov Today* 10(14):965–976, 2005.
13. Smith RA, Cokkinides V, Brooks D, et al: Cancer screening in the United States, 2010: a review of current American Cancer Society guidelines and issues in cancer screening, *CA Cancer J Clin* 60(2):99–119, 2010.
14. Pallis AG, Fortpied C, Wedding U, et al: EORTC elderly task force position paper: Approach to the older cancer patient, *Eur J Cancer* 46(9):1502–1513, 2010 Jun.

Assessment

Jeffrey Mariano and Lillian C. Min

Our nation is aging. By 2030, 20% of the population will be over the age of 65. It is estimated that 1.5 million new cases of cancer were diagnosed in 2009 and over 500,000 cancer-related deaths occurred. Of these, approximately 60% of cancer cases and 70% of cancer-related deaths will occur in individuals aged 60 years and older.[1] As the population ages, it is increasingly important that doctors and oncologists characterize the "functional age" of older patients with cancer in order to tailor treatment decisions and stratify outcomes on the basis of factors other than chronologic age, and develop interventions to optimize cancer treatments.[2,6,7]

CASE 4-1 **CASE STUDY: Mrs. S**

Mrs. S is an 80-year-old woman with a history of hypertension presenting to her primary care provider. She was recently hospitalized and discharged from a skilled nursing facility due to an ankle fracture received as a result of a car accident in which she was the driver. She completed rehabilitation and has since returned home. Prior to the accident, she was living alone. However, her son now checks in on her more frequently and calls her twice a day. At this point, she is also afraid of driving and has been relying on public transportation and family members.

Over the next year, Mrs. S becomes increasingly anxious and depressed. She describes "not feeling well" and weight loss. Lab tests are unremarkable. Her son brings concerns of depression to her primary doctor's attention and she is started on Citalopram. Repeat clinical breast exams reveal bilateral breast masses, the right greater than the left.

WHAT INFORMATION FROM A GERIATRIC ASSESSMENT WOULD HELP GUIDE TREATMENT?

Physiologic reserve, functional status, cognition, and comorbidity vary considerably among older adults as a result of the aging process. Given this heterogeneity of factors, a geriatric assessment (GA) may help in managing the older patient with cancer.[2,3,7]

OVERVIEW OF THE GERIATRIC ASSESSMENT

A geriatric assessment includes an evaluation of an older individual's functional status, medical conditions (comorbidities), cognition, nutritional status, psychological state, and social support, as well as a review of the patient's medications (Table 4-1). A meta-analysis of 28 controlled trials demonstrated that Comprehensive Geriatric Assessment (CGA), if linked to geriatric interventions, reduced early rehospitalization and mortality in older patients through early identification and treatment of problems.[74] The components examined in GA can predict morbidity and mortality in older patients with cancer, and can uncover problems relevant to cancer care that would otherwise go unrecognized.[2,8] This approach to cancer care can facilitate individualizing the options for cancer management, quality of life, and prognosis.[8,74]

Three fundamental concepts guide geriatric assessment and the resulting medical management. At the core of geriatric assessment is functional status, both as a dimension to be evaluated and as an outcome to be improved or maintained. The maintenance and restoration of functional status is an essential overriding objective of good geriatric and geriatric oncologic care.[2,5,6,7] A second overarching concept guiding geriatric assessment is prognosis, particularly life expectancy. Finally, geriatric assessment must be guided by patient goals.[2]

PHYSICAL FUNCTION

Functional Status

Functional status and disability reflect the interactions among multiple medical conditions, physiologic aging, psychosocial support, cognitive impairment, and the overall health and vitality of the individual.[4] Functional evaluation can add a dimension beyond the usual medical assessment, providing information on patient care needs and prognosis.[6,4]

The choice of functional assessment tool depends upon the characteristics of the population (community-dwelling, hospitalized, nursing home residents) and the level of function being assessed. Function can be assessed

TABLE 4-1	Components of the Geriatric Assessment

Functional Evaluation (Physical Function)
    Self report
    Performance-based
    Gait and balance evaluation
Comorbidity
Cognitive Function
Psychological State (Affective Assessment)
Social Support
Polypharmacy
Nutrition
Symptoms
Selected Geriatric Syndromes
Advanced Care Planning

by self-report, proxy report, performance-based testing, or a combination of these approaches.[1,3,5]

Self-Reported Tools to Measure Functional Status

Activities of Daily Living (ADLs and IADLs, Tables 4-2 and 4-3) [73].

Most commonly, older adults' functional status is assessed at two levels: activities of daily living (ADLs) and instrumental activities of daily living (IADLs). ADLs are self-care tasks, such as:

- bathing
- dressing
- toileting
- maintaining continence
- grooming
- feeding
- transferring

Questions about functional ability may be valuable if posed in reference to recent activities: for example, "Did you dress yourself this morning?" rather than "Do you dress yourself?"

An inability to perform basic ADLs alone implies a higher risk for functional decline, hospitalization, and poor outcomes leading to delirium and or death. Dependency in these tasks, which is present in up to 10% of persons aged 75 years or older, usually requires full-time help at home or placement in a nursing home.[72]

IADLs are tasks that are integral to maintaining an independent household, such as:

- using the telephone
- shopping for groceries
- preparing meals
- performing housework
- doing laundry
- driving or using public transportation
- taking medications
- handling finances

Asking "Did you drive here today?" or "When did you last drive? (rather than "Do you drive?") may elicit a more useful answer. IADLs are more likely than ADLs to be influenced by factors other than capacity, such as cultural and gender roles and learned skills.

Basic ADLs (BADLs) and IADLs are commonly reported as total scores (see Tables 4-2 and 4-3). The total score for BADLs is 0 to 6; for IADLs it is 0 to 8. In some categories of IADLs, only the highest level of function receives a 1; in others, two or more levels have scores of 1 because each describes competence at some minimal level of function. When these screens are used over time, they serve as documentation of a person's functional improvement or deterioration. It is worth noting that the description of the functional capabilities is more important than the number total score, especially when monitoring function over time.[73]

A longitudinal analysis of older adults that characterized functional states between independent in ADLs and mobility, dependent on mobility but independent in ADLs, and dependent in ADLs translated to diminished survival and more of that survival spent in disabled states. For example, the life expectancy of an ADL-disabled 75-year-old is similar to that of an 85-year-old independent person; thus the impact of the disability approximates being 10 years older with much more of the remaining life spent disabled.[30a]

Advanced Activities of Daily Living (AADLs).

Advanced activities of daily living represent the highest level of function and are comprised of vocational, social, or recreational activities that reflect personal choice and add meaning and richness to a person's life. The AADLs include employment, attending church, volunteering, going out to dinner or the theater, participating in physical recreational activities, and the like. Changes in these activities may reflect a precursor to IADL or ADL dysfunction.[72]

Karnofsky and Eastern Cooperative Oncology Group (ECOG) Performance Status (PS).

Traditionally, the oncologist's assessment of functional status includes an evaluation of Karnofsky or Eastern Cooperative Oncology Group (ECOG) performance status (PS), Table 4-4. In older adults, particularly those with multiple chronic diseases, the prognostic ability of ECOG-PS may not relate to the specific impact of cancer [2,6,8] and may be insensitive to functional impairment. Although 70% to 80% of older adults with cancer present with ECOG PS of 0 to 1 (normal or symptomatic but ambulatory), greater than half require assistance with IADLs.[5,21] Furthermore, studies have shown that physicians', nurses', and patients' assessments of performance status using these measures may be discordant.[10]

Use of Self-Reported Functional Status Measures in Cancer Patients

Older patients with cancer, both during initial diagnosis and as cancer survivors, are more likely to require functional assistance than those without cancer.[13,15] Functional

TABLE 4-2 Activities of Daily Living (ADLs)

In each category, circle the item that most closely describes the person's highest level of functioning and record the score assigned to that level (either 1 or 0) in the blank at the beginning of the category.

A. Toilet ____

1. Care for self at toilet completely; no incontinence	1
2. Needs to be reminded, or needs help in cleaning self, or has rare (weekly at most) accidents	0
3. Soiling or wetting while asleep more than once a week	0
4. Soiling or wetting while awake more than once a week	0
5. No control of bowels or bladder	0

B. Feeding ____

1. Eats without assistance	1
2. Eats with minor assistance at meal times and/or with special preparation of food, or help in cleaning up after meals	0
3. Feeds self with moderate assistance and is untidy	0
4. Requires extensive assistance for all meals	0
5. Does not feed self at all and resists efforts of others to feed him or her	0

C. Dressing ____

1. Dresses, undresses, and selects clothes from own wardrobe	1
2. Dresses and undresses self with minor assistance	0
3. Needs moderate assistance in dressing and selection of clothes	0
4. Needs major assistance in dressing but cooperates with efforts of others to help	0
5. Completely unable to dress self and resists efforts of others to help	0

D. Grooming (neatness, hair, nails, hands, face, clothing) ____

1. Always neatly dressed and well-groomed without assistance	1
2. Grooms self adequately with occasional minor assistance, e.g., with shaving	0
3. Needs moderate and regular assistance or supervision with grooming	0
4. Needs total grooming care but can remain well-groomed after help from others	0
5. Actively negates all efforts of others to maintain grooming	0

E. Physical Ambulation ____

1. Goes about grounds or city	1
2. Ambulates within residence on or about one block distant	0
3. Ambulates with assistance of (check one)	
a ( ) another person, b ( ) railing, c ( ) cane, d ( ) walker, e ( ) wheelchair	
1.___Gets in and out without help. 2.___Needs help getting in and out	
4. Sits unsupported in chair or wheelchair but cannot propel self without help	0
5. Bedridden more than half the time	0

F. Bathing ____

1. Bathes self (tub, shower, sponge bath) without help	1
2. Bathes self with help getting in and out of tub	0
3. Washes face and hands only but cannot bathe rest of body	0
4. Does not wash self but is cooperative with those who bathe him or her	0
5. Does not try to wash self and resists efforts to keep him or her clean	0

Scoring Interpretation: *For ADLs, the total score ranges from 0 to 6.* In the above-mentioned categories, only the highest level of function receives a 1; These screens are useful for indicating specifically how a person is performing at the present time. When they are also used over time, they serve as documentation of a person's functional improvement or deterioration.

From Lawton MP, Brody EM. Assessment of older people: self-maintaining and instrumental activities of daily living. *Gerontologist* 1969, 9:179-186. Copyright by the Gerontological Society of America. Reproduced by permission of the publisher.

status may be dependent on cancer stage, with observational studies showing this dependency is more commonly found in hospitalized patients with metastatic disease as compared with patients with nonmetastatic disease. IADL impairment predicted postoperative complications (P = .043) in a series of older adults undergoing cancer-related surgery[16] and functional status predicted risk of treatment-related toxicity in studies of ovarian cancer patients receiving standard cytotoxic chemotherapy.[28] In addition, the need for assistance in IADLs has been reported to correlate with psychological distress in older adults with cancer.[26]

The need for assistance with IADLs has been shown to have the same predictive capability for mortality among older adults with cancer.[11,12] Functional limitations in cancer survivors also persist.[11,13,14,19]

Because functional status changes over time and is affected by other conditions as well as cancer and by the patient's social needs, accurate assessments at multiple time points over the course of the cancer patient's life are valuable in monitoring response to treatment and can provide prognostic information that is useful in short- and long-term care planning. Acute or

TABLE 4-3	Instrumental Activities of Daily Living Scale (IADLs)

In each category, circle the item that most closely describes the person's highest level of functioning and record the score assigned to that level (either 1 or 0) in the blank at the beginning of the category.

A. Ability to Use Telephone _____
1. Operates telephone on own initiative; looks up and dials numbers — 1
2. Dials a few well-known numbers — 1
3. Answers telephone but does not dial — 1
4. Does not use telephone at all — 0

B. Shopping _____
1. Takes care of all shopping needs independently — 1
2. Shops independently for small purchases — 0
3. Needs to be accompanied on any shopping trip — 0
4. Completely unable to shop — 0

C. Food Preparation _____
1. Plans, prepares, and serves adequate meals independently — 1
2. Prepares adequate meals if supplied with ingredients — 0
3. Heats and serves prepared meals or prepares meals but does not maintain adequate diet — 0
4. Needs to have meals prepared and served — 0

D. Housekeeping _____
1. Maintains house alone or with occasional assistance (e.g., domestic help for heavy work) — 1
2. Performs light daily tasks such as dishwashing, bed making — 1
3. Performs light daily tasks but cannot maintain acceptable level of cleanliness — 1
4. Needs help with all home maintenance tasks — 1
5. Does not participate in any housekeeping tasks — 0

E. Laundry _____
1. Does personal laundry completely — 1
2. Launders small items; rinses socks, stockings, etc. — 1
3. All laundry must be done by others — 0

F. Mode of Transportation _____
1. Travels independently on public transportation or drives own car — 1
2. Arranges own travel by taxi but does not otherwise use public transportation — 1
3. Travels on public transportation when assisted or accompanied by another — 1
4. Travel limited to taxi or automobile with assistance of another — 0
5. Does not travel at all — 0

G. Responsibility for Own Medications _____
1. Is responsible for taking medication in correct dosages at correct time — 1
2. Takes responsibility if medication is prepared in advance in separate dosages — 0
3. Is not capable of dispensing own medication — 0

H. Ability to Handle Finances _____
1. Manages financial matters independently (budgets, writes checks, pays rent and bills, goes to bank); collects and keeps track of income — 1
2. Manages day-to-day purchases but needs help with banking, major purchases, etc — 1
3. Incapable of handling money — 0

Scoring Interpretation: *For IADLs, the total score ranges from 0 to 8.* In some categories, only the highest level of function receives a 1; in others, two or more levels have scores of 1 because each describes competence at some minimal level of function. These screens are useful for indicating specifically how a person is performing at the present time. When they are also used over time, they serve as documentation of a person's functional improvement or deterioration.
From Lawton MP, Brody EM. Assessment of older people: self-maintaining and instrumental activities of daily living. *Gerontologist* 1969, 9:179–186. Copyright by the Gerontological Society of America. Reproduced by permission of the publisher.

subacute changes in functional status are important to elicit as they may be a marker of underlying medical illness, including recurrence of cancer, cognitive losses, or other psychosocial issues.[3,6] Health care providers can promote their patients' autonomy by mobilizing appropriate medical, social, and environmental supports.

Performance-Based Instruments of Physical Function

Performance-based instruments can provide additional information beyond an older adult's self-reported perception of difficulty.[2,72]

Get-up-and-Go Test. Ambulation is an essential prerequisite for completing many of the activities of daily

TABLE 4-4	Karnofsky and Eastern Cooperative Group Performance Scales			
Percentage (%)	Karnofsky Performance Scale	Score	ECOG Performance Scale	
100	Normal, no complaints, no evidence of disease	0	Normal activity; asymptomatic	
90	Able to carry on normal activity; minor signs or symptoms of disease	1	Symptomatic; fully ambulatory	
80	Normal activity with effort; some signs or symptoms of disease			
70	Cares for self, unable to carry on normal activity or to do active work	2	Symptomatic; in bed <50% of time	
60	Requires occasional assistance, but is able to care for most of his/her needs			
50	Requires considerable assistance and frequent medical care	3	Symptomatic; in bed 50% of time; not bedridden	
40	Disabled, requires special care and assistance			
30	Severely disabled, hospitalization indicated; death not imminent		100% bedridden	
20	Very sick, hospitalization indicated; death not imminent	4		
10	Moribund, fatal processes, progressing rapidly			
0	Dead	5	Dead	

living and slowing of gait speed is an indicator of future morbidity. For example, gait speeds of 1 m/s or less, and especially those less than 0.6 m/s, predict hospitalization, cognitive impairment, and mortality.[70,71]

The "Get-up and Go Test" has been recommended.[3,5,6,7,8,9] This assessment tool does not require specialized equipment, but uses an armless chair and has the individual stand up from the chair, walk 3 meters and sit back down. (Table 4-5) It can be performed by the physician, nurse, or other trained health care provider. Severe abnormalities are considered present if the subject appears at risk for a fall at any time during the test. The time needed to complete this task is used to score the test; greater than 15 seconds is considered a positive screen. Also, ranges of times required to complete the task correlate with independence in some functional tasks. (Table 4-5)

COMORBIDITY

Survival rates from the 15 most prevalent invasive cancers have improved over the past 10 years,[79] with declining deaths due to colorectal cancer attributable to improvements in detection, risk-factor reduction, and treatment.[79] The Surveillance, Epidemiology, and End Results (SEER) study has shown that over one quarter of older patients with colon cancer have three or more chronic conditions, and over half of older patients have at least one chronic condition.[80] Furthermore, concurrent aging of the population is expected, many of whom survive into their oldest decades with a greater burden of chronic medical comorbidities. Having two or more chronic conditions is prevalent in two-thirds of older patients (age ≥65) in the general United States population; while the prevalence increases to three-fourths of the oldest patients (age ≥80).[81,82] These trends suggest that clinicians will face the increasing challenge of managing older cancer survivors with multiple comorbidities, each of which may be considered for recommended clinical guidelines, care processes, and medication regimens.[83-85]

TABLE 4-5	Timed Get-Up and Go Test*

Examiner asks the patient to:
- Stand up from a chair (without use of armrests, if possible)
- Stand still momentarily
- Walk 10 feet (3 meters)
- Turn around and walk back to chair
- Turn and be seated

Factors to note:
- Sitting balance
- Imbalance with immediate standing
- Pace (undue slowness) and stability of walking
- Excessive truncal sway and path deviation
- Ability to turn without staggering
- Observe and time the patient

Positive screen:
- Time of >15 seconds to complete test

		Timed Get Up and Go (secs)		
		10-19	20-29	30+
Tub or shower transfers	Self	59%	60%	23%
Climbs stairs	Self	77%	60%	4%
Goes outside alone	Yes	82%	50%	15%
Chair transfer	Self	100%	93%	62%

Adapted from Podsiadlo D, Richardson S. J Am Geriatrics Soc 1991;39:142-148 and from Susan Friedman, MD, MPH, University of Rochester.
*Proportion able to complete mobility tasks, according to "Timed Get Up and Go" times

There are no clinical guidelines that address specific combinations of malignancies and common noncancer comorbidities of aging. Rather, guidelines for the care of older cancer patients focus on determining overall life expectancy on the basis of functional status and the index malignancy.[86] The National Comprehensive Cancer Network (NCCN)[86] suggests that supportive, rather than curative, care be recommended for older patients with a serious comorbidity and at least one functional impairment.

In the absence of a guideline for this geriatric patient that addresses all of Mrs. Z's comorbidities in

CASE 4-2	CASE STUDY: Mrs. Z

Mrs. Z is a 76-year-old woman with rectal cancer (T1N1M0) who presents with a fall and a new compression fracture. She was diagnosed with rectal cancer 12 months ago, when she presented with rectal bleeding. She was treated initially with capecitabine and radiation because her oncologist felt she was frail and looked more like an 85-year-old. Her other past medical history is significant for essential hypertension and osteoarthritis of the knees. Last year, during the workup of her cancer, mild type 2 diabetes was discovered. She continues to have mild insulin resistance, which she has managed through diet modification resulting in some weight loss. Last week, she fell while reaching overhead in her kitchen, and landed on her right buttock. In the emergency room she was found to have a new compression fracture of S2 and a stable hairline fracture of the right ala. MRI of the spine and pelvis was negative for bony lesions. She was discharged with an abdominal brace and pain medications. She has had an excellent response to her cancer treatment and is being evaluated for definitive surgical treatment.

In light of Mrs. Z's cancer and comorbidities, what is her life expectancy?

combination (i.e., someone with rectal cancer, diabetes, hypertension, osteoarthritis, and a new fragility fracture), the challenge is to weigh the relative risks and benefits of recommended care for these conditions, the expected benefits of the care, and this patient's goals and preferences. The patient's overall life expectancy should be considered in light of the time required for the expected benefit to be gained ("time to benefit"). This approach has been suggested by diabetes guidelines from the American Diabetes Association,[87, 88] as well as by other authors.[83,89-91] Braithwaite et al.[92] have proposed a general (noncancer) framework to further consider the "payoff time," which is the time frame over which a recommended treatment's cumulative benefits exceeds its harms, and whether or not the patient's life expectancy according to his or her most serious condition exceeds this payoff time.

In this case of Mrs. Z, the decision whether to recommend treatment of her osteoporosis, hypertension, and diabetes depends on whether or not she will survive long enough to realize those benefits. A list of some of the instruments for assessing comorbidity is shown in Table 4-6.

Estimating Life Expectancy with Respect to Cancer

The SEER provides an online calculator (http://seer.cancer.gov/canques/survival.html) to estimate the life expectancy for many cancers. Specifically for this patient with colorectal cancer (variables entered were: race = white, site = colon and rectum, year of diagnosis 1999-2006, age at diagnosis = 75+, stage at diagnosis = regional), mortality risk over the next 5 years was estimated at 65%. This estimate did not take into account her chemotherapy and radiation, nor her comorbid conditions.

TABLE 4-6	Comorbidity Scales
Charlson Comorbidity Index (CCI)	A weighted index that takes into account the number and the seriousness of comorbid disease; a score over 5 is considered high and is usually associated with poor prognosis
Cumulative Illness Rating Scale-Geriatric (CIRS-G)	Classifies comorbidities by organ systems (13 or 14 according to the version) and grades each condition from 0 (no problem) to 4 (severely incapacitating or life-threatening condition)
The Adult Comorbidity Evaluation (ACE-27)	Measures the severity of comorbidity based on 26 disease systems; each condition is graded with a three-category severity system (mild, moderate, severe)

From References 75, 76, 41.

Estimating Life Expectancy by Age and Comorbid Conditions

Because this patient has a number of comorbidities, using age alone in this patient overestimates her life expectancy. Simple life tables based on age and gender available from the United States National Vitals Statistics[93] approximate this patient's life expectancy at approximately 10 years. A simple online life expectancy estimator on the basis of age alone is available at the American Association of Retired Persons website (http://www.ssa.gov/OACT/population/longevity.html).

One approach suggested by Walter et al. for decisions related to cancer screening in older patients is to first estimate whether a patient falls into the healthiest or sickest quartile of health in comparison to other similarly-aged patients.[91] Under the assumption that Mrs. Z is in the bottom quartile of health compared to other women in her age group, her life expectancy is only 4.6 years.[91]

One study of older colorectal cancer patients has considered the effect of common comorbid conditions on survival.[80] The comorbidities considered were chronic obstructive pulmonary disease, heart failure, diabetes, atrial fibrillation, cerebrovascular disease, myocardial infarction, peripheral vascular disease, hip fracture, ulcers, dementia, rheumatologic disease, chronic renal failure, paralysis, liver disease, and AIDS. Given that Mrs. Z had one of these conditions (diabetes) and that her rectal cancer was stage III, applying the results of this study would result in a predicted life expectancy of 5.8 (95% CI 5.5-6.2) years.

When a comorbid disease, rather than the cancer, is severe and life-threatening, it may dominate the life expectancy calculation. In the case of heart failure patients, an online calculator based on the Seattle Heart Failure Model can be found at: http://depts.washington.edu/shfm/. For liver disease, the Mayo Clinic has published the End Stage Liver Disease (MELD) Score available at: www.mayoclinic.org/meld/mayomodel7.html.

For chronic kidney disease in older adults, annual risks can be found by age group and disease stage.[94] For type 2 diabetes, the Cleveland Clinic has developed a multivariable calculator for 6-year risk at: www.lerner.ccf.org/qhs/risk_calculator. Predicted life expectancy for dementia patients has also been studied.[95] A palliative care website has been developed to provide various disease-specific and general calculators at www.pallimed.org/2007/05/prognosis-links.html.

Other Considerations

Although comorbidity is most commonly used to estimate survival, older patients' functional status plays a central role in predicting mortality and making medical decisions.[96,97] One screening tool, the Vulnerable Elders-13 Survey (VES-13),[98] is based on functional status and age, rather than comorbidities. It provides risks for both death and functional decline over specific time intervals.[99,100] The VES-13 estimates life expectancy of less than 5 years for older (age ≥ 75) patients with scores of 8 or less.[100] Expectation of further functional decline within 5 years can be predicted for older patients with scores of 4 or less.[100] For patients who value preservation of functional status, this tool might be more useful than using life-expectancy alone.

Recommended Care of Comorbidities In Older Patients with Limited Life Expectancy

Two geriatric-specific clinical guidelines and quality indicators that address broad areas of medical care across multiple comorbidities were published in 2007. Quality indicators from the Assessing the Care of Vulnerable Elders Study (ACOVE-3)[101] define the level of care performance below which quality of care is considered to be poor. These indicators were tailored to older patients' limited life expectancy and individual care preferences. Better performance on the ACOVE indicators has been shown to be associated with improved survival.[102] The Screening Tool to Alert Doctors to the Right Treatment (START)[103] uses chronic conditions to remind clinicians to recommend 22 medications that are commonly omitted in the care of older patients.

COGNITIVE

Cognitive impairment increases with age and confers an increased risk for all cause mortality.[37] Frequently, especially in its early stage, it goes unrecognized.[38] Studies that included a screening cognitive exam as part of the GA for older patients with cancer have found that up to 25% to 50% had abnormalities that warranted further evaluation.[5,26a] Assessment of cognitive status is essential to provide a basis for comparison in future encounters. Studies have shown that cognitive impairment affects diagnosis

and treatment options and can affect decision-making in the older cancer patient (both in accepting treatment and in prognosis).[40,41,42,43] Specifically, cognitive impairment is an important risk factor for the development of delirium.[39]

Mini-Mental Status Exam (MMSE) and Montreal Objective Cognitive Assessment (MOCA)

The MMSE is a brief quantitative measure of cognitive status in adults. It can be used to screen for cognitive impairment and to aid in estimating its severity. It is composed of tests of orientation, registration, calculation, recall, language, and visual-spatial skills. It is helpful in establishing a diagnosis of dementia (cognitive impairment severe enough to affect functional status). It can be used serially to follow the course of cognitive changes in an individual over time or to compare mental status in certain situations (for example, when hospitalized or after chemotherapy) with baseline. The Montreal Objective Cognitive Assessment (MOCA) is another screening tool that has been developed, and has been found to be more sensitive than the MMSE in detecting mild cognitive impairment in brain metastasis patients.[77,78] Abnormal scores in either screen may herald the need for more testing or for functional reevaluation to mobilize more care (medication management, caregiving).

Mini-Cog. This test involves a three-item recall and a clock drawing test. These scales are designed as screening tools; further evaluation is warranted when a screen is positive.[6,8]

Delirium and the Confusion Assessment Method (CAM)

Delirium is a geriatric syndrome that should be considered with any change in mental status and cognition. The hallmarks of delirium are acute onset, fluctuating course, impaired attention, and cognitive changes. It can be mistaken for dementia, depression, or another psychiatric problem. The onset of delirium in any cancer patient is important, as multiple causes that are more common in cancer, including brain metastasis or metabolic issues like hyponatremia or hypercalcemia, can predispose the already at-risk individual to develop delirium.

The Confusion Assessment Method (CAM) is an easy to assess, four-step diagnostic test (Table 4-7).[39]

Because dementia and cognitive impairment increase with age, if cognitive screening is abnormal, the physician should fully assess cognition or refer the patient for more detailed neuropsychologic assessment.[8]

AFFECT (AFFECTIVE ASSESSMENT)

An estimated 12% to 20% of community-dwelling persons aged 65 years and older experience significant depressive symptoms.[45] These patients present with weight loss, insomnia, memory loss, and functional decline. In older

TABLE 4-7	Confusion Assessment Method

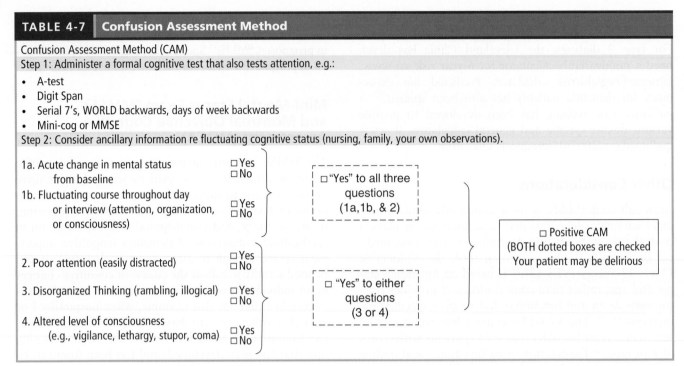

Confusion Assessment Method (CAM)

Step 1: Administer a formal cognitive test that also tests attention, e.g.:

- A-test
- Digit Span
- Serial 7's, WORLD backwards, days of week backwards
- Mini-cog or MMSE

Step 2: Consider ancillary information re fluctuating cognitive status (nursing, family, your own observations).

1a. Acute change in mental status from baseline — ☐ Yes ☐ No

1b. Fluctuating course throughout day or interview (attention, organization, or consciousness) — ☐ Yes ☐ No

☐ "Yes" to all three questions (1a, 1b, & 2)

2. Poor attention (easily distracted) — ☐ Yes ☐ No

3. Disorganized Thinking (rambling, illogical) — ☐ Yes ☐ No

4. Altered level of consciousness (e.g., vigilance, lethargy, stupor, coma) — ☐ Yes ☐ No

☐ "Yes" to either questions (3 or 4)

☐ Positive CAM (BOTH dotted boxes are checked Your patient may be delirious

Adapted from Inouye SK. The Confusion Assessment Method (CAM): Training Manual and Coding Guide 2003. Yale University School of Medicine. Accessed on 9/4/07 from http://elderlife.med.yale.edu/pdf/The%20Confusion%20Assessment%20Method.pdf

adults with depressive symptoms, 90% exhibit weight loss, compared to 60% of younger adults.[2,8] Cultural variation and overlap with major medical illness may influence how emotional states are expressed.[44] Affective assessment is particularly important in older adults with cancer; for example, symptoms of depression were associated with poorer progression-free survival, overall survival, and increased toxicity in older women with ovarian cancer treated with platinum-based regimens.[28] Some studies have shown that women diagnosed with depression and breast cancer receive less than definitive treatment and worsened survival.[2,8] Although cancer can elicit normal grief and bereavement, a suspicion of underlying depression should be considered by all members of the health care team. The GDS (Geriatric Depression Scale) and PHQ-9 are recommended as a depression screen in cancer patients.[46]

In one study, 20% of cancer patients were found to be depressed and in half of those, depression would have been missed without using the GDS. Given the consequences of depression and the options for treatment and support, screening for depressive symptoms should be part of the assessment in caring for older adults with cancer.[8,20,22]

Other elements of geriatric assessment account for issues that are rarely abnormal in younger adults (e.g., hearing, nutrition) but which may cause substantial morbidity in older persons and which are described later in this chapter. These geriatric issues are important in the management of older adults with cancer and are covered in other parts of this book. If these issues are present, they are often directly or indirectly worsened by the treatment and progression of cancer.[3] Affective disorders are discussed in greater detail in Chapter 15.

SOCIAL (SOCIAL ASSESSMENT)

Performance status, as measured by the ECOG-PS, represents a clinician's viewpoint and does not take into account the subjective psychosocial aspects of life that assume greater importance as one ages.[2,6] For cancer patients, the periodic assessment of social support allows the health care team to detect changes in care needs and prevent caregiver burnout. Informally, clinicians can probe systematically by themselves or with other members of the team (e.g., social workers or nursing staff).[48,49] For frail older cancer patients, the availability of assistance from family and friends may help inform the decision about cancer treatment strategy, including surgery or certain chemotherapies.[51]

CAREGIVER BURDEN

For many caregivers, there is value in the caregiving role, but it is a reality resulting in emotional and physical sacrifice, as well as profound economic difficulties. In one study, over half of caregivers reported not getting training they perceived as necessary in the management of treatment side effects; in helping manage pain, nausea, or fatigue; or in wound care. Twenty-five percent reported poor or fair health and low confidence in the quality of the care they provided. The inability of caregivers to meet the patients' needs for daily assistance may compromise patient well-being and result in hospitalization.[50,51]

The Zarit Caregiver Burden Index, a 22 item instrument, assesses the reaction of family members caring for older adults with chronic diseases, including cancer.[48,49] Shorter versions, including the Zarit-12, have been studied in breast cancer patients for evaluation and screening.[49] Studies are needed to determine how caregiver burden affects the pattern of health care resource utilization and older cancer patient outcomes, including adherence to treatment, survival, and quality of life.[50] Caregiver burden is discussed in more detail in Chapter 26.

POLYPHARMACY

Community-dwelling older Americans take an average of 2.7 to 6 prescription medications and 1 to 2.4 over-the-counter medications. Studies have shown that polypharmacy is associated with an increased risk of adverse drug reactions and falls.[8] Studies have shown that the number of drug-related problems is associated to the total number of prescriptions. These drug-related problems include drug-drug interactions, drug-disease interactions (NSAIDs and renal insufficiency), drug-nutrient interactions, or malnutrition caused by side effects causing anorexia, nausea, vomiting, altered taste, or mucositis. A complete review of prescription and nonprescription medications, vitamins, and supplements is important in all cancer patients.[52,53]

NUTRITION

Nutritional Screen and Malnutrition

Malnutrition is among the most serious manifestations of cancer and its treatment. Cancer-induced malnutrition may be more severe in older adults that have associated impaired body energy regulation, altered body composition and cell function with changes in body water and fat, and diverse dietary behaviors coupled to changes in taste and smell, medications, and multiple chronic illnesses. Cancer patients with a weight loss greater than 5% have a shorter median survival rate than cancer patients with stable weight.[54] Cancer and nutrition are discussed in greater detail in Chapter 20.

HEARING AND VISION

Both vision and hearing loss restrict activity, predict functional disability, foster dependency, diminish the sense of well-being, and increase stress in older adults.

Visual impairment is related to increased morbidity and increases risk for falls, hip fractures, and depression.[8]

Given that some vision and hearing impairment is treatable, a screen should be undertaken. For vision, this can be accomplished by use of a Snellen eye chart, and for hearing, with a whisper test.

SYMPTOMS

Pain and Nonpain Symptoms

Pain is one of the most frequent and disturbing symptoms associated with cancer. Older adults are more likely to experience pain, less likely to complain of pain, and more likely to have pain go unrecognized.[56,57,60,61] Pain may be minimized for various reasons, including expectations with aging,[58] its impact on increased family and caregiver involvement, and its being interpreted as a metaphor of death.[55]

Patient self-report is the most accurate and reliable way of reporting pain. Pain scales are usually used in the clinical setting. Numeric 0-10 scales, face pain scales, verbal scales in English and other languages can all be utilized. Furthermore, attaching pain to a functional outcome (e.g., how pain affects ambulation, sleep, or mood) adds value to the assessment. The American Geriatrics Society has guidelines on the management of persistent pain in older adults with cancer.[56] In addition to pain, the palliation of nonpain symptoms, including nausea, anorexia, insomnia, pain, dyspnea, and constipation, is critical in the management of cancer patients. Pain and nonpain management are discussed in greater detail in Chapters 16, 17, 18, and 19.

ADVANCED CARE PLANNING

Advance directives is a general term that describes legal documents (e.g., living wills and durable power of attorney for health care). These documents allow a person to give instructions about future medical care if an individual is unable to participate in medical decisions because of serious illness or incapacity.[63] Clinicians treating cancer patients need to make it clear that discussions of advance directives do not equate to stopping treatment.[2] Preferences for how aggressive to be in treating cancer are separate issues. As such, discussions regarding advance directives need to begin early in the course of treatment rather than in the days when incapacity or death is imminent. Clinicians should begin discussions with older patients about preferences for specific treatments while they have the cognitive capacity to make these decisions.[63] Patients should be asked to identify a spokesperson to make medical decisions if the patient cannot speak for herself or himself. This information should be conveyed through a durable power of attorney for health care (DPAHC), which also allows patients to specify treatments that they do not want. Many states have allowed the use of Physician Orders for Life-Sustaining Treatment (POLST), a specific advance directive that documents a patient's end-of-life treatment preferences and serves as an order sheet. The standardized form is signed by both the physician and the patient and must be honored across all settings of care. (See Chapters 28 and 29.)

PATIENT PREFERENCES AND GOALS

The creation of patient goals is instrumental in decision making. As people age, their current and future health may enter prominently into determining and achieving their life goals. Among the very old, the patient's goals may be limited to achieving a functional or health state (e.g., being able to walk independently), controlling symptoms (e.g., control of pain or dyspnea), maintaining his or her living situation (e.g., remaining in one's home), or short-term survival (e.g., living long enough to reach a personal milestone such as an upcoming holiday). Sometimes, patient and physician goals differ. For example, a patient may want a cure when the physician believes that only symptom management is possible, especially with cancer. Conversely, the physician may believe that a better outcome is possible but the patient declines to pursue the recommended path (e.g., mastectomy).

A STRATEGIC APPROACH TO ASSESSMENT IN THE OLDER PATIENT WITH CANCER

Typically, geriatric assessment is conducted in two stages: screening and further assessment of positive screens. Because of time constraints in the busy primary care and oncology practices, screening can be delegated to office staff and patients and their families through standing orders and forms for staff, as well as by previsit questionnaires.

Studies have shown that these screening questions and assessments, e.g., ADL or GDS/PHQ-9, can be applied to older cancer patients.[2]

In ambulatory clinical settings, self- or proxy-reported functional status is collected by questionnaires or by interview with patients or family. A functional status assessment that indicates a patient's ability to perform specific functional tasks *and* provides information about who provides help, if needed, is more valuable than merely assessing ability. An example is the pre-visit questionnaire used in the UCLA outpatient geriatric practice (http://www.geronet.ucla.edu/images/stories/docs/professionals/Geri_Pre-visit_Questionnaire.pdf). Another is proposed by the National Comprehensive Cancer Network (http://www.nccn.org).[2,5]

These questionnaires gather information about:

- past medical and surgical history
- medications/allergies
- social history, including available social support resources
- preventive services
- ability to perform functional tasks and need for assistance
- home safety
- advance directives.

In addition, the pre-visit questionnaire can include specific questions assessing:

- vision
- hearing
- falls
- urinary incontinence
- depressive symptoms.

CASE 4-1   COMPREHENSIVE ASSESSMENT CASE. PART 1

Mrs. S was subsequently diagnosed with ductal carcinoma in situ and lobular adenocarcinoma and was referred to an oncologist. Mastectomy was recommended, as well as chemotherapy and radiation.

Geriatric Assessment Results
Functional Status
ECOG: 0-1, Karnovsky score: 80-90
   5/6 BADL (Patient needs assistance in getting into tub to bathe.)
   4/8 IADL (Patient uses phone, still able to use stove, takes medication by setting it in her bathroom.)
   Timed Get-Up and Go: 13 seconds (<15 seconds normal); no history of fall

Comorbidity
Hypertension, no renal insufficiency

Cognition
2/3 recall with a normal clock, with ability to extrapolate hands at 10 minutes after 11.

Affective
Negative PHQ-9

Social
Good family support and good perception of care with 4-hour caregiver and son

Nutrition
BMI 23

Pain and Nonpain Syndromes
None

Hearing/Vision
Wears glasses for reading, denies hearing loss

Advanced Care Planning
Son established as DPOAHC. Functional goals of intact cognition and ambulation were important. Did not want to be a burden to her family and cherished her independence.

Clinical Course
The patient underwent mastectomy, with her family being informed about delirium risk, given the abnormal screening. The family anticipated the need for increased caregiving postoperatively as well. Postoperative day 2, she had a positive CAM (Confusion Assessment Method) and perseverated about needing to take care of her cats. She was found to have some urinary retention and UTI. She recovered and was sent to a skilled nursing facility, at which time she was able to ambulate with a walker >200 ft. She had outpatient physical therapy and graduated to a cane. She was treated with erlotinib (Tarceva) and did well.

CASE 4-1 **COMPREHENSIVE ASSESSMENT CASE. PART 2**

After 3 years of follow-up, she presents to the emergency department with a 1-month history of worsening mental status. Her son notices that her medications are not taken correctly and that she has been having episodes of insomnia, as well as a trip and near fall. He now visits her daily and has hired a caregiver to be with her during the nights. Lab workup reveals a sodium level of 125 and imaging reveals new metastatic lesions to the brain.

Functional Status
ADL survey filled out by son.
   2/6 BADL (Patient with all ADLs except feeding and transferring)
   0/8 IADL (Son has moved in to assist her)

Timed Get-up and Go Test
With walker, 25 seconds (<15 seconds normal) with nearby assistance of son. Two falls over past 1 month; no injuries, no syncope or seizure.

Comorbidity
Renal insufficiency, orthostatic hypotension

Cognitive Status
0/3 recall with an abnormal clock, with inability to place the numbers in the clock, perseverating on the number 12.

Affective
Unable to conduct GDS or PHQ-9 (deferred)

Social
Positive caregiver burden, as seen on 12-point Zarit Caregiver Burden Scale, also a financial burden.

Nutrition
Weight loss of 8 pounds

Pain Symptoms
Complains of dizziness and headache

Nonpain Symptoms
Constipation

Hearing/Vision
No change

Advanced Care Planning
Son decides, on the basis of prior discussions, that pursuing palliation of symptoms was more important than continuing treatment.

Plan
Patient transitioned to hospice at home with 24-hour care in light of prior goals of care.
   Ongoing monitoring for caregiver burden assisted by hospice social worker, volunteers, and health aide.

Summary

Geriatric oncology is defined by the multidimensional and multidisciplinary approach of the elderly cancer patients. Autonomy, beneficence, nonmaleficence, and justice are the four fundamental principles on which are based the treatment objectives and practical management of these patients. Studies have also shown that decisions on curative treatment, palliative chemotherapy, and surgery can be affected by the patient's chronologic age.[10,19,27] Furthermore, studies have shown that cancer and its treatment precipitate geriatric syndromes such as falls, malnutrition, and delirium both as a direct effect or indirect effect mediated by other comorbidities.[67,68] By using a geriatric evaluation, characterizing functional status (physical, cognitive, psychosocial) and comorbidities, and taking into account the patient's wishes, a more meaningful and proactive approach can be used to manage the patient's cancer.

Functional status and a geriatric evaluation also help in *prioritizing individual patient problems and deciding on the intensity and effectiveness of treatment.* Functional assessment should be accurately recorded so that the **degree of change** and the **speed of change** can be monitored. When multiple medical, psychosocial, and cognitive comorbidities are present, the control of chronic diseases like hypertension and diabetes is frequently less important than managing the symptoms of cancer, particularly in the more functionally frail. When there are ongoing declines in physical, cognitive, or psychosocial functioning, continuation of palliative chemotherapy or other options in the management of their cancer should be reevaluated.

CASE 4-1 **COMPREHENSIVE ASSESSMENT CASE. CASE SUMMARY**

In this case, a geriatric assessment characterized changes in Mrs. S's functional status that were associated with loss of independence, increased caregiver burden, and greater financial expenditures. At several time points, *changes in functional status* were an important *presenting symptom of illness, in this case of her breast cancer.*

For ongoing cancer treatment, prognosis for functional status improvement or decline become important factors *in determining treatment options and further transitions of care* (e.g., hospital to home with increased care vs. Skilled Nursing Facility). For the former, if the prior functional status is not known, how can recovery be framed after a major catastrophic event such as a new diagnosis of breast cancer? The primary care physician, oncologist, or other members of the health care team (i.e., physical therapist, nurse) must be able to convey specific knowledge of the person's previous level of function to assist in setting reasonable targets for recovery. For example, because Mrs. S's functional status was preserved at the time of her presentation with breast cancer, mastectomy and chemotherapy were appropriate and acceptable options.

Throughout patients' cancer care, establishing a "safe" environment that supplements their functional status is critical. This can be achieved by additional caregivers or other supported care settings (assisted living, nursing home, rehabilitation center). In this case, the family was informed of the need to anticipate increased care.

For the busy medical practice, the use of a modified geriatric evaluation specifically focusing on physical function, self-reported (ADLs) with ECOG and Karnofsky PS as well as performance-based, is recommended; cognitive evaluations, and more in-depth psychosocial evaluations should be pursued. Delegation of screening tests to other members of the healthcare team is important. As the cancer population ages, this approach will take on more importance as health care professionals move to describing a person's "functional age" rather than his or her "chronologic age."

Conducting careful, comprehensive, and periodic geriatric and functional assessments (initial, after treatments, and at other times), primary care and oncology providers can promote their patients' autonomy and mobilize appropriate medical, social, and environmental supports on their behalf.

 See expertconsult.com for a complete list of references and web resources for this chapter

SUGGESTED READINGS

1. Boyle DA: Delirium in older adults with cancer: implications for practice and research, *Oncol Nurs Forum* 33(1):61–78, 2006 Jan 1:Review.
2. Braithwaite RS, Concato J, Chang CC, et al: A framework for tailoring clinical guidelines to comorbidity at the point of care, *Arch Intern Med* 167(21):2361–2365, 2007.
3. Extermann M, Aapro M, Bernabei R, et al: Task Force on CGA of the International Society of Geriatric Oncology. Use of comprehensive geriatric assessment in older cancer patients: recommendations from the task force on CGA of the International Society of Geriatric Oncology (SIOG), *Crit Rev Oncol Hematol* 55(3):241–252, 2005 Sep:Review.
4. Fried LP, Kronmal RA, Newman AE, et al: Risk factors for 5-year mortality in older adults: the Cardiovascular Health Study, *Jama* 279(8):585–592, 1998.
5. Higginson IJ, Gao W, Jackson D, Murray J, Harding R: Short-form Zarit Caregiver Burden Interviews were valid in advanced conditions, *J Clin Epidemiol* 63(5):535–542, 2010 May.
6. Hurria A: Geriatric assessment in oncology practice: *J Am Geriatr Soc* 57(Suppl 2):S246–S249 2009 Nov.
7. Lawton MP, Brody EM: Assessment of older people: self-maintaining and instrumental activities of daily living, *Gerontologist* 9:179–186, 1969.
8. Management of cancer pain in older patients: AGS Clinical Practice Committee, *J Am Geriatr Soc* 45(10):1273–1276, 1997 Oct.
9. Naeim A, Reuben D: Geriatric syndromes and assessment in older cancer patients, *Oncology (Williston Park)* 15(12):1567–1577, 2001 Dec:1580; discussion 1581, 1586, 1591.
10. Overcash J: Prediction of falls in older adults with cancer: a preliminary study, *Oncol Nurs Forum* 34(2):341–346, 2007 Mar.
11. Raji MA, Kuo YF, Freeman JL, Goodwin JS: Effect of a dementia diagnosis on survival of older patients after a diagnosis of breast, colon, or prostate cancer: implications for cancer care, *Arch Intern Med* 168(18):2033–2040, 2008 Oct 13.
12. Reuben DB, Seeman TE, Keeler E, Hayes RP, Bowman L, Sewall A, Hirsch SH, Wallace RB, Guralnik JM: Refining the categorization of physical functional status: the added value of combining self-reported and performance-based measures, *J Gerontol A Biol Sci Med Sci* 59(10):1056–1061, 2004 Oct.
13. Rodin MB, Mohile SG: A practical approach to geriatric assessment in oncology, *J Clin Oncol* 25(14):1936–1944, 2007 May 10.
14. Saliba D, Elliott M, Rubenstein LZ, et al: The Vulnerable Elders Survey: a tool for identifying vulnerable older people in the community, *J Am Geriatric Soc* 49:1691–1699, 2001.
15. Satariano WA, Ragland DR: The effect of comorbidity on 3-year survival of women with primary breast cancer, *Ann Intern Med* 120:104–110, 1994.
16. Sawhney R, Sehl M, Naeim A: Physiologic aspects of aging: Impact on cancer management and decision making, part I, *Cancer J* 11:449–460, 2005.
17. Sehl M, Sawhney R, Naeim A: Physiologic aspects of aging: Impact on cancer management and decision making, part II, *Cancer J* 11:461–473, 2005.
18. Terret C: How and why to perform a geriatric assessment in clinical practice, *Ann Oncol* 19(Suppl 7):vii300–vii303, 2008 Sep.
19. van Ryn M, Sanders S, Kahn K, et al: Objective burden, resources, and other stressors among informal cancer caregivers: a hidden quality issue? *Psychooncology*, 2010 Mar 4.
20. Walter LC, Covinsky KE: Cancer screening in elderly patients: a framework for individualized decision making, *Jama* 285(21):2750–2756, 2001.
21. Wedding U, Roehrig B, Klippstein A, Steiner P, Schaeffer T, Pientka L, Höffken K: Comorbidity in patients with cancer: prevalence and severity measured by cumulative illness rating scale, *Crit Rev Oncol Hematol* 61(3):269–276, 2007 Mar:Epub 2007 Jan 4. PubMed.

Choosing the Right Oncologist and the Value of a Second Opinion

Melissa Cohen

A diagnosis of cancer is an overwhelming experience for patients and their family members; therefore choosing the "right" oncologist is often the most important decision they make. The oncologist has many roles, being involved in diagnosis, counseling, treatment, administration, support, and coordination of care. Often a patient is limited in his or her choice by location or insurance plan. Even within these limitations, there are still many decisions to make: tumor-specific versus general oncologist, oncologists associated with teaching hospitals versus those in the community, as well as a variety of personal characteristics. Ultimately, the patient and family will select an oncologist they feel comfortable with for a balance of reasons. Frequently, making such a decision requires meeting several doctors (first through third opinions) or whatever else is required until they find a doctor with the personality and clinical characteristics with which they are content.

The first step in choosing the right oncologist is finding one who has experience treating the type of cancer with which a patient has been diagnosed. The comparison of outcomes among general medical oncologists and tumor-specific oncologists remains a matter of considerable debate. In the oncology literature, there is little literature comparing outcomes between general versus tumor-specific oncologists. Who delivers the "best" care is more likely to be based on a number of factors such as patient volume, personal preferences, and differences

between academic and community setting. Oncologists who specialize in a particular tumor are more likely to be affiliated with large hospitals or academic teaching hospitals that may not be located in proximity to the patient's home and which can make receiving treatment involve considerable logistics and travel time. In a recent survey, specialist oncologists who practiced in a university setting were more likely to be aware of clinical trials and to enroll patients into them than oncologists who practiced alone or in private groups in the community by a ratio of 56:1.[1] In addition, academic oncologists were simultaneously more likely than community oncologists to report providing off-protocol therapy.[2] On the other hand, general medical oncologists can provide excellent care and achieve excellent outcomes. An advantage to community oncologists may be their increased availability to patients. Studies that show a benefit of one over the other usually use intermediate outcomes and there are many confounding factors, including referral biases, shared care, and illness burden.

ACADEMIC VERSUS COMMUNITY SETTING

Teaching hospitals are responsible for training medical residents and fellows in the United States. There are many studies that examine outcomes in teaching hospitals versus those in a community setting. Superior outcomes have been reported in some studies, but others claim the opposite. A systematic review of the literature demonstrated a great deal of variability, but overall there was no major difference in the effectiveness of treatment provided by teaching hospitals or nonteaching hospitals.[3] The most convincing arguments in favor of outcomes in teaching hospitals pertain to cancer patients undergoing complex surgical procedures who benefit from board-certified specialty surgeons, multidisciplinary teams, availability and use of sophisticated clinical amenities, and highly trained personnel.[4–6] A study of over 24,000 cases of breast cancer, comparing outcomes, suggests that patients with infiltrating ductal carcinoma treated at teaching hospitals had significantly better survival than those treated at high-volume centers or community hospitals, particularly in the setting of advanced disease.[7] A study in Great Britain of nearly 3000 women also suggests this trend, demonstrating that breast cancer patients treated in specialist units had 57% lower local recurrence rate and 20% lower risk of death.[8] However, the literature also highlights some less optimal aspects of receiving care in teaching hospitals. Often teaching or academic centers are not in proximity to the cancer patient's home, and travel may be a burden; this may be more significant as the condition deteriorates or if the treatment plan is quite intense. In addition, if patients do not live near the treating hospital, it is likely that in an emergency they will be hospitalized close to home, where their records may not be available and they will not be under the care of their primary oncologist or team. In addition, physicians in academic centers have additional responsibilities other than patient care that may make them less "available." There are many reasons why obtaining care in the community setting may be preferable. For instance, a community hospital is more likely to be close to a patient's home and convenient for emergencies. The doctor treating the patient's cancer is most likely going to be the one treating him or her on inpatient admissions and returning phone calls and answering questions. The doctors, nurses, and office staff are generally more available and have more flexible hours than those provided in a teaching hospital setting.

The optimal type of personality for an oncologist depends on who the patient is and what qualities are important to him or her.[10] For the most part, it is agreed upon that "effective" care requires a match between health care provider skills and the needs and expectations of the patient.[9] Table 5-l lists many of the characteristics that oncologists, ideally, should possess.

One of the most important characteristics of an oncologist is that he or she be an effective communicator (understandable, direct, and simple). When 100 patients at an Israeli cancer center were asked about doctor-patient communication, nearly 90% of patients felt strongly that eye contact was important.[10] Trust is a central element in the patient-physician relationship. Patients base this trust on physician behaviors such as

TABLE 5-1	Potentially Important Characteristics of an Oncologist
Effective communicator	
Trust	
Compassionate	
Patient	
Experienced	
Gender (if patient has a preference)	
Same cultural/language background	

competence, compassion, dependability, confidentiality, and communication.[11-13]

- Compassionate ("touchy-feely") or more reserved ("hands off")
- Experienced (young and with recent training, older and seasoned with more experience)
- Gender: Some patients feel that to have a physician of a specific gender will improve their ability to communicate.
- Culture: Just as with gender, a patient and his/her family concentrate their efforts on finding a physician with a similar cultural background, so that the diagnosis, prognosis, and treatment plan can be communicated in a culturally acceptable fashion.

CASE 5-1	CASE UPDATE

Not only did it take 2 hours to drive to the initial consultation, but the physician was running behind, spoke abruptly, and strongly argued for an aggressive treatment plan with combined hormone and chemotherapy. The daughter was hoping for a more informative encounter that would allow more discussion and more involvement with decision making.

VALUE OF A SECOND OPINION

Second opinions in oncology are common.[14-16] In 1992, 56% of 1500 cancer survivors in the United States reported to have obtained at least one second opinion.[17] It has been shown that a process of second opinion is of great value for the staging of tumors, which is the foundation for individual treatment decisions.[18,19] Second opinions are sought for many reasons. (Table 5-2.)

Denial/ Need for More Information

Denial occurs relatively frequently in patients with cancer, because of the life-threatening character of the disease. As stated by Bayliss, "Often the patient or patient's relatives are concerned at the diagnosis and

TABLE 5-2	Reasons for a Second Opinion in Oncology

Denial/Need for more information
Treatment is too aggressive or not aggressive enough
Interpersonal difficulties
Treatment failure

TABLE 5-3	Goals/Benefits of Multidisciplinary Team Cancer Meetings

Improved consistency, continuity, coordination, and cost-effective care
Improved communications between health professionals
Improved clinical outcomes
Increased recruitment into clinical trials
Educational opportunities for health professionals
Support in a collegial environment
Increased job satisfaction and psychological well-being of team members

From Fleissig A, Jenkins V, Catt S, Fallowfield L. Multidisciplinary teams in cancer care: are they effective in the UK? Lancet Oncol. 2006 Nov;7(11): 935-43.

CASE 5-1	CASE UPDATE

The family decides to get a second opinion. The second oncologist they consult offers a different opinion. Given her comorbid conditions, the oncologist believes that the addition of chemotherapy to hormone therapy would add less than 1% in overall 10-year survival. The patient had a strong preference against chemotherapy and feels reassured after the conversation that hormone therapy alone is the best choice for her, personally.

potential prognosis that the first opinion is unacceptable or not fully comprehended until confirmed by another expert."[20] Most patients report the reason for seeking a second opinion is their need for more information. This does not necessarily mean that the first specialist did not provide the patient with enough information. A plethora of research has shown that recall of clinical information and treatment in the medical encounter is suboptimal.[21-23] It has been hypothesized that the ability to recall this information predicts patient satisfaction.[24] Many studies suggest there are many factors that influence this ability such as age, gender, educational status, and prognosis, among others.[24]

Treatment

Cancer treatment is usually toxic and/or potentially disfiguring. The treatment offered by the first oncologist may be deemed too radical, or often, in the case of the older cancer patient, not radical enough, and some alternative treatment plans are hoped for in the second consultation.[20] Another reason for seeking a second opinion is when interpersonal difficulties occur. Dissatisfaction with the first specialist was observed in one third of cancer patients questioned regarding their motives for seeking a second surgical opinion, in a study in the Netherlands.[25] Treatment failure and clinical trial availability is a very common reason for a second opinion.

There are several important things to review in a second opinion. Patients usually have high expectations for this consultation. Asking at the outset of the visit for the patient's specific agenda and questions they want answered can improve patient and physician satisfaction.[26-28] The basis of the second opinion is a thorough reevaluation of the patient's case, including a review of diagnostic material such as diagnostic history, sequence of events, surgical record, radiographic images, pathology report, and, at times, the tissue itself.

In oncology, perhaps more than in other fields of medicine, diagnostic and treatment guidelines and protocols are well defined for most tumor types.[29] The variability of interpretation and weighing of older patients' clinical and personal characteristics, however, leads to considerable variability in the advice they receive, and therefore a second opinion may be more important.

THE ROLE OF CASE CONFERENCES AND TUMOR BOARDS

Caring for most cancer patients is a complex process utilizing multiple modalities of treatment that can be provided by a number of health care professionals; it therefore necessitates good coordination and communication throughout the entire process. Multidisciplinary team meetings are regularly scheduled meetings designed to review individual cancer patients prospectively, and form appropriate management plans using evidence-based medicine from multimodality input.[30] Global acceptance and implementation of multidisciplinary teams (MDTs) has been seen; they are standard of care in the United Kingdom, United States, continental Europe, and Australia. Participants at such meetings usually consist of medical oncologists, radiation oncologists, surgical oncologists, radiologists, nurses, and social workers. The main purpose of these meetings is to ensure all appropriate tests and treatment options are considered for each patient (Table 5.3)

Theoretically, MDT cancer meetings should increase adherence to guidelines, aid in decision making, and improve outcomes by ensuring a high-quality diagnosis, evidence-based decision making, optimal treatment planning, and timely delivery of care. It is felt that by bringing together multiple practitioners with diverse experience, knowledge, and skills, holistic evaluation of patients can occur and the most appropriate treatments will be considered. According to the literature, specific tumor types such as breast, rectal, head and neck cancers, and inoperable non-small cell lung cancer are the most common specialties within oncology wherein multidisciplinary team meetings occur.[31] This approach becomes exceptionally important when dealing with complex cases such as making treatment decisions for patients where there is little evidence to guide treatment. Elderly patients are a heterogeneous group, with multiple comorbidities and widely varying functional status, all of which make predicting their response to treatment difficult. This is where the strength of the MDT cancer meeting can be utilized, as decision making needs to combine the existing evidence, the available treatment options, and consideration of geriatric principles. Less obvious benefits to MDT cancer meetings include the opportunity to improve the coordination of services, as well as the learning opportunities

they provide for participants. MDTs provide the opportunity for team members to learn from each other. However beneficial MDT cancer meetings seem, there are many obstacles that make their coordination difficult. MDTs require substantial administrative, human, and technical resources in order to run successfully. They require consistent participation by physicians, which can take away from patient care. For instance, radiologists may work in many tumor types, making attendance at each specialty MDT difficult. Further critiques argue that participation in MDT cancer meetings may increase the time needed to process patients, and that they increase costs.

 See expertconsult.com for a complete list of references and web resources for this chapter

SECTION III

Treatment

Overview of Cancer Surgery in the Elderly

M. Margaret Kemeny and David M. Heimann

In the next 50 years, the number of Americans older than 65 is expected to double[1] from 35 million to 70 million. Because the incidence of cancer increases exponentially with advancing age, there will be a significant rise in the number of elderly patients diagnosed with cancer. It is projected that by the year 2050, the number of cancers in the elderly will reach 2.6 million.[1] Currently, people older than 65 account for 60% of newly diagnosed malignancies and 70% of all cancer deaths.[2]

Knowing that the life expectancy of a girl born in 2005 is 80.4 years, that for a boy it is 75.2 years,[3] and that life expectancies of a 75-year-old woman and man are 12.8 and 10.8 years, respectively,[3] should lead the cancer surgeon to be appropriately aggressive in the endeavor for 5-year survival in the elderly cancer patient.

Because surgery is the mainstay of treatment for solid tumors, the greatest dilemma for the oncologic surgeon is whether the use of radical surgery, with its accompanying morbidities, is justified in the very elderly. With advances in modern medicine, it is understood that any patient up to age 70 is eligible for the same degree of surgical intervention as a younger patient would be, unless the patient has very severe comorbidities. This chapter is dedicated to the discussion of treatment strategies for the patient age 70 or older. Unfortunately, scientific data from randomized studies is often not readily available for older populations because they are more likely to be excluded from clinical trials. Studies that are available are retrospective and often display considerable bias in the patients chosen for certain treatments, especially surgical procedures. Prejudices can arise from what is perceived as limited life expectancy, the presence of comorbid diseases, assumed decreased functional or mental status, limitations in economic resources, and assumed inability to tolerate treatment. The influences of these biases have affected the enrollment of patients into protocols and the treatment, and probably the survival, of elderly patients with cancer.

A study evaluating survival up to 10 years after the diagnosis of cancer in patients older than 65 years with various cancers revealed that not receiving definitive therapy for the patient's cancer was associated with a threefold greater death rate.[4] Inadequate treatment remained a significant factor, even after controlling for stage at diagnosis, socioeconomic factors, comorbidity, and physical functioning. Thus the evidence suggests that the withholding of appropriate treatment because of age will result in inferior survival.

The idea that the elderly, as a group, cannot tolerate extensive surgery has not been supported by the data. Over the past 30 years numerous publications have shown that surgical procedures can be performed safely in the elderly.[5-15] The balance between operative risk and expected cure or palliation is important when treating any patient with cancer. The elderly patient's age alone should not be an automatic contraindication to extensive surgery. The impact of treatment on the quality of life is extremely important and should always be kept in mind.

Data supports the rule that surgical morbidity and mortality rise with advanced disease states and emergency surgery. Because there is often a delay in cancer diagnosis in elderly patients, this can lead to more advanced cancers and a greater number of emergency presentations with the associated worse outcomes. Thus early diagnosis and treatment in the elderly should be encouraged. Not performing surgery in the elective setting may result in the same patient's need for life-saving emergency surgery several months later.

This chapter reviews the role of surgery in the management of elderly patients with the following common solid organ cancers: (1) breast cancer; (2) colon cancer; (3) liver metastases; (4) gastric cancer; (5) pancreatic cancer; (6) melanoma.

BREAST CANCER

CASE 6-1

A 79-year-old woman presented to her physician with a large palpable breast mass. She had a past medical history of congestive heart failure, poorly-controlled hypertension, poorly-controlled diabetes, morbid obesity, and bipolar disorder. She was a widow and lived by herself. Because of her significant comorbidities and the perceived risk of general anesthesia, she underwent a lumpectomy and sentinel lymph node biopsy under local anesthesia. Her pathology revealed a T3 lesion, 6 cm in size with clear margins and negative sentinel lymph node. The tumor was positive for both estrogen receptor (ER) and progesterone receptor (PR) and negative for HER-2/neu. After recovering from her surgery, the patient was able to receive standard postlumpectomy radiation by having transportation arranged for her by social services. She remains disease-free at this time on daily tamoxifen.

This case illustrates several points about breast cancer in the very elderly. Patients are often not screened after the age of 75 and can present with very large and sometime locally advanced cancers, like this woman. There are many elderly who are actually too frail to receive general anesthesia, yet for breast cancer these procedures can be done safely under local anesthesia. With the proper transportation support, the elderly, even those who live alone, can receive appropriate radiation. Tumors are overwhelmingly hormone-positive and hormonal therapy can be given safely to most of these patients.

The incidence of breast cancer rises with age. Nearly one third of breast cancers occur in women older than 70 years[16] and half the deaths are in women older than 65 years of age.[17]

Should the surgical treatment of breast cancer in the elderly be different than for younger women? Although the morbidity and mortality for breast surgery in the elderly is very low,[18] the fear of treatment morbidity and mortality sometimes prompts a minimalist approach in the elderly, whereas, paradoxically, at other times, mastectomy is offered with little if any discussion about the possible desire for breast conservation. In addition, reconstruction is rarely offered to elderly patients.

Despite the fact that the National Institutes of Health consensus conference found breast-conserving therapy (BCT) to be the preferable method of treating early-stage disease[19] it is still underutilized for all ages and particularly in the elderly. The elderly have also been found to have a lower rate of BCT in the treatment of ductal carcinoma in situ (DCIS).[20]

Hurria et al.[21] performed a retrospective study examining the factors influencing treatment patterns for women aged 75 and older with breast cancer. The goal of the study was to determine local and systemic treatment patterns for these patients. Even in this advanced age cohort, there was a difference in treatment seen between those patients aged 75 to 79 and those who were older. However, there was no difference in receiving hormonal therapy, which is generally viewed as a "less-toxic" treatment. Chemotherapy, radiation therapy, and axillary lymph node dissection, which are generally viewed as more "toxic" therapies were less likely to be used in the armamentarium for patients older than 80.

Patients with increased comorbidities were significantly less likely to receive radiation therapy, despite the findings of the Cancer and Leukemia Group B (CALGB)

study that radiation is beneficial in preventing locoregional disease in women, age 70 and older, who have undergone partial mastectomy. Other studies have also demonstrated that when breast conservation is performed, it is often done without axillary dissection or the use of postoperative radiation, as would be the standard for younger women.[18,22] In one retrospective series, the survival of elderly women was found to be lower for those treated with less-than-standard protocols.[22]

The relatively recent implementation of sentinel lymph node (SLN) biopsy instead of a full axillary dissection has resulted in decreased operative morbidity. Overall, SLN biopsy has been shown to be a safe procedure, with accuracies of 97% in randomized studies of all age groups.[23,24] Looking specifically at the older patient, one series of 241 patients 70 years or older identified the SLN in every one, with no major complications.[25] Another study of 730 breast cancer patients compared the rate of identification of SLN in the younger patients and the 261 (36%) patients who were at least 70 years of age. The overall sentinel node identification rate was statistically equivalent in the group younger than 70 (98.8%) versus the older group (97.1%).[26] These kinds of data support the dictum that SLN biopsy should be offered to all women diagnosed with invasive breast cancer who do not have palpable axillary disease, regardless of age. The combination of lumpectomy with SLN biopsy, which is now considered the standard of care, can be done as an outpatient procedure with limited if any morbidity and there should be no reason to deny this definitive treatment to the elderly.

Radiation therapy to the breast after BCT is considered standard therapy, yet radiation is often omitted in many elderly patients. In one series, only 41% of women older than 75 years had radiation, in contrast to 90% of women younger than 65 years and 86% of women between the ages of 65 and 74 years.[27] Concerns have been expressed about whether the elderly will tolerate radiation, whether they will have difficulty completing therapy because of physical restraints in getting to radiation facilities, and whether long-term outcomes are the same as in younger patients. However, many studies have provided evidence to refute these concerns.[28,29] Furthermore, studies show that local recurrence rates for breast cancer have been reported as high as 35% in the elderly when radiation is not given,[30] contradicting the theory that those patients will not benefit from radiation therapy. A randomized study from the CALGB compared 647 women older than 70 years with stage I estrogen-positive breast cancer that were randomized to receive lumpectomy plus tamoxifen or lumpectomy followed by tamoxifen and radiation therapy. The group given radiation had a significantly lower risk of locoregional recurrence (1% versus 7%; p<0.001) at a median follow-up of 7.9 years.[31] Surgeons who believe that radiation therapy is not possible in the elderly will not offer them the choice of lumpectomy, moving straight to mastectomy. Again, evidence has shown that this is not the correct way to treat these elderly patients, who should have the same choice for breast-conserving therapy as younger patients.

In the elderly patient who undergoes a mastectomy, very rarely is breast reconstruction performed or even offered. In one study, the single greatest predictor for a surgeon to recommend breast reconstruction was patient age younger than 50.[32] Yet experience with breast reconstruction in patients older than 60 demonstrates that it is safe, provides good long-standing results, and has acceptable complication rates when compared to younger patients. Age alone should not be a determining factor in selecting women for breast reconstruction, but this should be a discussion between the patient and physician.

In summary, surgical treatment of breast cancer in the elderly should follow the standard of care used for all women. Breast-conserving surgery and SLN biopsy with radiation has been shown to be safe and effective in treating breast cancer, with low morbidity and mortality in all age groups.

COLON CANCER

CASE 6-2

A 77-year old- man presented to the emergency department with acute onset of abdominal pain. A CT scan revealed a partial small bowel obstruction with a cecal mass. The patient had never had a colonoscopy and was not followed by a primary care physician. On follow-up abdominal films the next day, the oral contrast from the CT scan was noted in the left colon. Thus after a bowel prep, a colonoscopy revealed a near-obstructing large cecal adenocarcinoma. He was taken to the OR on the next day for a right hemicolectomy. Pathology showed a T3N2 (12/25LN+) stage IIIC colon cancer. Postoperatively, an abdominal fluid collection in the right lower quadrant developed, which required drainage by interventional radiology. After drainage, he did well. He received adjuvant chemotherapy, is doing well more than 1 year postoperatively, and is free of disease on radiographic studies.

This case illustrates three points about colon cancer in the elderly: (1) right-sided lesions are more common; (2) lesions are detected at more advanced stages; (3) emergency operations are often necessary at presentation, with increased morbidity.

The incidence of colorectal cancer increases with age, as 90% of patients are diagnosed after age 55.[33] Several studies report a difference in tumor location between the more elderly and the younger patients, with more right-sided lesions and fewer rectal lesions in the elderly.[34-38] Because patients with right-sided lesions are more likely to present later, due to fewer signs and symptoms compared to left-sided or rectal cancers, the older patients are more likely to fall into the late presentation category.

Several studies show that elderly patients are more likely to undergo emergency surgical procedures compared to a younger population. In one study from the British Colorectal Cancer Collaborative Group (CCCG), the incidence of undergoing an emergency operation more than doubled for patients 85 or older (11% for younger than 65 years vs. 29% for 85 years or older, p<0.0001).[39] The same study also revealed differences in both stage at presentation and the rate of curative surgery within the elderly population, with the "older of the old" presenting with more advanced disease and being less likely to undergo curative surgery.

Because of recent data from a number of studies demonstrating improved survival when at least 12 lymph nodes are examined in resection specimens for colon cancer, this number is now considered the gold standard for node removal. The data revealed a benefit in resecting at least 12 lymph nodes irrespective of the patient's age. The adequacy of number of lymph nodes removed in elderly patients was recently examined,[38] revealing that as age increased the number of nodes removed decreased. This might reflect a less extensive operation, possibly accounting for decreased survival in the elderly.

The mainstay of curative therapy for all nonmetastatic colon cancer is adequate surgical resection. It may even be required in many cases in the presence of disseminated disease to avoid or treat the complications of obstruction and bleeding. A number of retrospective series examined the influence of advanced age on the morbidity of colon cancer surgery. The risk of perioperative complications is generally reported to be higher in the elderly than in younger patients. In a meta-analysis, the cardiovascular complications were statistically significantly increased (p<0.001) in one series from 0.8% in patients older than 65 to 4% in patients older than 75.[39] Pneumonia and respiratory failure was seen in 5% of patients younger than 65 years, compared to 15% in those at least age 85 (p<0.001). However, the anastomotic leak rates in the meta-analysis were not statistically different in young versus elderly patients. A large study from the United Kingdom of more than 2500 patients 80 years old or older showed an increased mortality, but colectomy-specific complications, such as anastomotic leaks, were no different in the elderly versus younger patients. The 30-day overall mortality rate was 15.6%, but increased to 27.5% for those at least age 95. Multivariate analysis for this group of very elderly patients revealed the following independent risk factors for 30-day mortality: age; operative urgency; ASA grade; resection versus no resection; metastatic disease. Other studies support these conclusions that comorbid factors in the very elderly may increase multisystem-related complications, which are further exaggerated in the emergent situation, but there is no increase of anastomotic leaks due to advanced age.

Emergency operations are clearly associated with an increased mortality rate. Elderly patients presenting with malignant bowel obstructions are a high-risk cohort with increased postoperative complications and mortality. In the previously mentioned British study, approximately

25% of patients that underwent either a palliative stoma or a Hartmann procedure died within 30 days postoperatively.[40] These procedures are often done as an emergency in an end-stage patient, two factors known to contribute to an increased risk of morbidity and mortality.[7,41] Early intervention with semi-elective surgery would often avoid situations such as bleeding, perforation, and obstruction that require emergency surgical intervention.

Overall cancer-related survival was comparable when comparing patients aged 75 and older to those under 75, despite an increase in operative mortality for the older population.[42] One study showed that although the physical status and operative mortality were worse in the elderly undergoing surgery for colorectal cancer, for those elderly who were fit for surgery, who underwent curative resection, and who survived more than 30 days, the 5-year survival was comparable to younger patients by multivariate analysis.[36]

Age alone should never be a contraindication for colectomy, and whenever possible, the full curative treatment including adjuvant chemotherapy should be utilized as indicated by pathologic and operative findings.

LIVER METASTASES FROM COLON CANCER

CASE 6-3

An 85-year-old man who had a colon resection for a stage III colon cancer 7 years prior was noted on routine blood work to have an elevated CEA level at 7.1 ng/mL (normal <2.5). A CT scan showed a solitary lesion in the left lobe of the liver. These findings were confirmed by PET scan which revealed only the lesion in the left lobe of the liver. Treatment options were discussed with the patient and he opted to undergo a liver resection, a left lateral lobectomy. The patient required no blood transfusions. He was discharged home 5 days after surgery and has done well since.

Metastatic disease from colorectal cancer is predominantly (80%) found in the liver and often confined to the liver on presentation. For patients with liver-only disease that is deemed operable, liver resection can lead to a 21% to 48% 5-year survival.[43-48] The safety of performing liver resections has greatly improved in recent years owing to improvements in techniques of resection and intraoperative and postoperative care. Liver resections are now being routinely performed with mortality rates of less than 5%.[43,45,47-49]

Liver resections can also be performed safely in elderly patients. A number of series have looked at morbidity and mortality rates for older individuals. A study from Memorial Sloan-Kettering Cancer Center reviewing liver resections for colorectal metastases in 128 patients older than 70[13] found the perioperative mortality rate and the morbidity rate were the same as for patients younger than 70. In multivariate analysis, the three factors that

TABLE 6-1	Predictors of Survival from Liver Resection	
Variable	Zero Points	One Point
Age	≤60	>60
Tumor size	<5 cm	≥5 cm
Nodal involvement of primary tumor	No	Yes
Disease-free interval	≥2 years	<2 years
Number of liver lesions	<4	≥4
Resection margins	Negative	Positive
CEA level	<5	≥30
	Total Points	**Survival Rate**
2-year survival	0-2	79%
	3-4	60%
	5-7	43%

From Nordlinger B, Guiguet M, Vaillant JC et al. Surgical resection of colorectal carcinoma metastases to the liver. A prognostic scoring system to improve case selection, based on 1568 patients. Association Francaise de Chirurgie. Cancer 77(7): 1254, 1996.

were found to be important in predicting complications (male sex, resection of at least one lobe of the liver, and an operating time of greater than 4 hours) did not include age. Median hospital stay for patients aged 70 years and older was only 1 day longer than for patients younger than 70 years.

There are several prognostic scoring systems to estimate the prognosis after liver resection, and none of them has age as one of the significant prognostic variables. When deciding on the usefulness of a liver resection in an elderly patient one of these systems should be employed. The clinical risk score devised by Memorial Sloan-Kettering[50] used 5 factors to compute survival. They were: (1) nodal status of primary disease; (2) disease-free interval of less than 12 months between primary and metastases; (3) more than one hepatic tumor; (4) CEA level greater than 200 ng/mL; and (5) size of metastases greater than 5 cm. If all of the factors are good, then the projected 5-year survival is 60%. If a patient has all the negative factors, the survival drops to 14%. Another scoring system from France uses seven variables (Table 6-1) and computes 2-year survival. These systems should be used for all patients, including the elderly, because elderly patients can benefit from liver resection equally to younger patients.

GASTRIC CANCER

CASE 6-4

A 76-year-old man with a history of alcohol and tobacco abuse reported dark tarry stools and was noted by his primary care physician to be anemic. He underwent upper and lower endoscopy and was noted to have a large ulcer along the greater curvature of the stomach. A biopsy was performed, which revealed adenocarcinoma. The patient reported neither weight loss nor early satiety. He had a history of diabetes mellitus, hypertension, and obesity. A metastatic workup was negative, and the patient underwent a total gastrectomy with a D2 lymphadenectomy with Roux-en-Y esophagojejunostomy reconstruction. He recovered well and was discharged home 1 week postoperatively. Within a month of his surgery, he started chemoradiotherapy for his Stage II (T2bN1) gastric cancer.

Gastric cancer rates have been declining over the past 75 years in the United States[51], but the prognosis has not improved, with 5-year survival being 20% to 40%.[52] Despite the fact that the incidence of the disease has fallen in the past 75 years, the number of patients diagnosed at 75 years or older is actually increasing.[52] Gastric cancer in the United States is generally seen in the elderly, with nearly 50% of cases in males and 60% of those in females being in patients older than 70 years.[53] Surgery is the only curative modality available for gastric cancer. Palliative surgery is often needed for bleeding and obstruction. An important element in deciding about gastrectomy in the elderly is the impact on the quality of life. A study that addressed this question in a small series of patients older than 70 years undergoing total gastrectomy showed that 70% of patients returned to "normal life" after 1 year.[54]

In Asia, where gastric cancer is much more common, many investigators have examined the characteristics of gastric cancer in the elderly. Symptoms at presentation and location of disease in the stomach have been found to be similar in younger and older patients.[55,56] Also, studies have shown no difference with age in the incidence of lymph node metastases and stage at diagnosis, with most patients having T3 and T4 disease at the time of exploration.[55,56]

Curative surgery for gastric cancer requires either a subtotal or a total gastrectomy depending on the location and size of the tumor. The exact extent of lymph node dissection necessary remains a controversial subject, yet most surgical oncologists perform at least a D2 resection. There have been a number of reports on the morbidity and mortality rates of gastric resections in the elderly (Table 6-2). Although preoperative risk factors, particularly cardiac and pulmonary, are increased in the elderly with gastric cancer, most complications and deaths are caused by infections, anastomotic leaks, and pulmonary problems just as in younger patients.[6,57-59] A large study from Italy reviewing gastric resections for gastric cancer over a 15-year period reported that the overall postoperative surgical complication rate was 20% in the elderly group (age 75 and older) versus 17% in the younger. The postoperative mortality rate for both groups was 3%. Multivariate analysis revealed that age was not a risk factor for either postoperative morbidity or mortality.[52]

The 5-year survival for curatively-resected patients with gastric cancer is similar for younger and older patients (Table 6-3). In a recent Japanese study, the overall survival was significantly different between the two groups (p<0.0001), but the cause-specific survival was not statistically different (p=0.3447).[60] An American study found that 5-year survival was 17% for elderly patients (older than 70 years) compared to 21% for younger patients (p=0.45).

In summary, there is no data to support anything less than surgical resection for gastric cancer in the elderly, and it should be offered to patients irrespective of age as the only chance for cure.

PANCREATIC CANCER

CASE 6-5

An 81-year-old man with painless jaundice presented to the emergency department. Laboratory workup revealed a bilirubin level of 18.9 mg/dL and CA 19-9 of 117 U/mL (normal <37). A CT scan showed biliary dilation but no pancreatic mass. Endoscopic retrograde cholangiopancreatography (ERCP) was unsuccessful for both diagnosis and biliary stent placement. Thus the patient was taken for surgical exploration; the pancreas was found to be hard with no discrete mass seen. Pancreatic biopsies initially revealed pancreatitis, but further biopsies confirmed adenocarcinoma. A pylorus-sparing pancreaticoduodenectomy was performed. Final pathology demonstrated a 4.5 cm high-grade adenocarcinoma with negative margins. Out of 10 lymph nodes excised none were involved by cancer.

Postoperatively the patient did well but was discharged to a nursing home for 1 month because he lived alone and needed assistance with his care. He then was discharged home and received adjuvant chemoradiotherapy. He shows no evidence of disease (NED) 1 year later.

TABLE 6-2	Gastric Resections in the Elderly				
Reference (Year)	Country	Age	Number of Patients	Morbidity (%)	Mortality (%)
Wu (2000)[93]	Taiwan	≥65	433	21.7	5.1
Saidi (2004)[94]	US	≥70	24	33.3	8.33
Mochiki (2005)[95]	Japan	≥70	30*	13.3	0
		≥70	16†	25	0
Kunisaki (2006)[60]	Japan	≥75	117	29	0.85
Gretschel (2006)[96]	Germany	>75	48	48	8
Orsenigo (2007)[52]	Italy	≥75	249	29	3

*All laparoscopic-assisted gastrectomy
†All open gastrectomy

TABLE 6-3	Gastric Cancer Survival after Curative Resection: Young versus Elderly Patients (published since 2000)			
Reference (Year)	Number of Patients	Age	5-Year Survival (%)	P Value
Saidi (2004)[94]	24	<70	20.8	0.45
	24	≥70	16.6	
Mochiki (2005)[95]	73	<70	98.4*	0.48
	30	≥70	95.7	
Kunisaki (2006)[60]	625	45-65	73.6	0.0001
	117	≥75	59.2	
Gretschel (2006)[96]	148	<60	59	0.05
	167	60-75	46	
	48	>75	40	
Orsenigo (2007)[52]	869	<75	54	NS
	249	≥75	47	

*Laparoscopic-assisted distal gastrectomy for early gastric cancer only

Over two thirds of patients with pancreatic cancer are older than 65 years at diagnosis.[61-63] The overall survival of all patients who present with pancreatic cancer is dismal, with 5-year survivals of 5%, up from 3% in 1986.[51] This is attributed in part to the fact that most patients with pancreatic cancer are diagnosed late in the course of the disease when surgical resection is no longer feasible. Only 9% to 15% of pancreatic carcinomas are considered resectable at presentation.[61,63]

A pancreaticoduodenectomy, with or without sparing the pylorus, is the operation of choice for the most common pancreatic lesions, which are located in the head of the pancreas. This is also the surgical procedure for periampullary, duodenal, and distal common bile duct neoplasms. Until the early 1980s, pancreatic resection was associated with an extremely high complication rate, as well as a mortality rate as high as 26% in some centers. However, in more recent years, the morbidity and mortality rates associated with pancreaticoduodenectomy have decreased significantly at specialty centers[64-66] and mortality rates of between 0 and 5% are now the standard at high-volume centers.[64,65,67] In selected elderly patients, mortality rates for surgery are acceptable and even comparable to the younger group.[13,68-70]

A review of 138 patients older than 70 who underwent pancreatic resection for malignancy reported an operative mortality rate of 6% and a morbidity rate of over 40%.[13] No significant differences were found in length of hospital stay, rate of intensive care unit admission, and morbidity or mortality rates between patients younger than 70 years and those older than 70 years. Multivariate analysis found that the only factor that was a significant predictor of complications was a blood loss of more than 2 liters. Median survival was 18 months, and 5 year survival was 21%.

A study from Johns Hopkins evaluating pancreaticoduodenectomy in octogenarians showed that they had a longer postoperative length of stay and a higher complication rate compared to younger patients. The mortality rate, however, was similar between the two groups.[71] They reported a 5-year survival rate for pancreatic cancer of 19% in patients older than 80 years and 27% in patients younger than 80, which was not a statistically significant difference.[71]

For patients with pancreatic cancer whose tumors cannot be resected, biliary obstruction can be effectively managed with stents, placed either endoscopically or percutaneously using the transhepatic approach.[72-75] Mortality rates are lower for stent placement than for surgical bypass and hospital stays are shorter. Early complication rates are lower from this procedure, but long-term complication rates such as recurrent jaundice and cholangitis are more common than with surgical bypass. These complications may be considered acceptable in view of the high surgical morbidity and mortality for biliary bypass procedures.

As with other solid tumors, if an elderly patient presents with a resectable tumor, surgery is the best therapy because it offers the best chance for cure. Another benefit of surgery is that lesions may turn out to be ampullary or biliary in origin and therefore have better survival rates, but only if resected.

MELANOMA

CASE 6-6

An 84-year-old woman presented to the office with a painful, ulcerated pigmented lesion on her left foot. She had a history of diabetes mellitus, hypertension, and obesity. Under spinal anesthesia, the patient underwent a wide local excision of the lesion from the dorsal surface of the left foot. The defect was closed with a split thickness skin graft. She also underwent a left inguinal sentinel lymph node (SLN) biopsy. The pathology showed a tumor that was level 3, 1.2 mm in depth with negative sentinel lymph nodes. She did well with no further treatment.

The overall incidence of melanoma in the United States is increasing, and surgery continues to be the mainstay of therapy. The cumulative lifetime risk of developing melanoma in the United States in 2002 was 1 in 68 compared to 1 in 250 in 1980.[76] This increased incidence of melanoma is due to an increasing incidence in the older population, as the incidence in the younger populations appears to be leveling off or even declining.[77]

The characteristics of melanoma appear to be slightly different in the elderly. Although the extremities are the most common location for melanomas in females, head and neck melanomas become more frequent with advancing age.[78,79] In men, truncal melanomas are most common, but again, head and neck melanomas become more frequent and surpass truncal melanomas after the age of 70.[78,79] Older patients have been reported to have worse prognostic indicators with increased incidence of ulceration, thicker melanomas, and deeper levels of invasion.[80-82]

A study of more than 17,000 patients showed that for each 10-year increase in age there was a decrease in both 5-year and 10-year survival rates.[83] Whether this represents a delay in the diagnosis or a worse malignant potential of these lesions in the elderly population is unknown.

The treatment for malignant melanoma is surgical excision with adequate margins and there is no evidence to suggest that the treatment for the elderly should be any different. Controversies over the width of margins and need for regional lymph node dissection have been addressed in a number of randomized trials. These studies have shown that the necessary width of margins of resection is determined by the thickness of the primary melanoma. For lesions less than 1 mm thick, a 1 cm margin is adequate.[84,85] For lesions greater than 1 mm thick, a margin of 2 cm is advised, on the basis of the results of the Intergroup Melanoma Surgery Trial.[86,87]

Although age has not been used as a criterion for determining the margins of resection, one large retrospective series did report age to be a significant independent factor in the risk for local recurrence.[89] Patients older than 60 were found to have a local recurrence rate of 7.8%, patients between the ages of 30 and 59 had a local recurrence rate of 2.5%, and patients younger than 30 had a local recurrence rate of 1.2% at a median follow-up of 8 years.

The dissection of regional lymph nodes for melanoma treatment is routine for patients with clinically positive nodes; however, the value of elective node dissection for patients with clinically negative lymph nodes has long been debated. Because regional node dissections carry significant long-term complications it would be advantageous to avoid them in patients with known negative lymph nodes. The use of SLN biopsy technique, introduced by Morton[88] in 1992, has allowed an accurate evaluation of the lymph node basin without a complete dissection. However, complete dissections are still necessary for positive sentinel nodes and for palpable nodal disease. Patients are now routinely getting SLN biopsies for any lesion greater than 1 mm in thickness. The sentinel node can now be harvested with 98% accuracy.[90]

Morton[91] reported the findings of 1,269 patients with intermediate-thickness melanomas (1.2-3.5 mm) randomly assigned to wide local excision with or without SLN biopsy. Disease-free survival was significantly higher (P=0.009) in the patients undergoing SLN biopsy compared to the observation group at 5 years because potentially positive lymph nodes were not removed from this group. The overall rate of death from melanoma and melanoma-specific survival, however, was similar for both groups; however, for patients with positive nodal metastasis, the 5-year survival rate was higher in the SLN group (72% versus 52%). Also, the number of positive lymph nodes was lower in the SLN group (1.4 versus 3.3), showing disease progression during observation. This study led to the conclusion that SLN biopsy has staging, prognostic, and survival value in patients with intermediate-thickness melanoma.

In a large retrospective analysis of the national cancer data base for melanoma (comprised of a total of 84,836 cases), factors associated with decreased survival included more advanced stage at diagnosis, nodular or acral lentiginous histology, increased age, male gender, nonwhite race, and lower income. Five-year survival was worst, stage-for-stage, in patients 60 years or older. For early disease, the 5-year survival was 81.4% for the patients older than 60 versus 90.5% for those younger than 60. For late disease, the 5-year survival was 32% for the older patients versus 40.5% for the younger ones.[92]

Because surgical treatment of melanoma can be done with low risk, in fact under local anesthesia if necessary, no one should be denied it because of age or poor performance status. Treatment of melanoma for elderly patients should be as aggressive as in younger patients.

 See expertconsult.com for a complete list of references and web resources for this chapter

SUGGESTED READINGS

1. Heimann DM, Kemeny MM: Surgical Management of the Older Patient with Cancer. In Hurria A, Balducci L, editors: *Geriatric Oncology: Treatment, Assessment and Management*, New York, NY, 2009, Springer Science and Business Media, Inc, pp 157–200.
2. Hurria A, Leung D, Trainor K, et al: Factors influencing treatment patterns of breast cancer patients age 75 and older, *Crit Rev Oncol Hematol.* 46:121, 2003.
3. Gennari R, Rotmensz N, Perego E, et al: Sentinel node biopsy in elderly breast cancer patients, *Surg Oncol* 13(4):193, 2004.
4. Tan E, Tilney H, Thompson M, et al: The United Kingdom National Bowel Cancer Project - Epidemiology and surgical risk in the elderly, *Eur J Cancer* 43:2285, 2007.

5. Audisio RA, Bozzetti F, Gennari R, et al: Position paper: The surgical management of elderly cancer patients: recommendations of the SIOG surgical task force, *Eur J Cancer* 40:926, 2004.

6. Surgery for colorectal cancer in elderly patients: a systematic review, Colorectal Cancer Collaborative Group. *Lancet* 356:968, 2000.

7. Heriot AG, Tekkis PP, Smith JJ, et al: Prediction of postoperative mortality in elderly patients with colorectal cancer, *Dis Colon Rectum* 49:816, 2006.

8. Orsenigo E, Tomajer V, Palo SD, et al: Impact of age on postoperative outcomes in 1118 gastric cancer patients undergoing surgical treatment, *Gastric Cancer* 10:39, 2007.

9. Chang CK, Jacobs IA, Vizgirda VM, Salti GI: Melanoma in the elderly patient, *Arch Surg* 138:1135, 2003.

Radiation Therapy for the Older Patient

Jeffrey Wu, Susan McCloskey, and Michael L. Steinberg

Within 1 year of the discovery of x-rays by Wilhelm Roentgen in 1895, radiation was used for the treatment of malignancy.[1] Today, approximately 50% to 60% of cancer patients receive radiation therapy (RT) as part of their disease management.[2,3] The role of RT is particularly important for the geriatric population, given the association of aging with an increased incidence of cancer, as well as the often present comorbidities in the elderly that may preclude the delivery of more invasive or aggressive treatment alternatives.[4] Radiation therapy is an important treatment option as monotherapy or in combination with other treatment modalities for older patients with cancer.

This chapter will provide an overview of the basic mechanisms and rationale for the use of RT and discuss the process of care and toxicities associated with RT in the management of elderly patients with cancer. Radiation therapy alone is generally well tolerated in the aged, while concurrent chemoradiotherapy (CRT) requires considered patient selection due to increased treatment-related morbidity. External beam radiation delivered by linear accelerators is the treatment delivery method most often utilized by radiation oncologists for treatment of the elderly; however, other RT techniques such as brachytherapy and radiopharmaceuticals may also be useful. The increased precision of modern RT technology, which allows for significant increase in normal tissue sparing, will be discussed because of its potential import in tailoring treatment to the special needs of the aged. Radiation therapy, used in combination with other treatment modalities or as monotherapy, offers a powerful therapeutic tool for the management of the elderly patient with cancer, for both curative and palliative clinical circumstances.

MECHANISMS, RATIONALE, AND PROCESS OF CARE FOR RADIATION THERAPY

Radiation oncology deals with the therapeutic application of ionizing radiation to treat benign and malignant diseases. The most common approach used to deliver ionizing radiation is external beam radiation therapy (EBRT), which utilizes high-energy photons, or electrons produced by linear accelerators. Protons and other heavy particles, including neutrons and carbon ions, are less commonly used and continue to be studied. Radioactive isotopes generating beta particles and gamma rays are delivered by brachytherapy, the surgical implantation of radioactive sources into the body to treat cancer, and with systemic radiopharmaceutical treatments.

The benefit of radiation therapy stems from the biological fact that ionizing radiation directly and indirectly damages the genetic material of the cell, the DNA, which controls cell growth and replication. Although normal cells are also in the path of the radiation beam, they have superior DNA repair mechanisms and therefore can more readily repair damage sustained from irradiation. Cancer cells are more susceptible to this DNA damage-related disruption of cell replication and undergo cell death through necrosis or apoptosis. Laboratory studies examining the relationship of age and tumor radiosensitivity *in vitro* and within animal models are limited.[5] However, the relationship of age and radiation-induced normal tissue toxicity has been more extensively studied. From these studies, it is thought that the mechanism by which radiation affects normal tissue cells is similar in younger and older patients.[6,7]

When the cancer patient is evaluated for RT, the radiation oncologist determines whether radiation treatment is indicated in the particular clinical circumstance, establishes the specific intent of the treatment, and defines an overall treatment plan. Radiation therapy may be used alone or in combination with surgery or systemic therapies such as chemotherapy. In almost all cases, the aim of RT is to provide local control of a tumor for either a curative or palliative outcome. In the curative circumstance, a patient may accept a greater risk of toxicity associated with higher doses of RT or the addition of concurrent chemotherapy with or without surgery. In contrast, the goal of radiation therapy in the palliative setting is to ameliorate or prevent cancer-related symptoms without causing additional significant morbidity.

The decision to recommend RT and the aggressiveness of its application for elderly patients must be individualized to the clinical circumstance, the patient's overall functional status, and his or her general medical condition. Clinical experience and the medical literature have concluded that age alone should not preclude the use of RT.[8-13] The clinical discussion to follow will illustrate that the toxicities experienced by elderly patients receiving RT are not significantly different from or more severe than those of the general cancer patient population. However, other issues beyond age may be relevant to the consideration of radiation therapy in the elderly patient. For example, the patient's general medical condition, functional status, issues of quality versus quantity of life, logistical and social obstacles to treatment, comorbidities, polypharmacy, and neurocognitive status all must be factored into the treatment decision-making process. Tools such as the Comprehensive Geriatric Assessment (CGA) allow for a broad appraisal of the physical, mental, social, and functional capabilities and limitations of elderly adults. Such formal evaluation tools may enhance the medical decision-making process regarding the appropriateness of specific treatments, including RT, and also better inform inclusion criteria for clinical trials where older patients had traditionally been excluded solely on the basis of age.[6,13]

After the radiation oncology consultation, if radiation therapy is deemed indicated and appropriate, the patient undergoes a radiation treatment planning session called a simulation. During the simulation, the patient is positioned on a simulated treatment couch in the exact position that will be used during actual daily treatment on the linear accelerator (Figure 7-1). Immobilization devices, such as a custom face mask for head immobilization or body molds or casts, are often used to help provide stable and reproducible patient positioning to enhance the accuracy of the daily treatment. Patients who are able to cooperate with the simulation and the daily treatment setup are more likely to receive accurate and precise targeting of RT throughout their treatment course. However, patients with cognitive impairment, dementia, severe anxiety, or other functional deficits that may limit compliance offer challenges to the treatment management. Such circumstances may require modifications such as alteration of treatment field size, use of anti-anxiety medications, prescribing a shortened course of therapy, or even, rarely, anesthesia.

During the simulation, imaging with x-rays, fluoroscopy, or computerized tomography (CT), sometimes combined with positron emission tomography (PET) or magnetic resonance imaging (MRI) provide visualization of the region to be treated with radiation. The images obtained are electronically transferred to a specialized dedicated treatment-planning computer, where the tumor target is defined and surrounding normal structures are contoured by the radiation oncologist. The radiation oncologist then works with a team of physicists and dosimetrists to select the appropriate radiation dose, beam energy, and beam direction(s) required to

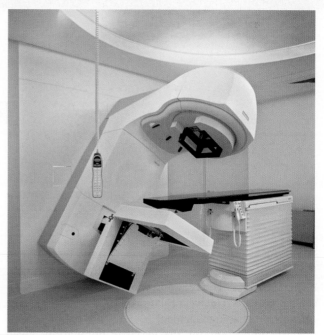

FIGURE 7-1 Linear accelerator. *(Courtesy of Siemens)*

effectively treat the tumor while limiting the dose to normal tissues and critical structures. Treatment planning can take anywhere from several hours to several days depending on the complexity of the case.

A course of RT is typically fractionated, meaning the total dose is delivered in smaller divided doses over time, typically over several days or weeks. Conventional curative courses of RT utilize a daily dose of 180 and 200 cGy given 5 days per week and lasting between 4 and 9 weeks in duration. Palliative courses of radiation are often shorter, ranging from a single treatment to 20 treatments over 4 weeks' time. Fractionation exploits a number of radiobiological principles that increase the therapeutic benefit of radiation therapy. Fractionation allows for normal tissues to repair sublethal DNA damage between fractions, which enhances the patient's tolerance of the treatment. In addition, fractionation allows for tumor cells to undergo redistribution into more radiation-sensitive phases of the cell cycle between fractions and for reoxygenation of tumor cells between fractions, making them more sensitive to RT.

A change in fractionation scheme alters the biological effect of radiation therapy. In some cases, such as hyperfractionation (two treatments per day separated by a minimum of 4 hours), the goal is intensification of dose to improve tumor control within the limits of acute and late toxicities. By achieving a higher total dose to the tumor within the same or shorter time period without a substantial increase in acute or late toxicity, the probability of tumor control can be enhanced. Selected elderly patients with head and neck cancer have been shown to tolerate variations of such aggressive regimens.[14]

In other instances, modifications in fractionation are made to accommodate patients with mobility or transportation issues while still providing effective tumor response, particularly in the palliative setting. An extended duration of RT can be problematic for some older patients with mobility issues, certain comorbidities, or other logistical issues hindering daily transport for treatment. In this regard, shortened treatment courses, called *hypofractionated*, made possible by advanced treatment planning methods, can enhance the applicability of RT to the unique needs of the elderly cancer patient. Hypofractionation without compromising tumor control requires an increase in the size of each fraction, and therefore will result in increased late normal tissue toxicity. However, late toxicity may not be of concern for the older patient who stands to benefit from the symptomatic relief and shortened treatment time offered by hypofractionated RT.

A review of the literature on short-course RT for aged cancer patients by Donato, et al.[15] describes various regimens used for malignancies of the brain, breast, lung, prostate, bladder, and rectum, demonstrating safe and effective palliation of symptoms in each organ system. One exception is hypofractionated palliative RT for head and neck cancers, in which the clinical benefits do not appear to outweigh toxicities. A special case of hypofractionation, called stereotactic body radiation therapy (SBRT), can be used with curative intent for a number of tumor sites and is discussed in the section on Cutting Edge RT Techniques.

BALANCING TOXICITY OF RADIATION THERAPY WITH THERAPEUTIC GOALS

The goal of radiation therapy is to maximize the probability of tumor kill while minimizing the risk of normal tissue injury. This risk-benefit analysis is influenced by the intent of treatment. For curative treatment, higher radiation doses are required to maximize tumor control. Such higher doses may be associated with increased normal tissue toxicity. For palliative cases, the aim is to deliver the minimum dose that is able to achieve durable improvement of the tumor-associated symptom while also minimizing the risks of RT-induced toxicity.

With the exception of the RT-associated symptom of treatment-induced generalized fatigue—which is not universal and most of the time does not occur—radiation toxicities and their associated side effects are local and site-specific. RT-related side effects can be categorized as acute (those symptoms occurring during the treatment course), subacute (those symptoms occurring within 3 months of treatment), and late toxicities (those occurring beyond 3 months of completion of RT).

Acute and Subacute Effects of Radiation Therapy

Acute toxicity occurs in normal epithelial tissues or other rapidly dividing cell populations within the treatment field. It demonstrates the equilibrium between cell

TABLE 7-1	Typical Acute Side Effects and Basic Management
Reaction	**Management**
Skin erythema/ desquamation	Aloe vera; hydrocortisone (0.5%, 1%) cream; silver sulfadiazine cream
Mucositis	Sodium bicarbonate oral gargle; diphenhydramine/viscous lidocaine/aluminum hydroxide mix; oral sucralfate suspension; amifostine
Odynophagia/ dysphagia	Hydrocodone/acetaminophen elixir, oral sucralfate suspension, nystatin suspension; preventative swallow exercises
Pneumonitis	NSAIDs, oral steroids
Nausea/vomiting	Prochlorperazine; ondansetron
Diarrhea	Loperamide; diphenoxylate/atropine
Cystitis/dysuria	Phenazopyridine; oxybutynin; tolterodine
Proctitis	Hydrocortisone (1%, 2.5%, 10%) ointment
Myelosuppression	Transfusion; brief treatment break
Fatigue	Exercise; psychosocial intervention; supportive care

death and stem cell proliferation in response to radiation damage. Clinically and histopathologically, the acute reaction is also characterized by inflammatory and immune responses to both radiation-induced tumor cell death and damage to normal tissue. Acute side effects are expected to occur to some degree in most curative courses of RT. Depending on the site of treatment, toxicities may include hair loss, dysphagia, odynophagia, skin erythema or desquamation, nausea, vomiting, oral mucositis, esophagitis, pneumonitis, enteritis, proctitis, and cystitis. Acute toxicities, if they are to occur, typically happen approximately 2 to 3 weeks after initiation of daily radiation therapy (Table 7-1), and are only infrequently of significant severity to warrant brief breaks in treatment or the discontinuation of therapy. The vast majority of acute side effects are managed by outpatient pharmacological interventions or nutritional modifications, are usually self-limited, and resolve within several weeks of completing the course of radiation treatment.

Acute Effects and the Suitability of Radiation Therapy in Treatment of the Elderly

The notion that elderly patients should be offered noncurative regimens or not offered radiation as a treatment option at all because they may not be able to tolerate a curative course of radiation therapy is not supported by clinical experience or the peer-reviewed literature.[6,12,16] Indeed, aging is associated with changes in molecular and biochemical pathways at the cellular level. However, experiments have been performed on mouse[17] and pig skin,[18] mouse lip mucosa,[19] and vascular smooth muscles cells *in vitro*,[20] all of which describe similar acute normal tissue radiosensitivity across varying host ages.

One study on the acute radiation response in skin of young and old rats reported a decrease in tissue radiosensitivity correlated with age.[21] Clinically, many retrospective studies support the view that RT alone does not cause significant differences in toxicity between younger patients and older patients without other severe comorbidities and reasonable performance status. Zachariah et al. retrospectively examined the records of 203 patients aged 80 or older who received RT at facilities associated with Moffitt Cancer Center over a 7-year period and found that more than 90% were able to complete treatment without significant complications.[22] This completion rate is similar to the overall population of patients treated with RT. A similar study by Wasil et al. also concluded that older patients safely tolerate radiation therapy both for curative and palliative intent, with more than 80% of patients able to complete their planned treatment course.[23] Even CRT can be offered to provide improved outcomes in the elderly population for such diseases as locally advanced head and neck cancer, lung cancer, and esophageal cancer. Such aggressive regimens do result in an increased acute side effect profile in all age groups. Elderly patients may be more vulnerable to such stresses; thus careful patient selection and aggressive supportive management may be required.[13]

During the course of radiation therapy, patients are scheduled to see the radiation oncologist a minimum of once weekly for assessment of acute toxicities, but can and should be seen more often depending on the needs of the patient. Most common side effects are easily managed with over-the-counter medications and skin care products, though some side effects may require prescription-strength medications, and at times more aggressive interventions (see Table 7-1). All cancer patients benefit from the multidisciplinary management by social workers, dieticians, transportation aides, and other support staff. This is particularly true for many geriatric patients who battle their disease with the added burdens of social isolation, a weakened support structure, self-denial of symptom severity, and decreased patient concern regarding the critical nature of self-care and personal advocacy. Straightforward side effects may be rationalized, ignored, and exacerbated by patient ennui resulting in an increased probability of more severe treatment-related sequelae such as dehydration with electrolyte imbalance and/or dysphagia leading to malnutrition and cachexia.[12,13,16] Although the results of a study reviewing 210 patients older than 74 years treated with a variety of aggressive RT regimens for varying sites of disease concluded that curative RT is well-tolerated in older patients, the authors, for reasons similar to those mentioned earlier, also recommended more vigilant management of mucositis and diarrhea in elderly patients, who are prone to dehydration.[14]

Not uncommon in the geriatric population is the use of pacemakers and implantable defibrillator devices. There is a rare possibility of radiation-induced malfunction of these devices when they are directly in or near the treatment beam. Caution should be taken by the radiation oncologist by consulting with the patient's cardiologist and a medical physicist to ensure that the treatment will not cause untoward effects on the function of these devices.[24,25]

Subacute Effects

The most common subacute side effect of RT is radiation pneumonitis, in patients whose normal lung is necessarily within the treatment field as required in the treatment of lung cancer or breast cancer. This side effect occurs in the days and weeks following treatment and is characterized by mild symptoms of breathlessness and a dry cough. It is usually managed conservatively. In patients taking long-term steroid medication for preexisting medical problems or in those patients with severe lung disease such as chronic obstructive pulmonary disease (COPD), radiation pneumonitis may be much more severe and require management by a pulmonary specialist to prevent a more serious progression of the symptoms.

Late Effects

Late effects developing in patients who have received radiation therapy are usually associated with damage to vascular, lymphatic, nervous, and/or connective tissues or other cell populations with a low mitotic rate. These effects can occur anytime from 3 months to many years after radiation exposure. Most such problems occur between 9 and 24 months after completion of treatment; they rarely occur beyond 5 years. Most late effects caused by radiation do not rise to a level that meaningfully affects the patient's quality of life.[26] Typically, signs and symptoms such as chronic skin changes of epidermal telangiectasia and tanning, subdermal fibrosis, and mild-to-moderate soft-tissue fibrosis comprise the majority of radiation-induced late side effects. These side effects tend not to cause significant morbidity for the patient. As with acute reactions, late toxicity must be localized to the treatment field and is dependent on total dose, fractionation, and volume of the critical organs irradiated, and rare idiosyncratic patient response to radiation. In contrast to acute effects, most late-effect damage is irreversible. However, the use of tocopherol (vitamin E) and pentoxifylline has been reported to improve late-effect changes of soft tissue fibrosis in symptomatic patients.[26,27] Hyperbaric oxygen therapy has also been shown to relieve several radiation-induced late side effects.[28] Infrequently, significant permanent decrement in the patient's quality of life can result. For example myelopathy, cataracts, xerostomia, gastrointestinal stricture, pulmonary fibrosis, lymphedema, nephropathy, osteoradionecrosis. and soft tissue scarring and/or necrosis are possible rare late outcomes, even in properly administered radiation therapy.

Laboratory data do not suggest that worse late toxicities of RT are related to host age. For example, several *in vitro* studies on fibroblasts, which are thought to be the principle cells involved in late radiation response, did not demonstrate a relationship between radiosensitivity and age.[29,30] Animal studies of individual organ systems do not correlate aging with more severe late reactions, and several studies even suggest older animals show a greater resistance to the late effects of radiation. In Ruifrok et al., the latency period between spinal cord irradiation and the development of myelopathy was significantly longer in older versus younger rats.[31] Another pair of experiments from separate laboratories, examining radiation-induced nephropathy, both demonstrated decreased renal radiosensitivity in older pigs[32] and rats.[33] In one clinical circumstance, the findings are less clear-cut. For CNS malignancies, some reports suggest elderly patients receiving brain irradiation to large treatment volumes are at greater risk of cognitive decline as a result of therapy.[34,35] However, in this case, vascular comorbidities such as hypertension, diabetes, and atherosclerosis, with a higher incidence in the elderly, confound the causal analysis between age and toxicity.[36] In addition, the conventional wisdom regarding cognitive changes associated with cranial irradiation has recently been augmented by the understanding that patients with CNS primary and metastatic disease often suffer preradiation neurocognitive problems. When baseline neurocognitive measures are made before RT, the imputed effects of RT fall away.[37] Nevertheless, due care to limit the amount of brain irradiation in young and older patients remains a current tenet of good radiation oncology practice.

The concern over late toxicity may also be less relevant for some elderly patients with shorter life expectancy. In general, the risk of late complications can be reduced by decreasing the per-fraction dose. However, in such a case, the total course of radiation must be extended in order to achieve a high enough dose to control the tumor. For some patients, improving present quality of life is the higher priority over minimizing the possibility of late effects. In such cases, which are usually palliative, a shortened or hypofractionated course of RT is often effective and may provide the benefit of both symptom relief and abridged treatment days.

Comorbidities and Radiation Therapy in the Elderly

As previously described, clinical and laboratory studies do not suggest that aging alone affects the mechanisms of acute or late radiation response. However, aging is associated with comorbid illnesses, as well as with a decline in physiologic reserve.[38] It is likely that these factors play the most relevant role in the selection of elderly patients for RT as well as their tolerance of it. Common medical conditions faced by the elderly such as hypertension, atherosclerosis, heart disease, and COPD are rarely, on

their own, contraindications to RT.[12] Rather, treatment and management decisions are influenced by a combination of factors including the anatomical region being irradiated, the volume of critical organs or structures in the treatment field, and the specific comorbidities and associated functional status of the patient. For example, because the older patient can be at increased risk for upper respiratory tract or urinary tract infections, special attention for the development of acute side effects in these organ systems may be warranted during their RT course. In another case, a patient with Parkinsonian tremor may pose a challenge because of his or her difficulty remaining still; however, appropriate immobilization and treatment field design usually obviates significant difficulties with delivery of RT in such patients. Finally, as elderly cancer patients already demonstrate high rates of fatigue and depression,[39] minimizing treatment-related fatigue is particularly important for such patients. Studies suggest the RT-induced fatigue is less severe and lasting than its chemotherapy[40] or combined modality counterparts,[41] and with modern RT techniques further shrinking the irradiated volume and course of therapy, even greater gains have been observed.[42] These examples highlight the heterogeneous composition of the elderly population, who despite comorbidities, with proper individualized assessment and treatment design, are still good candidates for RT. Considering the three major modalities of oncologic care, RT is often a reasonable option for the geriatric patient who may be unable to tolerate the physiologic stresses of surgery or chemotherapy.

CUTTING-EDGE TECHNIQUES IN RADIATION THERAPY

The two major factors moderating the effectiveness and toxicity of RT are dose and the volume of tissue being irradiated. The biological effect of a particular total dose of radiation is a function of the dose per fraction, the fractionation scheme, and the total time over which the dose is delivered. Refinement in dose fractionation has been studied since radiation was first applied to the treatment of cancer. In the past decade, the use of advanced imaging technologies for both tumor target delineation and intratreatment target localization, introduction of sophisticated treatment planning software, and enhanced treatment delivery instruments have vastly improved the ability to precisely irradiate tumors while sparing normal tissues. Several of these techniques are valuable for the treatment of the elderly cancer patient.

Improved Targeting

Radiation fields were once as basic as a single treatment field (port) or uncomplicated anterior/posterior opposed (AP/PA) treatment fields with or without simple blocking utilized to shape the treatment beams. These approaches may still be appropriate field designs for specific cases;

however, with the aid of improved imaging technology, especially CT, methods to deliver the dose to the target volume have dramatically improved the precision of radiation treatment. Intensity-modulated radiation therapy (IMRT), stereotactic radiosurgery (SRS), stereotactic radiotherapy (SRT), and stereotactic body radiation therapy (SBRT) are technologies used to treat tumors with the prescribed dose while at the same time dramatically minimizing irradiation of adjacent normal tissues to limit the short- and long-term side effects of treatment and maximize its therapeutic benefits.

A specific set of technologies called image-guided radiation therapy (IGRT) represents the latest advance in RT targeting. Utilizing imaging technologies of ultrasound, fluoroscopy, or CT combined with sophisticated localization techniques including stereoscopic shift technique, IGRT allows for daily localization of the treatment target, yielding increased precision of treatment and decreased normal tissue irradiation. IGRT is a critical aspect of improved targeting in RT.

IMRT

Traditionally, treatment planning decisions regarding beam angles and field shapes were made first during the isodose treatment planning process, followed by dosimetry calculations and modifications to achieve the prescribed dose to the intended target. This was called "forward" planning. Conversely, the initial step of IMRT defines the doses to the target volume and critical structures (also called organs at risk, OAR), followed by "inverse" treatment planning, which utilizes software that optimizes beam angles and shapes in order to produce the desired dose distribution. During the IMRT treatment, the patient, the treatment couch, and the beam all move, while at the same time the beam is mechanically spoiled or modulated. The result of this process is the mathematical equivalent of creating literally thousands of tiny microbeams aimed at the treatment target, producing a highly defined dose distribution irradiating the tumor while avoiding designated critical structures. (Figure 7-2)

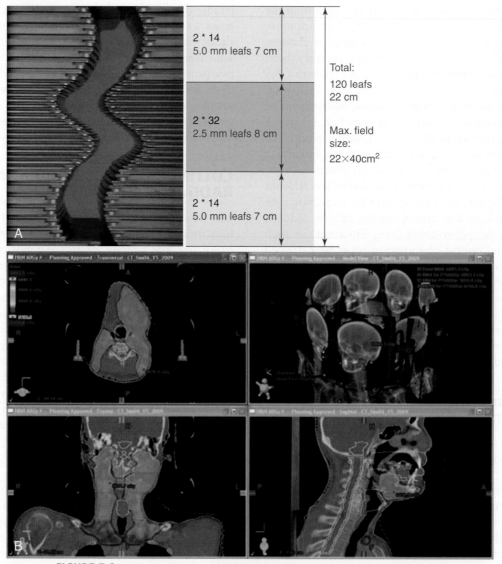

FIGURE 7-2 A, Multileaf collimator. **B,** IMRT plan for T2N2 oropharyngeal cancer.

In the mid-1990s, use of IMRT began experimentally at a few institutions worldwide, but the past decade has seen a rapid increase in its application. IMRT has been shown to reduce rates of xerostomia in head and neck irradiation,[43-45] permitted curative dose escalation in prostate cancer treatment while dramatically decreasing rectal and genitourinary treatment related morbidity,[46-48] and provided a retreatment option for recurrent disease in previously irradiated areas,[49-51] to name just a few examples of this technology's significant benefits to patients. IMRT has emerged as the standard of care for a number of disease sites including prostate cancer, head and neck cancer, many CNS tumors, breast cancer, anal cancer, and esophageal cancer. Many other disease sites are actively under investigation to define the potential benefits of the precision of IMRT.[52] IMRT's potential to decrease treatment-related morbidity should not be underestimated. While to our knowledge no studies have examined the application of IMRT specifically for the geriatric population, the benefit of increased normal tissue sparing in elderly patients with multiple comorbidities is intuitively apparent.

SRS

Stereotactic radiosurgery was first described by neurosurgeon Lars Leksell and radiobiologist Bjorn Larsson in 1951 as a method to treat intracranial lesions, avoiding open surgery by utilizing a machine called the Gamma Knife.[53] This technology, comprised of 201 Cobalt-60 sources focused on a single point, was developed to effectively treat a multitude of benign and malignant cranial lesions including arteriovenous malformations (AVM), acoustic neuromas, meningiomas, pituitary tumors, and primary and metastatic brain tumors. Today, a number of machines, including the Gamma Knife and modified or dedicated linear accelerators with SRS capability (e.g., Novalis TX, CyberKnife, XKnife, Trilogy, Synergy S), are able to treat cranial lesions.

The basic premises of SRS include: (1) a stereotactic frame of reference functioning to provide precise localization of an intracranial target; and (2) machinery capable of delivering one to five fractions of high dose radiation with very sharp dose fall-off gradients to minimize irradiation of surrounding tissues (Figure 7-3). A treatment course of more than five fractions to an intracranial (or extracranial) tumor in which stereotactic localization is utilized in the delivery methodology is commonly referred to as stereotactic radiotherapy (SRT).

The use of SRS has become common in the elderly patient for the treatment of primary and metastatic brain tumors, meningiomas, AVMs, trigeminal neuralgia, and primary and recurrent pituitary tumors. The procedure is minimally invasive in nature and of short duration—usually one day. Customarily, a head frame was attached to the patient's skull to ensure precision of treatment delivery, but recently technologies and techniques have been developed that allow completely noninvasive frameless

treatments, which enhances patient acceptance of the procedure (see Figure 7-3). SRS is widely used for the treatment of brain metastases due to excellent local control rates and the possibility of avoiding the need for whole-brain radiation therapy (WBRT).[54-56] The potential of avoiding WBRT, typically a 2 to 3 week course of treatment, may be important for the older patient facing difficulties with daily transportation or concerns of cognitive decline from RT.[42,57]

SBRT

Treatment of extracranial tumors utilizing the precision of stereotaxis is known as stereotactic body radiotherapy (SBRT). Using only one to five fractions for the entire treatment course, it can be used to treat a number of anatomical sites effectively. Radiobiologically, the high dose and hypofractionated nature of SBRT is thought to exploit different mechanisms of cell damage than conventional RT by causing endothelial apoptosis and the upregulation of unique inflammatory cascades.[58-60] SBRT's truncated treatment course coupled with its comparable or superior tumor control as compared to standard fractionation makes it logistically beneficial for the elderly. SBRT is also a noninvasive alternative to surgery, which is of particular utility in the treatment of the older patient with significant comorbid diseases. For example, medically inoperable patients with early stage non-small cell lung cancer (with comorbidities of COPD, coronary artery disease, or cerebrovascular disease) who have historically been treated with conventional RT (with local control rates of only 30% to 50%)[61-63] are now successfully managed with three to five SBRT treatments (Figure 7-4). SBRT for early stage lung cancer has demonstrated 3-year local control and overall survival rates of 88% to 92% and 42% to 60%,[64-66] respectively, establishing a superior alternative to conventional RT and a medically equivalent option to the surgical standard-of-care, lobectomy. The use of SBRT as the primary treatment for a number of tumors including prostate cancer,[67,68] liver metastases,[69] renal primary and metastatic disease,[70] and pancreatic cancer[71] is currently under investigation. For example, SBRT for early-stage prostate cancer was first examined prospectively by King et al.[68] where five fractions of SBRT delivered every other day resulted in favorable PSA response without severe late rectal toxicities. While longer-term evaluation is necessary, this technique is a prime example of how dose and targeting modifications stemming from advancements in medical physics and discoveries in radiobiology provide a safe, effective treatment option for younger and older patients alike.

Brachytherapy

The surgical application of a radiation source placed within a body cavity (intracavitary) or implanted directly in the tissue or tumor itself (interstitial) is called

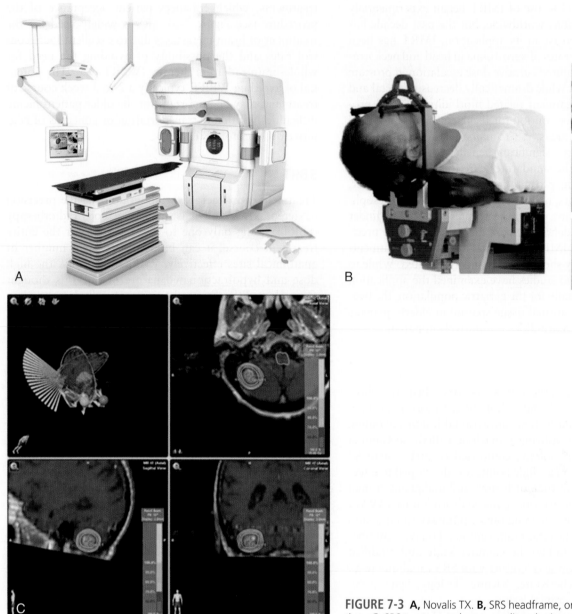

FIGURE 7-3 A, Novalis TX. **B,** SRS headframe, or frameless alternatives. **C,** SRS treatment plan on a solitary brain metastasis.

brachytherapy. Many of the technical advantages of SRS and SBRT including dose escalation, conformality, and short duration of treatment were first achieved by brachytherapy. Interstitial treatment is invasive and often requires local or general anesthesia or conscious sedation. It may have the concomitant risk of bleeding and infection associated with a surgical procedure. Nevertheless, in certain situations, brachytherapy allows for convenient and low morbidity treatment of tumors in the elderly.

Brachytherapy is used to treat malignant diseases throughout the body including the brain, eye, head and neck, breast, lung, esophagus, biliary tract, endometrium, cervix, prostate, and soft tissues. Two examples highlighting the usefulness of brachytherapy in the elderly are its application in the two most common malignancies in the geriatric population, breast and prostate cancer.

Postlumpectomy management of breast cancer customarily requires whole breast external beam RT over 5 to 7 weeks. Alternatively, accelerated partial breast irradiation (APBI) using brachytherapy delivers treatment in 10 fractions over the course of five days, with early clinical experience demonstrating favorable results.[72,73] ABPI is particularly applicable to the older cancer patient because of its short treatment duration. APBI compared to whole breast RT is being investigated prospectively by the large NSABP B-39 randomized trial, which is still in accrual.

Prostate "seed" interstitial brachytherapy involves the placement of radioactive isotopes directly into the prostate gland under ultrasound guidance. Due to the short half-life and lack of external penetration of the radioactive isotope, the radiation safety risks to medical personnel and the patient's family members are *de minimis*.

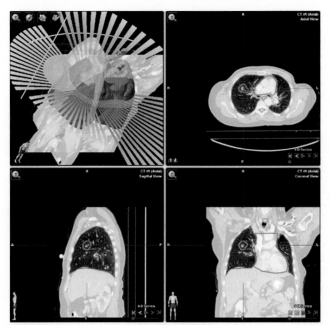

FIGURE 7-4 SBRT treatment plan of T2 non-small cell lung cancer.

It is a 1-day procedure done on an outpatient basis. It has equivalent tumor control in low-risk prostate cancer patients and low rates of toxicity similar to those associated with other RT procedures or radical prostatectomy, which is usually not offered to patients older than 70 years.[74,75]

Radiopharmaceuticals

Radiopharmaceuticals are used to treat systemic malignant disease. Given by oral, intravenous, or intraarterial routes, radioactive isotopes can be administered attached to pharmaceutical vehicles, as in radioimmunotherapy (RIT), or in an unattached soluble form, known as "unsealed source" RT.

Unsealed sources rely on the natural properties of the element to aggregate at the site of interest. For example, I-131 is absorbed and concentrated in follicular thyroid cells. As it decays, I-131 releases β particles, with a path length of 1 to 2 mm, which destroy normal thyroid and thyroid cancer cells. Other radionuclides including Sm-153 and Sr-89 are used to palliate widespread metastatic bone pain associated with metastatic breast, prostate, and lung cancer. These radioisotopes bind to hydroxyapatite, most actively at the tumor-bone interface of osteoblastic lesions, where they deliver therapeutic doses of radiation via beta decay. Myelosuppression is a possible side effect for all patients, which may be especially concerning in the aged, or when this treatment modality is used concurrently with other chemotherapeutics.[76]

Radioimmunoglobulins are monoclonal antibodies linked to a radioisotope. Y-90 and I-131 are favored because of their short half-lives, beta decay, and stability in complex with the antibody. Radioimmunotherapy is most successful in the treatment of certain lymphomas. An international phase III randomized clinical trial reported that consolidation with Y-90 ibritumomab tiuxetan compared to no additional therapy after first-line induction for follicular lymphoma improved progression-free survival from 13.3 months to 36.5 months.[77] Data from four clinical trials were pooled to examine the safety and efficacy of Y-90 ibritumomab tiuxetan in three age groups of non-Hodgkin lymphoma patients. Patients older than 70 years had similar rates of hematologic toxicity compared to the group of patients younger than 60, and rates and durations of response were similar in all age ranges.[78]

CLINICAL APPLICATIONS

Given the prevalence of cancer in the elderly, several publications have specifically examined tolerability of or alternatives to standard of care radiation regimens in the elderly. Several relevant publications by primary cancer diagnosis are discussed later in the chapter.

Glioblastoma

Glioblastoma (GB) is the most common primary central nervous system malignancy and is commonly diagnosed in the elderly. The standard of care for patients with glioblastoma is maximal surgical resection followed by fractionated external beam radiation, with concurrent and adjuvant temozolomide.[79] This regimen has been specifically studied in patients older than 65 years in two prospective single-arm trials that demonstrated a median overall survival of 11 months and acceptable toxicity.[80,81] However, a retrospective review of the same age population compared 19 patients treated with concurrent radiation and temozolomide to 20 patients treated with radiation alone and found 42% grade 3-4 toxicity among patients receiving concurrent CRT versus 0% in the patients receiving RT alone.[82] Such reports of increased toxicity in elderly patients receiving combined modality therapy have motivated the study of alternative regimens.

Radiation alone, delivered using either standard or abbreviated fractionation schemes, is associated with median survival of 4 to 8 months.[83-87] Roa et al. randomized 100 patients, age 60 or older, to postoperative standard RT (60 Gy in 30 fractions) versus abbreviated RT (40 Gy in 15 fractions) and found statistically equivalent overall survival of 5.1 versus 5.6 months.[86] Similarly, temozolomide alone has been investigated as an alternative strategy in elderly patients with glioblastoma, and median survival rates of approximately 6 months have been reported.[88-90] Minniti et al. prospectively treated 43 patients older than 70 with hypofractionated RT (six fractions of 5 Gy each delivered over 2 weeks) followed by adjuvant temozolomide, and achieved a median overall survival of 9.3 months.[91] Of note, a recent prospective trial randomized 85 patients older than 65 with newly diagnosed high-grade glioma to best supportive care versus RT (50 Gy in 28 fractions) and found significant improvement in median survival (29.1 versus 16.9 weeks) among patients receiving RT, with no associated decrements in quality of life or cognition.[87]

Head and Neck Cancer

Curative radiation-based treatment for head and neck cancer can be associated with significant acute and chronic toxicity which often gives reason for pause when considering tolerability in an elderly patient. Concurrent chemoradiation (CRT) is standard of care for most patients with locally advanced head and neck malignancies but has been minimally studied in the elderly. Turaka et al. compared quality-of-life outcomes among patients older than 60 and younger than 50 receiving concurrent CRT and found that patients older than 60 experienced greater decrement in physical, cognitive, emotional, and functional quality-of-life endpoints.[92]

Concurrent CRT may also be associated with increased chronic toxicities. In a case-control study of patients enrolled in three RTOG randomized trials of CRT, age was found to be a significant predictor of late toxicities, with 56% of patients older than 65 experiencing late toxicity versus 31% of patients younger than 50.[93]

Prior to the era of definitive concurrent CRT, several studies examined outcomes among elderly patients receiving definitive radiation and concluded comparable cancer control outcomes and acceptable toxicity.[11,94-97] Pignon et al.[11] specifically reported toxicity endpoints among patients older than 70 receiving definitive radiation on EORTC clinical trials and noted equivalent acute mucositis and weight loss. Older patients experienced significantly greater grade 3-4 functional acute toxicity, but this did not translate to differences in overall survival, or in frequency of late radiation damage.

Among younger patients who are not chemotherapy candidates, two alternative strategies have been evaluated: altered fractionation and concurrent radiation with cetuximab, a monoclonal antibody against the epidermal growth factor receptor. Allal et al.[98] retrospectively compared outcomes of 39 patients age 70 or older and 81 patients younger than 70 treated with altered fractionation RT (specifically accelerated concomitant boost), and found equivalent acute and late toxicities. While an unplanned treatment break was observed in 8% of the elderly group and in none in the younger group, all patients completed the planned RT schedule, and there was no difference in overall survival and locoregional control between the two groups. The authors conclude that this aggressive RT-alone regimen for curative intent is feasible for appropriately selected older patients. Although the strategy of concurrent radiation and cetuximab has not been specifically studied in the elderly, the

randomized trial of RT versus concurrent cetuximab and RT found a 10% improvement in 3-year overall survival with no added acute toxicities, other than acneiform rash, with the addition of cetuximab, suggesting that cetuximab may be a reasonable consideration in elderly patients able to tolerate RT.[99]

Non-Small Cell Lung Cancer

Definitive radiation is standard of care for early-stage medically inoperable non-small cell lung cancer (NSCLC), and concurrent CRT is standard of care for locally advanced NSCLC. Conventional external beam radiation has been the historical standard for patients with medically inoperable early stage NSCLC. However, rates of 5-year survival with definitive RT have ranged from 10% to 30%,[100,101] well inferior to rates of 65% to 70% achieved with surgery alone.[102] For elderly patients with early-stage medically inoperable NSCLC, recent advances in technology have allowed for alternative regimens that may be more tolerable, and potentially more effective, in the elderly. Yu et al. conducted a prospective multiinstitutional study of involved field IMRT in 80 patients with medically inoperable NSCLC and reported no grade 4 toxicity and minimal grade 3 toxicity (3.8% pneumonitis, 2.5% hematologic toxicity, and 1.3% esophagitis), with 36.7% experiencing elective nodal failure (i.e., recurrence in an initially uninvolved and untreated lymph node).[103] Stereotactic body radiation therapy, which involves the precise delivery of a limited number of high dose fractions (typically three to five fractions), has been a recent paradigm shift that has consistently achieved 3-year local control rates exceeding 85%, with minimal associated morbidity.[64-66] Delivery of fewer fractions and minimal associated morbidity may facilitate greater use of SBRT in elderly patients who have comorbidities or transportation limitations that would have precluded traditional daily fractionated RT delivery.

Movsas et al. examined the impact of age on outcome among 979 patients with locally advanced NSCLC who were enrolled on six prospective Phase II and III RTOG trials from 1983 to 1985, and found that patients younger than 70 had improved survival with more aggressive therapy (induction chemotherapy followed by standard RT, or concurrent CRT followed by hyperfractionated RT), while patients older than 70 achieved optimal quality-adjusted survival with standard RT alone.[104] Pignon et al. examined outcomes, stratified by age, among 1208 NSCLC patients who received definitive RT on one of six EORTC randomized trials and found comparable survival and acute and late toxicity, with the exception of increased weight loss in the older age groups[105]. Schild et al.[106] performed a secondary analysis of a North Central Cancer Treatment Group prospective trial of chemotherapy plus twice daily versus once daily RT to determine the impact of age on outcome. While patients older than 70 were found to have higher grade 4+ toxicity (81% vs. 62%), grade 4+ hematologic toxicity (78% vs. 56%), and grade 4+ pneumonitis (6% vs. 1%), no differences were noted in overall survival. Rocha Lima et al. similarly conducted a secondary analysis of patients with locally advanced or metastatic NSCLC enrolled on CALGB trials 8931 and 9130 to determine the impact of age on outcome and found no differences in treatment tolerance, response, survival, or continuation of treatment between patients older and younger than 70.[107] A secondary analysis of RTOG 94-10 performed by Langer et al. found that, although patients older than 70 experienced more grade 3-4 esophagitis and grade 3 neutropenia with concurrent CRT, CRT resulted in the longest survival for patients older than 70.[108] Taken together, the data for efficacy and toxicity of radiation regimens for elderly patients with locally advanced NSCLC would suggest that fit elderly patients may benefit from aggressive combined modality therapy; however, elderly patients should be monitored closely and receive optimal supportive therapy, given expected increases in associated toxicity.

Breast Cancer

Postlumpectomy radiation is standard of care for all patients undergoing breast conservation surgery for early-stage invasive breast cancer, and is recommended for patients with high-risk features (including positive nodes, positive margins, or tumor size exceeding 5 cm) in the postmastectomy setting. Data examining outcomes among women older than 70 undergoing postlumpectomy or postmastectomy radiation suggests tolerability and efficacy. However, recent data has emerged to suggest that omission of postlumpectomy RT in select patients older than 70 may be acceptable.

The Early Breast Cancer Trialists' Collaborative Group reported a meta-analysis of 23,500 women enrolled in prospective trials of RT versus observation in the postlumpectomy setting and found that a 19% absolute reduction in 5-year local recurrence associated with the addition of RT translated into an absolute 15-year 5% reduction in breast cancer-specific mortality.[109] However, many have argued that older women with favorable-prognosis breast cancer may not significantly benefit from the addition of postlumpectomy RT. Hughes et al.[110] randomized 636 women older than 70 with pathologic T1, estrogen receptor-positive, margin-negative invasive breast cancer status post lumpectomy to adjuvant RT and tamoxifen versus tamoxifen alone. No differences were noted in rates of distant metastases or overall survival. Although local recurrences were statistically significantly fewer in the RT arm (1% versus 4% at 5 years, and 1% versus 7% at 8 years[111]), the differences were small, leading the authors to conclude that omission of RT is a reasonable choice for women older than 70 with early-stage, estrogen receptor-positive

breast cancer. Because the rise in local recurrence rate in the tamoxifen-alone group (from 4% at 5 years to 7% at 8 years) would be expected to progress with longer follow-up, many practitioners maintain support for RT in the elderly patient with longer life expectancy.

When postlumpectomy radiation therapy is indicated, elderly women are acceptable candidates for hypofractionated RT, including whole- or partial-breast hypofractionated RT. Hypofractionated RT has been studied in three prospective trials that randomized patients with early-stage invasive breast cancer postlumpectomy to 50 Gy delivered in 25 daily fractions versus 41.6 Gy in 14 fractions, 39 Gy in 13 fractions, 40 Gy in 15 fractions, or 42.5 Gy in 16 fractions. The hypofractionated regimens were associated with equivalent locoregional control and survival, and equivalent or reduced morbidity.[112-114] Accelerated partial-breast RT (APBI) remains controversial, given the lack of randomized data with adequate follow-up to confirm equivalence. However, a recently released American Society for Therapeutic Radiation Oncology (ASTRO) Consensus statement concludes that women older than 60 with pathologic T1N0, estrogen receptor-positive, margin-negative, favorable-histology tumors are suitable candidates for partial breast irradiation.[115]

Randomized trials have established a survival advantage with the addition of postmastectomy radiation for younger patients with high-risk disease.[116-118] Given the exclusion of older women from these trials, Smith et al. used the SEER database to examine outcomes among women older than 70 who underwent mastectomy with or without adjuvant RT and found that postmastectomy RT was associated with a statistically significant survival advantage among patient older than 70 with high-risk disease (defined as T3/4 and/or N2/3).[119]

Gastrointestinal Malignancies

Pancreatic Cancer. The median age of diagnosis for pancreatic cancer in the United States is 72, and 42% of all patients diagnosed with pancreatic cancer are older than 75.[120] For medically operable patients with surgically resectable disease, surgery is standard of care, commonly followed by adjuvant concurrent CRT. Definitive concurrent CRT is recommended for patients with locally advanced unresectable pancreatic cancer. Miyamoto et al.[121] retrospectively examined toxicities associated with fluoropyrimidine-based concurrent CRT in 42 patients older than 75 and found that 19% required hospitalization; 17%, emergency room visits; 36%, RT treatment breaks; 7%, chemotherapy treatment breaks; and 21% failed to complete therapy. Survival outcomes were similar to those achieved in a younger patient population enrolled in prospective trials, leading the authors to conclude that the elderly may benefit equivalently from combined modality therapy, at the expense, however, of substantial treatment-related toxicity.

Rectal Cancer. Neoadjuvant or adjuvant CRT is recommended for patients with stage II or III rectal cancer. This regimen has not been prospectively evaluated in the elderly; however, the SEER database was recently examined to determine trends in utilization and completion of CRT and associated outcomes among 2886 patients older than 66 years with stage II or III rectal cancer. Completion of adjuvant CRT was associated with significant decreases in 5-year adjusted cancer mortality risk, thus highlighting the benefit of adjuvant CRT in the elderly. Only 37.5% and 54.2% of stage II and stage III patients initiated adjuvant CRT per NIH recommendations, and of those, only 47.6% and 67.5%, respectively, completed treatment. Presumably, physician expectation or patient experience of treatment-related toxicity may be significant enough to deter recommendation of and completion of therapy.[122] Existing data, however, do not demonstrate worse severity or tolerability of pelvic RT toxicities in older patients to support this line of reasoning,[10,123] and greater advocacy of CRT in fit elderly patients may be beneficial.

Although not specifically evaluated in the elderly, an alternative strategy for neoadjuvant RT delivery that has been prospectively studied and may have inherent advantages in the elderly is short-course RT, consisting of five fractions of 5 Gy each, delivered preoperatively.[124]

Esophageal Cancer. Most patients with primary esophageal malignancies will be recommended to receive CRT, either definitively or perioperatively. Mak et al.[125] retrospectively examined toxicities associated with CRT in 34 patients older than 75 and found that 50% completed CRT, 38.2% experienced grade 4 or worse acute toxicity, and 70.6% required hospitalization, emergency room visits, or RT treatment breaks. Two-year overall survival was 29.7%, leading the authors to conclude that CRT is associated with substantial morbidity in the elderly, survival is low, and future efforts should focus on improvement of treatment tolerability in the elderly. Of note, only seven patients were treated with IMRT techniques, which for esophageal cancer is becoming the treatment standard,[126,127] and which could potentially meet the needs of the geriatric patient population.

Prostate Cancer

The median age of diagnosis for prostate cancer is 68.[120] Given that elderly men with low-risk, early-stage prostate cancer will likely die with prostate cancer rather than of it, the NCCN Guidelines recommend that life expectancy be considered in management decisions and that active surveillance be discussed as a treatment option for patients with limited life expectancy. For patients who elect active treatment, external beam radiation therapy is a safe and effective option. Two retrospective series compared biochemical recurrence-free survival between patients older and younger than 75 and older and younger than 60, respectively, and found no differences in biochemical recurrence-free survival by age.[128,129]

The University of Chicago examined genitourinary and gastrointestinal toxicity outcomes after prostate cancer RT among four age cohorts: younger than 60, 60 to 69, 70 to 74, and 75 years and older. No significant differences were noted in acute or late GI or GU toxicity by age.[130] Brachytherapy, a procedure in which radioactive seeds are permanently implanted in the prostate gland in a single session under local or general anesthesia, is a treatment option for men with low-risk prostate cancer and has inherent logistic advantages in an elderly patient.

Radiation Therapy for Benign Conditions

Radiation therapy is an effective modality for the treatment of several benign conditions that may affect the elderly, including acoustic neuroma, pterygium, Graves disease, heterotopic ossification, meningioma, arteriovenous malformations, degenerative osteoarthritis, trigeminal neuralgia, and keloids.[131]

Palliative Radiation

Palliative radiation is effective in a variety of clinical circumstances. Symptoms that can be effectively palliated with radiation include pain from bone or visceral metastases[132,133]; cough, hemoptysis, and dyspnea from pulmonary malignancies[134]; dysphagia from head and neck cancers[135-137] or from obstructing gastrointestinal or pulmonary malignancies[138-141]; bleeding secondary to gynecologic, genitourinary, or gastrointestinal malignancies[142-144]; and neurological deficits from brain metastases or spinal cord compression.[145-148] Given that palliative radiation is commonly employed in patients with limited life expectancy, shorter course regimens have been investigated. Lutz et al.[149] recently published a comprehensive review of shorter course, or hypofractionated, palliative radiotherapy. The authors concluded that hypofractionated palliative radiation allows for "time-efficient, cost-effective, and minimally toxic" symptom palliation. This review included nine randomized trials of 8 Gy or 10 Gy delivered in a single fraction versus multiple fraction regimens for palliation of pain secondary to bone metastases and concluded equivalence. The randomized trials have repeatedly found equivalent pain relief and pain medication requirements among patients receiving a single versus multiple fraction regimen for palliation of pain from bone metastases. Higher rates of retreatment have been found among patients receiving single fraction radiotherapy, which is less of a concern among patients with limited life expectancy.

The review also examined studies of hypofractionated radiotherapy for patients with symptomatic lung cancer, pelvic malignancies, and head and neck cancer. Potential hypofractionated regimens available for patients with inoperable, advanced, symptomatic lung cancers include two- or five-fraction regimens.[150-154] For advanced symptomatic pelvic malignancies including gynecologic and

TABLE 7-2	Indications for Palliative Radiation Therapy and Rates of Improvement
Condition	**Percentage of Patients Experiencing Symptom Improvement**
Bone pain	73% - 93%
Brain metastases	56% - 75%
Superior vena cava syndrome	62% - 95%
Spinal cord compression	67% - 73%
Hemoptysis	48% - 88%
Dyspnea	40% - 64%
Vaginal bleeding	41% - 69%
Dysphagia	48% - 86%

Data from references 150, 156-162.

genitourinary malignancies, hypofractionated regimens have included one and three fraction regimens. Among patients with advanced head and neck cancers, quality of life improvements have been documented with a regimen known as "Quad Shot," referring to delivery of four fractions given twice daily for 2 days.[155] (Table 7.2)

CONCLUSION

Radiation therapy plays an essential role as monotherapy or in combination with other treatment modalities in the curative and palliative management of older patients with cancer. Laboratory data do not suggest that radiation-induced acute or late toxicities are age-dependent. Numerous clinical reports emphasize that age alone is not a contraindication to radiotherapy. CRT and other radical RT regimens may also be feasible in appropriately selected patients. Age-related access and medical issues such as comorbidities, logistical barriers to treatment, and waning social support can all be managed in the radiation oncology setting. In addition, modern RT technologies such as IMRT, SRS, and SBRT benefit patients of all ages, and are well-suited to address many of the management issues associated with treating the elderly cancer patient. With careful and personalized evaluation of the patient with tools such as the comprehensive geriatric assessment, elderly patients can often be offered optimal radiation therapy as part of their cancer care.

See expertconsult.com for a complete list of references and web resources for this chapter

Adjuvant Therapy for Elderly Patients with Breast, Colon, and Lung Cancer

Daniel Becker and Dawn L. Hershman

Cancer is the second leading cause of mortality in the United States and disproportionately affects the elderly. In 2009, breast, colorectal, and lung cancer together accounted for more than one third of the 1.5 million expected diagnoses of cancer, and for about 250,000 deaths.[1] The median age of cancer diagnosis in breast, colorectal, and lung cancers was 61 years, 71 years, and 71 years, respectively.[2]

Adjuvant therapy is defined by the National Cancer Institute (NCI) as "additional cancer treatment given after the primary treatment to lower the risk that the cancer will come back."[3] Adjuvant therapy is generally aimed at eliminating residual disease left behind at surgery. Decisions regarding the utility of adjuvant therapy weigh the likelihood of recurrence with the patient's life expectancy and susceptibility to short- and long-term toxicities. Over the past decade, increased screening with colonoscopy, mammography, and computed tomography (CT) of the chest has resulted in cancer detection at earlier stages.[4,5] Multiple different treatment modalities, including chemotherapy, radiation therapy, and biologic or targeted therapy may have a role in the treatment of early-stage cancer. Because elderly patients are often underrepresented in clinical trials, the benefits and risks in elderly populations are not well understood. However, even in settings of proven benefit, elderly patients are frequently not as likely to be offered or to receive curative therapy.[6-9]

The goals of this chapter are to introduce the major principles and fundamental practices of adjuvant therapy for breast, colon, and lung cancer in elderly patients. By the end, the reader should understand the factors that contribute to the decision to use or withhold adjuvant therapy. These factors include tumor and patient characteristics, as well as the benefits and toxicities associated with each therapy. Case presentations will highlight the challenges to providing appropriate cancer care for an individual patient. The specific cancer sections will explore prognostic factors and factors predictive of

response to therapy, both of which play important roles in decisions regarding adjuvant therapy. The cancer-specific section will also offer an overview of the therapies used to treat breast, colon, and lung cancer, with a focus on how the use of those therapies may be different in older patients.

PREDICTORS OF BENEFIT FROM ADJUVANT THERAPY

Decision making about the use of adjuvant therapy is influenced by tumor and patient characteristics.

Tumor Characteristics

A prognostic factor is defined by the National Cancer Institute (NCI) as an element that can be used to define the chance of recovery from a disease or the risk or relapse.[10] A predictive factor is used to estimate the likelihood that a patient will respond to a particular therapy. Many tumor characteristics have important prognostic and predictive value. Prognostic indicators in breast cancer include tumor stage and grade, lymphovascular invasion, and hormone receptor status.[11-14] Hormone receptor status and increased HER-2/neu expression also predict response to hormonal therapy and trastuzumab, respectively.[14,15] Prognostic indicators in colon cancer include tumor stage, grade, lymphovascular invasion, and preoperative serum carcinoembryonic antigen levels.[16-18] Stage and grade are unique in their almost universal prognostic value for varied tumor types. Additional prognostic and predictive factors will be reviewed in the cancer-specific sections.

The risk of relapse after primary surgical therapy is the main contributor to any decision regarding the benefit of adjuvant therapy; often a patient whose cancer is more likely to relapse is also more likely to benefit from adjuvant therapy. Stage of disease is one of the strongest predictors of relapse risk. Staging is defined by the TNM system, established by the American Joint Committee on Cancer (AJCC),[19] where T refers to the size of the primary tumor, N refers to the degree of lymph node involvement, and M refers to the presence or absence of distant metastases. The relationship between advancing age and stage varies by cancer. In multiple analyses, older breast cancer patients presented with more advanced-stage disease while older colon cancer patients presented at stages similar to younger patients, and older lung cancer patients presented with earlier-stage disease.[20-23] It is also noteworthy that changes in screening and medical care will influence the relationship between age and stage at diagnosis. Evidence suggests that both increased mammography and decreased use of hormone replacement therapy have contributed to the decrease in estrogen receptor-positive breast cancer in women in their 60s.[24]

The grade of the tumor is also an important determinant of relapse risk.[11,16] Although the specifics of tumor grade differ by tumor type, higher grade tumors are typically recognized by higher rates of cellular proliferation, increased invasion into surrounding tissue, and less similarity to their tissues of origin. As cancer cells acquire additional genetic changes that increase their potential to invade and metastasize, they frequently appear histologically to be less like their tissues of origin.[25] The relationship between advancing age and tumor grade is variable by tumor type.[12,26] Other tumor characteristics, including hormonal receptor status, lymphovascular space invasion, presence and absence of genetic alterations, and tumor genetic profiles influence relapse risk.[13,17]

Patient Characteristics

Patient characteristics, including life expectancy and the risk of treatment-related adverse outcomes, factor into any risk-benefit analysis about adjuvant therapy. Advanced age does not, by itself, predict toxicity from or poor response to therapy.[9,27] Advanced age is, however, associated with multiple other physiologic changes, including decreased performance status and increased numbers of comorbid conditions that may change the effects of therapy.

Pharmacokinetics. With advancing age, the body fat percentage increases, which decreases total body water and decreases the volume of distribution.[28] There is also an age-related decrease in glomerular filtration rate that prolongs the effects of medications excreted by the kidney, and which limits the use of medications with renal toxicity.[29] In addition, creatinine becomes a poor marker of glomerular filtration rate in elderly patients because of their decrease in muscle mass, which may not be recognized by the treating physician.[30,31]

Comorbidities. Coexisting renal or hepatic disease will change the half-life of administered medications, with resultant changes in the toxicity profile. Other comorbid conditions may influence the effects of therapy in ways that are less obvious. The Charlson comorbidity index was designed to predict 1-year mortality on the basis of a weighted composite score for the following categories: cardiovascular, endocrine, pulmonary, neurologic, renal, hepatic, gastrointestinal, and neoplastic disease.[32] One study of more than 1200 patients with non-small cell lung cancer noted that although a higher Charlson comorbidity score was associated with increasing age, only higher comorbidity score, and not age, was independently associated with decreased survival.[33]

Performance Status. Performance status is used to quantify the patient's functional capabilities. The two most widely used scales for performance status in oncology are the Karnofsky and Eastern Cooperative Oncology Group scales. Several studies have shown that poor performance status is associated with increased therapy-related toxicity and poor survival.[34,35] While predictive of outcome, there is evidence that these performance status scales may underestimate the degree of functional impairment in older patients, when compared with the activities of daily living (ADL) and instrumental activities of daily living (IADL) scales.[36]

Comprehensive Geriatric Assessment. The comprehensive geriatric assessment (CGA) generally includes functional status, comorbid medical conditions, cognitive status, psychological conditions, nutritional status, and medication review.[37] Functional status in a CGA may be assessed by the ADL and IADL, both of which focus on the patient's ability to complete specific daily tasks in and out of the home. The CGA predicts overall survival and toxicity of cancer treatment. It adds additional valuable information to assessments of performance status alone.[38,39]

Functional Reserve. Older patients may experience more severe toxicities than younger patients. For example, several studies have suggested significantly increased rates of neutropenia in patients older than 70 years who are receiving chemotherapy, after controlling for other risk factors.[40,41] Chemotherapeutics known to damage the heart have been shown to be more toxic in patients older than 65.[42,43] In many circumstances, the distinction between age as an independent predictor of toxicity or age as a marker for other changes that predict toxicity is unknown. Other studies have found similar rates of severe toxicity in younger and older patients treated with chemotherapy, albeit in highly selected patient populations.[7,44]

Therapy Characteristics

Each cancer-related therapy has a distinct toxicity profile, that may or may not be influenced by the patient's age, and which is weighed against the likelihood of benefit for the patient.

DISEASE-SPECIFIC ISSUES: BREAST CANCER

CASE 8-1	CASE PRESENTATION

A 74-year-old woman presents with a 4 cm mass in the left breast, discovered on her first mammogram in 5 years. Needle biopsy confirmed adenocarcinoma that expressed estrogen and progesterone receptors, but which did not overexpress the HER-2/neu protein receptor.

Pretherapy Evaluation
Comprehensive geriatric assessment reveals that the patient is completely independent by the IADL scale. Her only comorbidity is diabetes, which is controlled with oral medications; she shows no evidence of end-organ damage. She continues to work as an accountant, takes care of two grandchildren every Wednesday, and walks four mornings a week with her closest friends. The patient's cognitive function, nutritional status, and psychological state are excellent. Her medications include metformin and a daily baby aspirin.

Clinical Staging

On physical exam, the patient has a palpable 4 cm, firm, mobile nodule in the upper outer quadrant of the left breast, and a 2 cm palpable node in the left axilla.

Mastectomy versus Breast-Conserving Therapy

Total, or simple, mastectomy includes removal of the whole breast and the fascia overlying the pectoralis major. Breast-conserving surgery removes the tumor mass with specimen margins that are free of tumor. Prospective randomized trials have established the equivalence of mastectomy and the combination of breast-conserving surgery and radiation, while breast-conserving surgery without radiation results in a higher local recurrence rate and worsened survival.[45] The decision regarding appropriate breast surgery is challenging and personal. The absolute contraindications to breast-conserving surgery include multicentric disease, diffuse calcifications on mammogram, prior radiation to the chest wall, and inability to obtain clean margins.[46] Relative contraindications to breast-conserving therapy include connective tissue disease and large tumor size relative to breast size.[47] In addition, patients who are unable to receive radiation because of logistical issues may not be appropriate candidates for breast conservation surgery.

Older women are less likely to have breast-conserving surgery, and those who have it are less likely to have radiation therapy when compared to younger women.[48,49] A patient's decision as to whether to undergo a mastectomy versus breast-conserving therapy is strongly influenced by her physician's recommendation.[50]

Axillary nodal evaluation by sentinel node biopsy or nodal dissection is the standard of care for all women with invasive breast cancer.[51] Older women are significantly less likely to have axillary lymph node dissection.[52] For some, this may be appropriate, as there is evidence that women older than 70 years with estrogen receptor-expressing tumors and tumors less than 2 cm with no clinical axillary involvement may be safely treated with resection followed by tamoxifen, without axillary nodal exploration.[53] Guidelines suggest that axillary node evaluation should not be omitted in a patient who is being considered for any adjuvant therapy in addition to hormonal therapy, and specifically should be pursued in patients with higher-risk cancers.[54]

CASE 8-1	CASE CONTINUED

The patient proceeded to a lumpectomy and axillary lymph node dissection. Additional laboratory data and chest x-ray were unremarkable. The final staging is pathologic T2 (tumor >2 cm, but <5 cm), N1 (nodal involvement in 1 to 3 ipsilateral axillary nodes), M0 (no distant metastases), stage IIB. The patient had a normal echocardiogram with a left ventricular ejection fraction of 60%.

Prognostic and Predictive Factors Stage

As noted earlier, cancer stage is a universal predictor of the patient's overall prognosis. The cancer Surveillance, Epidemiology, and End Results (SEER) database tracks cancers in the US in a representative 26% of the population. In the year 2000, from the SEER database, 60% of breast cancer cases were diagnosed as localized disease with the cancer confined to the primary site; 33% were diagnosed as regional disease with spread beyond the primary site or into the local lymph nodes; and 5% were metastatic at diagnosis. The 5-year relative survival rate for localized disease was 98.3%; for regional disease, 83.5%; and for metastatic disease, 23.3%.[1] Older patients with breast cancer are more likely than younger patients to present with metastatic disease.[22]

Histology and Grade. Grade has been described earlier and represents a composite evaluation of the tumor's aggressiveness by histologic criteria. Grade is a well-established predictor of outcome.[11] Older patients tend to present with breast cancer with lower proliferative rates and lower incidence of lymphovascular invasion, both markers of less aggressive behavior.[12,55] Breast cancer may present with variable histologic patterns, and these histologic subtypes may have different clinical behavior. Approximately 75% of women with invasive breast carcinoma, a cancer of epithelial cell origin, have infiltrating ductal type carcinoma. Patients who have a component of invasive lobular carcinoma frequently present at a more advanced stage than those with purely infiltrating ductal carcinoma, and their tumors are more likely to be hormone-sensitive.[56]

Hormone Receptor Status. The expression of estrogen and progesterone receptors on the surface of breast cancer cells is both prognostic and predictive of response to hormonal therapy. Collectively, patients who are either estrogen- and/or progesterone-receptor positive live longer than patients whose tumors are hormone receptor-negative. This association holds true after accounting for age, stage, histology, and other demographic variables. The association is also maintained in both older and younger women.[13] Tamoxifen is a selective estrogen receptor modulator (SERM) that is an estrogen receptor antagonist in breast tissue and an agonist in other tissues, including bone and uterus. Estrogen receptor (ER) status strongly predicts response to tamoxifen therapy, with a 31% reduction in the annual breast cancer death rate in ER-positive patients and no effect on patients with ER-negative disease.[14] For postmenopausal women, aromatase inhibitor therapy, either alone or given sequentially with tamoxifen, has been shown in multiple clinical trials to be superior to tamoxifen therapy alone.[57,58]

HER-2 Status. HER-2 is a transmembrane glycoprotein receptor of the epidermal growth factor receptor family. Approximately 18% to 20% of breast cancer patients overexpress the HER-2 protein. Older women are less likely to express HER-2 than younger women.[12] HER-2 expression predicted poor cause-specific survival in both older and younger women prior to the use of trastuzumab, an anti-HER-2 antibody.[59] The benefit of trastuzumab is confined to those patients with immunohistochemically confirmed overexpression of HER-2 or fluorescence in situ hybridization-confirmed elevated gene copy number of HER-2/neu.[15]

Overall Prognosis

The overall prognosis of elderly women with breast cancer is the net effect of the biology of the tumor and the efficacy and tolerability of therapy. The overall prognosis of older women has been reported in some studies to be comparable to the prognosis for younger women and in other studies to be worse than the prognosis for younger women.[23,60] Differences in receipt of adjuvant therapy likely contribute to these disparate results. In a study of 407 women aged 80 years or older who were treated during the 1990s, 12% received no therapy; 32%, tamoxifen only; 7%, breast-conserving therapy only; 33%, mastectomy; and 14%, breast-conserving therapy with adjuvant radiation therapy.[61] The 5-year breast cancer specific survival for these groups were 46%, 51%, 82%, and 90%, respectively. Age was strongly associated with less-aggressive treatment after controlling for tumor type, general health status, and comorbidities.

Adjuvant Therapies: Radiotherapy

Adjuvant radiotherapy may be used in two settings: after breast-conserving therapy and after mastectomy. A review of almost 50,000 women age 65 or older treated for breast cancer in the 1990s found that approximately 76% of the patients who had lumpectomies also had radiation therapy. Receipt of postlumpectomy radiation

therapy was associated with later year of diagnosis, younger age, fewer comorbidities, nonrural residence, chemotherapy, white race, and no prior history of heart disease.[62] Older age has also been associated with longer delay between lumpectomy and radiation therapy.[63] In a randomized trial of 636 women older than 70 years with small, node-negative, ER-positive breast cancer who were assigned to either BCT with tamoxifen and radiotherapy or BCT with tamoxifen only, found that risk of local relapse was increased at 5 years, from 1% to 4% without radiation; however, survival was not significantly different between the groups.[53]

Adjuvant Therapies: Systemic

Chemotherapy. The National Comprehensive Cancer Network (NCCN) recommends adjuvant chemotherapy for all patients less than 70 years old with nodal involvement or with tumors larger than 1 cm.[51] The guidelines recommend consideration of chemotherapy for patients with tumors between 0.6 and 1 cm after evaluation of hormone receptor status, HER-2 status, and other unfavorable features including angiolymphatic invasion, high nuclear grade, or high histologic grade. Common chemotherapeutic drugs used include doxorubicin, cyclophosphamide, 5-fluorouracil, paclitaxel, and docetaxel. A meta-analysis of 194 randomized trials of adjuvant chemotherapy begun by 1990 found that anthracycline-containing compounds reduced the annual breast cancer death rate by 38% in patients younger than 50 years, and by 20% in patients aged 50 to 69.[14] Few patients older than 70 were included in these trials. Another meta-analysis established the survival benefit of adding a taxane to anthracycline chemotherapy, regardless of patient age.[64] In a dose-dependent fashion, anthracycline chemotherapy is associated with development of cardiomyopathy in elderly patients with hypertension.[43] In an effort to avoid the anthracycline toxicity, docetaxel and cyclophosphamide were compared to doxorubicin and cyclophosphamide for the treatment of early breast cancer. Sixteen percent of the trial participants were age 65 or older and, after 7 years of follow up, both disease-free survival and overall survival were better in the docetaxel/cyclophosphamide arm.[65]

In a single institution study of more than 1500 women aged 55 or older treated for breast cancer between 1997 and 2002, older age was a significant predictor of not receiving chemotherapy when indicated by guideline recommendations. This association remained after controlling for confounding factors such as stage, tumor characteristics, comorbidity score, and other demographic variables.[66] To assess the toxicity of chemotherapy for older patients in the community, one analysis of SEER-Medicare data from 1991 to 1996 found that the hospitalization rate for chemotherapy complications was 9%, which increased with increasing stage of cancer and increasing comorbidities, but did not differ by age category.[27] An evaluation of data from four randomized trials of adjuvant therapy that compared a higher dose or more intense chemotherapy regimen with a lower dose or less intense regimen suggested that more chemotherapy was associated with longer disease-free and overall survival. There was no association between age and disease-free survival. Older patients had more non–breast cancer-related deaths.[67]

Molecularly Targeted Therapy. Trastuzumab, a monoclonal antibody against the HER-2/neu receptor, is recommended for use in patients with HER-2/neu overexpression or gene amplification and tumors larger than 2 centimeters or lymph node involvement who are receiving adjuvant chemotherapy.[51] The benefit of trastuzumab was established in a combined analysis of two randomized trials that demonstrated a 33% decreased risk of death among patients who received trastuzumab.[68] Trastuzumab is typically started either with or after chemotherapy and continued weekly to complete 1 year of therapy. Major toxicities of trastuzumab include cardiomyopathy, allergic infusion reactions, and variable pulmonary toxicities.[68] Data on the use of trastuzumab in elderly patients are limited, but suggest that efficacy and toxicity are similar in all age groups.[69,70]

Hormonal Therapy. The goal of hormonal therapy for breast cancer is to reduce estrogen stimulation of the tumor. Three major modalities are used to reduce estrogen stimulation: ovarian ablation, by oophorectomy, with radiation, or by chemical means with luteinizing hormone-releasing hormone (LHRH); estrogen receptor blockade by a partial agonist (tamoxifen); and blockade of peripheral estrogen production by an aromatase inhibitor, in women without functioning ovaries. A meta-analysis of the effects of hormonal therapy in randomized trials of more than 60,000 patients demonstrated that for estrogen receptor-positive breast cancer, tamoxifen therapy for 5 years reduced the annual breast cancer death rate by 31% over 15 years, irrespective of patient age.[14] Aromatase inhibitors (AIs) decrease conversion of androgen precursors into estrogens, and have been shown to be superior to adjuvant tamoxifen therapy in postmenopausal women in a number of large randomized trials.[57,71] AIs are less likely to cause venous thromboembolic events and endometrial cancer, but are more likely to result in arthralgias and accelerated bone loss. Aromatase inhibitors are now recommended by the NCCN as first-line hormonal therapy for postmenopausal women.[51] Subgroup analyses of the older patients in the aromatase inhibitor trials confirm that AIs have similar efficacy and toxicity in older and younger postmenopausal patients.[72] A review of more than 1500 breast cancer patients treated at MD Anderson Cancer Center between 1997 and 2002 noted that, after accounting for comorbidities and stage, among only patients with good performance status, in situations where guidelines recommended hormonal therapy, women aged 75 and older were 90% less likely to be treated with hormonal

therapy than women aged 55 to 64.[66] Challenges to the effective use of adjuvant hormonal therapy include poor compliance and high cost.[73,74]

Decision Aids for Medical Therapy

Adjuvant! Online. The large amount of clinical and pathologic prognostic and predictive information is difficult to integrate into an overall assessment of prognosis for an individual patient. Adjuvant! Online is a program that synthesizes patient age, comorbidity, ER status, tumor grade, tumor size, and number of positive nodes to determine an overall risk of recurrence and death at 10 years.[75] The program has been validated in multiple cohorts.[76] The program also calculates the benefit of chemotherapy and hormonal therapy on the basis of data from large randomized trials. The results can be displayed in graphic form, printed, and given to the patient to help clarify the benefits of adjuvant therapy.

Oncotype. Traditionally, women with small, hormone-sensitive cancers have been most difficult to counsel regarding the risks and benefits of chemotherapy. Recently, a diagnostic tool has been developed, Oncotype DX, that quantifies the expression of 21 genes in a woman's tumor sample, and generates a numerical risk of distant recurrence assuming the patient were to take hormonal therapy alone.[77] The results characterize whether the patient has low, intermediate, or high risk of relapse, which corresponds to relapse rates of approximately 7%, 14%, and 31%, respectively. The results are independent of age. Retrospective studies show that tumors with high recurrence scores have a large benefit from chemotherapy and those with low recurrence scores have no benefit from chemotherapy.[78] Ongoing prospective studies are validating the predictive benefit of chemotherapy in patients with intermediate risk of metastatic recurrence

MammaPrint. The MammaPrint assay uses gene expression array technology on 70 genes to classify tumors as either good or poor prognosis. It was developed and validated on a cohort of women that included both hormone receptor negative and positive disease, as well as patients

---

CASE 8-1 | CASE CONCLUSION

In preparation for discussion of the risks and benefits of adjuvant therapies, the patient's profile was entered into the Adjuvant! Program[75] (Fig 8-1). According to the Adjuvant! algorithm, approximately 42 patients out of one hundred patients with this profile who receive no therapy will be alive in 10 years. Twenty-nine patients are expected to die from causes other than cancer, and 29 patients are expected to die from cancer. Adding hormonal therapy would be expected to decrease the cancer related mortality by approximately 7%, and adding chemotherapy to that would be expected to decrease the cancer-related mortality by an additional 14%. The patient decided that she would pursue treatment with adjuvant chemotherapy, radiation therapy, and hormonal therapy.

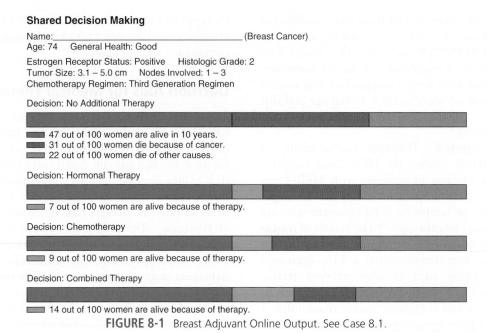

Shared Decision Making

Name:_____ (Breast Cancer)
Age: 74   General Health: Good

Estrogen Receptor Status: Positive   Histologic Grade: 2
Tumor Size: 3.1 – 5.0 cm   Nodes Involved: 1 – 3
Chemotherapy Regimen: Third Generation Regimen

Decision: No Additional Therapy

- 47 out of 100 women are alive in 10 years.
- 31 out of 100 women die because of cancer.
- 22 out of 100 women die of other causes.

Decision: Hormonal Therapy

- 7 out of 100 women are alive because of therapy.

Decision: Chemotherapy

- 9 out of 100 women are alive because of therapy.

Decision: Combined Therapy

- 14 out of 100 women are alive because of therapy.

FIGURE 8-1 Breast Adjuvant Online Output. See Case 8.1.

with and without nodal involvement.[79] The Mamma-Print Assay has also been validated in an older cohort (median age 62.5 years) of patients with node-negative breast cancer.[80] Prediction of response to chemotherapy is not known.

Summary

Decisions regarding adjuvant therapy for older patients with breast cancer are complex and involve consideration of all possible adjuvant options (radiation, chemotherapy, targeted therapy, and hormonal therapy). They must factor in the patient's priorities, medical conditions, functionality, and the likelihood of tumor recurrence. Therapy should not be withheld on the basis of chronological age alone.

Predictive and Prognostic Factors

Pathologic Stage. Colorectal cancers may spread by direct extension, or by hematogenous, or lymphatic routes.[81] Hematogenous dissemination from most of the colon typically follows the venous drainage to involve the liver prior to the lungs. A notable exception to this is distal rectal cancer which, because of venous drainage directly into the inferior vena cava, may metastasize to the lungs without involvement of the liver.[82] T stage in colon cancer is related to depth of invasion, without reference to the size of the mass. An evaluation of population outcomes in patients with colon cancer from the SEER database found 5-year stage-specific survival of 93.2% for stage I, 82.5% for stage II, 59.5% for stage III, and 8.1% for stage IV.[18] Number of nodes involved is an important

---

CASE 8-2 COLON CANCER

Case
A 76-year-old man with hyperlipidemia presents with black stool. On colonoscopy he is noted to have a 3 cm mass in the descending colon. The biopsy confirms adenocarcinoma.

Clinical Staging and Presurgical Evaluation
The patient's only comorbidities are hypercholesterolemia and hypertension. He takes atenolol and lovastatin. He lives with his wife of 18 years, retired 7 years ago from the U.S. Postal Service, and is an avid golfer. He routinely does the grocery shopping for the family. His weight is stable at 192 pounds and he is 72 inches tall. The comprehensive geriatric assessment suggests that his functional status, cognitive ability, nutritional status, and psychological profile are all adequate. The patient's laboratory analyses reveal a mild microcytic hypochromic anemia, and are otherwise normal. His CEA level is not elevated. CT scan of the chest, abdomen, and pelvis show no pathologic findings other than the mass in the descending colon.

Primary Therapy
The patient decides to proceed with hemicolectomy and lymph node dissection. Pathologic evaluation reveals an intermediate grade T3 (tumor invades through the muscularis into the subserosa), N2 (involvement of 4 or more lymph nodes) tumor, and the final stage is IIIC.

---

prognostic factor.[83] Interestingly the number of nodes sampled in colon cancer surgery is also an important predictor of survival for patients with cancer in stages 1 to 3, with at least 12 nodes removed predicting a better overall survival.[84] Prognosis in colon cancer has been reported to be similar in older and younger patients.[85,86]

Grade and Tumor Features. Tumor grade also predicts outcome in patients with colorectal cancers.[16] Older patients present with high-grade tumors as frequently as do younger patients.[26] Additional features of the biopsy specimen, including vascular invasion,[87] lymphatic invasion,[88] and positive surgical margins are also prognostic indicators.[89,90]

Histology. More than 95% of all colon cancers are adenocarcinomas.[91] One histologic subtype, signet ring cell carcinoma, which represents only approximately 1% of all adenocarcinomas of the colon, is associated with poorer prognosis.[18,92]

Biochemical and Molecular Markers. Carcinoembryonic antigen is a glycoprotein that is overexpressed in adenocarcinoma relative to normal colon epithelial cells. Its function has not been completely elucidated, but localization on the cell surface and homology with other adhesion molecules suggests a role in cell-cell interactions.[93] DNA microsatellite instability is a marker of poor DNA mismatch repair. Microsatellite instability in tumor tissue is used to screen for the genetic defects that cause hereditary nonpolyposis colorectal cancer (HNPCC), and is also found in 10% to 15% of sporadic colon cancers. For reasons that are not entirely clear, low microsatellite instability (i.e., effective DNA mismatch repair) is associated with poor prognosis in sporadic colon cancer.[94] The relationship between microsatellite instability and age remains poorly defined.

The ras intracellular signaling molecule plays a key role in growth signaling transfer from cell surface epidermal growth factor receptors (EGFR) and nuclear DNA targets. Activating mutations of the K-ras can decrease cancer dependence on external stimuli via the EGFR.[95] Mutant K-ras has also been shown to be an important determinant of poor response to therapy with anti-EGFR antibodies in advanced colorectal cancer.[96]

Adjuvant Therapy

Chemotherapy. A benefit for chemotherapy (5-fluorouracil [5-FU] and leucovorin) over observation was first established in a pooled analysis of three randomized trials that demonstrated a 22% decrease in mortality associated with the receipt of chemotherapy in patients with stage III colon cancer.[97] Subsequently, the MOSAIC trial showed an absolute 5% disease-free survival advantage at 3 years for patients with stage III colon cancer who received adjuvant infusional 5-FU, leucovorin, and oxaliplatin (FOLFOX) relative to those who received 5-FU and leucovorin alone.[98] Patients in the FOLFOX arm experienced more neuropathy, hematologic, and gastrointestinal toxicity. Elderly patients are underrepresented in clinical trials, but both observational and subset analyses confirm the benefit of adjuvant chemotherapy in older patients.[9,99-101] Sargent and colleagues pooled elderly patient data from seven phase III trials of adjuvant 5-FU based therapy and found an overall survival benefit of 24% compared to

no therapy in all age groups, including the 506 patients older than age 70.[9] A small prospective study reported increased, but tolerable, levels of neuropathy and neutropenia in patients aged 76 to 80 years old.[102] Similar benefit has been reported in multiple population-based studies.[100,103] An analysis of patients aged 65 or older in the SEER-Medicare database with stage III colon cancer reported that only 52% received adjuvant 5-FU; however, among those treated with 5-FU there was a 34% reduction in mortality.[99,104] The decision regarding the use and type of adjuvant chemotherapy is increasingly complicated with newer and often more toxic chemotherapy regimens.

Molecularly Targeted Therapy. Although bevacizumab is used in metastatic colon cancer,[105] no significant benefit for bevacizumab therapy was seen in a randomized trial of patients with early-stage colon cancer.

Decision Aids

As in breast cancer, the wealth of prognostic information from clinical, pathologic, and molecular features of each case is difficult to integrate into an adjuvant therapy benefit. The Adjuvant! program includes a prognosis and benefit estimator for colon cancer.[75] The colon cancer recurrence calculation incorporates patient age, gender, comorbidity, depth of invasion, grade, number of positive nodes, and number of examined nodes.

Recurrence Score. Early studies suggest that a recently validated 18 gene recurrence score may predict colon cancer recurrence and overall survival independent of mismatch repair, tumor grade, stage, lymphovascular invasion, and nodes examined.[106] The clinical implications of the recurrence score with regard to treatment benefits are unknown.

CASE 8-2	CASE CONTINUED

The Adjuvant! program estimates that for this patient who is in good health with a high T and N stage tumor that his likelihood of dying from cancer within the next 5 years is approximately 47% (Fig 8-2). The program estimates that using adjuvant 5-fluorouracil and oxaliplatin will reduce the likelihood of dying from the cancer by 17%. After discussion with his treating physicians and consideration of his independent performance of activities of daily living and ECOG performance status score of 0, as well as his strong desire to use all available therapy to maximize his chance of long-term survival, the patient decides that he would like to undergo treatment with adjuvant 5-FU and oxaliplatin.

Summary

Adjuvant therapy for colon cancer in the elderly should include consideration of stage, grade, CEA level, and anatomy; a geriatric assessment; and patient preference. Chemotherapy is the standard of care for patients with stage III colon cancer, but current regimens cause substantial toxicity for older and younger patients.

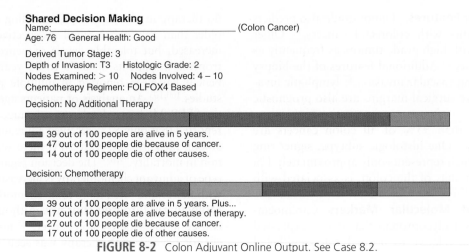

Shared Decision Making
Name:_____ (Colon Cancer)
Age: 76   General Health: Good

Derived Tumor Stage: 3
Depth of Invasion: T3   Histologic Grade: 2
Nodes Examined: > 10   Nodes Involved: 4 – 10
Chemotherapy Regimen: FOLFOX4 Based

Decision: No Additional Therapy

39 out of 100 people are alive in 5 years.
47 out of 100 people die because of cancer.
14 out of 100 people die of other causes.

Decision: Chemotherapy

39 out of 100 people are alive in 5 years. Plus...
17 out of 100 people are alive because of therapy.
27 out of 100 people die because of cancer.
17 out of 100 people die of other causes.

FIGURE 8-2 Colon Adjuvant Online Output. See Case 8.2.

LUNG CANCER

Lung cancer is broadly divided into small cell and non-small cell histologic types. In a recent review of the SEER database, the small cell lung cancers accounted for approximately 15% of all lung cancers, and incidence has been decreasing.[107] The histology, behavior, and therapy for these two types of lung cancer are significantly different. The section will focus on small cell type lung cancers.

CASE 8-3   CASE

A 68-year-old man with a 40 pack-year history of smoking is noted to have a 5 cm right upper lobe lung mass and enlarged right hilar nodes on a CT scan performed for evaluation of cough. Broncho-scopic biopsy reveals adenocarcinoma.

Clinical Staging and Pretherapy Evaluation
The patient reports that he has lost 10 pounds over the past 3 months. He stopped smoking 10 years ago and exercises three or four times weekly for 30 minutes to 1 hour. His medical history includes atrial fibrillation and an associated transient ischemic attack, for which he takes warfarin, and sciatic nerve pain for which he takes gabapentin. He has lived alone without assistance since his wife died of breast cancer in her 50s. He is active in the local senior center and spends about 2 hours there daily playing chess or exercising in the gym. He weighs 185 pounds, is 6 feet tall, and has a normal physical exam. The patient scores well on all components of the comprehensive geriatric assessment. Complete blood count, hepatic profile, and basic metabolic panels are within normal limits. Pulmonary function tests show no evidence of obstruction. Bronchoscopy is normal. PET/CT scan shows uptake in the mass and the right hilar nodes. Mediastinoscopy and biopsy confirms adeno-carcinoma in the right hilar nodes, without evidence of mediastinal nodal involvement. MRI of the brain is normal.

Surgery

A randomized trial of lobectomy versus wedge resection reported significant increases in recurrence and death rates for patients treated with wedge resection.[108]

Lobectomy or pneumonectomy are recommended by the NCCN as the standard of care for resectable non-small cell lung cancers; however, elderly patients are less likely to undergo curative surgery.[109,110] Studies on the outcomes of elderly patients after lung cancer resection have varied, with some studies reporting similar outcomes as younger patients,[111,112] and others reporting increased surgical mortality.[113]

CASE 8-3   CASE CONTINUED

The patient proceeded to right upper lobectomy and lymph node dissection. The final staging was T2 (tumor >3 cm and <7 cm), N1 (ipsilateral hilar nodes), M0, stage IIa.

Prognostic and Predictive Factors

Pathologic Stage. The AJCC staging system for lung cancer, updated in 2009, correlates well with prognosis, with 5-year overall survival ranging from 77% for small tumors without nodal spread to 2% for distantly meta-static disease.[104] Advancing age is associated with lower stage lung cancer at diagnosis.[21]

Histology. Adenocarcinoma and squamous cell carci-noma histologies comprise the majority of lung cancers, with similar histologic breakdown across age groups.[110] There is no clear consensus on the prognostic difference between the two predominant histologic subtypes.[114-116] Blood vessel invasion, however, is associated with a poor prognosis in multivariate analysis.[116]

Molecular Markers. A mutation of the epidermal growth factor receptor (EGFR) to a constitutively active form is an important predictor of response to EGFR inhibitors (i.e., gefitinib and erlotinib) in patients with metastatic cancer.[117] Studies suggested that patients older than 70 years may have similar rates of EGFR mutations to younger patients, and a similar response

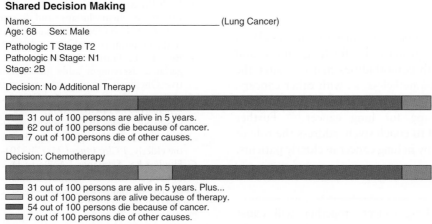

FIGURE 8-3 Lung Adjuvant Online Output. See Case 8.3.

to these therapies.[118] There is currently no proven role for molecularly targeted therapy in patients with limited-stage lung cancer. *RAS* is an oncogene whose protein serves to convey growth signals from surface receptors, including the EGFR, to the nucleus. Because the KRAS protein and EGFR are involved in the same oncogenic pathway, they are rarely mutated in the same patient's cancer. KRAS mutations predict nonresponsiveness to erlotinib.[119] Various studies have reported KRAS mutations to have either poor prognostic significance or no prognostic significance in different cohorts.[120,121] P53 is a tumor suppressor gene that is frequently mutated in lung cancer. P53 has been associated with worse prognosis and greater benefit from adjuvant therapy.[122]

Adjuvant Radiotherapy

A large French randomized trial failed to show a benefit to adjuvant radiation therapy following resection of an early-stage lung cancer.[123] A subsequent meta-analysis from 10 randomized trials confirmed this finding.[124] Survival and radiation toxicity in elderly patients were evaluated in a retrospective study of 1208 patients treated with thoracic radiation in trials of neoadjuvant, adjuvant, and definitive radiation.[125] There was no difference in survival or toxicity, including nausea, esophagitis, dyspnea, weakness, and performance status change, by age group.

Chemotherapy

A pooled analysis of five randomized trials showed that cisplatin in combination with another chemotherapy agent was associated with an 11% mortality reduction and a 5-year absolute survival benefit of 5.4%.[126] Several additional randomized trials have confirmed the benefit of adjuvant cisplatin.[127,128] Further analysis of these trials suggested that older patients received a decreased dose of chemotherapy, yet still had similar benefit relative to younger patients.[7] As mentioned previously, however,

older patients are consistently underrepresented in clinical trials, and therefore the results are often not generalizable to the large population of patients diagnosed with lung cancer.[129]

Combined Therapy

There is little support for using adjuvant chemoradiotherapy in lung cancer. Two phase II trials have evaluated the potential utility of neoadjuvant radiation and chemotherapy in locally advanced disease with mediastinal nodal involvement.[130,131] Neither has shown a benefit to chemotherapy in combination with radiation therapy followed by surgery. A secondary analysis of a randomized trial of chemotherapy with either daily or twice daily radiation as definitive therapy for stage III lung cancer noted that patients older than 70 years experienced worse toxicity, including myelosuppression and pneumonitis, with combined therapy.[40]

Targeted Therapy

There is currently no role for molecularly targeted adjuvant therapy for non–small cell lung cancer

Decision Aids

Adjuvant! has a program available to calculate the benefit of chemotherapy in non–small cell lung cancer.[75] The variables used in the analysis include age, gender, number of comorbid conditions, T stage, and N stage.

CASE 8-3 | **CASE CONCLUSION**

The patient has a discussion with his oncologist regarding the risk and benefits of adjuvant therapy (Fig 8-3). The patient understands that over 5 years he has an approximately 63% chance of dying from his cancer. He also understands that cisplatin combined with vinorelbine will likely decrease that likelihood by approximately 8%. He decides to have adjuvant cisplatin doublet chemotherapy.

Summary

Lung cancer is the number-one cause of cancer-related death. Smoking is the primary risk for lung cancer, and is also associated with comorbidities that can alter the benefits of therapy. Nonetheless, as with other cancers, elderly patients may benefit from surgery and standard adjuvant chemotherapy for lung cancer.[126] Further research is warranted to conclusively address the role of adjuvant chemotherapy in lung cancer in elderly patients.

CONCLUSION

Breast, colon, and lung cancers together will cause approximately one quarter of a million deaths in the United States in 2009. Adjuvant therapy with radiation, chemotherapy, hormonal therapy, and targeted agents offers the best chance of cure to patients diagnosed with localized disease. Elderly patients are often excluded from clinical trials, frequently have more comorbid medical illnesses, and can present with tumor characteristics that are different from those found in younger patients, all of which makes decisions regarding adjuvant therapy more challenging. Historically, older patients have been undertreated with adjuvant therapy. Prognostic and predictive features of the tumor, including stage, grade, lymphovascular invasion, and surface receptor expression should be evaluated, along with patient characteristics including a comprehensive geriatric assessment, performance status, and comorbid medical illnesses, to decide when to use adjuvant therapy for an individual patient. Validated decision aids including the Adjuvant! program and gene expression profiling can help integrate prognostic factors and stratify patients on the basis of risk of cancer recurrence.

See expertconsult.com for a complete list of references and web resources for this chapter

SUGGESTED READINGS

1. Neugut AI, Fleischauer AT, Sundararajan V, et al: Use of Adjuvant Chemotherapy and Radiation Therapy for Rectal Cancer Among the Elderly: A Population-Based Study, *J Clin Oncol* 20(11):2643–2650, 2002.
2. Sargent DJ, Goldberg RM, Jacobson SD, et al: A pooled analysis of adjuvant chemotherapy for resected colon cancer in elderly patients, *N Engl J Med* 345(15):1091–1097, 2001.

3. Early Breast Cancer Trialists' Collaborative Group (EBCTCG): Effects of chemotherapy and hormonal therapy for early breast cancer on recurrence and 15-year survival: an overview of the randomised trials, *Lancet* 365(9472):1687–1717, 2005.
4. Repetto L, Fratino L, Audisio RA, et al: Comprehensive geriatric assessment adds information to Eastern Cooperative Oncology Group performance status in elderly cancer patients: an Italian Group for Geriatric Oncology Study, *J Clin Oncol* 20(2):494–502, 2002.
5. Schild SE, Stella PJ, Geyer SM, et al: The outcome of combined-modality therapy for stage III non-small-cell lung cancer in the elderly, *J Clin Oncol* 21(17):3201–3206, 2003.
6. Hughes KS, Schnaper LA, Berry D, et al: Lumpectomy plus tamoxifen with or without irradiation in women 70 years of age or older with early breast cancer, *N Engl J Med* 351(10):971–977, 2004.
7. Bouchardy C, Rapiti E, Fioretta G, et al: Undertreatment strongly decreases prognosis of breast cancer in elderly women, *J Clin Oncol* 21(19):3580–3587, 2003.
8. Hershman DL, Wang X, McBride R, et al: Delay in initiating adjuvant radiotherapy following breast conservation surgery and its impact on survival, *Int J Radiat Oncol Biol Phys* 65(5):1353–1360, 2006.
9. Muss HB, Woolf S, Berry D, et al: Adjuvant Chemotherapy in Older and Younger Women With Lymph Node-Positive Breast Cancer, *JAMA* 293(9):1073–1081, 2005.
10. Thürlimann B, Keshaviah A, Coates AS, et al: Breast International Group (BIG) 1-98 Collaborative Group, A comparison of letrozole and tamoxifen in postmenopausal women with early breast cancer, *N Engl J Med* 353(26):2747–2757, 2005.
11. Paik S, Shak S, Tang G, et al: A multigene assay to predict recurrence of tamoxifen-treated, node-negative breast cancer, *N Engl J Med* 351(27):2817–2826, 2004.
12. Folprecht G, Cunningham D, Ross P, et al: Efficacy of 5-fluorouracil-based chemotherapy in elderly patients with metastatic colorectal cancer: a pooled analysis of clinical trials, *Ann Oncol* 15(9):1330–1338, 2004.
13. Sundararajan V, Mitra N, Jacobson JS, et al: Survival associated with 5-fluorouracil-based adjuvant chemotherapy among elderly patients with node-positive colon cancer, *Ann Intern Med* 136(5):349–357, 2002.
14. Jessup JM, Stewart A, Greene FL, Minsky BD: Adjuvant chemotherapy for stage III colon cancer: implications of race/ethnicity, age, and differentiation, *JAMA* 294(21):2703–2711, 2005.
15. Owonikoko TK, Ragin CC, Belani CP, et al: Lung cancer in elderly patients: an analysis of the surveillance, epidemiology, and end results database, *J Clin Oncol* 25(35):5570–5577, 2007.
16. Jackman DM, Yeap BY, Lindeman NI, et al: Phase II clinical trial of chemotherapy-naive patients >= 70 years of age treated with erlotinib for advanced non-small-cell lung cancer, *J Clin Oncol* 25(7):760–766, 2007.
17. Langer CJ, Manola J, Bernardo P, et al: Cisplatin-based therapy for elderly patients with advanced non-small-cell lung cancer: implications of eastern cooperative oncology group 5592, a randomized trial, *J Natl Cancer Inst* 94(3):173–181, 2002.

Chemotherapy

Sumanta Kumar Pal and Arti Hurria

Cancer and aging are related phenomena, as evidenced by the fact that 60% of cancer incidence and 70% of cancer-related mortality occurs in individuals older than 65.[1] Treatment of cancer in the older adult represents a multidisciplinary effort, frequently integrating medical oncologists, geriatricians, radiation oncologists, and surgeons. As chemotherapy is a commonly used anticancer strategy, collaboration between the former two groups is of critical importance. Physiologic changes that accompany aging may alter the tolerance of chemotherapy, and geriatricians, primary care providers, and medical oncologists may play a role in co-managing related side effects. There are two distinct scenarios in which chemotherapy is applied: (1) the metastatic setting, where the principal goals of treatment are maintenance of quality of life (QOL), prolongation of survival, and decreasing disease-related symptoms; and (2) the neoadjuvant and adjuvant setting, where the goals of treatment are to decrease the risk of disease relapse and disease-related mortality.

The decision to administer chemotherapy is always dependent upon the goals of treatment, as well as the potential risks and benefits to the patient. With these goals in mind, the decision is made to pursue a specific chemotherapy regimen. In the adjuvant setting, polychemotherapy regimens are delivered to eradicate residual microscopic disease through the use of multiple agents with distinct mechanisms of action. In the metastatic setting, the goal is to control disease while maintaining quality of life. The approach to metastatic disease varies on the basis of the disease one is treating. For example, in the setting of breast cancer, studies have demonstrated that combination chemotherapy in comparison to single-agent sequential therapy produces higher response rates but no difference in overall survival.[2-3] In contrast, even among adults older than 70, studies suggest that combination therapy represents a standard for metastatic lung cancer.[4] Patient-related factors, such as performance status, can also inform the decision between single-agent and combination therapy.[5] Numerous studies have also been performed across malignancies to optimize the dosing schedule of chemotherapy–notably, schedule may have a profound effect on efficacy.[6] In the older adult, where transportation and compliance are often key issues, the chemotherapy schedule is of even greater importance.

In this chapter, clinical vignettes (outlined in Table 9-1) are used to underscore general considerations for the use of chemotherapy in older adults.

CASE 9-1

G.R. is a 75-year-old man who presents to his primary care physician with persistent cough that has worsened over the course of 2 months. He is a nonsmoker, and has a past medical history notable only for mild hypertension, managed with a thiazide diuretic. A chest x-ray reveals multiple pulmonary nodules, up to 4 cm in size. He is referred to a medical oncologist, who orders further workup including imaging of the brain, chest, abdomen, and pelvis. CT of the chest reveals a 4 cm spiculated lesion in the right apex of the lung and several 1-2 cm lesions in the right lower, left lower, and left upper lobes. Other imaging studies show no evidence of distant disease. A CT-guided biopsy is performed of the 4 cm lesion in the right apex, and pathologic review of the specimen is consistent with non-small cell lung cancer, adenocarcinoma subtype. A biopsy is subsequently performed of a left lower lobe nodule, which confirms metastatic disease. The oncologist discusses with the patient the fact that the cancer is incurable and the goals of treatment are to prolong survival, minimize disease symptoms, and maintain quality of life. Ultimately, the patient elects to proceed with chemotherapy and receives a combined regimen of vinorelbine and gemcitabine. He visits his primary physician 1 week after his second cycle of therapy is completed and is neutropenic and febrile. He is admitted for IV antibiotics. Blood culture, urine culture, and chest x-ray finds no definitive source of the fever. Imaging of the chest after his second cycle suggests a response to treatment, with a decrease in size of all previously noted lesions.

DISCUSSION OF CASE 1

Older adults are largely underrepresented in oncology clinical trials, making it challenging in many scenarios to cite the benefit associated with chemotherapy within this demographic.[7] However, several datasets are emerging to allow for an evidence-based approach in this population. The benefits of chemotherapy and best supportive care in comparison to best supportive care alone were described in the Elderly Lung Cancer Vinorelbine Italian Study Group (ELVIS) trial.[8] In this study, 191 patients older than 70 with advanced non-small cell lung cancer were randomized to receive either best supportive care (BSC) or BSC along with vinorelbine chemotherapy.

TABLE 9-1	Overview of Case Discussions and Concepts		
Case	Malignancy	Chemotherapy	Considerations in the Older Adult
1	Lung cancer	Vinorelbine Gemcitabine	Use of systemic therapy in advanced non-small cell lung cancer Myelosuppression related to vinorelbine and gemcitabine Use of growth factor support
2	Breast cancer	Doxorubicin Cyclophosphamide	Benefit of adjuvant breast cancer therapy Risk of congestive heart failure with doxorubicin and cyclophosphamide
3	Ovarian cancer	Cisplatin Paclitaxel	Neuropathy related to cisplatin and paclitaxel Characterization of renal function Physiologic changes with age
4	Colon cancer	5-Fluorouracil Irinotecan	Management of diarrhea related to 5-fluorouracil and irinotecan
5	Breast cancer	Capecitabine	Polypharmacy/Drug interactions Hand-foot syndrome related to capecitabine

Patients receiving vinorelbine therapy were more likely to survive to one year (32% versus 14%). Toxicities commonly seen with vinorelbine (including neutropenia, anemia, constipation, and fatigue) were more frequent in the treatment group. Nonetheless, patients receiving vinorelbine were less likely to develop symptoms related to lung cancer and had less pain.

Once a decision to receive chemotherapy is made, then the specific regimen needs to be determined, as well as the decision of whether to give monochemotherapy or polychemotherapy. Prospective randomized trials reveal conflicting data. One prospective study randomized 120 patients aged 70 or older with advanced non-small cell lung cancer to either vinorelbine alone or gemcitabine with vinorelbine.[9] Combination chemotherapy resulted in superior median survival (29 weeks versus 18 weeks, P < 0.01). However, these results were not replicated in a much larger study. In the Multicenter Italian Lung Cancer in the Elderly Study (MILES), the combination of gemcitabine and vinorelbine was compared to vinorelbine or gemcitabine alone in 698 patients older than 70 with non-small cell lung cancer.[10] The study results demonstrated that combination chemotherapy did not improve survival as compared to use of a single agent. Furthermore, combination therapy led to increased rates of neutropenia, thrombocytopenia, vomiting, and fatigue. Notably, the side-effect profiles of gemcitabine and vinorelbine are slightly overlapping; as with vinorelbine, gemcitabine can lead to neutropenia, anemia and fatigue.

While the MILES study heralds caution for the combination of gemcitabine and vinorelbine, recent data from French Thoracic Oncology Intergroup trial 0501 (IFCT-0501) point to the potential efficacy of a distinct doublet regimen.[4] In this phase III study, 451 patients between the ages of 70 and 89 were randomized to receive single-agent therapy (with either vinorelbine or gemcitabine), or monthly carboplatin with weekly paclitaxel. The Eastern Cooperative Oncology Group (ECOG) performance status (a clinical tool used to grade the generalized

TABLE 9-2	The Eastern Cooperative Oncology Group (ECOG) Performance Status Scale
ECOG Performance Status	Description
0	Fully active and able to carry on all pre-disease performance without restriction.
1	Restricted in physically strenuous activity but ambulatory and able to carry out work of a light or sedentary nature.
2	Ambulatory and capable of all self-care but unable to carry out any work activities. Active more than 50% of waking hours.
3	Capable of only limited self-care, confined to bed or chair more than 50% of waking hours
4	Completely disabled. Cannot carry on any self-care. Confined to bed or chair.
5	Dead

functional status of a cancer patient; Table 9-2) ranged between 0 and 2. Toxicities of both carboplatin and paclitaxel are described in detail subsequently (Case 9-3), and the doublet did elicit more hematologic toxicity than single-agent therapy. However, unlike the MILES study, significantly longer survival was observed in those patients who received doublet therapy as compared to a single agent. Thus, emerging data suggest the benefit of combination therapy among patients with good performance status.

Recognizing the toxicity profile of chemotherapeutic agents allows for preemptive strategies to mitigate adverse effects. Given that both vinorelbine and gemcitabine are known to cause myelosuppression, growth factors could be used to decrease the risk of neutropenia and associated neutropenic sepsis. Several guidelines incorporate age-based risk stratification to aid the practitioner in appropriate use of growth factor therapy.[11] In the current scenario, given the occurrence of neutropenic fever after the first cycle of chemotherapy, growth factors are recommended with any further use of the same regimen. Neutropenic fever should be recognized by the practitioner as an oncologic emergency; prompt administration of empiric antibiotic therapy and relevant clinical examinations (including, but not limited to, blood cultures, chest x-ray, and urine culture/analysis) are essential.

CASE 9-2

A.L. is a 70-year-old woman with a history of mild hypertension and hypercholesterolemia, well-controlled with metoprolol and lovastatin, respectively. On a recent visit to her primary physician, she pointed out a lump in her right breast, which was biopsied and which revealed the presence of invasive ductal cancer. She had a lumpectomy and a sentinel node biopsy, which revealed cancerous involvement of an axillary node. An axillary dissection was performed. On pathologic analysis, the patient was found to have a 4.5 cm invasive breast cancer (hormone receptor-positive, HER-2 negative) with 5 out of 12 lymph nodes examined involving tumor. A staging work-up revealed no evidence of metastatic disease. After visiting with her oncologist, she elects to receive adjuvant chemotherapy to decrease the risk of relapse and mortality from breast cancer. She receives doxorubicin and cyclophosphamide. After two cycles of therapy, she presents to her primary physician for a routine follow-up appointment. There, she notes having increasing shortness of breath and dyspnea on exertion. On physical examination, she is noted to have increased jugular venous distension and 2+ pitting edema in her lower extremities, bilaterally. Fine crackles are auscultated on pulmonary exam.

DISCUSSION OF CASE 2

The patient described in this scenario has early stage (nonmetastatic) breast cancer; however, she has several risk factors placing her at a high risk of distant spread of the tumor, including lymph node positivity and tumor size. Adjuvant chemotherapy is given to decrease the risk of distant spread. In order to determine the magnitude of benefit from adjuvant chemotherapy, oncologists often turn to the Oxford Overview, a comprehensive meta-analysis of randomized trials of adjuvant chemotherapy in the setting of breast cancer.[12] This landmark meta-analysis includes data from 33,000 patients enrolled in 194 randomized clinical trials. Across all strata of age, there is a clinical benefit from use of multiagent adjuvant chemotherapy; however, the proportional benefit declines steadily with age. Limitations of these data include the low proportion of older adults included in randomized clinical trials (less than 7% older than 70 years); therefore, the authors acknowledge that there are too few women older than 70 to be reliably informative as to whether it confers a survival benefit. However,

over the past decade two prospective trials have been reported in older adults with breast cancer that have improved our evidence base. The French Adjuvant Study Group (FASG) 08 trial suggested that the combination of epirubicin and tamoxifen (as compared to tamoxifen alone) could delay recurrence of breast cancer in women older than 65 years with operable, node-positive disease.[13] A more recent trial, Cancer and Leukemia Group B (CALGB) 49907, examined whether single-agent oral chemotherapy (capecitabine) could be used in place of standard, multiagent infusional regimens in patients older than 65 years with early-stage breast cancer.[14] A survival advantage was found with use of standard polychemotherapy infusional regimens, suggesting this remains the standard of care.

Once the decision in Case 9-2 is made to proceed with adjuvant chemotherapy, the patient embarks on a regimen of doxorubicin and cyclophosphamide and develops clinical stigmata of congestive heart failure (CHF) shortly thereafter. The association between doxorubicin and CHF is well-documented, with a higher incidence of CHF at greater cumulative doses of doxorubicin.[15] The association between increasing age and anthracycline-associated cardiac toxicity was evaluated in an analysis of 630 patients treated with doxorubicin, which demonstrated that increasing age was a risk factor for doxorubicin-associated CHF at cumulative doses greater than 400 mg/m^2.[16] A SEER-Medicare analysis including patients with early breast cancer found that breast cancer survivors who had received an anthracycline-containing regimen had an increased risk of congestive heart failure in comparison to those who had not received an anthracycline or those who had not received adjuvant chemotherapy. Interestingly, this difference was most pronounced among women who were treated at ages 66 to 70, and was not observed in patients ages 71 to 90.[17] This SEER-Medicare analysis identified several other important predictors of cardiac toxicity in older women, including the presence of hypertension, diabetes, or peripheral vascular disease. In contrast, a longitudinal cardiac assessment of patients enrolled in Southwest Oncology Group (SWOG) trial 8897 (comparing adjuvant chemotherapy for breast cancer with or without doxorubicin) suggested no significant deterioration in left ventricular ejection fraction (LVEF) over time with anthracycline therapy.[18] The collective results of these studies can be incorporated into discussions with older patients considering anthracycline-based regimens. Furthermore, they may prompt a heightened awareness of potential cardiac toxicities in older adults and/or patients with specific comorbidities receiving these therapies.

Nonanthracycline alternatives to doxorubicin-cyclophosphamide adjuvant therapy are being studied. For instance, a randomized study (U.S. Oncology Trial 9735) compared doxorubicin-cyclophosphamide to docetaxel-cyclophosphamide (both regimens prescribed every 3 weeks for four cycles).[19] In this study, superior disease-free and overall survival was observed with docetaxel-cyclophosphamide, and an update of these data suggested similar efficacy in older and younger patients. Among patients with HER-2-overexpressing breast cancer, the addition of the monoclonal antibody trastuzumab to conventional chemotherapy has shown immense clinical benefit in the metastatic and adjuvant setting.[20] In the adjuvant setting, both anthracycline and nonanthracycline-containing regimens have been explored in combination with trastuzumab. A clinical trial compared adjuvant doxorubicin-cyclophosphamide followed by paclitaxel with or without trastuzumab to docetaxel, carboplatin, and trastuzumab.[21] Notably, both trastuzumab-based regimens produced similar disease-free and overall survival, although patients receiving doxorubicin-cyclophosphamide had a numerically higher incidence of congestive heart failure. As a result of these data, there is increasing interest in studying nonanthracycline chemotherapy regimens in combination with trastuzumab, particularly for patients with cardiac comorbidity.

CASE 9-3

G.M. is an 80-year-old woman with multiple medical comorbidities (including hypertension, hypercholesterolemia, mild renal insufficiency, and diabetes) who reports several months of abdominal bloating and cramping, unrelieved with laxative use. On pelvic examination, she is noted to have some mild adnexal tenderness. Pelvic ultrasound reveals bilateral ovarian masses, both measuring 8 cm. She is subsequently taken to the operating suite for a total abdominal hysterectomy and bilateral salpingo-oophorectomy, and receives several omental biopsies and pelvic washings. On final pathologic analysis, she is found to have epithelial ovarian cancer, grade 2, and has stage II disease (i.e., confined to the bilateral ovaries). She meets with an oncologist, who recommends that she receive six cycles of intravenous carboplatin and paclitaxel chemotherapy. She begins treatment, and visits her primary physician for a routine follow-up after receiving three cycles of therapy. She notes having decreased sensation in her toes, and on pinprick examination, she appears to have decreased tactile sensation. Her neurologic exam is otherwise unremarkable. Her glycated hemoglobin level is within normal limits.

DISCUSSION OF CASE 3

In Case 9-3, it is prudent to consider the patient's comorbidities in the context of her current complaints. Given a clinical history including diabetes, ruling out any metabolic disturbances is critical. Paclitaxel and related taxane compounds are coadministered with steroids to prevent hypersensitivity reactions, and this may contribute to impaired glycemic control and worsening of diabetic neuropathy. Alternatively, the neuropathy could be a direct consequence of paclitaxel, which inhibits microtubule depolymerization and results in direct axonal injury.[22]

The patient described in this case also has mild renal impairment. While renal impairment can certainly be associated with hypertension and diabetes, there is also an anticipated decrement in renal function with increasing age. Increasing age is paralleled by a decrease in renal blood flow, and a decrease in glomerular filtration rate of 0.75 mL/min per year is observed in most individuals older than 40.[23-24] Care should be taken to use appropriate metrics to estimate renal function in the older adult. Formulas such as the Cockcroft-Gault and Jeliffe equations were validated primarily in cohorts of younger patients without renal disease.[25-26] In contrast, formulas such as the Modification of Diet in Renal Disease (MDRD) equation incorporate age, and may therefore be more accurate in estimating renal function in this population.[27-28] Precise calculation of the creatinine clearance is particularly important in the setting of carboplatin therapy, as the drug is dosed in a manner distinct from most other chemotherapeutic agents. Specifically, the dosing of carboplatin is calculated by multiplication of the creatinine clearance and the area under the concentration-time curve (AUC).

Outside of declines in renal function, multiple other physiologic changes accompany increasing age. Gastrointestinal absorption of oral agents may be compromised by decreased splanchnic blood flow, decreased secretion of digestive enzymes, and mucosal atrophy.[29-30] Furthermore, hepatic metabolism may be affected by decreased levels of cytochrome P450.[31-32] Alterations in endocrine axes, impaired cardiac function, and decreased bone marrow reserve may further affect the tolerance for chemotherapy in the older adult.[24] Physiologic changes seen with aging may lead to intrinsic differences in pharmacokinetic profiles of chemotherapeutic agents in an older population. For instance, a study assessing paclitaxel (given at a standard dose every 3 weeks) demonstrated decreasing drug clearance with increasing age, and a concomitant increase

CASE 9-4

C.H. is a 72-year-old man who visits his primary physician for follow-up of hypertension. He is otherwise healthy, is still working as a concert pianist, and his only complaint on this visit is a decrease in stool caliber and increasing constipation. Physical examination is normal, but as it has been approximately 5 years since his last colonoscopy, he is referred to a gastroenterologist for repeat examination. Colonoscopy reveals a mass in the mid-sigmoid colon, and biopsy reveals colonic adenocarcinoma. A staging evaluation includes a CT scan of the chest, abdomen and pelvis, which reveals several lesions within the liver. After a colorectal surgeon suggests that the liver lesions are not resectable, only the colonic tumor is resected. Four weeks later, he is seen by a medical oncologist who wishes to initiate chemotherapy with a combination of infusional 5-fluorouracil (5-FU) and oxaliplatin. However, given his occupation, the patient is particularly concerned about the potential for neuropathy with oxaliplatin, and ultimately elects to receive 5-FU with irinotecan. Two months later, at a routine follow-up visit for hypertension, he notes having six to eight episodes of diarrhea daily.

TABLE 9-3	Selected Studies Assessing Pharmacokinetics of Standard Chemotherapeutic Agents	
Dosing Regimen	**Pharmacokinetic Changes**	**Toxicity in Older Adults**
5-Fluorouracil[38]	Clearance: ↔ with age; ↓ in female gender	Not reported
Capecitabine[49]	Clearance:↔ with age	Not reported
Docetaxel weekly[50]	Clearance: ↔ with age	Not reported
Docetaxel every 3 weeks[51]	Clearance: ↔	Severe neutropenia ↑ with age
Doxorubicin[52]	Clearance: ↓ with age	Not reported
Etoposide[53]	Clearance: ↔ with age	Moderate to severe neutropenia ↑ with age
Methotrexate[54]	Clearance: ↓ with age; ↑ with ↑ CrCl	Not reported
Oxaliplatin[55]	Clearance: ↔ with age; ↑ with ↑ GFR	Toxicity ↔ with age
Paclitaxel every 3 weeks[56]	Clearance: ↓	Moderate to severe neutropenia ↑ with age
Paclitaxel weekly[34]	Clearance: ↓ with age	Not reported
Temozolomide[57]	Clearance: ↔ with age	Neutropenia and thrombocytopenia ↑ in older women
Vinorelbine weekly[58]	Clearance: ↓ with age	Anemia and neutropenia ↑ with ↑ AUC
Vinorelbine every 3 weeks[59]	Clearance: ↔	Not reported

(Note: ↑ = increased, ↔ = unchanged, and ↓ = decreased.)
CrCl, creatinine clearance; GFR, glomerular filtration rate; AUC, area under the concentration-time curve

in the frequency of severe neutropenia.[33] Several other studies have assessed age-related changes in paclitaxel pharmacokinetics with age.[34-37] Table 9-3 summarizes these studies and others, which provide important insights into appropriate dosing of chemotherapy in older adults.

DISCUSSION OF CASE 4

Diarrhea is a side effect associated with multiple chemotherapeutic agents, including both 5-FU and irinotecan. 5-FU is an antimetabolite that can be administered in one of two schedules. When given as a bolus, the agent frequently results in myelosuppression. In contrast, when given on an infusional schedule, the dose-limiting toxicity of 5-FU is diarrhea. The pharmacokinetic properties of 5-FU have been studied extensively. In a cohort of 380 patients ranging in age from 25 to 91, it did not appear that clearance of 5-FU varied with age.[38] Separate studies have shown no difference in 5-FU toxicity or efficacy on the basis of age.[39-40]

Diarrhea is also associated with irinotecan, a topoisomerase I inhibitor, and may be either acute or delayed in onset. Acute diarrhea, caused by a cholinergic response to the drug, occurs during or within hours of treatment. In addition, a delayed-onset diarrhea often ensues 4 to 7 days after administration of irinotecan. Similar to studies of 5-FU therapy, a combined analysis of four clinical trials examined irinotecan-based chemotherapy regimens for colorectal cancer identified no difference in the risk of toxicity in comparing patients older or younger than 70.[41] In managing chemotherapy-related diarrhea, several pharmacologic strategies exist. Agents such as atropine may mitigate acute-onset diarrhea associated with irinotecan. For the later-onset diarrhea seen with infusional 5-FU, irinotecan, and various other agents, the practitioner may consider loperamide as an initial strategy. As the older adult may be more sensitive to changes in volume status, these symptoms should be followed closely with a low threshold for administration of intravenous fluids.[42]

CASE 9-5

J.R. is a 73-year-old woman who presents for follow-up evaluation of hypercholesterolemia, diabetes, and management of anticoagulation. With respect to the latter, she underwent valve replacement surgery 3 years ago for severe, symptomatic aortic stenosis, and has been maintained on warfarin since that time. Her medical history is also notable for stage II breast cancer diagnosed 6 years ago. On liver function tests, it is noted that she has a dramatically elevated alkaline phosphatase level, and transaminases are also elevated. The dose of her HMG-CoA reductase inhibitor has not been changed in several months; therefore a right-upper quadrant ultrasound is ordered for further evaluation. The study reveals multiple hypodense lesions in both lobes of the liver. Further CT evaluation of the chest, abdomen, and pelvis shows diffuse changes in the liver, suspicious for malignancy. CT-guided biopsy is performed, and pathologic analysis is consistent with metastatic breast cancer that is estrogen receptor-negative and HER-2-negative, consistent with the original tumor. The patient is referred to a medical oncologist, who initiates single-agent chemotherapy with oral capecitabine. Three weeks later, she presents for routine follow-up with a complaint of severe epistaxis, in addition to redness and burning overlying the palms of her hands and soles of her feet. A complete blood count is normal, but her INR is elevated to 5.0.

DISCUSSION OF CASE 5

Polypharmacy is a frequently encountered issue amongst older adults with cancer, increasing the risk for potential drug interactions.[43] In Case 9-5, the patient is concomitantly using warfarin and the oral prodrug capecitabine (converted systemically to the active metabolite, 5-FU). Pharmacokinetic interaction between these agents has been previously documented.[44] With cotreatment, the elimination half-life of warfarin increases by 51%, and the AUC increases by 57%. In a series of 21 patients with colorectal cancer taking this combination of medications, 30% of patients developed an INR greater than 3.0.[45] Furthermore, one third of the patients assessed experienced

TABLE 9-4	Examples of Interactions between Standard Chemotherapeutic Agents and Commonly Prescribed Drugs	
Chemotherapy	**Commonly Prescribed Agent**	**Nature of Interaction**
Capecitabine	Warfarin	Use of capecitabine with warfarin can lead to a prolonged prothrombin time.[60]
Etoposide	Glucosamine	Glucosamine may induce a relative resistance to etoposide and other topoisomerase II inhibitors, such as doxorubicin.[61]
Irinotecan	Phenytoin	Doses of phenytoin may need to be increased when irinotecan is administered concomitantly.[62]
Methotrexate	Amoxicillin	Penicillins may interfere with the renal tubular secretion of methotrexate, leading to increased methotrexate levels and consequent toxicity.[63]
Vinorelbine	Clarithromycin	Coadministration may lead to increased vinorelbine exposure and myelotoxicity.[64]

a clinically significant bleeding episode. Thus, in the scenario described, more vigilant monitoring of the INR and titration of the warfarin dose accordingly may have been warranted. Numerous potential interactions exist between standard chemotherapeutic agents and commonly used drugs; although not intended to be a comprehensive list, several of these interactions are listed in Table 9-4.

In addition to the bleeding diathesis, the patient in Case 9-5 also has redness and burning overlying the palms of her hands and soles of her feet. The latter symptoms are referred to as hand-foot syndrome, or palmoplantar erythrodysesthesia. This side effect is frequently encountered with capecitabine, as well as with several new inhibitors of angiogenesis used in anticancer therapy (i.e., sorafenib). Although no uniform guidelines exist for management of this syndrome, it has been suggested that emollients may be helpful in palliating associated pain.[46] In more severe forms of hand-foot syndrome, sloughing of the skin may be observed, and secondary infection may occur. As such, progression of hand-foot syndrome should be closely monitored. Toxicities should be reported immediately to the primary oncologist, so that dose reductions can be used when appropriate. Importantly, use of a lower dose of capecitabine has been assessed prospectively in a cohort of adults older than 70 years with metastatic breast cancer.[47] This lowered dose of capecitabine may ameliorate some of the adverse effects associated with capecitabine (including hand-foot syndrome), but appears to have preserved efficacy.

CONCLUSIONS

The current chapter is intended to provide the reader with an overview of general considerations surrounding the use of chemotherapy in the older adult. As the cases suggest, the practitioner is faced with a plethora of issues, beginning with the decision of whether to administer chemotherapy. Beyond this and the initial selection of treatment, an emerging literature may aid both the geriatrician and oncologist in recognizing toxicities related to chemotherapy. These age-specific studies frequently use a cutoff in the range of 65 to 70 years to define a population of older adults. As the field of geriatric oncology moves forward, there is increasing recognition that chronologic

age alone is not sufficient in characterizing older adults. Available guidelines advocate the use of clinical metrics to risk-stratify the older adult, such as the comprehensive geriatric assessment (CGA).[37] The CGA is currently being evaluated prospectively in trials conducted by the CALGB cooperative group.[48] More extensive use of these tools, which attempt to distinguish chronologic and physiologic age, may identify subpopulations of older adults who may yield particular benefit from chemotherapy.

See expertconsult.com for a complete list of references and web resources for this chapter

SUGGESTED READINGS

1. National Comprehensive Cancer Network Guidelines; Senior Adult Oncology Available at http://www.nccn.org
2. Hurria A, Lichtman SM: Clinical pharmacology of cancer therapies in older adults, *Br J Cancer* 98:517–522, 2008.
3. Gridelli C: The ELVIS Trial: A Phase III Study of Single-Agent Vinorelbine as First-Line Treatment in Elderly Patients with Advanced Non-Small Cell Lung Cancer, *Oncologist* 6:4–7, 2001.
4. Gridelli C, Perrone F, Gallo C, et al: Chemotherapy for Elderly Patients With Advanced Non-Small-Cell Lung Cancer: The Multicenter Italian Lung Cancer in the Elderly Study (MILES) Phase III Randomized Trial, *J Natl Cancer Inst* 95:362–372, 2003.
5. Frasci G, Lorusso V, Panza N, et al: Gemcitabine plus vinorelbine versus vinorelbine alone in elderly patients with advanced non-small-cell lung cancer, *J Clin Oncol* 18:2529–2536, 2000.
6. Smith TJ, Khatcheressian J, Lyman GH, et al: 2006 Update of Recommendations for the Use of White Blood Cell Growth Factors: An Evidence-Based Clinical Practice Guideline, *J Clin Oncol* 24:3187–3205, 2006.
7. Vestal RE: Aging and pharmacology, *Cancer* 80:1302–1310, 1997.
8. Lichtman SM, Wildiers H, Launay-Vacher V, et al: International Society of Geriatric Oncology (SIOG) recommendations for the adjustment of dosing in elderly cancer patients with renal insufficiency, *European Journal of Cancer* 43:14–34, 2007.
9. Camidge R, Reigner B, Cassidy J, et al: Significant Effect of Capecitabine on the Pharmacokinetics and Pharmacodynamics of Warfarin in Patients With Cancer, *J Clin Oncol* 23:4719–4725, 2005.
10. Pinder MC, Duan Z, Goodwin JS, et al: Congestive Heart Failure in Older Women Treated With Adjuvant Anthracycline Chemotherapy for Breast Cancer, *J Clin Oncol* 25:3808–3815, 2007.

Novel and Targeted Therapies

Marjorie G. Zauderer, Tiffany A. Traina, and Stuart M. Lichtman

A highly functional 83-year-old woman with early-stage breast cancer presents for follow-up. She has a history of controlled hypertension, and had coronary artery stents placed 3 years ago after an episode of unstable angina. Three months ago, routine mammography revealed a calcified lesion in her left breast. She underwent a biopsy that revealed invasive ductal adenocarcinoma. She had a lumpectomy and sentinel lymph node dissection, which revealed adenocarcinoma in 0 of 3 sentinel lymph nodes. On review of the pathology, her tumor was 1.3 cm, estrogen receptor (ER) positive, progesterone receptor (PR) positive, HER-2 positive, high nuclear grade, and moderately well-differentiated. She has no family history of breast cancer. She received radiation therapy to her left breast and is now ready to begin adjuvant treatment with an aromatase inhibitor and possibly trastuzumab. Cardiac evaluation consisted of an electrocardiogram showing nonspecific ST-T wave changes and an echocardiogram revealing an ejection fraction of 42% with segmental left ventricular wall motion abnormalities and mild mitral regurgitation. She is given a prescription for a 30-day supply of letrozole along with calcium and vitamin D supplements. It was decided to defer trastuzumab therapy because of the cardiac abnormalities. Three weeks later, she calls stating that she is completely out of medication. The pharmacy insists that she was given the correct number of pills. The patient uses a pill box which she herself fills weekly with her seven daily medications for hypertension, hypercholesterolemia, and hypothyroidism. It is unclear where the error occurred but there is significant concern that the patient may have consumed extra doses of the letrozole.

A 78-year-old man presented to his primary care physician complaining of weakness and fatigue. His physical examination was unremarkable except for guaiac-positive stools. The patient was referred for his first colonoscopy and was found to have a cecal mass; the biopsy showed adenocarcinoma. A CT scan revealed extensive pulmonary and liver metastases. His hemoglobin level was 8.9 gm/dL, with a ferritin level of 5 ng/mL. Past medical history was significant for hypertension. The patient had been hospitalized for a transient ischemic attack 3 months ago, which caused transient dysarthria. He is currently on aspirin. Because of extensive disease, he was started on systemic chemotherapy with FOLFOX (fluorouracil, leucovorin, oxaliplatin) and supplemental iron. Bevacizumab was deferred due to his recent arterial thrombotic event and hypertension.

Cancer is a disease of older adults, with approximately 60% of cancer diagnoses and 70% of cancer mortality occurring in individuals age 65 and older. As the population ages and life expectancy increases, there are more elderly adults with cancer and several unique challenges arise in caring for them. Specifically, the physiological changes associated with aging can affect the pharmacokinetics and pharmacodynamics of cancer therapies. Because the clinical trials that set the standards for oncology care have typically underrepresented the elderly and focused on a younger patient population,[1,2] the effects of age-related changes on drug dosing and tolerance have been understudied. In this chapter, the means by which these age-related changes may affect the safety, tolerability, and efficacy of novel and targeted therapies in the elderly will be reviewed. The challenges of polypharmacy and nonadherence in this population will also be explored. Finally, existing evidence regarding the safety and efficacy of targeted agents in elderly cancer patients will be discussed.

PHYSIOLOGIC CHANGES WITH AGING

While aging is a heterogeneous process, there are some characteristic changes in physiology and organ function that can have an impact on the pharmacology and toxicity of anticancer therapy. Several reviews discuss the pharmacology of chemotherapy in older patients,[3-5] and some of the key physiologic changes that occur with aging that may affect the pharmacokinetics and pharmacodynamics of anticancer therapies will be summarized (Table 10-1).

Renal Function

With increasing age, there is a decrease in renal mass and renal blood flow. While serum creatinine is often used to approximate renal function in younger adults, it is a poor indicator of renal function in older adults because of a decrease in muscle mass with age.[6] On average, the glomerular filtration rate decreases by approximately 0.75 mL/min/year after age 40. However, this decrease is not universal and approximately one third of all patients will have no change in creatinine clearance with age.[7] There

TABLE 10-1	Physiologic Changes with Aging	
Organ/System	**Physiologic Change**
Renal	Decreased creatinine clearance
Gastrointestinal	
• Decreased hepatic mass/ p450 system	Alterations in metabolism
• Mucosal atrophy	Decreased absorption
• Decreased secretion of digestive enzymes	Decreased absorption
• Decreased splanchnic blood flow	Decreased absorption
• Decreased gastric motility	Decreased absorption
Bone marrow	
• Anemia	Increased volume of distribution with hemoglobin-bound drugs
• Increased fat content	Decreased reserve
Body composition	
• Increased body fat	Increased volume of distribution for lipid soluble drugs
• Decreased body water	Decreased volume of distribution for water soluble drugs

are several equations that have been used to estimate glomerular filtration rate. The Cockcroft/Gault and Jeliffe formulas have primarily been validated in younger patients without renal disease.[8,9] For elderly patients with a glomerular filtration rate over 50mL/min, the Wright formula is more accurate.[10] For those with chronic renal disease, the modification of diet in renal disease (MDRD) formula is more accurate, as it takes into account age, sex, ethnicity, serum creatinine, blood urea nitrogen, and albumin.[11]

Absorption and Metabolism

As people age, they experience a decrease in splanchnic blood flow, gastrointestinal motility, and secretion of digestive enzymes, all of which, along with the mucosal atrophy that occurs with age, can alter drug absorption. In addition, hepatic mass and cytochrome P450 content decrease with increasing age. However, the consequences of these changes remain controversial.[12] As a result of changes in body composition involving an increase in body fat and decrease in total body water, the volume of distribution for drugs that are lipid-soluble increases and the volume of distribution decreases for water-soluble drugs. Many drugs are bound to albumin and, as a result, hypoalbuminemia can increase the volume of distribution of their bound drugs.

Bone Marrow

Bone marrow fat increases and bone marrow reserve decreases with increasing age. This decrease in reserve places older adults at increased risk for myelosuppressive complications from chemotherapy.[13] The American

Society of Clinical Oncology (ASCO) recommends primary prophylaxis with white blood cell growth factors for the prevention of febrile neutropenia in patients older than 65.[14] ASCO had suggested use of erythropoietin-stimulating agents. However, their use will be limited because of recent data and FDA recommendations (http://www.fda.gov/drugs/drugsafety/postmarketdrugsafetyinformationforpatientsandproviders/ucm109375.htm).[15] In addition, many drugs are bound to hemoglobin; anemia can therefore increase the volume of distribution of drugs, which in turn alters their metabolism.[5,16]

POLYPHARMACY

Polypharmacy means "many drugs" and is used to describe the use of more medication than is clinically indicated or warranted. While people older than 65 years represent approximately 15% of the population, they account for more than one third of all prescription drugs taken and an even larger percentage of nonprescription drugs. This often unnecessary use of many drugs can produce noxious results such as adverse drug reactions and drug-drug interactions and can lead to increased emergency room visits, hospitalizations, and nursing home admissions.[17] A recent drug evaluation reported that three medications accounted for about one third of emergency department visits for adverse drug events in older adults: warfarin (17.3%), insulin (13.0%), and digoxin (3.2%).[18] In addition, the elderly cancer patient often needs medications prescribed to treat possible side effects of other drugs.

NONADHERENCE

Adherence is defined by the World Health Organization (WHO) as the extent to which a person's behavior corresponds with agreed-upon recommendations from a health care provider. Issues related to adherence are not well understood, and it is difficult to measure accurately. Generally, clinicians assume that patients are taking medications as prescribed and believe their patients when they say they are doing so.[19] However, many studies have shown poor adherence with medications that have proven benefit when taken appropriately. A patient's choice to follow the clinician's advice is influenced by his or her assessment of risks and benefits.[19] Some of the major risk factors for poor adherence include cognitive impairment, treatment of asymptomatic disease, inadequate follow-up, poor provider-patient relationship, adverse effects of medications, and patient's lack of belief in the benefit of treatment.[20] Poor adherence has long been acknowledged as an obstacle in improving patient care. With the recently passed health care legislation reform, there is a desire to create an infrastructure for improving health outcomes through improved adherence.[21]

As many of the new anticancer targeted therapies are administered orally, they can be taken at home, eliminating the need for intravenous access; however, this shifts many of the responsibilities of managing the regimen from the oncologist to the patient. Even in clinical trials, a context in which the patients are highly motivated and receive extra supervision, adherence is quite variable, ranging from 20% to100%.[19] In addition, a study of anastrozole therapy adherence in early-stage breast cancer reported that approximately one in four women was not optimally adherent.[19] In 2009, at the San Antonio Breast Cancer Symposium, data from the British Columbia Cancer Agency, Vancouver, BC, Canada, were presented showing that only 40% of their population, all of whom receive medications free of charge, was compliant with hormonal therapy.

Despite the impressive efficacy of imatinib for chronic myelogenous leukemia (CML), treatment failure and suboptimal responses are seen and may be due to poor adherence.[22] From a study in Belgium evaluating imatinib adherence for CML, one third of patients were nonadherent, and those with suboptimal responses showed significantly less adherence.[23] Another prospective trial demonstrated a correlation between adherence to imatinib and major—and even complete—molecular responses.[24]

Clearly, further research focusing on strategies to improve adherence in the oncology setting is needed. One effective step to ensure appropriate prescribing and improve adherence is medication reconciliation with review of all medications at every visit. Patient and family education is another critical element in achieving medication adherence.[25] This is of particular importance in elderly patients, who often take multiple medications, and who may have difficulties managing complex regimens without assistance from caregivers.

TARGETED THERAPIES

There are three major classes of target drug therapy: endocrine therapy, monoclonal antibodies, and signal transduction inhibitor. Each class of medications and each specific drug has its own adverse reactions and safety profile. For none of these medications does enough data exist to routinely recommend dose alterations in the elderly (Table 10-2). However, many of these medications have specific side effects (Table 10-3) that are potentially more significant in an elderly population given their comorbid conditions, the prescription medications they often take, and the physiological changes associated with normal aging.

Endocrine Therapy

The oldest example of "targeted therapy" is perhaps the proposal of oophorectomy as a treatment for advanced breast cancer in 1889. Since then, drugs that inhibit estrogen signaling, whether by blocking the estrogen receptor, as with selective estrogen receptor modulators (SERM), or by inhibiting the production of estrogen, as with aromatase inhibitors, have become commonly used agents

TABLE 10-2	Recommended Dose Reductions		
Drug	**Elderly**	**Hepatic**	**Renal**
Tamoxifen	No	No	No
Aromatase inhibitor	No	No, but not studied with severe impairment	No
Bevacizumab	No	No	No
Cetuximab	No	No	No
Rituximab	No	No	No
Trastuzumab	No	No	No, unless creatinine > 2 mg/dL
Imatinib	No	Yes, severe impairment	Yes
Erlotinib	No	Yes	No
Sorafenib	No	Yes	Yes
Sunitinib	No	Not studied with severe impairment, no adjustment with mild or moderate impairment	Not studied
Temsirolimus	No	Not studied	No
Lapatinib	No	Yes, severe impairment	No
Bortezomib	No	Yes, moderate impairment	No

TABLE 10-3	Important Adverse Events
Drug	**Event**
Tamoxifen	Thromboembolism, ischemic cerebrovascular events, endometrial hyperplasia, endometrial cancer, and cataract development
Aromatase inhibitor	Musculoskeletal symptoms and osteoporosis
Bevacizumab	Thrombosis, bleeding, neutropenic fever, hypertension, and gastrointestinal perforation
Cetuximab	Diarrhea
Rituximab	Infusion reaction
Trastuzumab	Cardiac toxicity
Imatinib	Edema, rash, fatigue
Erlotinib	Rash, diarrhea
Sorafenib	Cardiac toxicity
Sunitinib	Cardiac toxicity
Temsirolimus	Thrombocytopenia
Lapatinib	Cardiac toxicity
Bortezomib	Thrombocytopenia

in the adjuvant and metastatic setting for older patients with hormone receptor-positive breast cancer. However, some data suggest that toxicities may vary within subgroups of older oncology patients and the impact of the different side effect profiles remains unclear.

Tamoxifen. Tamoxifen is a SERM that competes with estrogen for binding at the estrogen receptor. When used for 5 years in patients aged 70 or older with early-stage, ER-positive breast cancer, it has had a significant role in reducing the risk of breast cancer recurrence and death.[26] However, because tamoxifen has partial estrogen-agonist effects, its use is associated with an increased risk of thromboembolism, ischemic cerebrovascular events, endometrial hyperplasia, endometrial cancer, and risk of cataract development. Notably, the increased risk of endometrial cancer is almost exclusively seen in patients older than 50 and the absolute risk remains low.[27] Clearly, these risks may influence the safety and tolerability profile of tamoxifen in older women with breast cancer, especially those with other comorbid conditions.

Aromatase Inhibitors. Aromatase inhibitors (AIs) block the enzyme aromatase that is responsible for the peripheral conversion of androgenic substrates into estrogen. Several randomized trials demonstrated superior disease-free survival with AIs compared to tamoxifen for the adjuvant treatment of postmenopausal women with early-stage, hormone receptor-positive breast cancer. While AIs have been associated with an increased incidence of musculoskeletal symptoms and osteoporosis, there has been less endometrial cancer and hypercoagulability than with tamoxifen. Notably, in a study of 1,300 women aged 70 or older, they had significantly higher incidences of fracture, new osteoporosis, and heart disease relative to younger women but there was no treatment-related association.[28] However, a meta-analysis of several randomized AI studies suggested an increased risk for grade 3 and 4 cardiovascular complications (RR 1.31, p = 0.007) compared to tamoxifen.[29] There remains some ambiguity regarding specific toxicities in the elderly population, but for now the evidence favors use of aromatase inhibitors for hormone receptor-positive breast cancer in postmenopausal women.

Monoclonal Antibodies

Monoclonal antibodies are the most widely-used cancer immunotherapy. The first monoclonal antibodies were made entirely from mouse cells; this posed a problem when patients developed severe allergic reactions as their immune systems mounted attacks against the mouse antibodies because they were recognized as foreign. Over time, however, techniques have been developed to replace entire or significant portions of the mouse antibodies with human parts. These part-mouse and part-human antibodies are referred to as chimeric or humanized. Monoclonal antibodies function by either activating the immune systems of patients to recognize and then destroy cancer cells or by binding to parts of cancer cells or those cells that help them grow and blocking them from working.

Bevacizumab. Bevacizumab is a humanized monoclonal antibody that inhibits vascular endothelial growth factor (VEGF) from binding its receptor and thereby prevents downstream signaling events. It has been approved for use in multiple diseases. Rare but serious adverse reactions include hypertension, gastrointestinal perforation, and

proteinuria. Patients also commonly experience pancytopenia, diarrhea, and fatigue. Several studies have shown improved progression-free and overall survival with the incorporation of bevacizumab into first-line therapy in advanced colorectal cancer. Relative to younger patients, grade 3 to 4 leukopenia was 5% higher in the elderly.[30] In addition, a retrospective pooled analysis of five randomized studies in 1745 patients demonstrated an increased risk of arterial thromboembolic events in those aged 65 or older who received chemotherapy and bevacizumab.[31] From a community-based registry of 1953 patients receiving bevacizumab, the safety and effectiveness of bevacizumab in patients aged 65 or older was similar to those younger than 65.[32] In this cohort, age was not a significant factor in predicting targeted bevacizumab-related safety events. Additional studies have confirmed this finding.[33] Another analysis of elderly colorectal patients at the Mayo Clinic demonstrated an increased incidence of adverse events in the population age 75 and older relative to the group 70 to 74 years of age.[34] Thus, elderly patients appear to experience more adverse events but the nature of the association between these events and the addition of bevacizumab requires further study.

The role of bevacizumab in older patients with non-small cell lung cancer (NSCLC) has been examined. A retrospective analysis of the patients aged 70 and older showed a trend towards higher response rate and progression-free survival with the use of bevacizumab, but overall survival was similar.[35] Elderly patients did have a greater incidence of grade 3 to 5 neutropenia, bleeding, and proteinuria with bevacizumab. Bevacizumab was, therefore, associated with a higher degree of toxicity but no improvement in overall survival. Bevacizumab is also approved for use in the first-line treatment of metastatic breast cancer in combination with paclitaxel. A retrospective study of patients older than 65 who received bevacizumab with chemotherapy for advanced breast cancer revealed an increased incidence of thrombosis, bleeding, neutropenic fever, and gastrointestinal perforation.

On the basis of the data, bevacizumab is beneficial as first-line treatment in elderly patients with advanced colorectal disease. However, its role in the treatment of elderly patients with NSCLC and breast cancer is less apparent, especially in patients with underlying cardiovascular disease.

Cetuximab and Panitumumab. Cetuximab is a chimeric monoclonal antibody directed to the exodomain of the epidermal growth factor receptor (EGFR), which blocks downstream signaling. Panitumumab is a fully humanized antibody also directed against EGFR. After failure of standard therapies, cetuximab and panitumumab have shown activity against metastatic colorectal cancer.[36] However, retrospective subset analyses suggest that patients with KRAS mutations do not benefit from anti-EGFR therapy.[37,38] When used in combination with irinotecan in irinotecan-resistant patients, there is also some evidence suggesting drug-resistance reversal.[36]

Cetuximab is also approved for the treatment of head and neck cancer in combination with radiotherapy.

Unfortunately, very few data are available regarding cetuximab use in elderly patients. Common side effects include fatigue, rash, abdominal pain, weakness, and diarrhea. A retrospective review of elderly patients who received cetuximab for metastatic colorectal carcinoma revealed that 75% experienced rash, 11% grade 3; and 80% experienced diarrhea, 20% grade 3-4.[39] A prospective phase II study of first-line single-agent cetuximab in elderly patient with metastatic colorectal cancer, which excluded frail patients, demonstrated 12.2% grade 3 skin toxicity.[40]

Rituximab. Rituximab is a chimeric murine and human monoclonal antibody directed against the CD20 antigen of B-lymphocytes, and is used alone and in combination with cytotoxic chemotherapeutic agents to treat lymphomas. Despite the large proportion of elderly patients in the lymphoma population, few studies have evaluated rituximab in the elderly. Most adverse reactions are infusion-related and are usually mild after the first dose. The combination of rituximab with cyclophosphamide, doxorubicin, vincristine, and prednisone (CHOP) appears well-tolerated and effective in those older than 60 years with aggressive non-Hodgkin lymphoma[41] and, in fact, was first studied in the elderly population.[42] In addition, the role of maintenance rituximab after CHOP chemotherapy with or without rituximab was investigated in patients aged 60 or older. Overall, nonhematological toxicity was the same in the two groups of patients.[43] It therefore seems that the incorporation of rituximab into standard chemotherapy regimens for indolent and aggressive lymphoma in the elderly does not increase overall toxicity in a significant manner.

Trastuzumab. Trastuzumab is a humanized monoclonal antibody that targets the HER-2/neu receptor. In combination with chemotherapy, overall survival is improved in women with advanced and early-stage HER-2-amplified or overexpressed breast cancer.[44] Cardiac toxicity is a significant side effect, especially in patients who received concomitant anthracycline-based chemotherapy. For those older than 60 years, the risk of cardiac toxicity is higher (21% in those older than 60 years versus 11% in those 60 years or younger), but the overall survival advantage is maintained.[45] Because of the potential for cardiac toxicity, most patients with cardiac comorbidities were excluded from the adjuvant trials of trastuzumab. However, this restriction also eliminated many older patients, and thus the available data are limited regarding the benefit of adjuvant trastuzumab for women older than 60 years; at present, they suggest that the benefits outweigh the risks.[46]

Signal Transduction Inhibitors

Signal transduction inhibitors block signals passed between molecules; these signals are often involved in many functions of the cells including death, growth, and division. Many drugs have been developed to block particular signals in the hope of precluding cancer cells from rapidly multiplying and invading other tissues.

Imatinib. Imatinib is an orally administered tyrosine kinase inhibitor metabolized by the cytochrome P450 isoenzyme 3A4. Common toxicities include edema, fatigue, rash, nausea, diarrhea, muscle cramps, and pancytopenia. Nearly all patients with CML in chronic phase treated with imatinib achieve a complete hematologic response, which is defined as normalization of the white blood cell count with no immature granulocytes and less than 5% basophils, platelet count less than 450,000/μL , and a nonpalpable spleen.[47] Complete cytogenetic response, defined as no detectable Philadelphia chromosome-positive cells, occurs in 69% of those treated with imatinib for 12 months and 87% of those treated for 60 months.[48] The use of imatinib in elderly patients with chronic phase CML or Philadelphia-positive acute lymphoblastic leukemia has been studied and has shown efficacy similar to that in younger patients.

Although gastrointestinal stromal tumors (GISTs) are resistant to conventional chemotherapy, they are extremely sensitive to therapy with imatinib. Approximately 90% of patients with GIST experience tumor control with imatinib and prolonged overall survival. In a phase III trial of imatinib in patients with advanced or metastatic GIST, only the nonhematologic toxicities of edema, rash, and fatigue correlated with advanced age.[49]

Erlotinib. Erlotinib targets the tyrosine kinase domain of the epidermal growth factor receptor (EGFR). Rare but serious events such as gastrointestinal perforation, bullous and exfoliative rash, and corneal perforation have been reported. Common side effects include fatigue, rash, and diarrhea. Extreme caution is used in patients with abnormal liver function tests. In the National Cancer Institute of Canada Clinic Trials Group (NCICCTG) BR.21 study, the use of erlotinib improved survival in patients who had experienced treatment failure with first- or second-line chemotherapy for non-small cell lung cancer. A retrospective analysis of elderly patients in this trial revealed more toxicity overall and more severe toxicity.[50] In addition, tissue samples from participants in the BR.21 study were analyzed for EGFR mutations and EGFR copy number. Mutations and high copy number were predictive of a response to erlotinib and EGFR fluorescence, while EGFR fluorescence in situ hybridization (FISH) positivity and wild type were associated with a survival benefit from the use of erlotinib.[51]

Despite the paucity of randomized prospective studies to confirm the efficacy and tolerance of erlotinib in elderly patients, it is often used as a single agent in frail patients or those with poor performance status. Notably, a phase II study of erlotinib as first-line therapy for patients aged 70 and older with advanced non-small cell lung cancer showed that 12% of patients required discontinuation of therapy compared with 5% of those in the erlotinib arm of the BR.21 trial.[52] Additional open-label, nonrandomized studies have demonstrated tolerable toxicities with erlotinib use as first-line or subsequent therapy in elderly lung cancer patients. Erlotinib has also been studied in patients with end-organ dysfunction,[53] which may be applicable in the elderly population where end-organ dysfunction is more common.

Erlotinib, in combination with gemcitabine, for patients with unresectable pancreatic cancer has also been shown to modestly improve progression-free survival compared to gemcitabine alone.[54] Although this phase III trial did not focus specifically on elderly patients, the median age was 63.9 and ranged from 36.1-92.4. However, gemcitabine with erlotinib was associated with more toxicity including rash, death, and interstitial lung disease-like syndromes.

Sorafenib and Sunitinib. Sorafenib is an orally active multikinase inhibitor with effects on tumor cell proliferation and tumor angiogenesis. It has been shown to inhibit Raf kinase; vascular endothelial growth factor receptors 1, 2, and 3; platelet-derived growth factor receptor; FMS-like tyrosine kinase 3; c-Kit protein; and RET tyrosine kinase. It has been approved for use in renal and hepatocellular carcinoma, but seems to have activity in several other malignancies. In a subgroup analysis of a phase III trial (TARGET), adverse events were independent of age.[55] In addition, side effects caused by sorafenib were similar in both elderly and younger patients treated with the expanded access program in North America[56] and commonly included fatigue, hand-foot syndrome, diarrhea, thrombocytopenia, and neutropenia.

Sunitinib is an orally-administered, multitargeted tyrosine kinase inhibitor of VEGF receptors, platelet-derived growth factor receptors, FLT-3, c-Kit, and RET that improves progression-free survival in patients with clear cell metastatic renal cell carcinoma.[57] It is also used to treat imatinib-resistant GIST tumors.[58] Common toxicities include hypertension, decreased left ventricular ejection fraction, fatigue, diarrhea, and pancytopenia. However, there are no data regarding the toxicity in elderly cancer patients.

Most concerning in the elderly population is the potential cardiac toxicity associated with these medications.[59] Approximately one third of evaluable patients in a single observational study had a cardiac event while on these medications. All patients recovered and were able to continue treatment with a tyrosine kinase inhibitor, but almost 10% were seriously compromised and required escalation of care. The impact of this toxicity in the elderly population has not been examined.

Temsirolimus. Temsirolimus is an mTOR inhibitor that is approved for use in patients with advanced renal cell carcinoma (RCC). Because this drug is primarily metabolized in the liver, patients with moderate or severe hepatic dysfunction were excluded from clinical trials involving temsirolimus. In addition, most clinical studies of this drug have not included enough elderly patients to determine the safety and toxicity of this drug. Common

toxicities include edema, rash, hyperglycemia, mucositis, nausea, anemia, neutropenia, and thrombocytopenia. Given the significantly increased amount of thrombocytopenia in a study of patients with non-Hodgkin lymphoma with a median age of 70,[60] special consideration of this toxicity may be required in elderly patients. Notably, rare and sometimes fatal cases of bowel perforation, interstitial lung disease, and acute renal failure have occurred.

Lapatinib. Lapatinib is a dual HER-1 and HER-2 tyrosine kinase inhibitor that is approved in combination with capecitabine for the treatment of advanced HER-2-positive breast cancer after progression following trastuzumab-based chemotherapy. Common toxicities include fatigue, palmoplantar erythrodysesthesias, diarrhea, nausea, anemia, and neutropenia. In addition, rare but severe hepatoxicity, left ventricular dysfunction, and pulmonary toxicity have been reported. Dose reductions are recommended with severe hepatic compromise. There are no data regarding the effects of age on the pharmacokinetics of lapatinib, but thus far no differences in safety or effectiveness have been observed between patients older than 65 years and those 65 years and younger. There is also significant concern regarding the cardiac toxicity associated with this therapy. While the absolute incidence of cardiac toxicity is low at 1.6%, predictors of this toxicity include age older than 50, baseline cardiac dysfunction, and use of antihypertensive medications.[61]

Bortezomib. Bortezomib is a proteasome inhibitor used to treat multiple myeloma, and requires dose adjustment with moderate hepatic impairment. It is also active in mantle cell lymphoma and approved for use in relapsed/refractory disease.[62] Common toxicities include edema, nausea, thrombocytopenia, sensory neuropathy, and weakness. In a study of bortezomib in combination with melphalan and prednisone in elderly patients, overall toxicity was higher in patients aged 75 or older; however, this may have been related to the physical condition of these patients.[63] In addition, it is possible that the increased incidence of hematologic toxicities was due to melphalan and not to bortezomib. When compared to elderly subgroups from previous trials, the rates of serious adverse events were similar and were generally manageable.[64]

SUMMARY

The development of novel targeted therapies has helped improve survival for patients with cancer, but the toxicities differ from those associated with traditional cytotoxic chemotherapy and include more cardiovascular and cutaneous complications. In addition, as has been reviewed, differences in physiology, organ function reserves, and resilience in elderly patients seem to affect outcomes for this special patient population. Given the current state of evidence, the benefits seem to outweigh the risks for several medications such as aromatase inhibitors in postmenopausal women with hormone receptor-positive breast cancer, bevacizumab as first-line treatment in colorectal cancer, rituximab for indolent and aggressive lymphoma, trastuzumab for HER-2-overexpressing breast cancer, imatinib for GIST and CLL, and erlotinib to treat lung cancer. For some medications, such as sorafenib, sunitinib, and temsirolimus, there is a paucity of data. For yet other medications such as lapatinib and bortezomib, there is some evidence suggestive of increased toxicity, but its association with age as opposed to comorbid medical conditions is unclear. Clinical trials that characterize the needs and goals of therapy in elderly cancer patients are ongoing, but clearly disease-specific studies are needed to clarify the risk-benefit ratio of these newer targeted agents in the elderly population. Ultimately, the risk-benefit ratio must be considered for each individual patient to best minimize toxicity and maintain quality of life.

 See expertconsult.com for a complete list of references and web resources for this chapter

is unclear. Clinical trials that characterize the needs and goals of therapy in elderly cancer patients are ongoing but clearly disease-specific studies are needed to clarify the risk-benefit ratio of these newer targeted agents in the elderly population. Ultimately, the risk-benefit ratio must be considered for each individual patient to best minimize toxicity and maintain quality of life.

 Go to expertconsult.com for a complete list of references and web resources for this chapter.

aromatase inhibitors in postmenopausal women with hormone receptor-positive breast cancer, bevacizumab as first-line treatment in colorectal cancer, rituximab for indolent and aggressive lymphoma, trastuzumab for HER-2-overexpressing breast cancer, imatinib for GIST and CLL, and erlotinib to treat lung cancer. For some medications, such as sorafenib, sunitinib, and temsirolimus, there is a paucity of data. For yet other medications such as lapatinib and bortezomib, there is some evidence suggestive of increased toxicity, but its association with age as opposed to comorbid medical conditions

Clinical Trials in the Elderly

William Irvin Jr. and Hyman B. Muss

CASE 11-1

A 75-year-old man with a history of diabetes and hypertension presents with newly diagnosed colon cancer. He is diagnosed with stage IIIB cancer (T3N2A), with metastases found in 6 regional lymph nodes of 20 nodes sampled. He complains of baseline neuropathy in both his feet from his diabetes. His medications include aspirin, metformin, an acetylcholinesterase inhibitor, a multivitamin, a beta-blocker, a stool softener, a 5-alpha-reductase inhibitor, and "something to help sleep." He is retired, married to a healthy spouse, and capable of full activities of daily living (ADL) and instrumental ADL (IADL). Upon checking his laboratory values, everything is within the normal range, except for an elevated creatinine of 1.2 mg/dL. He says he wants the most "aggressive care possible" and asks for "cutting edge treatment." The oncologist to whom he was referred discussed with him a current national intergroup trial comparing several potentially toxic chemotherapy regimens and offered him participation. Outside of a trial, the oncologist suggested he consider 6 months of an oxaliplatin and 5-FU regimen, but his primary physician is worried about how he will tolerate it, because of concerns about preserving his quality of life and preventing a relapse. His primary physician wonders if the clinical trial offers him more effective treatment and a chance for improved survival. What are the major issues related to the trial and this patient's participation that are likely to influence his primary care provider's recommendation?

The patient in Case 11-1 typifies the complexity of cancer management in older patients. He has several comorbidities, is highly functional, and has a cancer that has a high risk for relapse but one for which adjuvant therapy confers a major improvement in survival.[1] Although in the United States the median age at diagnosis of cancer is 67 years and the median age of cancer death is 73 years, only a few percent of all adults are recruited to National Cancer Institute sponsored clinical trials and only a fraction of these are elders.[2] Accruing patients to cancer clinical trials, especially older patients, continues to be an ever more difficult challenge. In the past, few older patients were likely to be enrolled in clinical trials,[3,4] but recent studies suggest that about 30% of accruals to all Phase II and phase III National Cancer Institute (NCI) Cancer Cooperative Group trials are patients 65 years and older.[5,6] Although older patients are less likely to be offered trial participation, when trials are offered, the

rate of participation of about 50% is similar to younger patients.[7] Age bias plays a major role in whether a trial is offered, and few oncologists have been trained in the care of older patients. Options for clinical trials that focus on or include elders, overcoming barriers to accrual, and opportunities for research will be discussed in this chapter.

MAJOR ISSUES IN CLINICAL TRIAL DEVELOPMENT FOR OLDER PATIENTS

Major factors related to maximizing participation of older patients in clinical trials are listed in Table 11-1. Currently, there are at least 200 clinical trials currently enrolling patients that focus on cancer care in the elderly (www.clinicaltrials.gov). Over the past decade, there has been an increased awareness of the need for more clinical research in the older cancer patient. Clinical trials in the elderly population remain a challenge but as the general population ages, oncologists will be seeing larger numbers of elderly patients (many with poor function and substantial comorbidity) and will need data on appropriate management of these patients.

The age-related increased frequency of coexisting illnesses (comorbidities) and functional loss represents the major difference between older and younger patients with cancer. Our patient is typical of this scenario, having both diabetes and hypertension. Both comorbidity and functional loss contribute to a shorter life expectancy and may interfere with or worsen the effects of cancer treatment. Factoring the impact of comorbidities is important in both the curative and palliative setting. In the curative setting, treatments that have major negative effects on quality of life must be carefully weighed against their potential for improved survival benefit; in the palliative setting the use of surgery, irradiation, and systemic therapies should be primarily focused on preserving quality of life and improving symptoms. Clinical trials to date have not been successful in factoring comorbidity accurately into treatment decisions and have avoided dealing with these issues by excluding patients with major functional loss and comorbidities by the use of stringent eligibility criteria. Outside of a trial some internet-based programs such as Adjuvant!

TABLE 11-1	**Major Issues in Clinical Trial Development to Facilitate Inclusion of Older Patients**

Comprehensive Geriatric Assessment (CGA)
- Consider adding as an adjunct to eligibility; eliminate age bias
- Add as companion to trial helping to predict toxicity risk

Eligibility Criteria
- Minimize to essentials
- Organ function exclusion on the basis of metabolism of drugs used in trial

Statistical Considerations
- Consider increasing elderly cohort for positive trials with small sample of older patients.
  - Do after primary accrual goal reached (allows timely publication)
  - Use adaptive design based on elders' accrued and reported toxicity

Specific Trials for Older and/or Vulnerable and Frail Patients
- Define vulnerability and/or frailty using validated instruments.
- Aim to test effective treatments that may be less toxic.
- Use adaptive designs to minimize accrual.
- For oral agents, consider formal assessment or compliance with treatment.

Translational Research
- Consider adding biomarkers of aging or toxicity as part of trial
- Bank blood and tissue samples for future research purposes (add to consent)

(www.adjuvantonline.com) allow health care professionals to factor in the effect of comorbidity on survival for the adjuvant treatment of breast, lung, and colon cancer. Such programs, however, do not help clinicians estimate the increased risk of toxicity in sicker patients, restricting their use in treatment decisions in elders with cancer.

Comprehensive Geriatric Assessment and Clinical Trials

The key consideration in developing trials for elderly patients is the effect of treatment on the patient's overall function and well-being. Comprehensive geriatric assessment (CGA) provides as assessment of key domains related to quality of life and survival, including functional status, cognition, social support, psychological state (especially evaluation for anxiety and depression), nutritional status, and medication use.[8] The CGA is a set of validated instruments that include evaluation of the activities of daily living (ADL): eating, bathing, dressing, toileting, and getting in and out of bed; and instrumental activities of daily living (IADL): managing finances, cooking, shopping, taking medications, performing housework, traveling, and communicating with the telephone. These data can help identify vulnerable patients—those most likely to experience toxicity—and shorter versions of the assessment that can be

partially self-administered are now being tested in clinical trials.[9] Preliminary data show that they are feasible in the cooperative group setting, and studies are underway to determine what components of these instruments can help predict which patients are at greatest risk for side effects. Moreover, a recent trial showed that geriatric assessment in older breast cancer survivors was not only predictive of poor tolerance of treatment as self-reported by patients, but also of mortality at 7 years.[10] Further studies of this type are needed. Studies using the CGA as a research tool in elderly cancer patients have shown that it can independently predict survival, toxicity to chemotherapy, morbidity, and mortality.[11,12] Also, incorporating quality-of-life assessment tools such as the Functional Assessment of Chronic Illness Therapy questionnaires (www.facit.org) into research trials in the elderly will help measure the impact of treatment on quality of life.

Although when one hears the term clinical trials one thinks of treatment trials, important trials now in progress are testing whether geriatric assessment can help predict treatment toxicity. Two recent trials showed that geriatric assessment when added to standard clinical variables (for example performance status and hemoglobin) can help accurately predict toxicity for older patients receiving chemotherapy both in the adjuvant and advanced setting. Extermann and colleagues assessed 518 patients 70 years and older who were initiating chemotherapy for both early and late-stage cancer.[13] A score based on clinical and geriatric assessment data clearly predicted significant differences in hematologic and nonhematologic toxicity among cancer patients. A similar study by Hurria and colleagues in 500 patients also showed the added value of geriatric assessment data in predicting moderate and severe chemotherapy-related toxicity.[14] These trials, and others in progress like these, are important. For example, several large cooperative group trials are now incorporating geriatric assessment prior to treatment and may allow for more accurate prediction of treatment-related toxicity for older patients treated with newer state-of-the-art regimens.

Eligibility Criteria

Eligibility criteria must be carefully considered when designing trials for older patients, and in most instances should be as broad as possible[6,15]; that is, "let doctors be doctors" and let doctors and patients together decide on what level of risk is appropriate. There should be no upper age restrictions. Instead, for adjuvant trials, older patients who are otherwise healthy and have life expectancies greater than 5 to 10 years should be offered participation. Using life expectancy makes much more sense and can be reasonably estimated. For trials where improving the probability of cure is not the goal, eligibility criteria should not exclude elders on the basis of arbitrary criteria such as organ dysfunction unless the specific treatment being studied is metabolized by or has an toxic effect on the particular organ. For instance, creatinine clearance decreases linearly with increasing age; arbitrarily adding criteria with a threshold for renal function to a trial that does not include treatment that is renally excreted should be avoided. Hematologic, hepatic, and cardiac function thresholds should also be omitted when not related to the treatment being evaluated. It is estimated that by appropriately relaxing eligibility criteria, participation of the elderly in clinical trials can be increased by 60%.[6] Unless convincing data exist that support adding restrictive eligibility criteria on the basis of function, eligibility criteria should be as flexible as possible, allowing patients and their physicians flexibility in making decisions on trial participation.

Statistical Considerations

For state-of-the-art clinical trials, statistical considerations and getting an adequate sample size of older patients are also major concerns so as to make the outcome, and especially the toxicity data, generalizable to older patients. One strategy is to keep the elderly cohort open after the trial has met its major accrual goals so that one might reasonably determine that the major risks and benefits of any new treatments are similar for older and younger patients. A larger sample of older patients would be especially important in testing novel agents or procedures, as it would allow for adequate toxicity data to be gathered in this more vulnerable older population. Another strategy would be to require that a specific number of older patients be required in all phase II and III trials. This strategy, although tempting, might hamper completion of the trial, as extensive data show older patients are less likely to be offered clinical trials participation compared to younger patients. For these reasons, the strategy of leaving an elderly cohort open to evaluate a possible age-related treatment interaction appears a more practical and potentially more successful approach for future trials. Such a strategy could use an adaptive design based on the number of elders accrued to the trial and how many more elders should be accrued to better characterize any major toxicity among all the trial participants. For instance, if in a trial of 1000 patients, neutropenic fever was seen in 10% of the entire sample, and only 30 patients in the trial were 70 and older, one could leave the trial open for patients 70 and older to better determine a narrow confidence interval for this toxicity in the older age group.

Designing clinical trials specifically for the older cancer population should also be considered when there are potential differences in tumor biology with age (for example acute myelogenous leukemia, where the natural history of disease is different than in younger age groups), and where older patients—especially the frail and vulnerable—are not good candidates or are excluded from trials of regimens likely to be associated with major toxicity

and loss of function. An example of a successful trial designed specifically for older patients was performed by the Cancer and Leukemia Group B and restricted entry to women 65 years and older with early-stage breast cancer.[16] The plan made certain that an adequate sample of patients 70 and older would be accrued and used a novel adaptive Bayesian design[17] to optimize the sample size. In addition, two companion trials, one assessing compliance with oral chemotherapy and another evaluating the effect of the different treatments on quality of life, were made optional but highly recommended parts of the trial; both successfully met their accrual goals. The advantage of this approach is that such trials can focus on effective but potentially less-toxic treatments, can include specific assessments such as CGA instruments for identifying patients likely to be the most vulnerable to side effects, and can include or be restricted to the frail elderly. For trials focused on vulnerable or frail populations, it is important that clear and reproducible definitions be used to define the population at risk.[18]

Translational Research

Opportunities to further understand the effects of cancer treatment in the elderly may lie in evaluating biomarkers of aging, cytokine regulation, and the molecular interactions of cancer and age.[19] For example, there is evidence that interleukin-6 (IL-6 , an inflammatory cytokine that promotes differentiation of T cells and B cells, activation of T cells and macrophages, and secretion of immunoglobulin) increases during aging.[20,21] Increased IL-6 expression has also been found in certain cancers, such as multiple myeloma, lymphoma, Hodgkin lymphoma, renal cell carcinoma, chronic lymphocytic leukemia, and breast cancer.[22,23] Older patients with cancer and high IL-6 levels might be considered for clinical trials to determine their safety and efficacy in targeting cancer. In addition, IL-6 might serve as a marker of physiologic reserve and add to information obtained by geriatric assessment in predicting toxicity. Another exciting molecular marker of aging is p16 gene expression, which increases tenfold between ages 20 and 80 years.[24] Increased p16 expression is associated with cell senescence and may possibly prove to predict organ-related toxicity from radiation and chemotherapy.

Future studies might also address host factors related to drug activation and metabolism as related to clinical outcomes. Although these issues are not specific for older patients, they are of major importance. For example, the cytochrome P450 (CYP450) metabolic enzyme CYP2D6 has a major role in tamoxifen metabolism, activating tamoxifen to endoxifen, its most active metabolite.[25] The CYP2D6 gene is polymorphic, but even the wild-type variant is affected by many antidepressants, medications that are commonly used in older patients, and which cause a decrease in the conversion of tamoxifen to endoxifen.[26] These data point out the importance of trials that measure pharmacokinetic and pharmacogenomic parameters in older patients, especially in those taking medications that might interact with enzymes important in drug activation and metabolism.

IMPROVING ACCRUAL OF OLDER PATIENTS TO CLINICAL TRIALS

The major barriers to accrual of older patients to clinical trials are listed in Table 11-2. Identifying older patients who are eligible for trials and obtaining their consent to trials remains the major challenge in both community and academic settings and involves close collaboration with referring physicians. Oncology consultation shortly after the diagnosis of cancer allows for rapid assessment of the patient and identification of potential trials. A strong collaborative relationship with local primary care physicians who are interested in elder care will greatly facilitate this approach. Such relationships must include educating colleagues on the availability, goals, and importance of clinical trials in improving cancer care and require significant commitment by the investigator. If the focus is on accrual of vulnerable or frail patients, then close collaboration with the patient's primary care physician and establishment of relationships with geriatricians in the area will be essential for timely accrual. A strategy that includes periodic meetings to inform other health care professionals of available trials, a rapid means of seeing potential trial patients in consultation, and providing reminders of available trials, is likely to be worth the investment.

Physician-related obstacles remain a major barrier to accrual. Many physicians, even those in academic settings with strong clinical research support are unaware

of trials that might be available,[7] or, more likely, are too busy to think of them in the demanding clinics of today. A checklist or computerized reminder of available trials that is attached to the paper record, or shown in a reminder window in an electronic record when the patient is seen, is likely to be helpful in facilitating accrual. In one study of barriers to trials in older patients, the three major changes physicians felt would most likely lead to higher accrual were: (1) having available personnel in clinic to explain trials to eligible patients; (2) more physician education on toxicity issues; and (3) providing transportation to older patients for trial-related visits.[7] Of note, in the same study, is the finding that when older patients were offered trials, their rate of participation was similar that of younger patients at a level of about 50%.

Nursing and staff-related obstacles are usually related to time constraints and lack of support. Depending on resources, the most effective way to increase accrual is probably to assign a nurse or other well-educated staff member to screen patients, determine their eligibility, and, most importantly and with the help of the physician, discuss trial participation with patients and obtain their consent. Too often these tasks are added to an already full range of responsibilities, with the result being no time to devote to these key tasks. An increase in reimbursement for federally sponsored trials is desperately needed to provide financial support for the trial's mission. Patient-related obstacles are present all along the trajectory of enrollment. Because older patients are generally less educated than younger patients and require more time from professionals to explain the goal of the trial, and its treatments, toxicities, and logistics, family should be included in these discussions. In addition, older patients tend to have less financial resources and frequently must rely on others for transportation. Keeping trial designs simple, using decision-making aids during discussions, and using community resources to help with transportation can all help. Focusing trials on those most likely to participate may be the best strategy when resources are limited. Clinical trial participation is more common in patients who are positive about research, hope for a cure, are altruistic, are curious and enjoy novel experiences, want to be part of something important and help with research, and who feel close with their physicians and their staff.[27]

OPPORTUNITIES FOR RESEARCH

Major opportunities for research on older patients with cancer are available. Both the National Cancer Institute (http://www.cancer.gov/) and National institutes of Aging (http://www.nia.nih.gov/) have grant-funding opportunities for a broad range of interests. In addition, the American Federation for Aging Research (AFAR) has a list of useful links to companies, foundations, and organizations that support aging research, as well as its

TABLE 11-2	Major Barriers to Accruing Older Patients to Clinical Trials and Suggestions for Improvement

Identifying older patients who may be eligible for a trial
- Involves close collaboration with referring physicians and their nursing staff with focus on education about and availability of trials. Setting up an expedited consultation process is of great help.

Physician obstacles
- Educate colleagues on issues related to care of elders with cancer, including assessment of function and comorbidity, and risks of toxicity. Provide a checklist with of trials available that includes brief summary of eligibility criteria.

Nursing- and staff-related obstacles
- Identify a lead nurse or staff member to champion trials and provide funding and time for these individuals to screen and consent patients.

Patient-related obstacles
- Educate patients on rationale of trial, its goals, and its toxicity. Inform patients as to any added costs, both financial and logistic. Involve family in these discussions.

own grant-funding opportunities (http://afar.convio.net/site/PageServer?pagename=AFAR_Links). In addition, several NCI-funded cooperative groups have supported specific committees and infrastructure to facilitate trial development and accrual of older patients.[28]

CONCLUSIONS

Cancer clinical trials in older patients remain a challenge. Age bias persists and limits offering many older patients trial participation; also, many ongoing trials still inadvertently exclude older patients by virtue of stringent but frequently inappropriate eligibility criteria. Cancer trials focused on vulnerable and frail patients are few. Nevertheless, trial participation by older patients is improving, and a small but growing number of health care professionals are aware of and interested in developing new trials for elders, overcoming barriers to participation, and improving access. Funding remains a major problem and must be increased if there is to be substantial improvement in trials research in the aging population. Education of health care professionals and the public remains a key function in increasing awareness of cancer in the elderly and the complex decisions frequently needed in caring for this growing number of patients.

SUMMARY

Older persons comprise the majority of patients with cancer but continue to be underrepresented in clinical trials. Many of the most effective cancer treatments resulting from clinical trials have been inadequately studied in older patients, limiting the generalizability of the results to elders. Thus elders, when given state-of-the-art treatments, may suffer undue toxicity that interferes with their function and quality of life. There is an increasing awareness of the lack of participation of older patients in clinical trials and many health care professionals are now interested in improving accrual of elders to trials and in developing specific trials for the elderly, especially the vulnerable and frail.

This chapter focuses on issues related to trial design that affect the accrual of older patients such as comprehensive geriatric assessment, eligibility criteria, statistical considerations, specific trials for vulnerable and frail patients, and translational research. In addition, barriers to participation in clinical trials are addressed along with strategies to overcome them, including identifying older patients for trials, physician obstacles, nursing- and staff-related obstacles, and patient-related obstacles. New trials and increased accrual of elders are greatly needed and opportunities for research are available.

 See expertconsult.com for a complete list of references and web resources for this chapter

Communication and Treatment Decision Making

Arash Naeim

CASE 12-1   **CASE SCENARIO**

A 75-year-old woman with newly diagnosed breast cancer, who has received primary treatment with surgery and radiation, has a consultation with an oncologist to discuss the need for adjuvant treatment. She goes to her appointment with her husband of 50 years who has early dementia and hearing loss. Although she has a college education, she finds the information the oncologist provides to be too complicated and therefore does not ask any questions, leaves somewhat unsatisfied, and is not even sure what the doctor ultimately recommended.

PHYSICIAN-PATIENT COMMUNICATION

Physician-patient communication is a process by which information is exchanged between a physician and patient through a common system of symbols, signs, and behaviors.[1] Communication is a core clinical skill in the practice of medical oncology, and health literacy has a central role in cancer patients' ability to discuss their disease and prognosis with their oncologist in a meaningful way. The average clinical career of an oncologist is approximately 40 years and can involve up to 200,000 consultations with patients and their families. As with the general population, effective communication has many positive effects on cancer patients' adjustment to the disease and its treatment, whereas poor communication has negative consequences both for health care professionals and for patients.[2,3]

Effective communication between health care professionals and patients is essential for the delivery of high-quality health care. Communication issues are often a critical factor in litigation.[4] Research has suggested that effective communication during medical encounters positively influences patient recovery, pain control, adherence to treatment, satisfaction, and psychological functioning.[5,6] Because of the threat of mortality from the diagnosis of cancer, the uncertainty of therapy efficacy, and the physical and emotional stress of undergoing chemotherapy, patients must obtain a high level of complex information during communications with their treating physician.[7,8]

Older adults diagnosed with cancer are the population group considered to be at highest risk for poor communication with health professionals. The older patient is less likely to be assertive and ask in-depth questions. Overall physician responsiveness (i.e., the quality of questions, informing, and support) is better with younger patients than with older patients, and there is less concordance on the major goals and topics of the visit between physicians and older patients than between physicians and younger patients.[9,10]

COMMUNICATION BARRIERS IN THE ELDERLY

The literature suggests that evaluating such factors as memory decline and sensory deficits are essential in geriatric patient medical visits. These common age-related communication barriers are often overlooked in the oncology consultation and frequently compromise the quality of communications. There is a broad range of cognitive loss among individuals with dementia, and unless the physician is trained to uncover this problem, it can be missed in patients with mild or even moderate loss.[11] For example, the 1999-2001 National Health Interview Surveys (NHIS) indicate that 2.3 million (7.1%) community-dwelling people aged 65 and older are limited by memory impairment or confusion, while 800,000 (2.4%) are limited by senility and dementia.[12]

In addition to cognition, hearing and vision are important components of communication. Presbycusis, or decreased hearing of higher frequency sounds, is one of the most common and significant sensory changes that affect elderly people. The incidence of sensorineural hearing loss increases each decade so that by the seventh and eighth decades, 35% to 50% of older adults have hearing impairment.[13] Vision loss also has a significant impact on physician-patient interaction, because visual cues are vital in interaction. After age 65, there is a decrease in visual acuity, contrast sensitivity, glare intolerance, and visual fields. On the basis of the 1997-2002 NHIS, 15% to 25% of older adults had visual impairment.[13] The combination of both hearing and visual impairment among elders aged 65 to 79 was 7% and increased to 17% for individuals aged 80 and older.[13]

Physician visits for elderly patients with these functional impairments may be so difficult to coordinate that they result in frequently missed appointments. When these frail older patients finally do see the physician, the visits may be emotionally and physically stressful for them, limiting effective communication.[10,14]

HEALTH LITERACY

The Institute of Medicine defines health literacy as "the degree to which individuals have the capacity to obtain, process, and understand basic health information and services needed to make appropriate health decisions."[13] A patient's health literacy level, which includes such skills as the ability to comprehend prescription bottle labels, follow written and oral health instructions, and understand physician dialogue, may be significantly lower than his or her general literacy level.[15] The National Adult Health Literacy Survey (NALS) published in 2003 reported that more than 50% of the United States population older than 65 was either functionally illiterate or possessed marginal literacy skills.[16] The largest study of health literacy conducted to date in the United States found that 30% of patients at two public hospitals could not read or comprehend basic health-related materials. In addition, 42% failed to understand directions for taking medications, 60% could not comprehend a routine consent form, and 26% did not understand the information written on an appointment slip.[17]

NUMERACY (QUANTITATIVE LITERACY)

It is common for oncologists and other health care providers to use information about rates, percentages, and proportions when discussing treatment and prognosis. An important component of health literacy in the context of cancer treatment is the patient's ability to understand these basic probability and numeric concepts. Health numeracy can be defined as the degree to which individuals have the capacity to access, process, interpret, communicate, and act on numeric, quantitative, graphic, biostatistical, and probabilistic health information needed to make effective health decisions.[18] Although there is a correlation between prose or print literacy and numeracy, many patients have adequate literacy but poor quantitative skills. A cross-sectional study of 200 primary care patients demonstrated that only 37% of patients could calculate the number of carbohydrates consumed from a 20-oz bottle of soda that contained 2.5 servings.[19]

Decreased numeracy competency in cancer patients may have an impact on their ability to accurately assess their own health risks. Understanding numbers is essential to comprehend risk-benefit information. Patients need to: (1) acquire information from oral discussion, text, tables, and charts; (2) make calculations and inferences; (3) remember the information (short and/or long term memory); (4) weight the factors to match their own needs and values; and (5) make trade-offs to reach a health decision.[20] Cancer communication, especially risk communication, may be hard because the patient's knowledge relevant to cancer is often fragmented and inaccurate. Moreover, the education and everyday experience of an older cancer patient may not ensure the numeracy and health literacy required to evaluate the complex and uncertain benefits from treatment.[21]

INADEQUATE HEALTH LITERACY AND OLDER CANCER PATIENTS

A limited number of studies have focused on the prevalence and impact of health literacy in geriatric cancer patients. A survey of Medicare enrollees between June and December 2007 demonstrated that 34% of English-speaking and 50% of Spanish-speaking respondents had inadequate or marginal health literacy. Reading ability declined dramatically with age, even after adjusting for years of school and cognitive impairment.[22] One study in newly diagnosed prostate cancer patients with a mean age of 67 demonstrated that low health literacy limited patient understanding of complex information regarding treatment and quality-of-life issues.[23]

PHYSICIAN COMMUNICATION

The underpinning of effective verbal communication in the medical encounter is the interaction between a patient's health literacy level and the quality of dialogue between patient and physician. "Oral literacy demand" can be defined as the aspects of dialogue that challenge patients with low literacy skills.[24] During conversations, the general language complexity increases with the greater number of sentences in the passive voice and with faster dialogue pacing, both of which have negative effects on comprehension.[24]

The use of technical terminology is an important component of oral literacy demand. Research done on adult literacy of genetic information presented during genetic counseling sessions suggests that literacy demand was proportional to the use of technical terms.[25] A doctor's choice of vocabulary can affect patient satisfaction immediately after a general practice consultation, and if the doctor uses the same vocabulary as the patient, patient outcomes improve.[26] In addition, studies have found increased "dialogue density"—or the duration of uninterrupted speech by a physician—correlates with greater oral literacy demand.[27] A review of 152 prenatal and cancer pretest genetic counseling sessions with simulated clients found that the higher the use of technical terms, and the more dense and less interactive the dialogue, the less satisfied the simulated clients were and the lower their ratings were of counselors' nonverbal effectiveness.

In addition, patients with low health literacy are less likely to ask their physician to slow down the dialogue and repeat information when their understanding is compromised.[28] Interventions to modify health care provider use of technical terms, general language complexity, and structural characteristics of dialogue can enhance overall communication by decreasing patient oral literacy demand.[24]

DECISION MAKING

Low levels of health literacy present challenges to any decision-making paradigm,[29,30] especially in the case of complex cancer treatment decisions in the elderly. Complexity in the cancer-treatment decision process originates from the fact that selection of therapy is unique to every patient. Typically, several treatment options are possible and the oncologist and patient must together carefully weigh the risk of toxicity against the potential benefit. Patient preferences, quality of life, and social responsibilities must be considered along with the stage of disease, biologic characteristics of the tumor, and comorbid illnesses.

One important factor in decision making is "self-efficacy," or confidence in one's ability to understand and communicate with physicians. Patients with high self-efficacy have been found to have fewer episodes of depression and develop more realistic goals.

An important aspect of self-efficacy is the sense of control and involvement in the treatment, which has been associated with several desirable outcomes including greater patient satisfaction, increased adherence to treatment, and positive treatment outcomes in elderly patients. Evidence suggests that cancer patients who report greater self-efficacy are better-adjusted and experience better quality of life than those with low self-efficacy.[31]

Older patients are often less assertive in communicating with physicians, less likely to ask questions, and less inclined to take a controlling role in their health care decision making.[32] Self-efficacy is a predictor of how the patient perceives and reacts to the encounter with the physician.[33] Studies in older breast cancer patients have shown that patients with higher self-efficacy are more likely to report that discussions with their physicians are helpful.[34]

CAREGIVERS/COMPANIONS AND TREATMENT DECISIONS IN OLDER CANCER PATIENTS

The effect of family caregivers and companions on cancer treatment decisions is a frequently overlooked, yet significant influence. An estimated 20% to 50% of geriatric patients are accompanied by a family caregiver or companion during their routine medical visits.[35] Most cancer patients share their diagnosis and current condition with a family member or companion. These members of the patient's "social support network" are often highly motivated to help patients manage information related to their cancer treatment.[36] They play key roles

in interpretations of medical diagnosis, offering explanations, and encouraging patients to comply with their treatment plan. Their level of health literacy and actions during the medical visit are critical to defining these roles.

Patients with lower health literacy are likely to be more influenced by a caregiver or companion.[37] Specifically directed physician interactions with these individuals, including assessing their level of health literacy and providing them with appropriate written cancer information during the oncology visit, are important opportunities to optimize communication and medical decision making.[38]

The consequences of companion behavior on patient autonomy and its impact on the decision-making process during the medical visit are important areas of investigation. Several studies have found definite benefits when a family member is present, such as an increase in the amount of medical information provided.[39] Other researchers have determined a negative, intrusive effect of a third party on patient autonomy during a medical visit.[40] A study of 93 patients and companions during geriatric primary care visits found more autonomy-enhancing behaviors (facilitating patient understanding, patient involvement, and doctor understanding) than autonomy-detracting behaviors (controlling the patient and building alliances with the physician). They also found that while nonspousal companions are not as active in decision making, they are more likely to facilitate patient involvement in the visit than spouses.[35] (Figure 12-1.)

DECISION MAKING IN OLDER CANCER PATIENTS

The "shared decision model" has gained consensus as the preferred method of making treatment decisions, especially in the situation where many different therapeutic strategies are equivalent. Patient autonomy is prioritized and the physician's obligation is to provide factual information and execute the patient's selected intervention.[41,42] A systematic review of studies has shown variability in older patients' desire to actively participate in their cancer treatment.[43,44] One study looking specifically at an older individual's participation in medication-related decision making identified perceived lack of knowledge, low self-efficacy, and fear as the major impediments to shared decision making.[45] Moreover, a very recent study demonstrated that statistical illiteracy (understanding the meaning of numbers) impeded both risk communication and shared decision making, and that interventions directed at changing the way information is presented could be helpful.[46]

These findings suggest that elderly patients may view their involvement in treatment decisions differently than younger patients, who are more homogeneous in their preference of the shared decision-making model. A study of hospitalized patients with advanced cancer and a palliative treatment goal demonstrated that younger age and higher Karnofsky index were significantly associated with active involvement in making treatment decisions.[47] Furthermore,

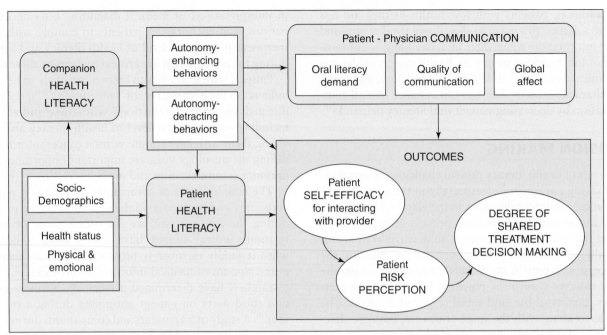

FIGURE 12-1 Impact of Three Key Variables on Outcomes The conceptual model above shows the effects of three variables (patient health literacy, patient-physician communication, and the role of the companion) on three outcomes (patient self-efficacy for decision making, risk knowledge, and satisfaction with the decision-making process). *(Reprinted with permission from Amalraj et al. Oncology 2009;23(4):369-75.)*

research in patients 70 years and older with a recent diagnosis of metastatic colorectal cancer found that relatively few (44%) wanted information about expected survival when they made a treatment decision, and 52% preferred a passive role in the treatment decision-making process.[48]

For older patients with advanced cancer, preferences for prognostic information and for an active role in treatment decision making are not easily predicted. Many factors including lower health literacy, socialized belief in the "traditional patient" role, and age bias among physicians who view older patients as passive participants can contribute to older patients assuming this passive role. Also, there may be a natural developmental tendency for older patients to want less responsibility for medical decisions and to rely on the expertise of others.[31] Explicit communication about decision-making preferences and the desire for specific facts such as prognostic information will help the oncologist distinguish which patients would benefit most from the shared decision-making model.[42, 49]

 See expertconsult.com for a complete list of references and web resources for this chapter

SUGGESTED READINGS

1. A First Look at the Literacy of America's Adults in the 21st Century: In U.S. Department of Education NCfES, ed: U.S. Department of Education, 2003.
2. Adelman RD, Greene MG, Ory MG: Communication between older patients and their physicians, *Clin Geriatr Med* 16:1–24, 2000.
3. Barnato AE, Llewellyn-Thomas HA, Peters EM, et al: Communication and Decision Making in Cancer Care: Setting Research Priorities for Decision Support/Patients' Decision Aids, *Medical Decision Making* 27:626, 2007.

4. Charles C, Gafni A, Whelan T: Decision-making in the physician-patient encounter: revisiting the shared treatment decision-making model, *Soc Sci Med* 49:651–661, 1999.
5. Charles C, Gafni A, Whelan T: Shared decision-making in the medical encounter: what does it mean? (or it takes at least two to tango), *Soc Sci Med* 44:681–692, 1997.
6. Clayman ML, Roter D, Wissow LS, Bandeen-Roche K: Autonomy-related behaviors of patient companions and their effect on decision-making activity in geriatric primary care visits, *Soc Sci Med* 60:1583–1591, 2005.
7. Elkin EB, Kim SH, Casper ES, et al: Desire for information and involvement in treatment decisions: elderly cancer patients' preferences and their physicians' perceptions, *J Clin Oncol* 25:5275–5280, 2007.
8. Fischhoff B: Why (Cancer) Risk Communication Can Be Hard, *J Natl Cancer Inst Monogr* 1999:7–13, 1999.
9. Gazmararian JA, Baker DW, Williams MV, et al: Health literacy among Medicare enrollees in a managed care organization, *Jama* 281:545–551, 1999.
10. Mandelblatt J, Kreling B, Figueuriedo M, Feng S: What is the impact of shared decision making on treatment and outcomes for older women with breast cancer? *J Clin Oncol* 24:4908–4913, 2006.
11. Peters E, Hibbard J, Slovic P, Dieckmann N: Numeracy Skill And The Communication, Comprehension And Use Of Risk-Benefit Information, *Health Aff* 26:741–748, 2007.
12. Sparks L, Nussbaum JF: Health literacy and cancer communication with older adults, *Patient Educ Couns* 71:345–350, 2008.
13. Roter DL, Erby LH, Larson S, Ellington L: Assessing oral literacy demand in genetic counseling dialogue: preliminary test of a conceptual framework, *Soc Sci Med* 65:1442–1457, 2007.
14. Roter DL, Hall JA, Katz NR: Relations between physicians' behaviors and analogue patients' satisfaction, recall, and impressions, *Med Care* 25:437–451, 1987.
15. Tennstedt SL: Empowering older patients to communicate more effectively in the medical encounter, *Clin Geriatr Med* 16:61–70, 2000.

SECTION IV

Supportive Care

Chemotherapy-Induced Myelosuppression in the Elderly

Bindu Kanapuru, Jerome W. Yates, and William B. Ershler

CASE 13-1

A 72-year-old man with a 40 pack-year smoking history is diagnosed with advanced lung cancer. His past medical history includes only hypertension. His creatinine level is 1.5 mg/dL. He lives with his daughter and is employed part-time as a volunteer in a gift shop. His daughter, a nurse, is concerned about the risks of myelosuppression with chemotherapy drugs and wonders about the benefit of chemotherapy at his age.

A 65-year-old woman with a diagnosis of node-positive breast cancer has been recommended to receive chemotherapy after surgery. She also has a history of diabetes, controlled with drugs, and she still maintains an active lifestyle. She wants to be treated with a regimen that offers her the maximum benefit, but is concerned that her age may increase the risk of infections and fatigue from the drugs.

Their primary physician decides to review the myelosuppressive toxicity of chemotherapy drugs in the elderly to help these patients make an informed decision.

PHYSIOLOGY OF AGING AS IT RELATES TO BONE MARROW FUNCTION AND RESERVE

Aging is a universal phenomenon that affects all normal cells, tissues, organ systems, and organisms. Accordingly, the bone marrow undergoes changes with age. Age-related hematologic changes are reflected by a decline in bone marrow cellularity, an increased risk of myeloproliferative diseases[1] and anemia,[2,3] and a declining adaptive immunity.[4,5]

The percentage of marrow space occupied by the hematopoietic tissue declines from 90% to 50% over the first 30 years of life and levels off thereafter, followed by a second decline to 30% at age 70, with the remaining space being taken up by fat.[6,7] A similar change occurs in the thymus, where involution begins at an earlier age and is reflected anatomically by a reduction in lymphoid mass with an increase in fat, and functionally by a steady decrease in the production of naive T cells.[8] Thus, fat infiltration into the bone marrow and thymus is associated with a reduced capacity to make new blood cells and diminished adaptive immune responses in late life.

Although age-related change in the bone marrow is well described, the exact mechanisms that regulate these changes remain speculative. For example, it remains unclear whether the age-associated expansion of marrow fat is a cause or an effect of aging and whether the changes seen in bone marrow and thymus are intrinsically related. All blood cells are derived from marrow pluripotent stem cells, which comprise 10% of the cellular fraction of cord blood but less than 1% of all adult bone marrow. Hematopoietic stem cells have a unique ability to self-renew, proliferate, and differentiate into every lineage of mature blood cells. Hematopoietic stem cells then give rise to two distinct multipotent stem cells within the bone marrow. Myeloid stem cells are precursors of granulocytes, monocytes, erythrocytes, and platelets; lymphoid stem cells are precursors of lymphocytes and plasma cells. There is always a large pool of maturing progenitors for each lineage within the bone marrow, allowing for rapid recruitment and release of cells in times of stress. The factors responsible for the constant turnover of these mature cells both inside the bone marrow and in the peripheral blood are poorly understood. However, there is evidence to support a role for both cell-intrinsic genetic programs and several hematopoietic growth factors within the bone marrow microenvironment in the regulation of hematopoiesis. Although a number of measureable changes occur in the stem cell compartment with aging, these changes do not compromise hematopoiesis in the absence of disease. Even when bone marrow is donated from a 65-year-old person to an HLA-matched younger recipient, the transferred marrow supports hematopoiesis for the life of the recipient.

Unlike the commonly held notion that stem cell compartments diminish either in number or function with age, ultimately resulting in an inability to meet homeostatic demands, age-related hematopoietic stem cell (HSC) changes appear to be an exception, at least for murine species in which this question has been most directly addressed. Early work demonstrated that marrow serially-transplanted could reconstitute hematopoietic function for an estimated 15 to 20 life spans.[9] Furthermore, the capacity for old marrow to reconstitute proved superior to that of young marrow.[10] Subsequently, a number of investigators using a variety of techniques have concluded that HSC concentration in old mice is approximately twice that found in the young.[11-14] Some evidence suggests that the intrinsic function of HSCs changes somewhat with age, most notably with a shift in lineage potential from lymphoid to myeloid development. This may contribute to an observed relative increase in neutrophils and decrease in lymphocytes in the peripheral blood of older people.[15]Although no significant change is seen in the peripheral blood leukocyte count with aging,[16,17] several qualitative neutrophil defects have been described. For example, a decreased respiratory burst response to soluble signals,[16] defective phagocytosis,[17] and impaired neutrophil migration to sites of stress[18] have been described. Although the exact cause for these functional changes has not been clarified, it may be associated with an age-related alteration in actin cytoskeleton and receptor expression in leukocytes.[19] There is a decrease in the peripheral lymphocyte count that is first noticeable in the fourth decade, with a gradual progression thereafter throughout the remainder of the life span.[20] Studies have also demonstrated qualitative alterations in T-lymphocyte function in the elderly.[21] Although the HSC compartment is sufficient to maintain normal blood counts in older individuals who are healthy, there is now a substantial literature indicating that bone marrow reserve is diminished in the older compared to younger cancer patient, and this becomes of clinical importance for patients receiving chemotherapy or radiation.

CLINICAL OBSERVATIONS: MYELOSUPPRESSION IN OLDER CANCER PATIENTS

According to the 2002-2006 Surveillance, Epidemiology, and End Results (SEER) data from the National Cancer Institute, more than 50% of cancers are first diagnosed in patients older than 65 years. Furthermore, this group sustains approximately 70% of all cancer deaths (Figure 13-1).[22] Physicians tend to defer referring older patients for chemotherapy as compared to younger patients[23,24,25] despite evidence showing that the majority of the elderly are willing to accept cytotoxic treatment for possible benefit. Elderly patients who are referred to treatment are also likely to receive attenuated treatment when compared to younger patients. In the Annual Report to the Nation on the Status of Cancer, 1975-2002, Featuring Population-Based Trends in Cancer Treatment published in the Journal of National Cancer Institute in 2005, evaluation of cancer care delivery consistently showed that the elderly were less likely to receive standard therapy despite adjusting for comorbidities.[26] The perceived risk-benefit effect of chemotherapy, particularly concerns

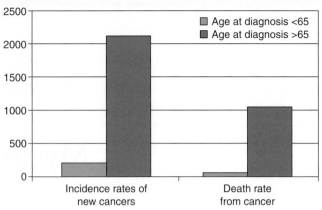

FIGURE 13-1 Age-adjusted incidence and death rates for all invasive cancers, 2002-2006. *(Adapted from SEER data.)*

about increased myelosuppressive toxicity in the context of advanced age and declining health status, may influence this decision. Understanding the risk of hematological toxicity, the mechanisms related to its possible increased frequency in the elderly, and its best management may further improve treatment outcomes in the geriatric population.

BENEFIT TO OLDER PATIENTS FROM CHEMOTHERAPY

Several studies in different types of cancer including colon, lung, breast, and lymphoma have shown that older patients treated with standard intensive regimens derive similar benefit in terms of response. EORTC conducted a MEDLINE review of phase III and phase II studies of chemotherapy in the adjuvant and metastatic treatment setting of colon cancer. They recommended that cytotoxic combination chemotherapy regimens (5-FU with irinotecan or oxaliplatin) offered similar benefits in older patients and should be considered standard therapy for fit older patients.[27] In lung cancer, both the European Organisation for Research and Treatment of Cancer (EORTC) Elderly Task Force and the International Society for Geriatric Oncology found elderly patients seem to derive the same benefit from adjuvant chemotherapy as younger patients.[28] Elderly patients who receive standard-dose intensive treatments during treatment for non-Hodgkin lymphomas[29] (NHL) and breast cancer[30] also have comparable rates of response. Most of these studies also revealed that the chemotherapy tolerability is similar among the older and younger patients. In addition, despite a significant decrease in functional status during treatment, most elderly return to their pretreatment levels after completion of therapy. However, greater hematological toxicity is seen in most studies in the elderly compared to the younger patients.[30]

One of the earliest papers published evaluating the effects of chemotherapy on the elderly was a review of 19 Eastern Cooperative Oncology Group studies of advanced

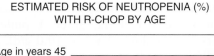

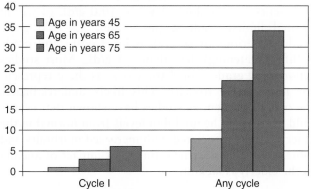

FIGURE 13-2 Estimated rates of neutropenia in an 80 kg subject with no risk factors. *(Adapted from Pettengell et al. Br J Haematol 2009;144(5):677-85.)*

cancer in eight disease sites. This study compared response rates and toxicity among 5459 patients younger than 70 to 780 patients older than 70. It reported that the elderly patients have similar response rates and survival expectancy as compared to the younger patients. Hematological toxicity was the most frequent side effect observed and was higher in those older than 70 years. Severe or worse toxicities (leukocytes less than 2000/mm^3, platelets less than 50,000/mm^3, neutrophils less than 1000/mm^3, or necessity for transfusions) was related to type of cancer, being more prevalent in patients with head and neck, ovarian, or gastric carcinomas; melanoma; and sarcoma.[31] Since then, advanced age has been consistently shown to predict an increased incidence of neutropenia, anemia, and infectious complications in multivariate regression risk models in a number of tumor types. In non-Hodgkin lymphoma patients, a risk model incorporating increasing age (10-year increments), increased dose, prior chemotherapy, recent infection, and low baseline albumin (less than 35 g/L) predicted higher risk of first-cycle febrile neutropenia with a sensitivity of 81% and a specificity of 80%.[32] Increasing age also was predictive for risk of febrile neutropenia in any cycle in this model (Figure 13-2). Pharmacokinetic studies of drugs in the elderly also demonstrate increased risk for neutropenia despite a failure to demonstrate an age-associated change in clearance.

MYELOSUPPRESSION IN ELDERLY LUNG CANCER PATIENTS

The majority (more than 50%) of non-small cell lung cancer (NSCLC) patients are older than 65 years. Chemotherapy protocols including platinum, non–platinum-based treatments like gemcitabine and vinorelbine, and taxane-based chemotherapy are widely used in treatment in either the adjuvant or advanced setting. Several retrospective analyses have found that elderly lung cancer

patients benefit equally from treatment in the adjuvant setting but at the expense of increased hematological toxicity. Toxicity analysis in pooled studies of cisplatin for adjuvant treatment of lung cancer identified grade 3 neutropenia in more than 50% of patients older than 65 years.[33]

Anemia and neutropenia are the two most common short-term toxicities reported in elderly patients undergoing chemotherapy for advanced lung cancer, occurring in up to 20% of patients.[34] A recent prospective study in stage III or IV lung cancer patients also demonstrated a higher incidence (8% versus 2%) of febrile neutropenia in elderly patients older than 75 years as compared to those younger than 55 years.[35] Treatment of advanced lung cancer with combination chemotherapy regimens can also cause increased myelosuppression in the elderly. More than 80% of patients older than 65 years experienced grade 3/4 neutropenia in the TAX-326 study, which evaluated three platinum-based regimens with docetaxel/vinorelbine. In another study in which more than 15% of those enrolled were older than 70 years, cisplatin/paclitaxel or etoposide chemotherapy was associated with greater than grade 3 leukopenia in more than 70% of the elderly and anemia in more than 25%.[36] Incidence of grade 3/4 thrombocytopenia is usually low in most studies, around 10%, but this is significantly increased in regimens incorporating gemcitabine and/or carboplatin, where rates as high as 35% have been reported in the elderly population.[37] Combination regimens used in the treatment of small cell lung cancer also have a high incidence of anemia (28%), neutropenia (77%), and thrombocytopenia (26%) when evaluated in the elderly population.

MYELOSUPPRESSION IN BREAST CANCER PATIENTS

Older patients treated with chemotherapy for breast cancer have a higher risk of being hospitalized for hematological complications, including febrile neutropenia.[38] Increased hematological toxicity has been observed in the metastatic setting in elderly breast cancer patients. The Piedmont Oncology Group published their experience of hematological toxicity in the elderly in five trials conducted between 1974 and 1989 and reported twice the rates of severe neutropenia for those older than 70 who were treated with cyclophosphamide/doxorubicin regimens for advanced breast cancer. In the adjuvant setting, combination regimens of cyclophosphamide and doxorubicin, with or without paclitaxel have high rates of grade 4 neutropenia, ranging from 8% to 42% in elderly patients.[39] Fluorouracil-based combinations with methotrexate/doxorubicin and cyclophosphamide (CMF/CAF) appear to be associated with a slightly decreased risk of hematological toxicity in the elderly. For instance, in the International Breast Cancer Study Group Trial VII, which evaluated addition of CMF to tamoxifen in the adjuvant setting, grade 3 neutropenia (neutrophil count < 750/µL) was seen in only 2.6% of patients and thrombocytopenia (< 50,000/µL) in 4.0%.[40] Very low rates of neutropenia and thrombocytopenia were also seen in the CALGB trial 8641, which tested different doses and durations of the CAF regimen.

Studies of toxicity in other solid tumors replicate findings in breast and lung cancer, with high rates of hematological toxicity in the elderly.

MYELOSUPPRESSIVE TOXICITY IN MALIGNANT LYMPHOMAS

Myelosuppressive toxicity is very common during treatment of hematological malignancies, as patients may start treatment with decreased values secondary to bone marrow invasion. In one study of 359 patients treated for malignant lymphoma ranging in age from 18 to 87 years and with 63% older than 50 years, more than 34% had hemoglobin levels less than 12 g/dL before starting chemotherapy, increasing to 49% during chemotherapy. Interestingly 53% of patients with grade 1 anemia by NCI criteria had anemia-related symptoms but were not offered any intervention.[41] Incidence of grade 4 neutropenia ranged from 4% to 91% in an analysis of 11 trials of elderly patients treated for non-Hodgkin lymphomas. The trials differed in the type of regimens used and also in the schedules administered, which most likely explains this wide range in incidence.[42] A subanalysis of a phase II trial in non-Hodgkin lymphoma in patients older than 60 years treated with CHOP (cyclophosphamide, doxorubicin, vincristine, and prednisone) therapy, reported severe neutropenia in 24% of cycles in patients aged 61 to 69 years and in 73% of cycles in patients aged 70 years or older. There was also a higher rate of neutropenic fever occurring in 8% of patients aged 61 to 69 years and in 42% of patients aged 70 years or older. Severe thrombocytopenia (<20,000/mL) was seen in 5% of patients aged 61 to 69 years and in 42% of patients aged 70 years or older.[43]

It is clear from the these data that myelosuppressive toxicity is definitely increased in the elderly as compared to the younger population. However, these retrospective analyses are hampered by limited representation of the elderly population, and the use of different definitions to evaluate the "elderly." It has been estimated that only 22% of patients in clinical trials are older than 65 years, and only about 10% are older than 70 years. Data on myelosuppressive effects of individual chemotherapy drugs in the elderly are very limited. Accordingly, we may be both overestimating efficacy and underestimating toxicity in the elderly on the basis of these trials.

Toxicities in clinical trials are generally assessed by WHO criteria, or more recently the NCI criteria, with grades from 1 through 4. However, these may be simplistic in their representation of the profound functional effects that can occur. For instance, by NCI Common Toxicity Criteria, grade 1 (mild) anemia represents a hemoglobin level of 10.0 g/dL to within normal limits; grade 2 (moderate), 8.0-10.0 g/dL; grade 3 (serious or severe), 6.5-7.9 g/dL; and grade 4 (life-threatening), less than 6.5 g/dL. Most studies report only grade 3 or 4 toxicities, as these represent the most severe toxicity. This likely underestimates the overall burden, as studies have shown that even a mild decrease in hemoglobin levels from normal in the elderly can be associated with increased morbidity and mortality.[44] Thus a true estimate of impact of anemia in the elderly is lacking.

CONSEQUENCES OF MYELOSUPPRESSIVE TOXICITY

One of the major consequences of increased hematological toxicity is that it increases the risk of suboptimal chemotherapy delivery in this group. Dose reductions are frequently employed upfront to reduce the risk of toxicity. Although this strategy has been successful in reducing myelosuppressive toxicity in the elderly population,[45] it is clearly associated with inferior outcomes and is probably one of the major factors contributing to increased mortality from cancer among the elderly.[46,47] Still, hospitalizations and mortality from febrile neutropenia are greater for elderly patients than for younger patients despite decreased dose intensity.[48] Myelosuppressive toxicity may also be persistent and decrease quality of life even long after completion of chemotherapy. Analysis of the Medicare SEER database to evaluate the incidence of chemotherapy toxicity-related conditions for 14 chemotherapy agents in elderly patients with non-small cell cancer revealed that the incidence of anemia increased from 20% to 35.9% during chemotherapy, and further increased to 30.7% to 37.6% when evaluated 3 months after chemotherapy. In a multivariate analysis, carboplatin, cisplatin, vinorelbine, paclitaxel and gemcitabine were significantly associated with development of long-term neutropenia and thrombocytopenia.

The economic burden in terms of supportive care during inpatient and outpatient hospitalization for febrile neutropenia is substantial, particularly in the management of hematological malignancies. Neutropenia has also been shown to influence the incidence and duration of nonhematological toxicities and to substantially decrease quality of life. Worsening or new-onset anemia during the course of chemotherapy significantly correlates with decreased performance status, increased fatigue, and overall decreased quality of life. Anemia also correlates with decreased survival in patients being treated for lymphomas and solid tumors. Major bleeding episodes associated with thrombocytopenia can lead to treatment delays and hospitalization, with resultant morbidity.

PREVENTING AND MANAGING MYELOSUPPRESSION IN THE OLDER CANCER PATIENT

Clearly, the hematological toxicity and adverse consequences from the same are increased in the elderly. Attempts to reduce this side effect include identifying and modifying treatment-related and patient-related factors that contribute to this increase.

MODIFICATION OF CHEMOTHERAPY TO REDUCE TOXICITY

Reduction in dose intensity has long been adopted as a way of reducing myelosuppression in the elderly population. For instance, in a retrospective nationwide survey of 567 oncology practices involving 4,522 patients with aggressive NHL treated with cyclophosphamide, doxorubicin, vincristine, and prednisone (CHOP); CHOP-rituximab (CHOP-R); or cyclophosphamide, mitoxantrone, vincristine, and prednisone (CNOP) elderly patients (older than 60 years) were more likely to receive less than 85% of the planned dose intensity, with an increased proportion of patients receiving this reduced dose for successive cycles.[49] However, as mentioned earlier, any benefit from reduced toxicity is countered by the reduced survival outcomes observed with decreased dose intensity or dose reductions.

Some chemotherapy regimens or drugs may be more myelotoxic than others in the elderly population. In a retrospective analysis of 132 patients aged 65 years or older with primary invasive breast cancer who received one of three different chemotherapy protocols: cyclophosphamide, methotrexate, fluorouracil (CMF); doxorubicin and cyclophosphamide (AC); or AC plus paclitaxel or docetaxel (AT-T); patients who received AC-based regimens were more likely to experience grade 3 or 4 hematological toxicity (32% versus 18%) and/or grade 3 neutropenic infection (29% versus 2%) as compared to those on the CMF regimen. The type of chemotherapy regimen (anthracycline compared to CMF) was a better predictor for toxicity than increased age or comorbidity score.[30] In the recent adjuvant CALGB trial (49907), breast cancer patients 65 years and older with a performance score of 0 to 2 were randomized to receive either "conventional therapy" (doxorubicin/cyclophosphamide or cyclophosphamide/methotrexate/fluorouracil [CMF]) or capecitabine. Approximately 50% of patients in the combination arm experienced severe hematological toxicity compared to less than 5% in the arm treated with capecitabine alone. However, response rates and survival were significantly better for those receiving combination therapies.

Similarly, in lung cancer patients, both docetaxel and vinorelbine demonstrated comparable efficacy in a phase III trial in older patients in terms of median survival but docetaxel was associated with more grade 3 to 4 neutropenia (82.9% vs. 69.2%).[50] Thus in a patient in whom occurrence of neutropenia will be life-threatening, vinorelbine is a reasonable option.

Incidence of specific myelosuppressive toxicities may also differ among regimens. In the elder specific subanalysis of the TAX-326 trial, patients with IIIB-IV NSCLC were randomized to docetaxel and cisplatin, docetaxel and carboplatin, or vinorelbine and cisplatin. The incidence of grade 3-4 thrombocytopenia and neutropenia was much higher in the elderly population on the docetaxel/carboplatin arm as compared to those on the other two arms. Grade 3-4 anemia was higher in the vinorelbine arm, occurring in 25% of those older than 65 years, as compared to 13.3% in the docetaxel/carboplatin arm and 5.4% in the docetaxel and cisplatin arm.[51]

Recently, a number of new drugs have been evaluated in the first-line and second-line treatment of lung cancer. Pemetrexed,[52] liposomal doxorubicin, and the newer targeted agents like erlotinib or gefitinib[53] may be less myelosuppressive and regimens incorporating these agents may be used more frequently to reduce the incidence of myelosuppression in the elderly. Interestingly, in a large analysis of advanced lung cancer patients older than 65 years, patients treated in combination with bevacizumab had a 60% rate of more than twofold increase in neutropenia within 2 months after chemotherapy. Another caveat with the use of targeted treatments in the elderly is that although hematological toxicity is reduced, nonhematological toxicity may be significantly enhanced, limiting the use of some of these drugs in this population.

Elderly patients with advanced lung and breast cancer also may be better served with a single chemotherapeutic agent than with combination regimens. A large randomized phase III trial (the Multicenter Italian Lung Cancer in the Elderly Study) of 700 elderly patients showed that the combination of vinorelbine plus gemcitabine was no more effective than single-agent vinorelbine or gemcitabine in the treatment of elderly patients with advanced NSCLC. Combination chemotherapy resulted in more thrombocytopenia (3%) than single-agent vinorelbine (<1%) and more neutropenia (13%), than single-agent gemcitabine (7%).[54]

Management of cancer in the elderly requires a careful consideration of the ultimate goal of treatment (cure versus palliation) and appropriate use of regimens to avoid further harm in this subgroup of patients.

Elder-specific trials with a gentler treatment-based approach have been proposed to improve management of older cancer patients (Table 13-1).[55,56] A pooled analysis of toxicity and outcomes in 118 elderly patients treated in two elderly-specific (inclusion criteria ≥ 65 years) and two nonspecific trials was conducted by the North Central Cancer Treatment Group. Grade 3 or worse hematological toxicity was seen in 68% of the elderly in age-unspecified trials as compared to 10% in the elderly-specific trials (neutropenia in 56% and 9% of patients, and thrombocytopenia in 14% and 1% of

TABLE 13-1	Myelosuppressive Toxicity (%) Reported in Patients in Elder-Specific Lung Cancer Trials					
	Anemia		Neutropenia		Thrombocytopenia	
Regimen	Grade 3	Grade 4	Grade 3	Grade 4	Grade 3	Grade 4
Gemcitabine/Vinorelbine	4	0	18	5	6	2
Vinorelbine [54]	1	0	14	3	4	1
Cisplatin/Gemcitabine	5		13.3	6.7	8.3	1.7
Cisplatin/Vinorelbine [55]	4.9		14.7	8.2		
Gemcitabine/Vinorelbine	2	0	16	13	3	<1
Vinorelbine	3	<1	14	11	<1	
Gemcitabine [56]	2		7	1	2	1
Docetaxel	2.3	1.1	26.1	56.8	0	0
Vinorelbine [50]	8.8	1.1	30.8	38.5	0	0

patients, respectively). There were no statistically significant differences with regard to treatment efficacy. However, conclusions from these trials are limited because of the small number of participants in the elder-specific trials.

PATIENT-SPECIFIC FACTORS AND MANAGEMENT

It remains unclear why some older individuals are predisposed to myelotoxicity and others are not. Certainly, age-related changes occur in other organs and tissues other than bone marrow that may contribute to this predisposition, particularly with regard to alterations in clearance and pharmacodynamics of potentially myelotoxic chemotherapy drugs. Awareness of these changes and appropriate adjustments for individuals with a reduced capacity to metabolize or excrete an active drug can eliminate or reduce myelosuppressive toxicity.

AGE-RELATED PHYSIOLOGICAL CHANGES

Changes in the Renal System

Age-associated changes in the kidneys including a decrease in glomerular filtration rate (GFR) and decreased concentrating ability predispose the elderly to a greater prevalence of chronic kidney disease, fluid and electrolyte imbalances, and impaired handling of drugs cleared by the kidneys with an increase in toxicity. It is estimated that GFR decreases at a rate of 1 mL/minute/year after the age of 40. Adjusting the dosage of drugs cleared by the kidneys may reduce the risk of toxicity. Assessing renal function using serum creatinine may be inaccurate as a result of decreased muscle mass in the elderly. An increased risk of hematologic toxicity was seen in older postmenopausal women with breast cancer and serum creatinine values of 1.5 mg/dL or less receiving adjuvant CMF compared to their younger counterparts. The creatinine clearance provides a more accurate estimate of renal function and can be used to predict toxicity. A retrospective study of 1,405 patients aged 65 years or older with breast cancer who were treated with CMF between 1998 and 2000 demonstrated increased hematological toxicity for those with a calculated creatinine clearance of less than 50 mL/min.[57] Increased myelosuppression associated with renal insufficiency has been observed with melphalan, fludarabine, cisplatin, etoposide and topotecan in those older than 70. Dose modifications are recommended on the basis of creatinine clearance, particularly for elderly patients being treated with these drugs. Another prospective study in older breast cancer patients showed that hematological toxicity was substantially decreased by treating with modified dosing of cyclophosphamide and methotrexate on the basis of the estimated creatinine clearance.[58] Many methods of calculating creatinine clearance are available, but the most commonly used is the Cockcroft-Gault formula, which calculates clearance on the basis of age and weight. However, this formula may also underestimate creatinine clearance in the elderly.

Changes in the Gastrointestinal System

Altered hepatic enzyme function leads to abnormalities in the metabolism of selected drugs. Decreased intracellular water, increased fat content, and low albumin in the elderly can significantly alter the volume and distribution of drugs. The pharmacokinetics and pharmacodynamics of the drugs may be influenced by their bound and unbound fractions. Both paclitaxel and docetaxel are extensively protein bound and are metabolized by the cytochrome P450 enzymes in the liver. No dose modification on the basis of age alone is recommended, but care should be exercised in elderly patients with indicators of poor nutritional status and who are on multiple drugs. Increased hematological toxicity due to altered gastrointestinal drug absorption secondary to age-associated decreased motility and decreased blood flow may be seen with oral cancer drug therapy.

TABLE 13-2	**Special Considerations for Chemotherapy Drug Dosing in the Elderly**			
Chemotherapy	Malignancy	Effect of Age on Pharmacokinetics	Modifying factors	Side Effects
Cyclophosphamide	Lymphomas; breast cancer	No change	No dose reduction for renal or hepatic dysfunction	Increased myelosuppression in secondary to toxicity at the cellular level; hemorrhagic cystitis
Cisplatin	Head and neck, lung cancers	No change	Kidney function	Myelosuppression, renal toxicity, ototoxicity, neuropathy
Carboplatin	Head and neck, lung cancers	No change	AUC based on Calvert formula	Myelosuppression but generally well tolerated
Doxorubicin	Breast cancer; lymphomas	No change	Dose reduction in patients with hypoalbuminemia	Cardiac toxicity and myelosuppression
Vinorelbine	Lung cancer	No change	Severe liver dysfunction, highly bound to platelets	Myelosuppression
Docetaxel Paclitaxel	Lung, prostate, and breast cancers	Conflicting data on clearance in older population; no dose adjustment for age alone	Metabolized by cytochrome P450 system, highly protein-bound; high interpatient variability; caution in patients with liver dysfunction	Neutropenia, fatigue
Gemcitabine	Lung and pancreatic cancers	Small increase in mean half-life with age; no dose changes on the basis of age alone	Caution in patients with renal and hepatic impairment	Neutropenia and thrombocytopenia
Etoposide	Lung cancer, lymphomas	Increase in free etoposide levels seen with oral therapy; minor dose reductions are recommended even in elderly with normal organ function	Hypoalbuminemia, increased bilirubin, and renal dysfunction can increase toxicity	Myelosuppression
Oxaliplatin	Colon cancer	No change	Severe renal dysfunction	Neuropathy and myelosuppression
Irinotecan	Colon cancer	Reduced dose recommended in patients older than 70 years and poor performance status	Toxicity increased with severe liver dysfunction	Diarrhea and myelosuppression

PHARMACODYNAMICS OF DRUGS AND AGING

Most of the commonly used chemotherapeutic drugs do not show changes in their clearance with age (Table 13-2) in the presence of functioning renal and gastrointestinal systems. Serum concentrations from oral etoposide are known to increase with age and correlate with nadir neutrophil counts after the first cycle. The Cancer and Leukemia Group B conducted a trial (CALGB 9762) and found a significant decrease in total body clearance of paclitaxel in the cohort of patients aged 75 years or older compared with those aged 55 to 64 and 65 to 74 years, with a resultant increase in grade 3-4 neutropenia of 49%. However, other studies have failed to show any change in paclitaxel clearance with age, and dose reduction is not recommended on the basis of age. Age alone is not a basis for dose reduction for many of these drugs in an otherwise healthy elderly patient.

PHYSIOLOGICAL VERSUS CHRONOLOGICAL AGE

Although aging is associated with physiological changes that may predispose the elderly to increased toxicity, the rate of aging is not the same in all individuals. Assessments on the basis of chronological aging may not be accurate enough to determine the tolerance to chemotherapy. The number of comorbid conditions increases with age. An NIA/NCI study estimated that the mean number of comorbidities increases with age: 2.9 for those 55-64 years, 3.6 for those aged 65-74 years, and 4.2 for those 75 years or older. At least 30% of those older than 75 were estimated to have six or more comorbid conditions.[59] Increasing number and severity of comorbidities both predict for increased hospitalization from hematological toxicity during chemotherapy in elderly cancer patients and also correlate with decreased survival.[38,59,60] (Figure 13-3). Several indices of comorbidities have been developed to evaluate the risk of treatment toxicity in elderly patients; however, they all have limitations in their application.[61] The most commonly used is the Charlson Comorbidity Index (CCI), an instrument that has been validated in cancer patients; it can predict the ability of elderly cancer patients to tolerate chemotherapy and can assist in planning treatment options.[62,63]

The general decline recognized as "frailty" is a multifactorial syndrome characterized by diminished physiological reserve and decreased ability to withstand stress. There are now objective criteria to better define this syndrome. One set of criteria, established as a component of the Cardiovascular Heart Study (CHS) included assessment of grip strength, walking speed, weight loss, exhaustion, and physical activity to define the frail phenotype. It is clear from multiple studies that frail subjects have increased comorbidities, disabilities, falls, institutionalization, and mortality. It would seem likely, but is yet unproven, that frailty would be associated with increased chemotherapy toxicity, including myelosuppression. Oncologists are familiar with functional assessment, having grown accustomed to either or both the Karnofsky or ECOG Performance Status (PS) evaluations. Nonetheless, it has been shown that nearly 40% of patients with ECOG performance status less than 2 (the level traditionally used in clinical trials) could have limitations in their activities of daily living (ADLs) and independent activities of daily living (IADLs).[64]

Because of different variables involved in predicting tolerance, the National Comprehensive Cancer Network (NCCN) has recommended a multidisciplinary approach to evaluate tolerance to chemotherapy in the elderly. A typical Comprehensive Geriatric Assessment (CGA) provides information relating to the comorbidity, functional status, cognition, mental status, social support, nutritional status, and medications of older adult patients in an effort to identify unsuspected conditions that may have an impact on the potential success of cancer therapy. This concept has been tested in older breast cancer patients in whom use of the CGA identified three or more functional deficits and poor tolerance to chemotherapy in nearly 60% of patients who had been rated by their physicians as "not ill." CGA was also used in 83 advanced ovarian carcinoma patients older than 70 years who received carboplatin AUC 5 and cyclophosphamide. Patient autonomy (functional status), comorbidities, daily medications, nutritional status, cognitive function, and the presence or absence of clinical symptoms of depression was assessed prior to starting chemotherapy. Depression symptoms and poor functional status (living at home with assistance, living with medical assistance in a specialized institution), were predictive of chemotherapy-induced severe toxicity including febrile neutropenia and early treatment withdrawal because of toxicity.[65] Despite these advances, there is no standardized method of CGA available at the present time for elderly cancer patients.

MANAGEMENT OF CHEMOTHERAPY-INDUCED TOXICITY

> After reviewing the available evidence and patient assessment, the 72-year-old advanced lung cancer patient is treated with single-agent gemcitabine on the basis of the results of the MILES study.
>
> The node-positive postmenopausal breast cancer patient is treated with dose-dense adriamycin, cyclophosphamide, and sequential paclitaxel in order to maximize her treatment outcome with a curative intent.
>
> Is there a role for prophylactic white blood cell growth factor support in these patients?

Role of Granulocyte-Stimulating Growth Factors

Retrospective review of clinical studies utilizing granulocyte colony-stimulating factor (G-CSF) and erythropoetin have shown that the elderly can respond to growth factors quickly and with a comparable increase in cell counts to younger patients. These agents are in the forefront of managing neutropenic toxicity in patients receiving chemotherapy both in primary and secondary prophylaxis and in the treatment setting. G-CSF has been shown to reduce the incidence of febrile neutropenia, hospitalization, and the need for intravenous antibiotics in metastatic breast cancer patients by more than 80%.[66] The preponderance of evidence shows that these agents are very beneficial in the elderly population as well. In elderly NHL patients, randomized trials have shown that the use of G-CSF can reduce the incidence of neutropenic infection by almost 100%. Similarly, use of G-CSF in elderly patients with acute myeloid leukemia was associated with significantly shorter duration of neutropenia and decreased use of antibiotics. Granulocyte-macrophage colony-stimulating factor (GM-CSF) also

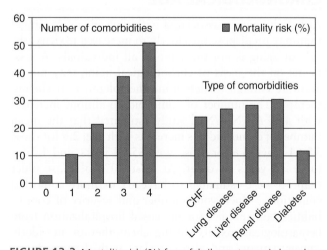

FIGURE 13-3 Mortality risk (%) from febrile neutropenia based on the number and type of comorbid illnesses. *(Adapted from Kuderer et al. Cancer 2006;106(10):2258-66.)*

has been shown to reduce time to neutrophil recovery as compared to placebo in elderly patients with acute myeloid leukemia (AML). Specifically, prophylactic use from the first cycle has been recommended because of the high frequency of first-cycle neutropenia seen in patients who did not receive G-CSF. In a large randomized controlled trial of elderly patients treated for solid tumors, pegfilgrastim use during the first cycle of chemotherapy decreased the incidence of grade 3 or 4 neutropenia from 68% to 26%, reduced antibiotic use and hospitalizations due to febrile neutropenia, and reduced the frequency of dose delays and dose reductions.[67] A recent systematic review and meta-analysis of randomized controlled trials comparing primary prophylactic G-CSF with placebo or untreated controls in adults with solid tumors or malignant lymphomas reported a 40% reduction in febrile neutropenia with the use of G-CSF in patients older than 65 years. Use of G-CSF in all patients regardless of age nearly halved the relative risk of infection-related and early mortality in solid tumor trials.[68] The NCCN Guidelines for Senior Adult Oncology and the American Society of Clinical Oncology (ASCO) recommend the prophylactic use of white blood cell (WBC) growth factors in clinical situations where the risk of neutropenia is greater than 20%.[69] Age older than 65 years was identified as an important patient characteristic that identified individuals for the receipt of prophylactic growth factor treatment. WBC growth factors are also recommended in older patients receiving curative therapy in the treatment of NHL or for adjuvant breast cancer treatment, where maintenance of dose intensity is essential to achieve a good outcome. Retrospective review of four randomized trials in adjuvant breast cancer reported a better overall survival in those who received more chemotherapy than in those who received less, regardless of age. The reduction in hazard of failure from more chemotherapy was 40% for those older than 65 years and 18% in those 50 years and younger.

The use of CSF therapy is also appropriate in this group when the risk of neutropenia from individual regimens is less than 20%, if other patient-related factors suggest a high risk of morbidity and mortality from neutropenia (Table 13-3). Treatment with CSF can be used to reduce the duration of neutropenia and the incidence of hospitalizations in these patients. Prophylactic antibiotic use with or without G-CSF has shown similar beneficial effect in some studies but no clear recommendation has been made about their use in elderly patients for prophylactic or secondary use for chemotherapy-induced neutropenia.

The risk of administration of growth factors is minimal, although a slight increase in thrombocytopenia has been reported with the use of GM-CSF. An increased incidence of bone and musculoskeletal pain has also been reported with use of G-CSF or GM-CSF. One note of concern, however, is that a greater number of breast cancer patients treated with white cell hematopoietic growth

TABLE 13-3	Indications for Prophylactic WBC Growth Factors in the Elderly

Risk of febrile neutropenia from chemotherapy ≥ 20%

Risk of febrile neutropenia from chemotherapy 10% to 20% and presence of additional risk factors for infectious complications:
- Previous episode of febrile neutropenia
- Advanced disease
- Heavily pretreated patients
- Presence of cytopenias due to bone marrow involvement
- Malnutrition
- Current infections
- Liver or renal dysfunction
- Multiple comorbidities
- Poor performance status

To support the administration of planned doses of chemotherapy on schedule in patients undergoing treatment with curative intent (CHOP or CHOP-like regimens)

factors were subsequently diagnosed with myelodysplastic syndrome or acute myeloid leukemia. The exact association with this outcome is unclear as older AML patients treated with these agents did not show progression of leukemia or worse outcomes.

> The patient with lung cancer does not receive prophylactic WBC growth factors, as the risk of febrile neutropenia with this regimen is less than 10%. He tolerates the treatment well except for increasing fatigue. Complete blood count reveals a hemoglobin level of 10 g/dL.
>
> The 65-year-old breast cancer patient is given prophylactic filgrastim to prevent neutropenia, as the regimen is associated with a greater than 20% risk of febrile neutropenia. She also maintains dose intensity and schedule. She is noted to have a hemoglobin level of 11.5 g/dL after three cycles and reports mild fatigue.
>
> Do they require any intervention at this time for the anemia?

Management of Chemotherapy-Induced Anemia

Anemia during cancer chemotherapy is associated with significant changes in quality of life. Recombinant erythropoietin has been used widely in the management of anemia during treatment of cancer. Although specific trials in the elderly are lacking, numerous randomized studies have shown a correlation between an increase in hemoglobin levels to 12 g/dL or more and improvement in fatigue and quality of life. Treatment with epoetin alfa and darbepoetin has also been shown to reduce the risk of blood transfusion by 18% in patients receiving chemotherapy; however, the use of these agents has come under severe scrutiny recently because of some published studies on their use with breast and head and neck cancers. In these trials of recombinant erythropoietin, an increased risk of thromboembolic events and possibly of tumor progression, with a reduction in chemotherapy response, was reported. The use of erythropoietin-stimulating agents

(ESA) is contraindicated in patients who are undergoing chemotherapy with a curative intent. Their use is also prohibited in patients with cancer-related anemia not related to chemotherapy. Although most of these trials targeted hemoglobin levels of 13 g/dL, the FDA reported that there was insufficient evidence to conclude that these agents do not decrease survival or promote tumor progression at hemoglobin (Hb) levels between 10 and 12 g/dL. The American Society of Hematology and the American Society of Clinical Oncology recommend the use of epoetin or darbepoetin for patients with chemotherapy-associated anemia and a hemoglobin concentration that is near to or less than 10 g/dL, with the primary goal of treatment being to increase hemoglobin and decrease transfusions. They recommend caution in the use of erythropoietin in patients receiving chemotherapy for hematological malignancies and those with an increased risk of thromboembolism. In patients with lymphomas, additional causes of anemia such as hemolytic anemia and bone marrow suppression should be ruled out. If patients do not respond with an increase in hemoglobin after initiating treatment, ESAs may be considered with the intent of reducing the transfusion requirement. In patients with milder degrees of anemia, the decision about the early use of erythropoietin should be made on the basis of individual circumstances and clinical situations. Priority should be given to identifying reversible causes of anemia including evaluating for deficiencies in iron, folate, or vitamin B12. Intravenous iron has been shown to increase hemoglobin response to erythropoietin, as well as to decrease the duration of treatment required to achieve the response, independent of iron stores, and may be used effectively in cancer patients.

> Initial physical examination and history reveal no other cause for the anemia in these patients.
>
> The ferritin level in the older gentleman was 250 μg/L. As he is receiving palliative chemotherapy and is symptomatic, a trial of epoetin alfa at 40,000 units weekly was started, to see if the hemoglobin levels will increase and his symptoms improve. The patient was also given intravenous iron. He responded to treatment, with an increase in his hemoglobin level to 11.5 g/dL after 8 weeks and an improvement in symptoms.
>
> In the postmenopausal breast cancer patient, ESAs should not be used to manage anemia as her anticipated treatment outcome is cure. No specific cause was identified in this patient and there was no intervention. The patient should be followed regularly to assess her symptoms and any requirement for transfusion.

Management of Chemotherapy-Induced Thrombocytopenia

Besides treatment dose reductions or dose delays, platelet transfusions are the only effective way to manage thrombocytopenia associated with chemotherapy. The appropriate threshold for platelet transfusion during chemotherapy recommended by the ASCO is a platelet count less than 10×10^9/L.[70] The risk of major hemorrhage is very rare above this level, and the risk of

TABLE 13-4	Recommended Domains for Research to Reduce Myelosuppressive Toxicity in Older Cancer Patients
1. Comprehensive Geriatric Assessment in elderly patients with cancer
2. Age-appropriate dose modification
3. Accurate assessment of renal and hepatic functions
4. Use of less myelosuppressive chemotherapy regimens
5. Single-agent rather than combination regimens in appropriate patients
6. Elder-specific clinical trials to assess response and tolerance to chemotherapy

alloimmunization and platelet refractoriness can be reduced. However, these levels may have to be modified in the elderly population who may have other risk factors for bleeding including use of anticoagulant drugs and poor performance status. Interleukin-11, the only growth factor approved for management of chemotherapy-induced thrombocytopenia, is effective in reducing the requirement for platelet transfusions but is associated with fluid retention and other cardiovascular side effects that may be problematic in the elderly population.[71] The thrombopoetin receptor agonists romiplostim and eltrombopag are currently undergoing phase I and II trials for management of chemotherapy-induced thrombocytopenia.

CONCLUSION

Myelosuppression is an important complication of chemotherapy in elderly cancer patients and requires careful appraisal and treatment (Table 13-4). Chronological age is not the only consideration when estimating the ability of a patient to tolerate chemotherapy. The Comprehensive Geriatric Assessment evaluating multiple geriatric domains should be used when possible to help identify elderly patients likely to benefit from chemotherapy. Appropriate use of growth factors in the elderly will reduce myelosuppressive toxicity while maintaining dose intensity and can improve treatment outcomes in the elderly.

 See expertconsult.com for a complete list of references and web resources for this chapter

SUGGESTED READINGS

1. Lipschitz DA, Udupa KB, Milton KY, Thompson CO: Effect of age on hematopoiesis in man, *Blood* 63(3):502–509, 1984.
2. Pallis AG, Papamichael D, Audisio R, et al: EORTC Elderly Task Force experts' opinion for the treatment of colon cancer in older patients, *Cancer treatment reviews* 2009.
3. Pallis AG, Gridelli C, van Meerbeeck JP, et al: EORTC Elderly Task Force and Lung Cancer Group and International Society for Geriatric Oncology (SIOG) experts' opinion for the treatment of non-small-cell lung cancer in an elderly population, *Ann Oncol* 2009.

4. Crivellari D, Bonetti M, Castiglione-Gertsch M, et al: Burdens and benefits of adjuvant cyclophosphamide, methotrexate, and fluorouracil and tamoxifen for elderly patients with breast cancer: the International Breast Cancer Study Group Trial VII, *J Clin Oncol* 18(7):1412–1422, 2000.

5. Muss HB, Woolf S, Berry D, et al: Adjuvant chemotherapy in older and younger women with lymph node–positive breast cancer, *JAMA* 293:1073–1081, 2005.

6. Chrischilles EA, Pendergast JF, Kahn KL, et al. Adverse events among the elderly receiving chemotherapy for advanced non-small-cell lung cancer, *J Clin Oncol* 28(4):620–627.

7. Gridelli C, Perrone F, Gallo C, et al: Chemotherapy for elderly patients with advanced non-small-cell lung cancer: the Multi-center Italian Lung Cancer in the Elderly Study (MILES) phase III randomized trial, *Journal of the National Cancer Institute* 95(5):362–372, 2003.

8. Lichtman MS, Wildiers H, Chatelut E, et al: International Society of Geriatric Oncology Chemotherapy Taskforce: Evaluation of Chemotherapy in Older Patients—An Analysis of the Medical Literature, *J Clin Oncol* 1832-1843, 2007 may 10.

9. Repetto L, Fratino L, Audisio RA, et al: Comprehensive geriatric assessment adds information to Eastern Cooperative Oncology Group performance status in elderly cancer patients: an Italian Group for Geriatric Oncology Study, *J Clin Oncol* 20(2):494–502, 2002.

10. Freyer G, Geay JF, Touzet S, et al: Comprehensive geriatric assessment predicts tolerance to chemotherapy and survival in elderly patients with advanced ovarian carcinoma: a GINECO study, *Ann Oncol* 16(11):1795–1800, 2005.

11. Vogel CL, Wojtukiewicz MZ, Carroll RR, et al: First and subsequent cycle use of pegfilgrastim prevents febrile neutropenia in patients with breast cancer: a multicenter, double-blind, placebo-controlled phase III study, *J Clin Oncol* 23(6):1178–1184, 2005.

12. Smith TJ, Khatcheressian J, Lyman GH, et al: 2006 update of recommendations for the use of white blood cell growth factors: an evidence-based clinical practice guideline, *J Clin Oncol* 24(19):3187–3205, 2006.

13. Rizzo JD, Lichtin AE, Woolf SH, et al: Use of epoetin in patients with cancer: evidence-based clinical practice guidelines of the American Society of Clinical Oncology and the American Society of Hematology, *Blood* 100(7):2303–2320, 2002 Oct 1.

14. Schiffer CA, Anderson KC, Bennett CL, et al: Platelet transfusion for patients with cancer: clinical practice guidelines of the American Society of Clinical Oncology, *J Clin Oncol* 19(5):1519–1538, 2001.

15. Kuderer NM, Dale DC, Crawford J, et al: Mortality, morbidity, and cost associated with febrile neutropenia in adult cancer patients, *Cancer* 106(10):2258–2266, 2006 May 15.

Nonhematologic Complications of Systemic Treatment of Cancer in the Older-Aged Person

Lodovico Balducci

The management of cancer in the older-aged person is an increasingly common problem, because the population is aging and cancer is largely a disease of aging.[1] Aging involves a progressive loss in functional reserve of multiple organs and consequently increased susceptibility to the complications of cancer treatment. These are important for several reasons. First of all, they may cause discomfort, disease, and death. Second, they may prevent the administration of effective cancer treatment. Third, they may lead to functional dependence that is associated with poorer quality of life and higher management cost. In this chapter, the nonhematological complications of systemic cancer treatment are examined, including descriptions of both the acute and chronic complications of hormonal, cytotoxic, and targeted therapy. At the end of the chapter, the unsolved issues related to the management of cancer in the older-aged person are outlined and a research agenda to address these issues is proposed.

CASE 14-1

A 75-year-old woman is diagnosed with early-stage breast cancer. After lumpectomy and radiation, she meets with her medical oncologist who discusses adjuvant treatment; the decision is made to treat her with hormone therapy alone, and she is placed on an aromatase inhibitor. Two months later she visits her primary care provider stating that she seems to be tolerating her new medication, but asking for pain medications for her worsening arthritis. She also mentions that she had a fall about 2 weeks ago but luckily did not break any of her bones. However, the emergency department physician noted that she appeared to have some "bone weakness" on her x-ray.

HORMONAL TREATMENT

Hormonal manipulations are the mainstay treatment of prostate and breast cancer. In this section the complications of luteinizing hormone-releasing hormone (LHRH)

analogs, estrogen, aromatase inhibitors, and selective estrogen receptor modulators (SERMs) are addressed.

LHRH Analogs

For more than 20 years, these agents have been used to induce chemical castration in patients with prostate cancer. The definitive benefits of this treatment have been demonstrated in only two circumstances: in the presence of metastatic disease confirmed by imaging[2] and in combination with radiation therapy for the management of locally advanced disease (stage C or III).[3] The benefits of adjuvant hormonal treatment in patients at high risk of recurrence are controversial.[4] Despite a lack of any evidence, it has become common practice to induce chemical castration in patients experiencing so-called chemical (PSA) recurrences.

In addition to loss of libido, chemical castration is complicated by hot flushes, fatigue, and possibly anemia.[5-7] It is not clear whether it may also cause cognitive decline. Fatigue is particularly ominous, as it has been associated with an increased risk of functional dependence and of death in older individuals.[8-10] Likewise, anemia has also been associated with death, functional dependence, and geriatric syndromes including falls and dementia.[11]

The best established long-term complication of castration is osteoporosis.[12-14] Treatment with LHRH analogs for longer than 1 year has been associated with increased risk of fracture that increases directly with treatment duration.[12] Other potential complications include diabetes and increased incidence of coronary events in patients with a preexisting history of coronary artery disease.[15-16]

The best management of complications from LHRH analogs is prevention, which includes avoiding the unwarranted use of these compounds. Hot flushes may respond to progesterone, to gabapentin, and to antidepressants, but these medications carry their own set of complications. Fatigue may be ameliorated with exercise.[17] The benefit of provigil in these situations is controversial.

Bone loss may be reversed by bisphosphonates or RANK ligand inhibitors (denosumab). These compounds are recommended in patients who already have osteopenia and in those for whom treatment with LHRH analogs for longer than 1 year is planned.[13-14]

A number of alternative approaches may also obviate some of the complications of LHRH analogs. These include: intermittent castration, use of androgen antagonists in lieu of LHRH analogs, LHRH inhibitors, and novel compounds such as abiraterone and more specific androgen antagonists.

Intermittent castration has become increasingly popular,[18] though it has not been conclusively demonstrated that it is as effective as continuous castration. In one study, bicalutamide in high doses was found to be as effective as castration in patients with metastatic prostate cancer.[19] This approach may allow some patients to preserve their libido, but it is expensive and associated with painful gynecomastia (that may be prevented by prophylactic breast irradiation). It is not clear whether long-term treatment with this compound may also lead to osteoporosis, diabetes, and coronary artery disease. Direct LHRH antagonists have only recently been introduced in the management of prostate cancer.[20] Their main indication is in treatment of patients with critical metastases (such as impending spinal cord compression or urinary obstruction) for whom LHRH analogs are contraindicated. At least theoretically, the complications of these agents should be similar to those of LHRH analogs.

Two types of drugs appear particularly promising in the management of hormone-sensitive prostate cancer: abiraterone[21] and highly selective androgen antagonists.[22] Both types of compounds were found active in "hormone-refractory prostate cancer," as they antagonize the effect of dihydrotestosterone synthesized within the cancer. Abiraterone is a selective inhibitor of androgen synthesis that prevents the synthesis of dihydrotestosterone within the gonads, the adrenals, and the tumor.[21]

Estrogen

Though seldom used nowadays, estrogen may provide effective and inexpensive treatment of both prostate and breast cancers. In metastatic prostate cancer, diethylstilbestrol (DES) appears to be at least as effective as LHRH analogs.[23] Unlike LHRH, estrogen does not cause loss of libido, osteoporosis, or hot flushes. Complications include painful gynecomastia and deep vein thrombosis. A never-solved controversy is whether DES in low doses (1 mg/daily) is as effective as and less risky than the most commonly used dose of 3 mg per day. Retrospective

studies suggest that this may be the case. Despite low cost and safety, the use of estrogen in metastatic prostate cancer has almost disappeared in the USA as a result of the aggressive marketing of LHRH analogs.

In metastatic breast cancer, DES at high doses (15 mg daily) is as effective as tamoxifen and may prove effective in 15% of patients whose cancer progressed while they were receiving tamoxifen.[24] The complications of this treatment include deep vein thrombosis, fluid retention, and congestive heart failure, and the risk of these increases with patient age.

Selective Estrogen Receptor Modulators (SERMs)

These include tamoxifen, toremifene, and raloxifene. Fulvestrant (Faslodex), although a pure estrogen antagonist, will also be discussed in this group.

Until recently, tamoxifen has been the mainstay treatment of hormone receptor-rich breast cancer.[25] This agent has reduced by 40% the systemic recurrence of breast cancer after surgery. Recent pharmacogenomic studies showed that tamoxifen is effective in women who are rapid metabolizers, that is, women in whom the activity of CYP2D6 is increased, because this enzyme converts the inactive parent compounds into active metabolites.[26] The concomitant prescription of tamoxifen and CYP2D6 inhibitors, such as paroxetine, should then be avoided. Toremifene has comparable activity as tamoxifen. Raloxifene is untested in the management of breast cancer. Tamoxifen and raloxifene reduce by approximately 50% the incidence of hormone receptor-rich breast cancer in women at risk.[27] Other beneficial effects of SERMs include prevention of osteopenia and osteoporosis and decreased serum cholesterol levels.[28] SERMs cause hot flushes, vaginal secretions, and deep vein thrombosis (DVT). In rare instances, tamoxifen and toremifene, but not raloxifene, cause endometrial cancer. Risk factors for DVT and endometrial cancer include age 70 or older and obesity.[29]

Hot flushes may be ameliorated by antidepressants and gabapentin.[29] The benefit of serial gynecologic exams for early diagnosis of endometrial cancer is controversial.

Being a pure antiestrogen, fulvestrant does not cause either DVT or endometrial cancer. The effect of this compound on the bone is not well understood, as it has not been studied in the adjuvant setting where long-term complications are expected.

Aromatase Inhibitors

These compounds have largely superseded SERMs in the treatment of breast cancer, in both the adjuvant and the metastatic setting.[30] Like tamoxifen, they may cause hot flushes. An especially troublesome complication is arthralgias, whose pathogenesis is poorly understood.[31] Arthralgia may represent a cause of functional limitations in older women. Unlike the SERMs, these compounds cause osteoporosis.[30] Early treatment with bisphosphonates such as zoledronic acid did prevent bone loss in the Z-fast study[32] but it has not been proven yet that this treatment prevents bone fractures. Current recommendations for the management of osteopenia and osteoporosis include assessment of bone density at the beginning of treatment and serially thereafter and institution of bisphosphonate therapy in the presence of bone loss.[33] Prophylactic bisphosphonate treatment in all women receiving aromatase inhibitors is not recommended.

Aromatase inhibitors have also been associated with an increase in serum cholesterol, but there is no evidence that they cause increased incidence of coronary artery disease or stroke.

In conclusion, hormonal treatment is the safest form of systemic cancer therapy for older individuals. Osteoporosis and increased risk of bone fractures are common complications of chemical castration for prostate cancer and of aromatase inhibitors, but these complications may be offset by bisphosphonates or RANK ligand inhibitor. Except in its application for chemical castration in patients with a preexisting history of coronary artery disease, there is no proof that LHRH analogs may cause coronary death. Deep vein thrombosis complicates treatment with estrogen and to a lesser extent with SERMs. Age and obesity are risk factors for these complications. Aromatase inhibitor-associated arthralgia may be a cause of disability for some older women.

As is the case for any medications, hormonal treatment should not be used in conditions when the risks supersedes the benefits. That seems to be the case for chemical castration in presence of chemical recurrence of prostate cancer.

CASE 14-2

A 75-year-old woman is diagnosed with early-stage breast cancer. After lumpectomy and radiation, she meets with her medical oncologist who discusses adjuvant treatment; the decision is made to treat her with both adjuvant chemotherapy and hormone therapy. Prior to starting therapy, she visits her primary care provider with concerns about the side effects of chemotherapy, as one of her friends mentioned that it is bad for the brain and the heart. She wants to know whether she should go through with it and if there is anything that she can do to avoid these complications.

CYTOTOXIC CHEMOTHERAPY

The risk of both acute and long-term complications of cytotoxic chemotherapy increases with age. Acute complications include mucositis, cardiotoxicity, and peripheral neuropathy. Chronic complications include chronic subclinical cardiac dysfunction, peripheral neuropathy, acute leukemia, myelodysplasia, and, possibly, dementia and functional dependence.

Acute Complications

Mucositis. The risk of mucositis from fluorinated pyrimidines and anthracyclines increases with age.[34] Mucositis may lead to volume depletion because of diarrhea and dysphagia. This complication is more rapid and more severe in older than in younger individuals because the total body water decreases with age.[34] It is not clear why mucositis is more common and more severe in older individuals. A possible explanation is found in aging rodents, in whom the proliferation of cryptal cells increases with age while the reserve of mucosal stem cells is diminished.[34] This condition would predispose to mucositis by a twofold mechanism. The increased proliferation would render the cryptal cells more susceptible to destruction by cycle-active agents while the depletion of mucosal stem cells would delay the repair of the mucosal damage.

In addition to age, other risk factors for mucositis include female sex, ethnic group, and genetics, including hereditary deficiency of enzymes involved in drug metabolisms.[35] New insight in the pathogenesis of mucositis reveals that the administration of cytotoxic drugs leads to oxidative damage, activation of stress-response genes, and increased production of nuclear factor KB and inflammatory cytokines that maintain and amplify the mucosal damage.[35] In addition, chemotherapy-induced alterations in the oral and intestinal flora may also play a role in the pathogenesis of mucositis.[35]

The management of mucositis is unsatisfactory.[36-37] The only medication that was proven to reduce the incidence and severity of mucositis in randomized controlled studies has been the keratinocyte growth factor.[38] This compound has not received widespread acceptance, however, because it is expensive and requires administration over several days. Recently, oral spray of human intestinal trefoil factor has ameliorated the risk of mucositis in a double blind phase II randomized study.[39] Physiologically, trefoil factor binds to mucin and prevents mucosal damage. It is produced by goblet cells, which are destroyed by cytotoxic chemotherapy.

The substitution of intravenous fluorinated pyrimidines with capecitabine has reduced the risk of mucositis, but capecitabine in full doses is not well tolerated for other complications, especially the hand-foot syndrome. Furthermore capecitabine is contraindicated in patients with renal insufficiency, which is an almost universal condition of age and is associated with interaction with drugs metabolized through the cytochrome p450 system. The use of these drugs, such as warfarin, increases with age.

Aggressive fluid resuscitation should be initiated without delay in patients who cannot drink because of diarrhea.

Neuropathy. Peripheral neuropathy is a common complication of alkaloids, epipodophyllotoxins, taxanes, epothilones, cisplatin, and oxaliplatin.[40] The risk of this complication increases with age. In older patients, these complications are also longer-lasting and more debilitating. Loss of sensation in the fingers may prevent the performance of basic ADLs including dressing, feeding, and toileting. Loss of sensation in the toes is associated with ambulatory difficulties and falls.

No antidote to peripheral neuropathy is available. Early discontinuance of the offending medication is the only effective prevention. In general, docetaxel appears to cause less neuropathy that other taxanes, but it is more myelotoxic.

Cardiomyopathy. The incidence of this often irreversible anthracycline complication increases with age and with medication dose.[41] The interaction of the medication with intracellular iron causes the production of free radicals that lead to a progressive damage of the cardiac sarcomeres. Cardiomyopathy may be prevented with the administration of doxorubicin by continuous intravenous infusion or with the administration of desrazoxane. This agent prevents the production of free radicals by chelating the cellular iron and preventing its interaction with the anthracyclines. Unfortunately, desrazoxane may reduce the antineoplastic effectiveness of doxorubicin[41] and is associated with increased risk of mucositis and myelotoxicity, which also become more common with age. The substitution of doxorubicin with pegylated liposomal doxorubicin (PLD) may reduce the risk of cardiomyopathy and other anthracycline complications including nausea and vomiting, alopecia, and myelotoxicity. The cancers for which the effectiveness of PLD has been proven include multiple myeloma, metastatic breast cancer, ovarian cancer, and AIDS-associated Kaposi sarcoma.[41] PLD is effective in lymphoma, although it is not clear whether it is as effective as doxorubicin. The most common strategy to prevent cardiomyopathy involves the discontinuation of doxorubicin when the patient ejection fraction decreases by at least 14% on the basis of serial measurements by MUGA or echocardiogram.

In the last few years, it has become clear that patients treated with anthracycline may experience a delayed subclinical cardiac dysfunction, whose incidence increases with age and is progressive in time. The Surveillance Epidemiology and End Result (SEER) data suggest that this complication may eventually lead to clinical cardiac insufficiency, because the diagnosis of congestive heart failure becomes more common with time among breast cancer patients who have received adjuvant chemotherapy than among those treated without chemotherapy.[42-43] It is not clear at present whether this complication may be prevented.

Dementia. An important and yet unresolved question is whether the common complication known as "chemobrain" may lead to dementia in older individuals, whose cognitive reserve is more limited than that of younger people. Reviewing the SEER data, Henke et al. reported that the diagnosis of dementia increased among older

women treated with adjuvant chemotherapy for breast cancer.[44] Other authors failed to confirm these findings.[45] Perhaps the most important question is not whether the diagnosis of dementia increases after chemotherapy but whether a degree of cognitive decline occurs that leads to functional dependence, and whether it may be prevented or ameliorated. This question can only be addressed with a prospective study.

Functional Dependence. In addition to the prolongation of survival, prolongation of active life expectancy is a major goal of geriatrics. Unfortunately, at present there are few data related to the functional consequences of cancer treatment. Studies conducted at the authors' institution suggested that:

- Functional dependence was more common among older breast cancer survivors who had been treated with chemotherapy.[8,46-47]
- Fatigue, which is almost universal in older cancer patients,[48] may be an important harbinger of functional dependence.[8] The interaction of fatigue and functional dependence has been reported in the geriatric population by other authors.[9-10]

The issue is one of the most important in geriatric oncology and needs to be studied prospectively. The most urgent questions to address include:

- Does functional dependence increase with time in older individuals treated with chemotherapy?
- Is functional dependence reversible?
- Which intervention may prevent or reverse functional dependence?

Delayed Complications

Secondary Leukemia and Myelodysplastic Syndrome. Chemotherapy related acute myeloid leukemia (AML) and myelodysplastic syndromes (MDS) account for 10-20% of all cases of AML.[49,50] Based on registry data, the incidence of AML occurring as a second malignancy, among patients whom treatment is feasible, is about 5%.[51] The high incidence of AML has been attributed to the increasing use of cytotoxic drugs causing DNA damage, and to longer survival of many treated patients.

The majority of secondary leukemias resulting from the use of cytotoxic drugs can be divided into two well-defined groups depending on whether the patient has received alkylating agents (melphalan, cyclophosphamide, nitrogen mustard, etc.), or drugs binding to the enzyme DNA-topoisomerase (etoposide, doxorubicin, daunorubicin, mitoxantrone, etc.).[52-54]

AML secondary to alkylating agents are frequently associated with MDS. These typically develop 5 to 7 years after initial cancer treatment, are associated with abnormalities in chromosomes 5 or 7; and have a poor prognosis. AML secondary to a topoisomerase II reactive drug are not associated with MDS. These typically occur within 5 years of therapy, and are frequently associated with an 11q23 cytogenetic abnormality.[55]

TARGETED THERAPY

This form of therapy was recently introduced and the complications in older individuals are poorly known. The following is a brief summary; for more detailed information, please see Chapter 10.

The incidence of *cardiomyopathy* from trastuzumab increases with age.[56] This complication, which is reversible in most cases, is caused by interference with myocardium trophism. In most cases, treatment with trastuzumab may be resumed without risk once the cardiac function is reversed.

Older individuals may be at increased incidence of *hypertension, thrombosis, and bleeding* when treated with angiogenesis inhibitors, especially bevacizumab.[57-61] Age should not be considered a contraindication to this treatment, but may suggest closer monitoring.

The incidence and severity of *skin toxicity* from tyrosine kinase inhibitors (TKI) may also increase with age.[62] This complication may be ameliorated with early treatment with clindamycin lotion and systemic tetracyclines. If the eczema progresses in spite of these measures, the tyrosine kinase inhibitor should be discontinued to prevent severe desquamative dermatitis that may even be lethal.

It should be emphasized again that the information related to these products and aging is scarce.

A LOOK AT THE FUTURE

With the aging of the population, treatment-related decisions for the management of cancer in older individuals will become more and more common. The basic questions of these decisions involve the balance of benefit and risks. For this purpose, it is essential to know:

- what are these complications;
- how common they are;
- how preventable they are;
- which patients are at increased risk.

As most cancer patients are older than 65, it is mandatory to have an adequate representation of individuals from this age group in all clinical trials, especially in those involving new drugs. The current scarcity of information in this segment of the population is unforgivable. It means that physicians treat most older cancer patients without knowing whether the treatment is beneficial or detrimental.

In the author's opinion, these provisions would go a long way to improve our knowledge and our decision-making process:

- **Phase II studies of all new drugs in patients aged 70 and older, to study the pharmacological**

changes occurring with age. It is known that after age 70, intestinal absorption, renal excretion, hepatic metabolism, and total body water all decline. In addition, the functional reserve of some systems that are targets of toxicity, such as the hemopoietic system and the mucosa may also decline. Thus it is legitimate to expect both pharmacokinetic and pharmacodynamic changes in older individuals.

- **Nationwide (or worldwide) databases of older individuals treated with systemic cancer treatment.** Given the diversity of the geriatric population, important information related to the consequences of these treatments can only be obtained with well-controlled descriptive studies. These studies may also allow the investigators to identify risk factors and to generate predictive models of benefits and risks of cancer treatment. The SEER data, coupled with the Medicare database, have been extremely helpful to identify long-term complications of cancer treatment in people aged 65 and older. These include the increased risk of bone fractures and coronary artery disease in patients treated with LHRH analogs for longer than 1 year; myelodysplasia, acute myeloid leukemia and chronic cardiomyopathy in individuals treated with anthracyclines;[12,42-44,63,64] and possibly the association of dementia and chemotherapy. Unfortunately, the SEER data do not include other variables besides chronologic age and comorbidity. Future databases should include functional dependence, degree of comorbidity, basic laboratory information (hemoglobin, albumin), and presence or absence of geriatric syndromes, and should involve periodic evaluation of function, cognition, nutrition, falls, and other problems that may compromise a person's survival and function. In this way, it may be possible to establish whether cancer treatment is a cause of accelerated aging, a key question in clinical decisions.

- **Utilization of the current predictive model of toxicity to generate new models applicable to the ever-enlarging cancer pharmacopeia.** The Chemotherapy Risk Assessment Scale in High Risk Patients (CRASH) was developed in our institution from the prospective observation of more than 500 patients aged 70 and older. This model predicts both hematological and nonhematological toxicity on the basis of the treatment regimen and individual patient characteristics, and will be presented at ASCO 2010. This model may represent a frame of reference for future study.

- Because functional dependence and cognitive impairments are likely complications of cancer chemotherapy, interventional studies aimed to prevent these complications should be performed with all determinate speed.

- The interaction of frailty and cancer treatment is poorly understood. Since frailty is a key concept in geriatrics, future studies should address the following questions: Is frailty a risk factor for treatment toxicity? Is frailty a complication of treatment? Is frailty reversible?

See expertconsult.com for a complete list of references and web resources for this chapter

SUGGESTED READINGS

1. Alibhai SM, Duong-Hua M, Sutradhar R, et al: Impact of androgen deprivation therapy on cardiovascular disease and diabetes, *J Clin Oncol* 27(21):3452–3458, 2009 Jul 20.
2. Balducci L: Supportive care in elderly cancer patients, *Curr Opin Oncol* 21(4):310–317, 2009 Jul.
3. Blijlevens N, Sonis ST: Palifermin (recombinant keratinocyte growth factor-1): a pleiotropic growth factor with multiple biological activities in preventing chemotherapy- and radiotherapy-induced mucositis, *Annals of Oncology* 18(5): 817–826, 2007.
4. Clarkson JE, Worthington HV, Eden OB: Interventions for treating oral mucositis for patients with cancer receiving treatment, *Cochrane Database Syst Rev*, 2007 April 18 (2): CD001973.
5. Heck JE, Albert SM, Franco R, Gorin SS: Pattern of dementia diagnosis in Surveillance, Epidemiology and End Results breast cancer survivors who use chemotherapy, *J Am Geriatr Soc*, 2008 Aug 4.
6. Floyd JD, Nguyen DT, Lobins RL, et al: Cardiotoxicity of cancer therapy, *J Clin Oncol* 23(30):7685–7696, 2005 Oct 20:Review.
7. Morales L, Pans S, Verschueren K, et al: Prospective study to assess short-term intra-articular and tenosynovial changes in the aromatase inhibitor-associated arthralgia syndrome, *J Clin Oncol* 26(19):3147–3152, 2008 Jul 1.
8. Shahinian VB, Kuo YF, Freeman JL, et al: Risk of fracture after androgen deprivation for prostate cancer, *N Engl J Med* 352(2):154–164, 2005 Jan 13.
9. Smith MR, Egerdie B, Hernández Toriz N, et al: Denosumab in men receiving androgen deprivation therapy for prostate cancer, *N Engl J Med* 361(8):745–755, 2009 Aug 20.
10. Walker M, Ni O: Neuroprotection during chemotherapy: a systematic review, *Am J Clin Oncol* 30(1):82–92, 2007 Feb
11. Leone G, Pagano L, Ben-Yehuda D, Voso MT: Therapy-related leukemia and myelodsplasia: susceptibility and incidence, *Hematologica* 92(10):1389–1398, 2007.
12. Patt DA, Duan Z, Fang S, Hortobagyi GN, Giordano SH: Acute Myeloid Leukemia After Adjuvant Breast Cancer Therapy in Older Women: Understanding Risk citation, *JCO* 25(25):3871–3876, 2007.

Depression and Anxiety in the Older Patient with Cancer: A Case-based Approach

Randall Espinoza

Emotional reactions to and psychological distress from cancer illness are very common and not all are pathological. Included in these frequent responses to cancer are fear, disbelief, apprehension, and rumination, as well as other concerns about the future, disability, disfigurement, cost of care, and being a burden to others. These reactions can occur not only at the time of receiving a cancer diagnosis, but upon learning that a relapse has occurred or that treatment has failed. Distinguishing normal distress, grief, and suffering from psychiatric complications requiring systematic assessment and specific intervention is a daunting task for both the general medical physician and the specialist oncologist. Knowing when to begin a psychiatric treatment or recommend a mental health referral may not always be obvious. These challenges of assessment and treatment are, in general, even more difficult in the older patient who often contends not just with cancer alone, but concurrently with a host of other medical problems, effects of multiple treatments, and accumulating life experiences and personal losses. Among the most common psychiatric complications in cancer, depressive and anxiety disorders are also among the most difficult to manage because of the heterogeneity of presentation and presence of multiple confounds. This chapter discusses the comprehensive evaluation and management of the geriatric oncology patient with depression and anxiety and presents in a case-based approach recommendations for mental health screening and surveillance, psychotropic management, and psychological intervention.

OVERVIEW

With the aging of the population and with the advent of improved cancer detection and advances in oncologic treatment leading to higher survival rates, greater numbers of older adults are at risk for developing cancer and are also living longer with cancer. Indeed, current

---

CASE 15-1   PART 1

Judith is a 76-year-old cancer survivor. She was first diagnosed with breast cancer 8 years ago and underwent a left mastectomy followed by irradiation therapy. She did well until 3 years ago when, after a fall, she was found to have bone metastasis and was started on adjuvant chemotherapy. Her cancer was "in check" and she remained very active and socially engaged. However, over the past year she began to complain of unremitting fatigue and seemed to lose interest in many of her usual activities. Now, for the past 3 months, she is more worried about minor matters, focuses on irrelevant details, and frets over being late for appointments. Her family has noted mood changes, loss of appetite with some weight loss, and an inability to follow conversations. Judith thinks her tiredness and distractibility are the result of poor sleep as she lies awake worrying about her cancer. She adamantly denies feeling depressed or sad, saying instead, "it's my cancer again." She is angry with her oncologist for not finding another regimen to address her recurrence.

Question 1: What is the psychological impact of cancer in the elderly?

Question 2: What are the mental health care needs of the older cancer patient and of the family?

Question 3: What is the prevalence of psychiatric disorders in late-life cancer?

---

estimates are that about 60% of all malignancies occur in persons 65 years or older and, if current population trends persist, by 2020 nearly 70% of all malignancies will occur in the older age group. Importantly, cancer is a leading cause of disability and distress worldwide, yet the psychosocial impact of cancer in the elderly is poorly understood or sufficiently recognized. Consequently, more attention must be focused on the psychological issues in cancer that affect management of the older patient.

As stated, psychological distress can present at any stage of management, and while it should not necessarily be considered pathological, it should be assessed for and addressed proactively. Manifestations of distress are varied and individualized according to the person's unique coping style and strengths, among other factors. Symptoms of psychological distress include somatic complaints such as poor sleep, general aches and pains, stomach upset, lower gastrointestinal distress, and muscle tension, and psychological complaints like inability to focus or concentrate, distractibility, irritability, sadness or feeling blue, or worry about the future. The oncologic provider and treatment staff should be aware of these symptoms, as direct and active supportive measures are quite useful in helping patients adjust and successfully cope, and some research suggests, may prevent further behavioral complications. Helpful interventions include active listening, acknowledgment of distress, validation of concerns, explanation of symptoms or care processes, problem-solving, and reassurance. Importantly, many symptoms are time-limited and resolve spontaneously. However, it is critical that psychological distress be screened for and documented since unusually severe or prolonged distress may lead to ineffective coping and poor decision making, and may indicate that the patient is at high risk for an adverse behavioral outcome or development of a psychiatric disorder. The National Cancer Comprehensive Network (NCCN) recommends use of the "Distress Thermometer" as a simple but very effective tool for assessing patients for distress and following symptoms over time and as a way of determining when further evaluation may be needed.

At the same time that the older patient is being queried for psychological distress, it can be useful to inquire about family and social support, trying to determine if it is available and adequate. The lack of extended support has been identified as a risk factor for psychological complications and possibly poorer adherence to treatment. For example, widowhood and social isolation are established risk factors for depression and substance abuse, which then themselves may lead to missed appointments. The older patient often presents with and relies upon close family and friends and may worry that a cancer illness may place an undue burden on them. Specific needs may include transportation to appointments, in-home help or safety evaluations, assistance with simple household chores or meal preparation, or referral to social service agencies. If the older patient's spouse is also ill, the care burden may fall upon adult children who may be poorly prepared for the additional time commitment required, the financial costs incurred, and the associated schedule disruptions. In addition, for the elderly who are more frail, who are cognitively impaired, or who come from a non-Western or different cultural background, involvement of family and an extended network of friends and caregivers may be instrumental and expected. Coordination of care, identification of key family spokespersons, and family meetings are often essential in the care of the older patient

in general, and with a serious illness like cancer, these communications assume greater importance. When family or caregiver dynamics are ineffectual or impaired, a distressed caregiver network or family may inadvertently contribute to the dismay and worry of the older patient. Finally, family and others may have their own concerns or misconceptions concerning cancer and may be unsure of what to expect or how to assist.

In general, depression and anxiety are not normal consequences of aging. In fact, studies of the prevalence of depression in community-dwelling healthy elderly indicate that the prevalence of major depressive disorders is lower in this age group than in the younger adult population. However, as illness burden accumulates, the prevalence of depression or anxiety in older age groups rises dramatically, whether measured by number, severity, or duration of condition(s). In the cancer population, up to 50% of patients report symptoms of psychiatric disturbance. Yet, determination of the exact prevalence of specific psychiatric disorders is difficult and prevalence estimates have varied widely because of multiple variables such as specific cancer type, study design, or demographics. Overall, prevalence of any psychological disturbance, meaning depression, anxiety, or adjustment disorder, has averaged around 30%. As no studies have focused on the epidemiology of depressive or anxiety disorders in older cancer patients, specific data for the elderly are not available. Nonetheless, a few general comments can still be made. There appears to be a strong association between depression and certain cancer types, notably head and neck, lung, and pancreatic cancers, although the exact mechanism of association is undetermined. While breast cancer in younger women may carry a higher depressive risk because of concerns about attractiveness, fertility, or general self-image, for the older female patient, especially at increasing age, the association appears to diminish. Conversely, the availability of a supportive spouse or partner diminishes the risk of developing depression or other psychological disturbances, so that widowed or single women with breast cancer may carry a higher risk of depression. However, effects of antihormone treatment with age may be another factor for which studies have not adequately controlled. Similarly, for men, prostate cancer appears to carry a higher depressive burden, with younger age at onset, degree of sexual impairment, or complications of intervention or antihormone treatment being other cofactors. As before, the availability of a supportive spouse or partner lowers the risk. In contrast, a high level of caregiver distress seems to be a risk factor for the development of psychiatric problems in older medical patients. Finally, other neurobiological factors of aging likely interact with specific cancer processes to mediate the expression and risk for development of psychiatric disturbances. In particular, acute or chronic stress, effects of tumor markers, immune responses in aging, and general systems resiliency may all play a role.

CASE 15-1	PART 1 SOLUTION

Judith's physician administers the Distress Thermometer and decides to monitor Judith's complaints. She is referred for social service assistance, because she needs transportation when her daughter is not available, and for an in-home occupational therapy safety evaluation. Since she feels alone, she is also referred to a local community breast cancer support group available through her church. Finally, to address her insomnia, she will learn yoga to try to relax before bed.

SCREENING AND DIAGNOSIS OF DEPRESSIVE DISORDERS IN GERIATRIC ONCOLOGY

CASE 15-1	PART 2

Judith comes for a routine appointment 1 month later. Despite general supportive measures, she continues to seem irritable and withdrawn. Her family reports that she no longer attends bridge games or seems to enjoy visits with her grandchildren. Judith still denies feeling depressed or sad. She says, "I'm just frustrated with life."

Question 4: How should assessment for depression be approached?

Question 5: What is the differential diagnosis of depression in an older cancer patient?

Question 6: What tools can be used screening and diagnosis?

While many patients may endorse some types of depressive symptoms, not all are willing to do so; thus determining who may be clinically depressed, or more precisely, who meets formal criteria for a depressive disorder is not always clear. Clinical depression affects physical, behavioral, psychological, and cognitive domains, each to a varying degree and leading to heterogeneity of presentation. Further complicating assessment are age effects and illness-related factors. However, the current diagnosis of a depressive disorder, using DSM-IV TR criteria, does not take into account this multidimensional nature of depression or recognize particular age-related or illness contributions, resulting in the overdiagnosis, underdiagnosis, and misdiagnosis of depression, especially in the elderly or medically ill populations. Criteria for Major Depressive Disorder, according to DSM-IV TR nomenclature used by psychiatrists and most mental health professionals, are listed in Table 15-1 and are outlined following a simple mnemonic "Sig E Caps." Note that symptoms must be present most days for at least 2 weeks continuously, and one symptom must include either depressed mood or anhedonia.

As indicated, when assessing an older patient with cancer, age-related factors should be taken into account; these include individual beliefs about mental illness and expectations about what life might be or mean in one's later years. Some older cohorts of patients view any expression of psychological distress as a sign of personal

TABLE 15-1	DSM-IV TR Criteria for Major Depression

- Diagnosis requires five of nine symptoms present for at least 2 weeks, nearly every day.
- To use the mnemonic one symptom must be:
  - depressed mood **OR**
  - decrease in interest/pleasure

S: suicidal thoughts
I: interest decrease
G: guilt; worthlessness
E: energy decrease
C: cognitive problems
A: appetite/weight change
P: psychomotor changes
S: sleep disturbance

TABLE 15-2	Challenges to Assessing Depression in Older Patients

- Gender differences
  - Men: anger, apathy, anhedonia but not sadness
  - Women: somatic symptoms, dysphoria
- Overexpression of somatic complaints
- Minimization of psychological problems
- Presence of medical comorbidity
  - Symptoms: fatigue, anorexia, insomnia, psychomotor slowing, pain
  - Cognitive impairment: detection and expression
  - Medication side effects
  - Competing time demands
- Presence of psychiatric comorbidity
- Rationalization: by patient, family and/or provider
  - "Reasons to be depressed . . ."
  - Nihilism

weakness or character flaw or with shame. Societal and cultural views often relegate older people to the background or discount their value. Sex differences in expression of psychological distress also exist. Women, because of cultural acceptance and social custom, are more open to disclosing their feelings and emotional concerns and are more accepting of psychological assistance. On the other hand, men generally tend to deny inner mental turmoil, and instead, may display distress in a culturally-sanctioned way such as with anger or aggression or may engage in risky behaviors or turn to substance abuse. Table 15-2 lists factors that confound the assessment of depression in an older person. One critical issue not to overlook is the role of therapeutic nihilism, where patient, family, and/or care provider may collude to try to "explain away" depression as a reasonable consequence of grave illness coupled with life circumstances. If this stance becomes accepted, many patients will likely suffer needlessly; depression contributes to disability and lessens quality of life, but once identified, depression is imminently treatable. Finally, patients older than 75 years who are diagnosed with a serious illness for the first time, those with preexisting cognitive impairment, those with lower levels of education, and those with a

TABLE 15-3	Diagnosing Major Depression in Physically-Ill Elderly

Depression criteria should emphasize:
- change of mood or interest with at least 2 weeks duration;
- nonphysical symptoms;
- social regression or incapacity.

Anorexia, sleep disturbances, fatigue, and motor retardation:
- These should only be considered if they accompany the aforementioned depressive symptoms and cannot be explained by physical illness or its treatment.
- If present at the outset, these symptoms **get worse with mood** and are out of proportion to symptoms expected from medical illness.

past history of depression or substance abuse (usually alcohol) also appear at greater risk for developing clinical depression.

Similarly, illness-related factors can affect each domain separately or in combination, and an identified psychiatric complaint may be due to the cancer illness itself, a complication of the illness, or the effect of a cancer treatment. For example, a brain tumor may affect an area involved with drive or pleasure, pain from cancer may disrupt sleep, or use of steroids may promote irritability. Furthermore, given the prominence of certain symptoms in cancer, to wit, anorexia, fatigue, sleep disturbance, and psychomotor slowing, knowing how and when to attribute a specific symptom to depression or to cancer can be daunting. Thus when approaching any patient with cancer who presents with a psychological or behavioral concern, it is useful to try to undertake an analysis of what may be driving the complaint in order to arrive at the correct diagnosis and best solution. There are clues to help guide when a depressive symptom may be caused by a psychiatric disorder rather than to cancer or a related cancer treatment. One of the most important is the temporal relationship between the psychiatric complaint and physical illness. In most cases, a mood or behavioral change will precede a worsening of any physical component, and to add further support to a diagnosis of a depressive disorder, physical symptoms will co-vary with depressive symptoms in a proportional relationship: as depressive symptoms worsen, so will physical complaints. Table 15-3 lists additional clues to help make the diagnosis of depression when serious medical illness is present and confounds assessment. It is also worth noting that it is the degree of functional impairment resulting from illness that appears to be the greater risk factor for development of depression, especially if the older person loses a fair degree of independence or mobility and if this change occurs abruptly with little time to adjust to or accept this change. How the caregiver or spouse responds to this impairment is another critical factor. Caregivers who become anxious or distressed about the cancer diagnosis or with complications of cancer treatment can often adversely affect the mood and

well-being of the patient. Having involved the caregiver at the outset of management may provide an opportunity either to assess the caregiver for treatment or to recommend a separate referral.

DIFFERENTIAL DIAGNOSIS OF DEPRESSION IN THE OLDER PATIENT WITH CANCER

While the previous discussion has focused on the diagnosis of major depression, it is important not to overlook what is involved, generally speaking, in the differential diagnosis. Included here are other medical illnesses and effects of medications or treatments, other depressive and psychiatric disorders, and life circumstances. Table 15-4 lists some considerations.

When a medical problem is found to be etiologically related or causal to the mood disorder, a diagnosis of Mood Disorder due to General Medical Condition is made. Treating the underlying medical problem may address the mood components, although frequently additional psychotropic or psychological management will be needed. However, another main point is that while major depression can present with physical complaints, many medical conditions also present with depressive symptoms, that is, depressive symptoms are not pathognomonic, and thus a careful history is critical to determining which problem is primary. For the older patient, while much of the focus will necessarily be on the management of cancer, new medical conditions can arise and exacerbations of preexisting problems may occur. Furthermore, depression can coexist with cancer, or any other medical problem, and often does. In the older patient, particular mention must be made of dementia and delirium, both of which occur more commonly with age and with increasing medical stressors or use of multiple medications. Since dementia prevalence rises with age and given that a longer life span also exposes people to a greater risk of cancer and to living with cancer, it is reasonable to expect that more patients will be afflicted with both dementia and cancer. How each condition might affect the other in terms of assessment or management is poorly understood. What is known is that the presence of dementia may influence the expression of depression, obscure its detection, or may confuse assessment. Alzheimer disease (AD), the most common type of dementia in later life, is often accompanied by a depressive complication, and indeed, up to 40% of AD patients by some estimates will experience depression over their course of illness. Importantly, studies show that depression in dementia is treatable with medications and with behavioral or psychological approaches, although the extent of improvement and durability of response varies, as would be expected in a neurodegenerative process. With regard to delirium, the main risk is in overlooking this important diagnosis. Untreated delirium carries a high mortality risk and may be a poor prognostic sign in a frail

TABLE 15-4	Differential Diagnosis of Depression in the Older Cancer Patient

Medical	**Medications**

Medical
- Endocrinopathies
- Metabolic derangement
- Infections
- Cardiopulmonary disease
- GI disorders
- Inflammatory processes
- Hematological conditions
- Musculoskeletal problems
- Delirium

Neurological
- Cerebrovascular disease
- Primary or metastatic tumor
- Basal ganglia disease
- Dementia

Medications
- Antihypertensives
- Analgesics (opiates)
- CNS depressants
- Chemotherapeutics

Psychiatric
- Adjustment disorder
- Anxiety disorder
- Substance-induced disorder
- Substance Abuse or Dependence disorder

Life Circumstances
- Grief and bereavement
- Social isolation/loneliness
- Poverty

GI, gastrointestinal; CNS, central nervous system.

TABLE 15-5	Common Chemotherapeutic Agents Associated with Depressive Symptoms

Corticosteroids
Vinblastine
Vincristine
Vinorelbine
Interferon
Procarbazine
Asparaginase
Tamoxifen
Cyproterone

older patient, especially if it does not clear and becomes chronic. From a psychiatric perspective, the concern for delirium is highest in medically ill patients with an abrupt onset of depressive symptoms, the presence of psychosis or acute suicidal ideation, or a history of substance abuse or polypharmacy. In addition, delirium should be considered in the differential diagnosis of patients who are hospitalized, who present to the emergency room, or whose cognitive profile appears at odds with their baseline.

When a medication or substance is thought to explain the mood disturbance, a diagnosis of Substance-Induced Mood Disorder is made, and removing the offending agent may result in improvement of the underlying behavioral problem. However, separating specific agents to see which is related to particular mood symptoms is often daunting if not impossible. With regard to the older patient, age-related changes in pharmacokinetics and pharmacodynamics are also relevant but remain understudied where cancer is concerned. The best clue again derives from history and determining whether the drug, when given, was temporally associated with induction of the observed mood or behavioral change. When a medication that seems to promote depressive feelings must be used to treat an underlying medical problem or manage a symptom, it is worth trying to find a drug with the desired effect but a different side-effect profile, from a different class or with a different mechanism of action. Similarly, other iatrogenic causes of depression cannot be overlooked; these situations usually involve polypharmacy, where drug-drug interactions are most likely a result of the sheer number of medications prescribed, and where drug monitoring is often inadequate and is more challenging the more providers are involved in a given patient's care. In management of an older patient, it may be unusually challenging to separate out the effects of

narcotics on mood, cognition, and behavior, especially in the presence of pain, which, if inadequately treated, is itself a risk factor for depression. Here clinical judgment must be used and careful attention placed on the goals of pain management. Determining if and when pain control has been achieved and has led to the desired outcomes can be a helpful guide. Encouraging the use of alternative and complementary forms of pain management may be another option for the older patient with cancer. Importantly, narcotics should never be withheld for fear of promoting addiction or dependency in a patient with cancer, especially in the terminal phase of illness. Finally, it is critical not to overlook that untreated depression can amplify the perception of pain or other distressing physical symptoms, so that effectively treating any underlying depressive disorder may also result in improvement in pain.

The previous list does not include specific concerns about chemotherapeutic agents. These are listed in Table 15-5. However, much controversy surrounds this association and the causal links have yet to be definitively proven. Nonetheless, caution should be followed when a cancer patient on one of these medications develops depressive symptoms for the first time after commencement. Further study is needed.

Other depressive disorders are possible in the older cancer patient and should be considered when symptoms are either of short duration or inadequate in number to meet DSM-IV-TR criteria for major depression. Importantly, while falling short of the full syndrome, these symptoms remain clinically meaningful and can adversely affect health outcomes, increase cost of care, and lower quality of life. If unresolved, these disorders also place patients at increased risk of developing major depression over the next year. Included in this category are the DSM-IV-TR diagnoses Subsyndromal Depression, which encompasses Minor Depression, Non-Dysphoric Depression, and Brief Reactive Depression; Dysthymia, which is diagnosed when symptoms of low-grade depression last for 2 years or longer; and Adjustment Disorder with depressed, anxious, or mixed mood. With regard to the last, adjustment disorder is an abnormal excessive reaction to a life stressor such as a new serious illness like cancer, getting divorced, or death of a loved

TABLE 15-6	Screening Instruments for Depression in Older Patients						
	Sensitivity	Specificity	Inpatient	Outpatient	Physically Ill	Cognitively Impaired	Responsiveness to Change
1 or 2-Question Screen	97%	67%	No	Yes	Yes	No	Limited
GDS 30, 15 item	94%	81%	Yes	Yes	Yes	Variable	Good
CSDD (19-item)	90%	75%	Yes	Yes	Unknown	Yes	Good
CES-D (20-item)	93%	73%	No	Yes	Yes	No	Good
PHQ-9	88%	88%	No	Yes	Yes	Unknown	Very Good

one, and usually begins within 3 months of onset of the stressor. Once the stressor or its consequences has terminated, symptoms resolve and should not persist beyond 6 months. Closer surveillance of these patients is suggested. Treatment of adjustment disorder is supportive and usually psychosocial and behavioral in nature rather than pharmacological.

It can be very difficult to separate out an anxiety disorder from clinical depression, given the overlap of symptoms between the two conditions. Indeed, anxiety can be a component of depression in some patients, and a certain subtype called Mixed Anxiety Depression or Anxious Depression may be more common in the elderly. Furthermore, a person can have both an anxiety disorder and a depressive disorder. Anxiety may also be a normal reaction to the diagnosis of cancer and may be part of a normal stress response. However, anxiety is not a disorder of mood, so depressed and sad feelings are absent, and anxiety does not affect interests or ability to derive pleasure. The section that follows more fully discusses assessment and management of anxiety disorders in older patients with cancer.

An often overlooked consideration in the older patient is substance abuse or dependence, either from a common substance such as alcohol or from prescription medications. When cancer enters into consideration, assessment can be confusing and management can quickly become problematic. A patient who is actively abusing cannot be reliably assessed, and every effort should be made to have the patient abstain for a sufficient period to allow for a more accurate accounting of symptoms. However, this area is controversial and not sufficiently studied in the older population or, specifically, in the situation of older cancer patients. Importantly, older patients with a past history of substance abuse or dependence appear to be at higher risk for developing depression in the context of serious illness.

Finally, life circumstances themselves may be demoralizing and discouraging, and separating out appropriate responses to these types of challenges can be daunting but should not be overlooked, minimized, or deemed pathological. Personal losses begin to accumulate and

grief and bereavement, which are unavoidable, should be recognized first as normal reactions. Financial difficulties may mount, especially when faced with expensive medical treatment on a fixed income. After children and despite the availability of Medicare and Social Security, the elderly have the highest poverty rates, with older single women being most at risk for impoverishment due to a catastrophic illness. To help defray the cost of care, an older person may be forced to move from a longtime home or into a new living arrangement. With aging, a person may undertake a life review and think of past deeds, of lost opportunities, or of poor choices made and look back with regret or sadness. Finally, with age, awareness of mortality and of limited time remaining enters into consciousness, which may precipitate an existential or spiritual crisis with anxiety, panic, and despair as prominent symptoms. Thoughts of death begin to appear and enter into usual discussion, not as a symptom of suicidal ideation, but as recognition of this final stage of life. If resolved successfully, distressing symptoms subside to be replaced with peace, gratitude, and calmness.

Screening and Assessment Tools

For all the issues discussed previously, depression can be challenging to detect and diagnose in older patients with cancer. While the "Distress Thermometer" provides a simple and systematic way of identifying patients who may require heightened surveillance for psychological distress, it has yet to be effectively compared to other "gold standard" self-report or clinician-administered depression screening or diagnostic instruments that are often recommended for use in older patient samples. However, a further question is whether these latter instruments, while validated in groups of older medically ill patients, have been specifically studied in older patients with cancer. The short answer is no. Notwithstanding the lack of studies, given the importance and prevalence of depression, it remains reasonable to suggest use of screening measures and other diagnostic tools in this population until data become available. These instruments and some psychometric properties are listed in Table 15-6.

Applying the one- or two-item Patient Health Questionnaire (PHQ) screens, along with the Distress Thermometer, can be an efficient strategy to identify the patient at risk for depression. The one-item question is, "Do you often feel sad or depressed?" and can be easily asked by staff at check-in or during a routine visit. The PHQ-2 screen asks, "Over the past 2 weeks, how often have you been bothered by: (1) a lack of interest; or (2) feeling sad or depressed?" These questions are rated on a scale of 0 to 3 (range from 0 to 6) with a positive score being 3 or greater. However, if the patient screens positive on one of these questions, further assessment should follow with a diagnostic instrument such as the Center for Epidemiological Studies-Depression Scale (CES-D), Geriatric Depression Scale (GDS, various forms available), Patient Health Questionnaire-9 (PHQ-9), or, if the patient is cognitively impaired, with the Cornell Scale for Depression in Dementia (CSDD). Most of these scales can be administered in about 3 to 10 minutes. A unique feature of the CSDD is the incorporation of observer or caregiver feedback on the patient. Lastly, except for the one- or two-item screeners, most can be used both to gauge severity of depression and to follow change from treatment, so that systematic use of the tools over time, e.g., weekly or monthly, can help guide the effectiveness of interventions or the need for additional specialist mental health referral. However, it is critical to keep in mind that a number of scale attributes should be considered when using these in a geriatric cancer setting. These include the time period assessed (past week or 2 weeks, for example), completion time and item length, variable assessment of multiple mood symptoms, impact of concomitant cognitive impairment, and phrasing of individual items such as hopelessness, which may have contextual importance and differing meaning depending on the patient's age or stage of illness. Except for the PHQ-9, which queries for all depressive symptom domains according to current DSM-IV-TR criteria, the advantage of the other identified tools is the reliance primarily on the psychological symptoms of depression.

CASE 15-1 PART 2 SOLUTION

Because Judith scored positive on the PHQ-2 screen, her physician administers the full PHQ-9 to assess her depression severity and obtain a baseline score. A review of her medication list does not reveal any apparent association between her mood complaints and her current medications. In fact, it appears that as her mood has worsened, her pain and fatigue symptoms have worsened. Her chart shows that she had an episode of depression about 8 years ago when she underwent her mastectomy and worried about disfigurement; thus she is at high risk of recurrence now that she has experienced a cancer relapse. However, since she will be starting a new chemotherapy regimen, the decision is made to follow her closely and reassess whether there was any change in her mood in a couple of weeks.

TREATMENT AND MANAGEMENT OF DEPRESSION IN THE OLDER PATIENT WITH CANCER

CASE 15-1 PART 3

Judith returns to her physician's office, still feeling terrible and complaining of pain. She is not sleeping well and feels more hopeless about her condition. She asks about euthanasia and moving to a locale where physician-assisted suicide is available.

Question 7: What are the serious consequences of depression?

Question 8: What treatment options are available? How are these chosen?

Question 9: What approach should be used for medication selection and monitoring?

Complications of Depression

Many of the same complications that can occur in depression are also possible in an older cancer patient. Morbidity increases, as does the risk of mortality from both medical and psychiatric causes. For example, depression is associated with increased mortality from heart disease, stroke, and cancer. Management of pain, insomnia, fatigue, and anorexia, common symptoms in cancer in general, becomes more challenging in the presence of comorbid depression. Furthermore, untreated depression adds to overall health care burden, increases cost of care, and lowers quality of life, the latter being of particular concern in the oncologic population, especially when entering chronic management phases or the terminal stage of illness. Depression is also associated with increased prescription drug use and an increased risk for substance abuse, especially alcohol, which may be overlooked in the elderly population. Depression alters motivation and outlook, so that adherence to medication, treatment, or office visits may decline. Among the most serious psychiatric consequences of depression in the elderly are inanition, catatonia, psychosis, dementia of depression, and suicide. Table 15-7 lists features of these complications in the older oncologic patient and some suggested treatment options will be discussed.

While development of any of these complications will likely prompt a psychiatric referral for evaluation, the primary care or oncologic provider should be aware of their presentations since these providers, rather than mental health professionals, will be the first to encounter these patients. In a more serious or gravely ill patient, states of inanition from depression can be difficult to identify, especially in the presence of aggressive interventions or particularly toxic chemotherapy. Similarly, catatonia can occur in patients with marked metabolic derangements or other primary medical problems, so a thorough evaluation will be needed in this situation before deciding that catatonia is a complication of a serious mood disorder. Patients who are psychotic may not overtly or spontaneously endorse this material,

TABLE 15-7	Complications of Depression in the Older Oncologic Patient		
		Treatment Options	
Condition	**Presentation**	**Somatic**	**Hospital**
Inanition	Marked by dehydration, weight loss, and severe functional impairment; appears delirious	Medications; ECT if no improvement	Medical or psychiatric depending on status
Catatonia	Marked by mutism, extreme withdrawal, negativism, motoric blunting or excitement, refusal of food or drink	ECT is first choice treatment	Likely psychiatric
Psychosis	Involves delusions of poverty, jealousy, nihilism, loss of body parts, fear of poisoning, paranoia, illusions, or frank hallucinations May be subtle and hard to detect if not specifically asked	Antidepressant plus antipsychotic; ECT if no improvement	Outpatient if support is available Psychiatric if refusing care or behavior is compromised
Dementia of Depression	Manifests with slowed information processing, confusion, poor attention and concentration, retrieval memory deficits, poor executive function	Medications; cognitive retraining; close surveillance	Likely outpatient unless other symptoms or caregiver stress
Suicide	Passive thoughts of death and dying, hopelessness, no future Active ideation may involve plans as well as intent	Medications; ECT if acute; requires frequent assessment	Depends on acuity and seriousness. Likely psychiatric

*ECT, electroconvulsive therapy

so specific query must be made about any unusual or uncharacteristic thoughts. Often, fear prevents patients from talking about these ideas, so that a sympathetic and trusted ear may facilitate uncovering of psychotic thinking. The older medically compromised patient is also at greater risk of developing significant cognitive impairment when seriously depressed, so that the patient may appear to be demented. This problem is worrisome for at least two reasons. First, older patients are at increased risk of developing dementia, so that a misdiagnosis or missed diagnosis of one or the other condition is possible. Second, should an older depressed patient develop this extent of cognitive impairment, the chances of converting to dementia over the next 3 to 5 years is high. However, unlike cognitive impairment due to dementia, which is rarely if ever reversible, the dementia of depression responds to appropriate depression treatment with a full recovery and ensuing improvement in cognitive deficits.

Of particular concern is the development and management of suicidal thinking. Most patients who completed suicide were never seen or treated by mental health practitioners, and some studies show that the majority of patients were in contact with their primary care physician within the last month of their life. Suicide rates are highest in the elderly population; both acute and chronic risk factors have been identified. These are listed in Table 15-8. Apart from identifying sociodemographic risk factors of suicide, which cannot be modified or easily corrected, it is critical to know those acute risk factors that are amenable to treatment and on which quick action and intervention can be lifesaving.

Sociodemographic risk factors include older age; white race followed by Native American ethnicity; and male sex, especially when single, divorced, or widowed. Other

TABLE 15-8	Acute and Chronic Risk Factors for Suicide in the Older Patient with Cancer
Acute	**Chronic**
Active symptoms: • Suicidal ideation • Impulsivity • Insomnia or sleep disturbance • Restlessness or agitation • Anxiety, fear or panic • Psychosis • Intoxication • Poorly controlled pain • Delirium • Hopelessness Organized or lethal plan Recent loss or widowhood Recurrence of cancer Failure of cancer treatment	Social isolation Financial strain Past psychiatric history (mood, schizophrenic, substance abuse, or personality disorder) Past history of suicide attempt Family history of suicide Past use of opioid analgesics, CNS depressants, or benzodiazepines Poorer physical functioning or impairment Chronic or multiple medical illness Chronic pain Prior brain injury Metastatic or advanced oncologic disease

risk factors include social isolation, poor or ambivalent family relationships, and financial strain. Being aware of or asking about a precipitating event can also be helpful. Inquiring about access to lethal means, especially firearms, is a critical part of any suicide assessment.

However, protective factors buffer individuals from suicidal thoughts and behavior. To date, protective factors have not been studied as extensively or rigorously as risk factors in older oncologic populations. Identifying and understanding protective factors is, nonetheless, equally as important as researching risk factors. Protective factors include effective clinical care for mental, physical, and substance abuse disorders; easy access to a variety of clinical interventions and support for help-seeking; family and community support and support from ongoing medical and mental health care relationships; skills in problem solving, conflict resolution, and nonviolent ways of handling disputes; and cultural and religious beliefs that discourage suicide and support instincts for self-preservation. Finally, patients who require immediate intervention or psychiatric assessment are those with a formed plan with a high degree of lethality and with high intent. That is, providers should take into account the chances of success of a suicide plan. The older patient with cancer may be frailer or more physically impaired, so that chances of survival from even a seemingly minor attempt may be diminished. Highly lethal means include gunshot wounds, overdose on multiple medications, hanging, and jumping.

A difficulty can arise, however, in distinguishing between the patient who is less acutely or actively suicidal with no firm plan or denial of intent from the patient in the terminal phase of illness who views life as essentially complete and desires a hastened death. Here the prior relationship with the primary care or oncologic provider can be extremely useful in determining whether the ideas: (1) relate to suicide (whether actively or passively pursuing actual death albeit with a measure of ambivalence); (2) are part of a normal developmental stage in late life; or (3) reflect a realistic assessment of terminal treatment stage. In the first situation, patients are generally distressed and ashamed of having suicidal thoughts and seek refuge and understanding from a provider who they know, and they fear rejection, abandonment, or being labeled psychologically impaired. Furthermore, in the older oncologic patient, who may have already faced many personal losses, the idea of death itself may be less sinister or tragic, but the fear of painful dying may remain quite real. The expression of suicidal thinking or of wanting to die may then be a way of communicating with the medical team and seeking reassurance that pain can and will be controlled. In this case, a measured empathetic response with more frequent monitoring and specific query about suicide is useful and usually sufficient. A patient who experiences sharing of distressful thoughts in a safe and nonjudgmental manner is more likely to call or make contact should his or her suicide plan or intent change. Thus, a relationship of trust and empathy, while no guarantee of avoidance of an adverse outcome from suicide, can be essential in a patient disclosing these suicidal ideas in the first place or in agreeing to contact the provider should the intensity or quality of ideation worsen. In the second scenario, with increasing age, awareness of mortality and death may lead to an existential or spiritual crisis that is not necessarily abnormal. An older person may have general thoughts of wanting to die or being ready to die, which are not always synonymous with suicidal thinking. Successful navigation of this psychological developmental stage results in acceptance and satisfaction with prior life choices and manifests as peace and calmness and an openness to discussion of life and its personally held meaning. Fear and distress are typically absent here and there is no devised plan of exit. Spiritual counseling, if the patient is so inclined, can be extremely comforting. In the last case, an older patient in the terminal phase of illness with thoughts of wanting to die or forgoing treatment may be expressing a wish to maintain ultimate control over intolerable pain or suffering and a desire to preserve dignity. Management includes maintaining a supportive relationship, assuring the availability of comfort care and conveying the attitude that much can be done to improve quality of life. It is critical to actively solicit and treat specific symptoms. Involvement of family or friends can make the experience less lonely and less dreadful. Open and frank discussion of poor prognosis shows patients they are valued, encourages their participation in treatment planning to the extent possible, and fosters dignity.

MANAGEMENT OF DEPRESSION

Before deciding upon an intervention, the patient should be assessed for past history of depressive episodes and substance abuse, family psychiatric history including history of depression and/or suicide, concurrent life stressors, losses due to cancer, and availability of social support. Assessment of the patient's experience with cancer deaths, of the meaning of illness, and of the patient's understanding of his or her illness and its prognosis is also important. Depression in older cancer patients can be treated with nonpharmacologic approaches such as psychotherapy or behavioral therapy, as well as with pharmacotherapy. The decision on which intervention to pursue is made on the basis of patient or family preference, severity or duration of illness, past history of response, and possibly, cancer prognosis. Usually, a combination of approaches provides the best chance for optimal improvement. However, it is important to recognize that adequate randomized controlled trials of depression treatment in the older patient across all stages of cancer illness are lacking and much of what is recommended is extrapolated from metanalyses or from studies in other medical groups or younger populations of cancer patients.

PSYCHOTHERAPY

In general, the goals of psychotherapy are to reduce emotional distress and to improve morale, coping ability, self-esteem, sense of control, and resolution of problems. Psychotherapy may be delivered on an individual basis, in group settings, or in couples or family sessions. Various forms of psychotherapy as listed in Table 15-9 have been studied in the general oncologic population; psychotherapy can be considered for use as a stand-alone treatment and not just as an adjunct to medication. Psychotherapy providers include psychiatrists, psychologists, nurses and

TABLE 15-9	Psychotherapy Treatment Models for Older Cancer Patients	
Model	**Goals**	**Sample Techniques**
Psycho-education	Provide explanation of illness and treatment processes.	Describe illness stages. Discuss treatment options.
Supportive	Strengthen self-esteem and sense of control.	Allow ventilation and validation of concerns. Model active listening.
Cognitive-behavioral (CBT)	Alter maladaptive coping skills or negative thoughts.	Identify underlying emotions and triggers. Reframe negative thoughts. Correct distortions.
Problem-solving	Address specific concerns and impediments to wellness.	Define and formulate problem. Generate alternative solutions.
Insight-oriented	Understand threat to self and meaning of illness.	Explore meaning of illness. Delineate defense mechanisms.
Grief	Adapt to loss and functional decline.	Identify role changes and challenges. Attach new meaning to experiences.
Existential	Provide meaning in life.	Search for meaningful activities and endeavors. Seek context for illness.
Complementary medicine	Access all available means of support and benefit.	Try music, meditation, yoga, acupuncture, and/or massage.
Spiritual counseling	Address spiritual concerns.	Discuss religious views on suffering and death.

social workers, although there may be limitations on the availability of adequately trained geriatric therapists with experience in treating medically ill populations. However, many useful techniques, such as active listening with encouraging comments, can be done by staff in the primary care or oncologic setting. It may be helpful to set aside some time during an office visit to specifically address emotional concerns and apply these supportive measures. The decision on whether to pursue psychotherapy is made on the basis of several factors including patient preference or values, concerns about polypharmacy, and severity or type of depression. Some patients may prefer to talk about their emotional problems rather than take a mind-altering drug, which may reflect a generational attitude about psychotropic treatment. Older patients with multiple medical problems may already be on several medications so that drug-drug interactions or sensitivity to drugs may be of concern. Finally, in the older patient with milder or briefer forms of depression and with limited functional impact, response to medication may be limited or modest and response to psychotherapy superior along with producing longer sustained improvement.

BEHAVIORAL APPROACHES

Recently, interest in other nonpharmacologic treatments for depression in older patients has grown amid reports that somatic symptoms like fatigue, insomnia, and pain, in particular, may be more amenable to these treatments. These options are listed in Table 15-10. Benefits include better acceptance, improved socialization, fewer adverse effects, and avoidance of polypharmacy. Notably, these options can be combined safely with medications if needed.

TABLE 15-10	Behavioral Approaches for Management of Depression in Older Cancer Patients
Strategy	**Comments**
Exercise	Includes both cardiovascular fitness and strength/resistance training
CBT-I	Specific form of CBT that addresses insomnia, fatigue and pain
Meditation	Helpful for both patient and caregiver; used in different settings
Yoga	Helpful for both patient and caregiver; used in different settings
Acupuncture	Limited but promising studies in older patients

Cognitive-behavioral therapy for insomnia (CBT-I), a specific form of CBT, has recently been developed and looks to be very promising in the treatment of cancer-related fatigue and insomnia, although specific study in the older oncologic population is lacking. The benefits of exercise appear to be greater in mild to moderate forms of depression, in patients with sedentary or inactive lifestyles and significant medical comorbidity including cardiac disease and dementia, and for those residing in long-term care facilities. Caregivers who experience depression because of increased stress and care burden also appear responsive to yoga and meditation.

PHARMACOLOGIC OPTIONS

Although there are many reports on the efficacy of antidepressants in depressed patients with cancer, there are no randomized, placebo controlled trials in the older oncologic population. This observation reflects the difficulty in conducting controlled studies of drugs in medically ill cancer patients. Nonetheless, there is much clinical experience with antidepressant drugs in this population. A specific antidepressant is often chosen on the basis of its side-effect profile, as on the whole, all medications are equally efficacious in treating depression and there is as yet no definitive evidence that newer drugs have any greater efficacy than older drugs in treatment of most forms of depression. The antidepressant agents that are better tolerated in patients with comorbid depression and medical conditions, including cancer, are the newer agents, which encompass the serotonin reuptake inhibitors (SRIs) and the novel or mixed action antidepressants. Tricyclic antidepressants (TCAs) and psychostimulants are reserved for use in selected patients. Mood stabilizers and monoamine oxidase inhibitors (MAOIs) will not be discussed here. Table 15-11 lists antidepressant drugs and some dosage recommendations, along with broad comments on their use. Note that antidepressants obtainable in the United States are only available in oral or possibly sublingual-dissolving form, so that it is not feasible to use them for patients who cannot take anything by mouth.

In general, SRIs are considered first-line treatment of depressive disorders in the older adult because of their better tolerability, ease of use, and general safety, especially in overdose. All SRIs are equally efficacious, with depressive symptoms improving after 4 to 8 weeks of a therapeutic dose. However, some studies suggest that in older populations the full effect may not be seen until after 12 or 16 weeks, so it is critical to assure patient adherence to medication. The most common class side effects are nausea, loose stool, headache, sleep disturbance (either somnolence or insomnia), sexual dysfunction, and a brief period of increased anxiety, restlessness, or even akathisia. This brief period of restlessness or increased anxiety usually occurs at the initiation of treatment, especially if the dosage is begun too high. These drugs may cause appetite suppression lasting a period of several weeks, which may be of concern in the older and frailer patient who may not have any excess weight to lose. Interestingly, after a period of weight loss or reduced appetite, some patients then experience carbohydrate craving and weight gain, but the amount is difficult to predict and is not seen uniformly in older populations. Other potential side-effects that may be more worrisome in the older patient include hyponatremia due to SIADH, sinus bradycardia, and bleeding due to an antiplatelet effect. Specific SRIs, as listed in Table 15-11, are also more prone to drug-drug interactions via cytochrome P450 mechanisms.

Although the SRIs share a similar side effect profile, there are some clinically relevant differences. Fluoxetine, for example, has the longest half-life (5 weeks) and an active metabolite norfluoxetine, which results in little, if any, risk of SRI discontinuation syndrome with abrupt cessation. Because of the relative short half-life (24 hours) of the other SRIs, patients are at risk for developing significant psychiatric, neurologic, gastrointestinal, or flu-like symptoms after abrupt withdrawal. Paroxetine causes the most anticholinergic side effects of the SRIs and causes the most weight gain. Fluvoxamine and paroxetine are more sedating, whereas fluoxetine can be activating. The former are often chosen for highly anxious patients, whereas fluoxetine is used for patients with apathy or low energy. Sertraline, citalopram, and escitalopram have fewer drug interactions, whereas fluvoxamine has the most, and this feature often limits its use.

While not specifically addressing the older oncologic patient, studies of citalopram, sertraline, fluoxetine, and mirtazapine have been shown to treat interferon-α–induced depression in clinical trials of patients with hepatitis C or cancer.

The novel and mixed-action antidepressants (venlafaxine, desvenlafaxine, duloxetine, bupropion, nefazodone, trazodone, and mirtazapine) differ from the SRIs in their mechanism of action, resulting in their different side effect profiles. Venlafaxine, desvenlafaxine, and duloxetine are serotonin/norepinephrine uptake inhibitors, with venlafaxine inhibiting serotonin reuptake at lower doses, thereby sharing some of the side effects of the SRIs while inhibiting norepinephrine reuptake at higher doses. Both duloxetine and venlafaxine have been shown to improve neuropathic pain and peripheral neuropathy in cancer patients. However, venlafaxine, desvenlafaxine, and duloxetine in a dose-dependent manner may contribute to diastolic hypertension. Bupropion is primarily a noradrenergic agent that increases dopamine reuptake at higher doses. Its stimulating effects may be beneficial to the depressed cancer patient with fatigue or excessive daytime sedation. Bupropion has fewer gastrointestinal side effects than the SRIs, but can induce diastolic hypertension in a dose-dependent manner. It increases the risk for seizures at higher doses, typically above 450 mg total, and should be avoided or used with caution in patients with seizure disorders, traumatic brain injury, or CNS pathology. Interestingly, it can assist in smoking cessation and has minimal effect on weight or sexual functioning. Although rare, it may contribute to confusion or psychotic symptoms because of its effect on dopamine. Venlafaxine, trazodone, mirtazapine, and some SRIs are useful in managing hot flashes. Trazodone may be used for its sedating properties and in low doses (50-100 mg at bedtime) is helpful in the treatment of the depressed cancer patient with insomnia. At higher doses, trazodone can cause orthostatic hypotension, thereby increasing the risk for falls. It has also been associated with priapism, and therefore should be used with caution in men. Concern about possible liver toxicity with nefazodone often limits its use, although it has mild calming effects, may promote better sleep architecture, and has less orthostatic risk compared to trazodone. Mirtazapine is a noradrenergic and specific serotonergic antidepressant. It has low affinity for muscarinic, cholinergic, and dopaminergic receptors, but a high affinity for H_1 histaminic receptors. It also antagonizes 5-HT$_3$ receptors. On the

TABLE 15-11	Antidepressant Medications used in Older Cancer Patients			
Drug (Generic Name)	**Starting Dosage mg (p.o.)**	**Therapeutic Range mg (p.o.), dosing***	**CYP450 Effects**	**Comments (See Text for Details)**
SRI Class				
Citalopram	5-10	10-60, qam or qhs	Not likely	Generally well-tolerated; expect fewer drug interactions
Escitalopram	2.5-5	5-20, qam or qhs	Not likely	Not yet generic; may be activating; fewer drug interactions
Fluoxetine	2.5-5	10-60, qam	2D6	Long half-life; available in elixir; moderate drug interactions
Fluvoxamine	12.5-25	50-300, bid or qhs	3A4 inhibitor	More sedating; expect more drug interactions
Paroxetine	5-10	10-60, qhs	2D6	More sedating; more anticholinergic; more weight gain?
Sertraline	12.5-25	25-200, qam or qhs	2C9, 2D6	Can be activating; possible Parkinsonism; drug interactions
Dual Action or Mixed Agents				
Bupropion extended release	75-100	100-450, qam	2D6 inhibitor	Activating; used in smoking cessation; risk for seizures
Desvenlafaxine	50	50-100, qam	3A4 substrate	Activating; not generic; may elevate diastolic BP
Duloxetine	20	40-120, qam to bid	2D6 inhibitor	Activating; not generic; may elevate diastolic BP
Mirtazapine	7.5-15	15-60, qhs	3A4 substrate	Less sedating at higher dosages; may promote weight gain
Nefazodone	25-50	150-600, bid or qhs	3A4 inhibitor	Generic only available; potent inhibitor; possible liver toxicity
Trazodone	12.5-50	25-300, qhs	3A4 substrate	Sedating; orthostasis at higher doses limits antidepressant use
Venlafaxine extended release	37.5	75-225, qam	2D6 inhibitor	Activating; IR form not well-tolerated
Tricyclic Antidepressants				
Tertiary amines				
Amitriptyline	10	25-150, qhs	2D6 substrate	Many side effects limit use in elderly
Imipramine	10	50-300, qhs	2D6 substrate	Many side effects limit use in elderly
Secondary amines				
Desipramine	10	25-200, qam	2D6 substrate	Usually activating; must follow blood levels and EKGs
Nortriptyline	10	25-150, qhs	2D6 substrate	Mildly sedating; must follow blood levels and EKGs
Psychostimulants				
Dextroamphetamine	2.5-5	5-60, bid to qid	Unknown	Best in two divided doses (AM, noon); analgesic adjuvant
Methylphenidate	2.5-5	5-60, bid to qid	None	Best in two divided doses (AM, noon); analgesic adjuvant
Modafinil	50	50-400, qam to bid	2C19 inhibitor	No generic, costly; similar side-effect profile to others
Armodafinil	50	50-250, qam	2C19 inhibitor	Isomer of modafinil; no generic, costly; similar side effects

*Dosing: Range listed is to maximum; thus divided dosing, if listed, is also to reach stated maximum.

basis of these properties, common features of mirtazapine include sedation, anxiolysis, appetite stimulation, and antiemesis. Because it can cause weight gain, it may be advantageous in the palliative care setting for anorectic-cachectic cancer patients, but it may not a good choice for those who are gaining unwanted weight from steroids or chemotherapy.

Tricyclic antidepressants (TCAs) antagonize muscarinic, cholinergic, H_1-histaminic, and α-adrenergic receptors, contributing to side effects of confusion, dry mouth, constipation, urinary retention, sedation, weight gain, and orthostatic hypotension. These side-effects are most prominent with the tertiary amines (amitriptyline and imipramine) and less so with the secondary amines (nortriptyline and desipramine). Thus, of the TCA class, the secondary amines are preferred in the older population. TCAs are still used in the oncology setting, especially when neuropathic pain is present. TCAs also exert

TABLE 15-12	**Matching Antidepressant Drug to Depressive or Physical Problem**	
	Drug Strategy	
Symptom or Concern	**Use**	**Avoid**
Anxiety/agitation	Mirtazapine; calming SRI; or mixed agent	Activating agent especially high dose at start
Insomnia	Mirtazapine; sedating agent	Activating agent especially at night
Daytime sedation/apathy	Bupropion; psychostimulant	Sedating agent during day or a high dose
Fatigue	Bupropion; psychostimulant	Sedating agent during day or a high dose
Pain	Mixed agent; TCA; psychostimulant	High doses if using opiates concurrently
GI upset	Mirtazapine; TCA	Some SRIs empty stomach
Anorexia/weight loss	Mirtazapine; paroxetine, TCA	Some SRIs, (des)venlafaxine, bupropion
Confusion/dementia	Citalopram, mixed agent, mirtazapine	TCA, some stimulants
Hot flashes	Venlafaxine; trazodone, mirtazapine	Some SRIs
Dry mouth/stomatitis	SRIs; psychostimulant	Mirtazapine; paroxetine, TCA
Difficulty swallowing	Dissolving or elixir form	
Slow gut motility	SRI, mixed agent	TCA, agents with anticholinergic effects
Polypharmacy	Citalopram; Mirtazapine	TCA; nefazodone, some SRIs

SRI, serotonin reuptake inhibitor; TCA, tricyclic antidepressant

cardiac conduction effects, so serial EKGs should be followed when they are used. TCAs are also more lethal in overdose. Finally, it is important to follow TCA drug levels, specifically with nortriptyline which may have a therapeutic window.

In cancer patients, the psychostimulants and the newer wakefulness-promoting agents (modafinil and armodafinil) promote a sense of well-being, decrease fatigue, improve concentration and attention, and may stimulate appetite. However, anorexia may develop at higher doses. These agents are not considered antidepressants per se. An advantage of these drugs is their rapid onset and relative effectiveness, and thus they are often preferred over traditional antidepressants in the depressed patient in the terminal phase of illness or with advanced cancer. In cases where traditional antidepressants have not yet worked or achieved the desired results, psychostimulants may be used adjunctively, although data on efficacy, tolerance, and safety in the older oncologic population are largely anecdotal. Psychostimulants can potentiate the analgesic effects of opioid analgesics and are commonly used to counteract opioid-induced sedation. Also, psychostimulants can cause tremor, anxiety, agitation, delirium, nightmares, insomnia, and even psychosis, and these agents may lower seizure threshold. At higher doses, they can produce tachycardia, other arrhythmias, or hypertension. These same side effects can occur with modafinil or armodafinil but possibly less frequently. Patients can be maintained on psychostimulants for long periods, e.g., 6 months to 1 year or longer, and if tolerance develops, dose adjustments can be made accordingly.

The decision on which medication to choose hinders on several aspects. Past history of positive response to an agent or a family history of response to a particular drug may be considered. However, usually other factors to take into account include the patient's overall health, cognitive status, financial resources, other concurrent medications, and concomitant psychiatric problems such as substance

abuse or psychosis. Prominent features of the depressive disorder, i.e., somatic presentation or needs, may drive drug-matching. Similarly, medication side effects may help guide selection, for example, choosing a sedating drug to address an insomnia complaint or choosing an activating drug to combat fatigue or excessive daytime sedation. Treatment of psychotic depression requires use of both an antidepressant and an antipsychotic. Possible strategies to consider in drug-matching are listed in Table 15-12 and may serve as a guide, with recognition of the need to individualize ultimate medication choice.

Should the initial drug fail after an adequate dosage and duration trial, it may be worth switching to a drug from a different class. However, if there has been a partial response to the initial drug challenge, options include: (1) increasing the dose further until the recommended maximum is reached and tolerance continues; (2) adding a second antidepressant and monitoring more closely for drug interactions; or (3) referring for psychotherapy. In any case, it is also important to assure medication adherence and to assure that the correct diagnosis has been made.

Finally, it is important for primary care and oncologic providers not to overlook the availability of and benefit derived from electroconvulsive therapy (ECT) in the older patient with severe major depression. Anecdotal reports of safety and benefit in medically ill and cancer populations do exist. Table 15-13 lists advantages and disadvantages of ECT that may help guide its implementation.

Indications for ECT include serious, life-threatening mood disorders; treatment failures; need for rapid definitive response (e.g., acute suicidality, states of inanition or catatonia); chronic depression with significant psychosocial, functional, and cognitive impairment; and psychotic depression, where ECT is probably the treatment of choice. A typical index ECT series is comprised of between 6 and 12 sessions, usually administered three times per week, although in elderly patients a frequency of twice per week is possible. Once a patient responds

TABLE 15-13	Electroconvulsive Therapy Considerations in Older Patients
Advantages	**Disadvantages**
• Superior efficacy (80% - 90%) in severe depression compared to antidepressant medication (when used as first-line choice) • Good efficacy (50% - 60%) in medication-resistant depression • More rapid onset of action • Good safety profile: very low mortality and low morbidity • Absence of medication side effects • Age may be a predictor of response	• Repeated general anesthesia • Cognitive and memory effects • Minor treatment side effects: headache, muscle aches, falls (especially in the elderly) • Acute relapse if a maintenance plan is not instituted • Cost of series

TABLE 15-14	Assuring an Adequate Medication Trial in Depression

- Discuss commonly experienced side effects.
- Be sensitive to patient concerns, e.g., weight gain, constipation or loose stools, lethargy, mental dulling, sedation, or sexual dysfunction.
- Know how to intervene to address side effects:
  - Reduce medication dosage temporarily to allow for acclimation or
  - Slow titration or
  - Change timing of use.
- Ask patients to repeat back what they have heard about the selected medication.
- Bring the patient back in 1-2 weeks for a medication and symptom review.
  - Ask patients to keep a log of symptoms and side-effects.
  - Specifically query about suicidal ideation.
  - Use a mood scale, e.g., PHQ-9, to follow response.

to ECT, it is essential that a maintenance plan to prevent relapse of depression be implemented. Maintenance plans can include combination pharmacotherapy, maintenance ECT (which occurs at decreasing frequency of weekly to monthly, for example), or a combination of medications and ECT. There presently are no data or studies of other brain stimulation therapies (vagus nerve stimulation [VNS] or transcranial magnetic stimulation [TMS]) in older cancer patients, and deep brain stimulation (DBS) remains experimental.

MONITORING PATIENTS DURING DEPRESSION MANAGEMENT

While it seems obvious, it is important to have the correct diagnosis so that the appropriate intervention, whether psychological or pharmacological, is selected. It is also recommended to have the patient and/or family share their expectations of treatment and gain a clear understanding of what the treatment is intended to do or provide. Unrealistic goals or misunderstanding of benefits can lead to poorer adherence and avoidable disappointments. Given the complexities noted, it is helpful to have a plan of care for management of depression that, besides systematic assessment of clinical symptoms with a mood scale, includes scheduled follow-up of treatment benefit and adherence. If considering a psychotherapy referral, then asking the patient or family about the outcome of the visit(s) will convey the importance of making the connection. It is also appropriate to request brief periodic reports from the therapist. Having this relationship and ease of communication allows for the provider and therapist to share useful information and identify obstacles or complications to treatment should these arise. With regard to drug management, after choosing a medication it is critical to follow through with dosage titration and to reach the recommended dosage range. Underdosing of medication is very common in primary care and among elderly depressed patients. Finally, to be effective, medication must be used for the indicated

amount of time. It may take 4 to 6 weeks for maximal effect to be seen, although it may be possible to see some initial improvement after 2 weeks. However, some studies suggest that full antidepressant effects in the elderly population may take as long as 8 to 12 weeks, so it is imperative that patients remain on the medication for a sufficient duration. Additional helpful pointers for assuring an adequate medication trial are listed in Table 15-14. Repeating mood scales periodically helps to gauge the extent of response and may give direction on when a change in treatment plan or review of diagnosis is needed. Finally, it is critical that the goal of any depression treatment be full symptom remission.

Duration of treatment of depression depends on several factors including whether there was a past history of depression. In general, patients who have had more than three previous episodes of depression before the age of 50 may require continuous lifetime treatment. At a minimum, a patient should be treated for at least 6 months after having achieved full symptom remission. As alluded to earlier, patients who do not reach full symptom remission and who continue with residual symptoms of depression are at higher risk of relapse, experience more functional impairment, and have a lower quality of life.

CASE 15-1	PART 3 SOLUTION

Judith still scores high on the PHQ-9, sleeps poorly, and indicates that she has great difficulty completing her daily tasks because of pain. However, she specifically denies suicidal ideation. While she found support groups helpful for general discussion, she would like to see an individual therapist and also would like to review medication options. On the basis of her symptom profile, a dual-action agent is chosen, along with a benzodiazepine for about a week; she will follow up in about 2 weeks. However, she is asked to call should she have any problems with her antidepressant or should she feel worse. Her family feels secure in being with her and expresses understanding of what to do should her thinking change to suggest suicidal intent.

ANXIETY IN OLDER PATIENTS WITH CANCER

Although anxiety is experienced by most cancer patients at some point during the course of their illness and treatment, anxiety is not well-studied in the geriatric oncologic population. In general, prevalence studies of anxiety in adult cancer cohorts place the range at between 20% and 25%. Anxiety is often seen at crisis points such as the initial diagnosis or discovery of a relapse after treatment. This anxiety can be viewed

---

CASE 15-2 | **PART 1**

Thomas is an 86-year-old retired music professor with a history of prostate cancer for the last 20 years. He initially underwent a radical prostatectomy and suffered postsurgical incontinence and sexual dysfunction, which has been distressing. He had been maintained on antihormonal therapy and was doing well until recently when repeat PSAs began to elevate. He presented twice to the emergency department with panic attacks and his wife is concerned about his behavior.

Question 10: How does anxiety manifest in a patient with cancer?
Question 11: How is anxiety diagnosed and what anxiety scales can be used to aid in diagnosis?
Question 12: What is the differential diagnosis?

---

as a normal reaction to a stressful and traumatic event and may even be a positive effect if anxiety motivates a patient to gather the information and support that helps inform decision making. However, it can be difficult to determine when a patient's anxiety lies out of the normal range and requires specific intervention. In general, anxiety that persists beyond the immediate period of a stressor and anxiety that causes impairment in functioning should prompt further evaluation. Anxiety may also be a component of other complications such as pain, delirium, and depression. While many patients will express anxiety symptoms, the rate of anxiety disorder and its subtypes is comparable to that in the general population. Most studies of psychiatric symptoms in cancer patients have reported a higher prevalence of mixed anxiety and depressive symptoms than anxiety alone. Correlations between measures of depression and anxiety on both clinician-rated and self-report measures are high. In all likelihood, this observation indicates that these measures tap common psychological traits such as negative affect or neuroticism. Anxiety increases with the diagnosis of cancer, peaks before surgical interventions, and frequently remains high thereafter, declining gradually during the first postoperative years. Anxiety increases as cancer progresses, and psychological health declines along with the decline in physical status. Chemotherapy administration is a source of anxiety that may develop into a conditioned anticipatory response, i.e., phobia, which may persist for years after the cessation of the chemotherapy. Radiotherapy is also

associated with increased anxiety, accompanied by concerns about increased bodily vulnerability and worries about whether the radiation will cause further bodily damage. The anxiety experienced during chemotherapy and radiation therapy may paradoxically increase at the termination of treatment, as patients feel unprotected, see their physician less often, and worry about the effectiveness or durability of treatment. Patients who are participating in clinical trials and feel that they have been randomly assigned to a less-aggressive treatment modality may also experience increased anxiety.

DIAGNOSIS OF ANXIETY

In the older cancer patient, the diagnosis should be approached comprehensively, but judiciously. Systematic assessment is paramount and includes a careful history, review of medications or treatments, review of past psychiatric and family psychiatric history, assessment of current family or social support, and review of basic laboratory results. In some cases, older patients may have a pre-existing anxiety disorder and, in fact, anxiety disorders are generally more prevalent than depressive disorders in older population cohort studies. In addition, older patients with anxiety may be at higher risk of current or past abuse of alcohol, benzodiazepines or other CNS depressants. Symptoms of anxiety may be grouped, as are depressive symptoms, into both cognitive and somatic domains. The cognitive or psychological symptoms can encompass fear of death, loss of control, thoughts of impending doom, hypervigilance, overgeneralizing, and catastrophizing. The somatic symptoms are often found in panic attacks and can include hyperarousal, tachycardia, shortness of breath, sweating, nausea, abdominal upset or distress, loose stools, trembling, and dizziness. Screening tools such as the single Anxiety Question, Beck Anxiety Inventory, Hospital Anxiety and Depression Scale and the Memorial Anxiety Scale for Prostate Cancer are examples of measures that might be routinely given to older patients and applied in office or hospital practice. The single anxiety question "Are you anxious?" while simple to use, nonetheless in a palliative care sample showed insufficient specificity to exclude patients who were not anxious.

DIFFERENTIAL DIAGNOSIS OF ANXIETY

The differential diagnosis of anxiety in an older patient with cancer can be challenging, as several factors may interact to contribute to anxiety. As shown in Table 15-15, medical conditions, medication or treatment effects, psychiatric disorders, and life circumstances must be considered.

Patients who are delirious may appear anxious, restless, and agitated and may exhibit marked impulsivity. Severe pain can make patients appear anxious, and when

TABLE 15-15	Differential Diagnosis of Anxiety in the Older Cancer Patient

Medical	Medications
• Delirium	• Asthma agents
• Endocrinopathies	• Steroids
• Pulmonary disease (COPD, emboli)	• Chemotherapeutics
• Cardiac disease (Arrhythmia, MI, CAD)	**Psychiatric**
• Gastrointestinal disorder (IBS)	• Generalized Anxiety Disorder
• Metabolic derangement	• Panic Disorder
• Pheochromocytoma	• Phobias
Neurological	• Posttraumatic Stress Disorder
• Seizure disorder	• Substance-Induced Anxiety Disorder
• Brain tumor	• Adjustment Disorder with anxiety
• Paraneoplastic syndrome	• Mood Disorder
Cancer-related	**Life Circumstances**
• Type	• Financial strain
• Initial diagnosis	• Disruptive family or social relationships
• Recurrence	• Housing problems or changes
• Treatment failure	
• Pain	

COPD, chronic obstructive pulmonary disease; MI, myocardial infarction; CAD, coronary artery disease; IBS, irritable bowel syndrome.

the pain is adequately treated, patients usually experience a marked reduction in anxiety symptoms. Patients with diseases of the respiratory system, such as lung cancer, or patients in respiratory distress can present with anxiety and restlessness. This anxiety can set off a cycle of worsening shortness of breath followed by more anxiety. An acute event such as a pulmonary embolus may also initially present with a patient appearing quite anxious. The symptoms of anxiety in these cases may respond initially to an anxiolytic medication, but the patient's anxiety will ultimately better respond to the proper medical intervention. Sepsis, endocrine abnormalities, hypoglycemia, hypercalcemia, and hormone-secreting tumors may all be associated with anxiety symptoms. There is some evidence that depression, anxiety, and panic attacks can occur in patients with pancreatic cancer, although the mechanism is not entirely clear. Several medications or treatments are associated with anxiety. Examples include medications used for their antiemetic properties. Steroids and other antiemetics can cause anxiety or akathisia, which is a motor restlessness accompanied by subjective feelings of distress and hyperactivity. In addition, withdrawal from alcohol, benzodiazepines, or other CNS depressants is associated with rebound anxiety.

From a psychiatric perspective, DSM-IV-TR describes a variety of anxiety disorders. A patient may have a pre-existing anxiety disorder or may develop an anxiety disorder after a cancer diagnosis. The spectrum of anxiety disorders includes diagnoses such as generalized anxiety disorder, panic disorder, and posttraumatic stress disorder. It also includes phobias, such as a fear of needles or claustrophobia. These may have great impact on cancer patients who must undergo multiple tests and procedures such as magnetic resonance imaging, injections, and intravenous treatments. An anxiety response may also be conditioned. Patients may have anxiety symptoms emerge as an anticipatory response to a repeated aversive treatment such as chemotherapy, to difficult procedures, or to places associated with painful experiences. When associated with an acute stressor such as news of illness or treatment failure, an adjustment disorder with anxiety can be diagnosed, especially if the symptoms are time-limited. As previously noted, depressive disorders are often accompanied by anxiety symptoms and deciding which is primary can be very complicated. The importance of diagnosing an anxiety disorder accurately is that evidence suggests greater and more sustained benefit from particular psychotherapies like CBT or problem-solving therapy (PST) over medications, which take a longer time to work and to which some anxious patients appear more sensitive. Finally, as in mood disorders, general life circumstances can be associated with anxiety or stress, and anxious reactions to these situations should not necessarily be deemed pathological, especially if anxiety helps to motivate a person to adopt more effective coping strategies, to make needed changes, or to seek appropriate help.

CASE 15-2	PART 1 SOLUTION

Further workup is ordered which reveals that he now has bone metastases. However, a brain MRI is negative for masses or worrisome lesions. While he has a history of depression, he denies any mood-related or other symptoms and instead reports that he primarily feels nervous, ruminates about his relationship with his wife, and worries about how he might respond to new treatments, given the bad outcomes previously experienced. Given the apparent association with news about recurrence, his physician diagnoses an adjustment disorder with anxious mood and will reassess periodically.

TREATMENT OF ANXIETY IN THE OLDER CANCER PATIENT

The most effective management of anxiety in cancer patients incorporates all modalities, that is, psychotherapy, behavioral therapy, and pharmacologic management. During the initial evaluation of the patient's symptoms, both emotional support and information are given to the patient. Exploration of the patient's fears and apprehensions about disease progression, upcoming procedures, or psychosocial concerns often alleviates a substantial degree of anxiety. Patient concerns usually include death, physical suffering, increased

On follow-up, it is learned that he again presented to the emergency department with another panic attack but fortunately, workup for acute medical problems was negative. Despite explanation of his condition and the available treatment options, he remains worried and feels overwhelmed; however, he again denies symptoms of depression and is not hopeless or suicidal.

Question 13: What treatment options are available for anxiety disorders?

Question 14: When and how should medications for anxiety be used?

dependence, loss of dignity, changes in social role functioning, spiritual matters, and worry about finances or employment.

PSYCHOLOGICAL TREATMENTS

The same types of psychological interventions previously mentioned in management of depression can be useful in addressing most anxiety situations or disorders. These have been shown earlier in Table 15-9. General measures involve showing support, acceptance and positive regard toward the patient; placing an emphasis on working together to achieve desired results; communicating a hopeful attitude that the goals of care will be achieved; showing respect for how the patient adapts to or handles difficulty; and focusing on the patient's strengths and acknowledging how successful the patient has been on his or her own, thereby promoting a sense of mastery and control. Each of these measures communicates to the patient one's active concern and continued involvement in his or her care. Patients with anxiety may benefit from specific cognitive-behavioral interventions including reframing negative, irrational thought processes; progressive relaxation; distraction; guided imagery; meditation; biofeedback; and hypnosis. These techniques are also used to treat the anxiety symptoms associated with painful procedures, pain syndromes, office visits, waiting for results, and anticipatory fears of chemotherapy and radiation therapy. Other psychotherapeutic techniques such as supportive and insight-oriented therapy may be helpful to reduce anxiety symptoms and allow for better coping with the cancer.

PHARMACOLOGICAL MANAGEMENT

The decision to use medication to manage anxiety is typically guided by the degree and pervasiveness of symptoms and the associated functional impairment. In mild cases of anxiety, supportive or behavioral measures should be pursued first, although formal psychotherapy referral may also be considered. In more severe cases of anxiety, while medications can be very useful, it is important to understand which symptoms will respond best and over what time frame, and to explain to the patient what to expect from a drug intervention and what the treatment plan for medication management will include. Somatic symptoms of anxiety are especially amenable to treatment and respond quickly. However, judicious use is necessary, particularly in the older patient for whom concerns about side effects or drug-drug interactions are high. Commonly used medications for anxiety are listed in Table 15-16.

For patients who experience persistent apprehension and anxiety, the first-line drugs are the benzodiazepines. Lorazepam and alprazolam are useful for anxiety, nausea, and panic. Both lorazepam and alprazolam have been shown in controlled trials to reduce postchemotherapy nausea and vomiting, as well as anticipatory nausea and vomiting. Benzodiazepines have amnestic properties; when given before chemotherapy or a procedure, this effect may reduce the likelihood that a conditioned aversion will develop. A longer-acting benzodiazepine, such as clonazepam, may provide more consistent relief of anxiety symptoms and have mood-stabilizing effects as well. The short-acting to medium-acting benzodiazepines, as well as the nonbenzodiazepine hypnotics (zolpidem, zaleplon, eszopiclone or ramelteon) may be effective for insomnia. Low-dose antipsychotics, such as haloperidol, olanzapine, and risperidone, may be more effective for the patient who is both anxious and confused. For patients with compromised hepatic function, the use of intermediate-acting benzodiazepines, such as lorazepam, oxazepam, and temazepam, is preferred. These drugs are metabolized by conjugation with glucuronic acid and have no active metabolites, and thus may be considered for use in patients with liver disease. Drowsiness and somnolence are the most common adverse effects of benzodiazepines. Reductions in dose and the passage of time eliminate these effects. Mental status changes may result from benzodiazepine use and are more common in elderly patients and in those with advanced disease, comorbid cognitive impairment, and impaired hepatic function. For the treatment of panic disorder and agoraphobia, the benzodiazepines and antidepressant medications (TCAs and SRIs) have demonstrated effectiveness. Although alprazolam rapidly blocks panic attacks, withdrawal can be difficult after prolonged use. In anxious patients with severely compromised pulmonary function, the use of benzodiazepines that suppress central respiratory mechanisms may be unsafe. A low dose of an antihistamine, nonbenzodiazepine or antipsychotic medication can be useful for these individuals.

Note that antidepressant medications have also been used in the management of anxiety disorders although, as stated before, no randomized controlled trials exist in the older cancer patient population. The same concerns regarding antidepressants pertain when used for treatment of anxiety instead of depression, but a few features are different. First, the lowest dose possible should be used when initiating an antidepressant drug, especially if it has

TABLE 15-16	Antianxiety and Sedative-Hypnotic Medications Used in Older Cancer Patients	
Drug	**Starting Daily Dose, Oral**	**Comments**
Benzodiazepines		*Higher risk of falls, confusion*
Alprazolam	0.125 to 0.5 mg tid to qid	Short acting, helps nausea
Lorazepam	0.25 to 0.5 mg bid to tid	Intermediate, no active metabolites
Oxazepam	10 mg bid to tid	Intermediate, no active metabolites
Temazepam	15 mg qhs	Intermediate, no active metabolites
Diazepam	2-5 mg bid to tid	Long acting, has metabolites
Clonazepam	0.25-0.5 mg bid to tid	Long acting
Nonbenzodiazepines		*Minimal cognitive problems*
Buspirone	5-10 mg bid to tid	May take 4-8 weeks for effect
Hypnotics		*May cause confusion, falls*
Zolpidem	5-10 mg qhs	
Zaleplon	5-20 mg qhs	
Eszopiclone	1-2 mg qhs	
Ramelteon	8 mg qhs	Possible P450 effects
Antihistamines		*May cause confusion, sedation*
Hydroxyzine	10-25 mg bid to tid	
Diphenhydramine	25-50 mg bid to tid	Do not use in dementia
Neuroleptics		*Possible cardiac risk? Monitor QTc*
Aripiprazole	2-5 mg qam or qhs	Not sedating, less EPS
Haloperidol	0.25-0.5 mg bid to qhs	Not sedating, more EPS
Risperidone	0.25-0.5 mg bid to qhs	More EPS, mild sedation
Olanzapine	2.5-5 mg bid to qhs	Metabolic changes, sedation
Quetiapine	12.5-25 mg bid, tid or qhs	Orthostasis, sedation
Others		
Trazodone	12.5-50 mg bid to qhs	Orthostasis, sedation

EPS, extrapyramidal symptoms

| CASE 15-2 | **PART 2 SOLUTION** |

Because this patient has now presented to the emergency department on several occasions, it is necessary to offer treatment. It is learned that he previously saw a therapist, and that he is interested in revisiting issues related to his marriage and to his concerns about aging and mortality; thus he agrees to undergo psychotherapy. In addition, because his anxiety symptoms are now more frequent, he is offered low-dose lorazepam to use as needed when he has a panic attack; it is also suggested that he begin an antidepressant for more sustained benefit and to avoid cognitive side effects from lorazepam, a concern of his. As he expresses psychological distress with gastrointestinal disturbances, a medication is chosen that has fewer GI side effects. A follow-up appointment is scheduled in 2 weeks, and he is instructed to call his physician should he worsen or have any medication difficulties or exacerbation of his anxiety.

"activating" properties, in an anxious patient, or when the patient expresses many somatic complaints. These patients tend to fixate on and misinterpret body sensations, so that any possible side effect quickly becomes worrisome. Second, the dose should be increased gradually at modest increments of a quarter or half pill. Third, the medication should be adjusted slowly, every 1 to 2 weeks, or when the patient has acclimated. Fourth, the dosage needed to treat an anxiety disorder may ultimately be higher than what is needed to manage depression; this

may present a problem, as some side effects occur in a dose-dependent manner. Lastly, given the slow titration, immediate effects may not be available, so it is important not to let the patient get discouraged. To help during this slow initiation and gradual titration phase, temporary use of a benzodiazepine may be considered. Also, while waiting for anxiolytic medication to take effect, other supportive or behavioral measures can be used concomitantly.

SUMMARY

With the aging of the population and the success of cancer treatments, there are increasingly more elderly patients diagnosed with, being treated for, and likely living with cancer. Comprehensive oncologic management must recognize and address the psychological distress and possible psychiatric sequelae experienced at each stage of illness or associated with treatment. Mental distress and psychiatric complications should not be seen as unavoidable consequences of cancer in later life. Management should also take into account the distinctive challenges and needs of the older-age patient. Discussed in this chapter are the diagnosis and management of depression and anxiety in the older cancer patient. Issues to consider in the geriatric population include presence of comorbid medical or psychiatric conditions, effects of concurrent treatments, probable polypharmacy, consequences of aging on drug metabolism, and unique later-life psychosocial and developmental perspectives. Each of these, singly or in combination, can influence the presentation and management of psychiatric disorders. Successful treatments for depression and anxiety in the older cancer patient encompass psychological, behavioral, and pharmacological interventions, and optimal outcomes often require a combination of approaches. Primary care and oncologic providers should be aware of the criteria for diagnosis, availability of and indications for treatment, options for drug management, commonly experienced drug side effects, and strategies to assure adherence and the best outcomes. Despite a large body of experience, however, more specific research on older cancer patient populations is needed to better assess the efficacy, safety, and effectiveness of these interventions.

SUGGESTED READINGS

1. Akechi T, Okuyama T, Onishi J, et al: Psychotherapy for depression among incurable cancer patients, *Cochrane Database Syst Rev* (2), 2008 Apr 16:CD005537.

2. Akechi T, Okuyama T, Sugawara Y, et al: Major depression, adjustment disorders, and post-traumatic stress disorder in terminally ill cancer patients: associated and predictive factors, *J Clin Oncol* 22(10):1957–1965, 2004 May 15.

3. Block SD: Assessing and managing depression in the terminally ill patient. ACP-ASIM End-of-Life Care Consensus Panel. American College of Physicians - American Society of Internal Medicine, *Ann Intern Med* 132(3):209–218, 2000 Feb 1.

4. Breitbart W, Rosenfeld B, Gibson C, et al: Meaning-centered group psychotherapy for patients with advanced cancer: a pilot randomized controlled trial, *Psychooncology* 19(1):21–28, 2010 Jan.

5. Carlson LE, Garland SN: Impact of mindfulness-based stress reduction (MBSR) on sleep, mood, stress and fatigue symptoms in cancer outpatients, *Int J Behav Med* 12(4):278–285, 2005.

6. Chochinov HM, Hassard T, McClement S, et al: The landscape of distress in the terminally ill, *J Pain Symptom Manage* 38(5):641–649, 2009 Nov.

7. Chochinov HM, Hack T, Hassard T, et al: Dignity therapy: a novel psychotherapeutic intervention for patients near the end of life, *J Clin Oncol* 23(24):5520–5525, 2005 Aug 20.

8. Dale W, Bilir P, Han M, Meltzer D: The role of anxiety in prostate carcinoma: a structured review of the literature, *Cancer* 104(3):467–478, 2005 Aug 1.

9. Goodwin JS, Zhang DD, Ostir GV: Effect of depression on diagnosis, treatment, and survival of older women with breast cancer, *J Am Geriatr Soc* 52(1):106–111, 2004 Jan.

10. Griffith JL, Gaby L: Brief psychotherapy at the bedside: countering demoralization from medical illness, *Psychosomatics* 46(2):109–116, 2005 Mar-Apr.

11. Hoffman KE, McCarthy EP, Recklitis CJ, Ng AK: Psychological distress in long-term survivors of adult-onset cancer: results from a national survey, *Arch Intern Med* 169(14):1274–1281, 2009 Jul 27.

12. Holland JC, Andersen B, Breitbart WS, et al: NCCN Distress Management Panel. Distress management, *J Natl Compr Canc Netw* 8(4):448–485, 2010 Apr.

13. Holland JC, Reznik I: Pathways for psychosocial care of cancer survivors, *Cancer* 104(Suppl 11):2624–2637, 2005 Dec 1.

14. Jehn CF, Kuehnhardt D, Bartholomae A, et al: Biomarkers of depression in cancer patients, *Cancer* 107(11):2723–2729, 2006 Dec 1.

15. Jin Y, Desta Z, Stearns V, et al: CYP2D6 genotype, antidepressant use, and tamoxifen metabolism during adjuvant breast cancer treatment, *J Natl Cancer Inst* 97(1):30–39, 2005 Jan 5.

16. Kast RE, Foley KF: Cancer chemotherapy and cachexia: mirtazapine and olanzapine are 5-HT3 antagonists with good antinausea effects, *Eur J Cancer Care (Engl)* 16(4):351–354, 2007 Jul.

17. Kelly B, McClement S, Chochinov HM: Measurement of psychological distress in palliative care, *Palliat Med* 20(8):779–789, 2006 Dec.

18. Kugaya A, Akechi T, Okuyama T, et al: Prevalence, predictive factors, and screening for psychologic distress in patients with newly diagnosed head and neck cancer, *Cancer* 88(12):2817–2823, 2000 Jun 15.

19. Kurtz ME, Kurtz JC, Stommel M, et al: Predictors of depressive symptomatology of geriatric patients with colorectal cancer: a longitudinal view, *Support Care Cancer* 10(6):494–501, 2002 Sep.

20. Kurtz ME, Kurtz JC, Stommel M, et al: Predictors of depressive symptomatology of geriatric patients with lung cancer: a longitudinal analysis, *Psychooncology* 11(1):12–22, 2002 Jan-Feb.

21. LeMay K, Wilson KG: Treatment of existential distress in life threatening illness: a review of manualized interventions, *Clin Psychol Rev* 28(3):472–493, 2008 Mar.

22. Lewis FM, Fletcher KA, Cochrane BB, Fann JR: Predictors of depressed mood in spouses of women with breast cancer, *J Clin Oncol* 26(8):1289–1295, 2008 Mar 10.

23. Loprinzi CL, Levitt R, Barton D, et al: Phase III comparison of depomedroxyprogesterone acetate to venlafaxine for managing hot flashes: North Central Cancer Treatment Group Trial N99C7, *J Clin Oncol* 24(9):1409–1414, 2006 Mar 20.

24. Marcus NJ: Pain in cancer patients unrelated to the cancer or treatment, *Cancer Invest* 23(1):84–93, 2005.

25. Masand PS, Tesar GE: Use of stimulants in the medically ill, *Psychiatr Clin North Am* 19(3):515–547, 1996 Sep.

26. McDonald AA, Portenoy RK: How to use antidepressants and anticonvulsants as adjuvant analgesics in the treatment of neuropathic cancer pain, *J Support Oncol* 4(1):43–52, 2006 Jan.

27. McPherson CJ, Wilson KG, Murray MA: Feeling like a burden to others: a systematic review focusing on the end of life, *Palliat Med* 21(2):115–128, 2007 Mar.

28. Menzies H, Chochinov HM, Breitbart W: Cytokines, cancer and depression: connecting the dots, *J Support Oncol* 3(1):55–57, 2005 Jan-Feb.

29. Miller M, Mogun H, Azrael D, et al: Cancer and the risk of suicide in older Americans, *J Clin Oncol* 26(29):4720–4724, 2008 Oct 10.

30. Miovic M, Block S: Psychiatric disorders in advanced cancer, *Cancer* 110(8):1665–1676, 2007 Oct 15.

31. Nelson C, Jacobson CM, Weinberger MI, et al: The role of spirituality in the relationship between religiosity and depression in prostate cancer patients, *Ann Behav Med* 38(2):105–114, 2009 Oct.

32. Nelson CJ, Cho C, Berk AR, et al: Are gold standard depression measures appropriate for use in geriatric cancer patients? A systematic evaluation of self-report depression instruments used with geriatric, cancer, and geriatric cancer samples, *J Clin Oncol* 28(2):348–356, 2010 Jan 10.

33. Nelson CJ, Weinberger MI, Balk E, et al: The chronology of distress, anxiety, and depression in older prostate cancer patients, *Oncologist* 14(9):891–899, 2009 Sep.

34. O'Mahony S, Goulet J, Kornblith A, et al: Desire for hastened death, cancer pain and depression: report of a longitudinal observational study, *J Pain Symptom Manage* 29(5):446–457, 2005 May.

35. O'Rourke RW, Diggs BS, Spight DH, et al: Psychiatric illness delays diagnosis of esophageal cancer, *Dis Esophagus* 21(5):416–421, 2008.

36. Okamura M, Akizuki N, Nakano T, et al: Clinical experience of the use of a pharmacological treatment algorithm for major depressive disorder in patients with advanced cancer, *Psychooncology* 17(2):154–160, 2008 Feb.

37. Onitilo AA, Nietert PJ, Egede LE: Effect of depression on all-cause mortality in adults with cancer and differential effects by cancer site, *Gen Hosp Psychiatry* 28(5):396–402, 2006 Sep-Oct.

38. Pitceathly C, Maguire P, Fletcher I, et al: Can a brief psychological intervention prevent anxiety or depressive disorders in cancer patients? A randomised controlled trial, *Ann Oncol* 20(5):928–934, 2009 May.

39. Postone N: Psychotherapy with cancer patients, *Am J Psychother* 52(4):412–424, 1998:Fall.

40. Reiche EM, Morimoto HK, Nunes SM: Stress and depression-induced immune dysfunction: implications for the development and progression of cancer, *Int Rev Psychiatry* 17(6):515–527, 2005 Dec.

41. Rodin G, Lo C, Mikulincer M, et al: Pathways to distress: the multiple determinants of depression, hopelessness, and the desire for hastened death in metastatic cancer patients, *Soc Sci Med* 68(3):562–569, 2009 Feb.

42. Roth AJ, Massie MJ: Anxiety and its management in advanced cancer, *Curr Opin Support Palliat Care* 1(1):50–56, 2007 Apr.

43. Roth AJ, Breitbart W: Psychiatric emergencies in terminally ill cancer patients, *Hematol Oncol Clin North Am* 10(1):235–259, 1996 Feb.

44. Savard J, Simard S, Giguère I, et al: Randomized clinical trial on cognitive therapy for depression in women with metastatic breast cancer: psychological and immunological effects, *Palliat Support Care* 4(3):219–237, 2006 Sep.

45. Savard J, Simard S, Ivers H, Morin CM: Randomized study on the efficacy of cognitive-behavioral therapy for insomnia secondary to breast cancer, part I: Sleep and psychological effects, *J Clin Oncol* 23(25):6083–6096, 2005 Sep 1.

46. Schwartz AL, Mori M, Gao R, et al: Exercise reduces daily fatigue in women with breast cancer receiving chemotherapy, *Med Sci Sports Exerc* 33(5):718–723, 2001 May.

47. Seruga B, Zhang H, Bernstein LJ, Tannock IF: Cytokines and their relationship to the symptoms and outcome of cancer, *Nat Rev Cancer* 8(11):887–899, 2008 Nov.

48. Sherman AC, Pennington J, Latif U, et al: Patient preferences regarding cancer group psychotherapy interventions: a view from the inside, *Psychosomatics* 48(5):426–432, 2007 Sep-Oct.

49. Spoletini I, Gianni W, Repetto L, et al: Depression and cancer: an unexplored and unresolved emergent issue in elderly patients, *Crit Rev Oncol Hematol* 65(2):143–155, 2008 Feb.

50. Stommel M, Kurtz ME, Kurtz JC, et al: A longitudinal analysis of the course of depressive symptomatology in geriatric patients with cancer of the breast, colon, lung, or prostate, *Health Psychol* 23(6):564–573, 2004 Nov.

51. Söllner W, DeVries A, Steixner E, et al: How successful are oncologists in identifying patient distress, perceived social support, and need for psychosocial counselling? *Br J Cancer* 84(2):179–185, 2001 Jan.

52. Waern M, Rubenowitz E, Wilhelmson K: Predictors of suicide in the old elderly, *Gerontology* 49(5):328–334, 2003 Sep-Oct.

53. Waern M, Rubenowitz E, Runeson B, et al: Burden of illness and suicide in elderly people: case-control study, *BMJ* 324(7350):1355, 2002 Jun 8.

54. Walker J, Waters RA, Murray G, et al: Better off dead: suicidal thoughts in cancer patients, *J Clin Oncol* 26(29):4725–4730, 2008 Oct 10.

55. Walker LG, Köhler CR, Heys SD, Eremin O: Psychosocial aspects of cancer in the elderly, *Eur J Surg Oncol* 24(5):375–378, 1998 Oct.

56. Wasteson E, Brenne E, Higginson IJ, et al: European Palliative Care Research Collaborative (EPCRC). Depression assessment and classification in palliative cancer patients: a systematic literature review, *Palliat Med* 23(8):739–753, 2009 Dec:Epub 2009 Oct 13.

57. Williams S, Dale J: The effectiveness of treatment for depression/depressive symptoms in adults with cancer: a systematic review, *Br J Cancer* 94(3):372–390, 2006 Feb 13.

58. Wilson KG, Chochinov HM, Skirko MG, et al: Depression and anxiety disorders in palliative cancer care, *J Pain Symptom Manage* 33(2):118–129, 2007 Feb.

Cancer Pain in Elderly Patients

Bruce Ferrell

Pain is the most feared aspect of cancer for most patients and families. For cancer patients, pain often means the cancer is getting worse and death may be imminent. Pain is the most common source of both physical and existential suffering and often leads patients to functional decline, anxiety, depression, and social isolation. These facts are ironic, given the current availability of highly effective drugs and other interventions for pain relief. Ample evidence exists to indicate that cancer pain can be controlled and suffering effectively reduced for almost all cancer patients.

The approach to cancer pain assessment and management is different in elderly versus younger persons. Older persons may underreport pain for a variety of reasons, despite functional impairment, psychological distress, and needless suffering related to pain. They often present with concurrent illnesses and multiple problems making pain evaluation and treatment more difficult. Elderly persons have a higher incidence of side effects to pain medications and a higher potential for complications and adverse events related to many cancer and pain treatment procedures. Despite these challenges, pain can be effectively managed in most elderly patients. Moreover, clinicians have an ethical and moral obligation to prevent needless suffering and provide effective pain relief, especially for those near the end of life.

PHYSIOLOGY OF CANCER PAIN

Cancer may be nociceptive or neuropathic. Identification of the physiologic process by which pain is perceived may help guide clinicians' choice of pain management strategies. Treatment aimed at specific pathophysiologic pain mechanisms may be more effective. Nociceptive pain is largely the result of stimulation of somatic or visceral pain receptors. Nociceptive pain may arise from tissue injury, inflammation, or mechanical deformation. Examples include tissue injury by tumor enlargement, organ obstruction, ischemia, inflammation, or injury related to diagnostic or treatment procedures such as surgery. Pain from nociception usually responds well to common analgesic medications, relief of the underlying cause, and tissue healing. Neuropathic pain results from pathophysiologic processes that arise in the peripheral or central nervous system. Examples include tumor

pressure or infiltration of nerves, neurotoxicity due to chemotherapy, and posttraumatic neuralgia (after amputation or mechanical nerve injury). Neuropathic pain mechanisms may be identified by association with known disease processes (e.g., postherpetic neuralgia or chemotherapy neurotoxicity), by neuroanatomical location (e.g., a dermatomal pattern), or specific descriptions of the character of the pain. Neuropathic pain may cause a radiculopathy, a pain sensation that travels along a nerve pathway. Common characteristics may include allodynia (a light touch elicits a painful sensation) or hypersensitivity (a painful sensation or pinprick elicits a hyperactive response), as well as descriptions of anesthesia, "pins and needles," or "like electricity." In contrast to nociceptive pain, neuropathic pain syndromes have been found to respond frequently to nonconventional analgesic medications such as anticonvulsant and antidepressant drugs. Some pain syndromes are thought to have multiple or unknown pathophysiologic mechanisms for which treatment is more problematic and unpredictable. Examples include fibromyalgia, recurrent headaches, and some vasculitic syndromes.

It is important to remember that all pain perception is modified by individual memory, expectations and emotions. These psychological mechanisms may enhance or diminish pain perception at the cortical level. Pain perception related to a purely psychological mechanism appears to be extremely rare in older people. These disorders akin to conversion reactions are more often related to somatoform disorders where nociceptive or neuropathic pain mechanisms become deeply entwined in psychological and behavioral pathology. Thus the assessment and treatment of pain should always take into consideration the psychological aspects of pain perception, and professional psychological and psychiatric interventions should be included in the multidimensional approach to pain management when appropriate.

Age-related changes in pain perception have been a topic of interest for many years. Elderly persons have been observed to present with painless myocardial infarction and painless intraabdominal catastrophes. The extent to which these observations are attributable to age-related changes in pain perception remains uncertain. Studies of pain sensitivity across the life span have shown mixed results. Decreased pain sensitivity (increased threshold) with aging can be supported by evidence of decreased numbers of receptors and changes in nerve conduction. Increased pain sensitivity (decreased threshold) with aging can also be supported by evidence of alterations in spinal cord and central nervous system processing (poorer endogenous analgesia). If these observations are correct, overall pain perception may not change much with aging. Clearly, additional studies are needed to define age-related changes specific to nervous system function and pain perception.

ASSESSMENT AND MEASUREMENT OF PAIN IN OLDER PATIENTS

Accurate pain assessment includes an estimate of pain intensity. Pain intensity can be estimated using a valid and reliable pain scale. Pain scales can be grouped into multidimensional and unidimensional scales. In general, multidimensional scales with multiple items often provide more stable measurement and evaluation of pain in several domains. For example, the McGill Pain Questionnaire has been shown to capture pain in terms of intensity, affect, sensation, location, and several other domains that are not possible to evaluate with a single question. The Brief Pain Inventory is a two-dimensional scale that includes intensity and interference with activities. This instrument, originally established for evaluation of cancer pain, has recently been validated in elderly patients, as well as in those with other causes of pain, and has been translated into several foreign languages (Figure 16-1).

Unidimensional scales consist of a single item that usually relates to pain intensity alone. These scales are usually easy to administer and require little time or training to produce reasonably valid and reliable results. Examples include the verbally administered 0 to 10 scale, a single-item visual analog scale, or one of several word descriptor scales that are available. These scales have found widespread use in many clinical settings to monitor treatment effects and for quality assurance indicators. It is important to remember that unidimensional pain scales often require framing the pain question appropriately for maximum reliability. Subjects should be asked about pain in the present tense (here and now). For example the interviewer should frame the question "How much pain are you having right now?" Alternatively the interviewer can ask, "How much pain have you had over the last week?" or "On average, how much pain have you had in the last month?" The latter questions require accurate memory and integration of pain experiences over time that may be more difficult for patients. Recent studies in those with cognitive impairment have shown that pain reports requiring recall are influenced by pain at the moment. Thus it may be more useful to use unidimensional scales to assess pain frequently at the moment while evaluating pain reports over time, much the way vital signs are used.

This is especially true for those with some cognitive impairment.

Pain Assessment in Those with Cognitive Impairment

Cognitive impairment, Alzheimer disease, stroke, or dementia can present substantial challenges to pain assessment. Fortunately, it has been shown that pain reports from those with mild to moderate cognitive impairment are no less valid than other patients with normal cognitive function. Weiner and associates have shown that these reports are usually reliable (stable over time) as well. Experience has shown that commonly available instruments are feasible for use in most patients with cognitive impairment. Thus most elderly patients with mild to moderate cognitive impairment appear to have the capacity to report pain accurately and reliably using commonly available methods.

Patients with severe cognitive impairment may represent substantial challenges for which no generalizable methods for pain assessment have been identified. Although it has been assumed that those in deep coma do not experience pain, it is not clear that such brain damage necessarily results in complete anesthesia. Patients with "locked-in syndrome" (having intact perception and cognitive function but no purposeful motor function and no means of communication) may suffer severely. Unfortunately no reliable methods exist to assess pain in these individuals. Health care providers must be aware of these situations and provide analgesia empirically, especially during procedures or for conditions known to be uncomfortable or painful. More often, most of those with severe cognitive impairment can and do make their needs known in simple yes or no answers communicated in various ways. For example, those with profound aphasia can often provide accurate and reliable answers to yes and no questions when confronted by a sensitive and skilled interviewer. For these patients it is important to be creative in establishing communication methods for the purpose of pain assessment.

Although pain is an individual experience, the use of family and caregivers in the assessment of pain can sometimes be helpful. Among patients with cognitive impairment, the history is often only obtainable from family or close caregivers. Family and caregivers are an excellent source of qualitative information about general behavior, medication usage, actions that seem to reduce pain, and actions that seem to aggravate pain. It is important to remember, however, that family and caregivers are limited in their interpretation of events and behaviors. In fact, evidence has suggested that when it comes to estimating pain intensity, proxies are not always very accurate or reliable. Our studies of elderly cancer patients suggest that caregivers may overestimate pain intensity and distress. It is often distressing to family and other caregivers who feel helpless in managing severe pain. Both physicians and nurses have been found to underestimate pain and to provide inadequate pain medication. In the final analysis, family and close caregivers can be valuable sources of qualitative information, but they probably should not be relied on entirely for quantitative assessment of pain intensity or distress, especially among those patients able to communicate their pain experiences.

MANAGEMENT OF CANCER PAIN

A variety of both drug and nondrug methods are available and effective in cancer pain management. Data clearly shows that patients benefit most from a multimodal approach incorporating both drug and nondrug strategies along with requisite patient and caregiver education, follow-up, and support. Patients should be given an expectation of pain relief, but it may be unrealistic

STUDY ID# ________ HOSPITAL # ________

DO NOT WRITE ABOVE THIS LINE

Brief Pain Inventory (Short Form)

Date: ____/____/____ Time: ____

Name: ____________ ____________ ____________
Last First Middle initial

1. Throughout our lives, most of us have had pain from time to time (such as minor headaches, sprains, and toothaches). Have you had pain other than these everyday kinds of pain today?

1. Yes 2. No

2. On the diagram, shade in the areas where you feel pain. Put an X on the area that hurts the most.

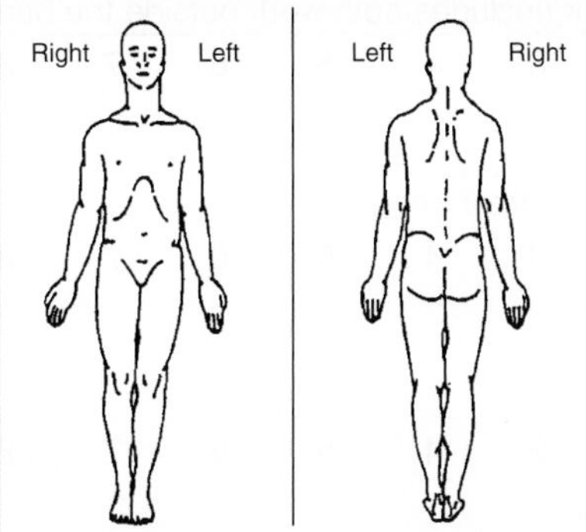

3. Please rate your pain by circling the one number that best describes your pain at its worst in the last 24 hours.

0 1 2 3 4 5 6 7 8 9 10
No Pain — Pain as bad as you can imagine

4. Please rate your pain by circling the one number that best describes your pain at its least in the last 24 hours.

0 1 2 3 4 5 6 7 8 9 10
No Pain — Pain as bad as you can imagine

5. Please rate your pain by circling the one number that best describes your pain on the average.

0 1 2 3 4 5 6 7 8 9 10
No Pain — Pain as bad as you can imagine

6. Please rate your pain by circling the one number that tells how much pain you have right now.

0 1 2 3 4 5 6 7 8 9 10
No Pain — Pain as bad as you can imagine

FIGURE 16-1 Brief Pain Inventory (Short Form).

7.   What treatments or medications are you receiving for your pain?

_____

_____

8.   In the last 24 hours, how much relief have pain treatments or medications provided? Please circle the one percentage that most shows how much relief you have received.

0%	10%	20%	30%	40%	50%	60%	70%	80%	90%	100%
No Relief										Complete Relief

9.   Circle the one number that describes how, during the past 24 hours, pain has interfered with your:

A.   General Activity

0	1	2	3	4	5	6	7	8	9	10
Does not Interfere										Completely Interferes

B.   Mood

0	1	2	3	4	5	6	7	8	9	10
Does not Interfere										Completely Interferes

C.   Walking Ability

0	1	2	3	4	5	6	7	8	9	10
Does not Interfere										Completely Interferes

D.   Normal Work (includes both work outside the home and housework)

0	1	2	3	4	5	6	7	8	9	10
Does not Interfere										Completely Interferes

E.   Relations with other people

0	1	2	3	4	5	6	7	8	9	10
Does not Interfere										Completely Interferes

F.   Sleep

0	1	2	3	4	5	6	7	8	9	10
Does not Interfere										Completely Interferes

G.   Enjoyment of life

0	1	2	3	4	5	6	7	8	9	10
Does not Interfere										Completely Interferes

FIGURE 16-1, cont'd

to suggest or sustain an expectation of complete relief for some patients with persistent pain. The goals and trade-offs of possible therapies need to be discussed openly. Sometimes a period of trial and error should be anticipated when new medications are initiated and titration occurs. Review of medications, doses, use patterns, efficacy, and adverse effects should be a regular process of care. Ineffective drugs should be tapered and discontinued. Patients and caregivers benefit from the empowerment often associated with "patient-controlled analgesia;" encouragement in the use of physical methods such as heat, cold, massage, and distraction; and the use of other cognitive behavioral techniques. Patient and caregiver education and instruction for these "self-help" interventions should be a part of the pain management plan for every patient with serious pain.

ANALGESIC DRUGS FOR CANCER PAIN

Any patient who has pain that impairs functional status or quality of life is a candidate for analgesic drug therapy. Analgesic medications are safe and effective in elderly people. All analgesic interventions carry a balance of benefits and burdens. For some classes of pain-relieving medications (opioids, for example) elderly patients have been shown to have increased analgesic sensitivity.

However, elderly people are a heterogeneous population, thus optimum dosage and known side effects are difficult to predict. Recommendations for age-adjusted dosing are not available for most analgesics. In reality, dosing for most patients requires beginning with low doses with careful upward titration, including frequent reassessment for dosage adjustments and optimum pain relief.

The use of placebos is unethical in clinical practice and there is no place for their use in the management of acute or chronic pain. Placebos, in the form of inert oral medications, sham injections, or other fraudulent procedures are only justified in certain research designs where patients have given informed consent and understand that they may be receiving a placebo as a part of the research design. In research, placebos help identify and measure random or uncontrollable events that may confound results of some research designs. In clinical settings, placebo effects are common, but they are neither diagnostic of pain nor indicative of a therapeutic response. The effects of placebos are short-lived and most patients eventually learn the truth, resulting in loss of patient trust and more needless suffering.

Acetaminophen

Acetaminophen is the drug of choice for elderly persons with mild to moderate pain, especially that of osteoarthritis and other musculoskeletal problems. As an analgesic and antipyretic, acetaminophen acts in the central nervous system to reduce pain perception. Despite the lack of anti-inflammatory activity, studies have shown that acetaminophen is as effective as most nonsteroidal anti-inflammatory drugs (NSAIDs). Given in a dose of 650 mg to 1000 mg four times a day, it remains the safest analgesic medication for most patients compared to traditional NSAIDs and other analgesic drugs. Unfortunately, acetaminophen overdose can result in irreversible hepatic necrosis. Therefore, the maximum daily dose should never exceed 4,000 mg per day. Some authors have suggested that the maximum dose of acetaminophen should be reduced in hepatic insufficiency. Unfortunately, evidence to identify a level of hepatic impairment justifying a dose adjustment has not been validated.

Nonsteroidal Anti-Inflammatory Drugs

Nonsteroidal anti-inflammatory drugs (NSAIDs) have analgesic activity both peripherally and centrally. They are potent inhibitors of cyclooxygenase and prostaglandin synthesis that have effects on inflammation, pain receptors, and nerve conduction and may have central effects as well. Clinical trials have found no advantage of COX-2–specific inhibitors compared to traditional non-specific COX-inhibiting NSAIDs in terms of peak pain relief, total pain relief, and in indices of joint inflammation in patients with arthritis. Safety profiles of these agents have been impressive in reduction of gastrointestinal injury, renal toxicity, and bleeding diathesis, but concerns about a higher risk of cardiovascular events have reduced their overall appeal. Moreover, COX-2–specific inhibitor NSAIDs appear to have similar problems compared with traditional NSAIDs with respect to the incidence of both drug-drug and drug-disease interactions.

NSAIDs are appropriate for short-term use in inflammatory conditions such as gout, calcium pyrophosphate arthropathy, acute flare-ups of rheumatoid arthritis, and other inflammatory rheumatic conditions. They have also been reported to relieve the pain of headache, menstrual cramps, and other mild to moderate pain syndromes. Individual drugs in this class vary widely with respect to anti-inflammatory activity, potency, analgesic properties, metabolism, excretion, and side-effect profiles. Moreover, it has been observed that failure of response to one NSAID may not predict the response to another. A disadvantage of NSAIDs is that they all demonstrate a ceiling effect, that is, a level at which increased dose results in no further increase in analgesia. A large number of NSAIDs are now available; however, there is no evidence to support a particular compound as the NSAID of choice. Several are available over-the-counter without a prescription.

Use of high-dose NSAIDs for long periods of time should be avoided in elderly patients. The concomitant use of misoprostol, histamine-2 receptor antagonists, proton pump inhibitors, and antacids is only partially successful at reducing the risk of significant gastrointestinal bleeding associated with NSAID use. Also, the side-effect profiles of gastroprotective drugs in this population must be weighed against their limited benefits. For those with multiple medical problems, NSAIDs are associated with an increased risk of drug-drug and drug-disease interactions. NSAIDs may interact with antihypertensive therapy. Thus, the relative risks and benefits of NSAIDs must be weighed carefully against other available treatments for older patients with chronic pain problems. For some patients, chronic opioid therapy, low-dose or intermittent corticosteroid therapy, or many other nonopioid analgesic drug strategies may have fewer life-threatening risks compared to long-term, high-dose NSAID use.

Opioid Analgesic Medications

Opioid analgesic medications act by blocking receptors in the central nervous system (brain and spinal cord) resulting in a decreased perception of pain. Selected opioid analgesic medications are listed in Table 16-1. Opioid drugs have no ceiling to their analgesic effects and have been shown to relieve all types of pain. Short-term studies have suggested that elderly people, compared to younger people, may be more sensitive to the pain-relieving properties of these drugs. This has been shown for acute postoperative pain and chronic cancer pain. Advanced age is associated with a prolonged half-life and prolonged pharmacokinetics of opioid drugs. Thus,

TABLE 16-1	**Selected Opioid Analgesic Medications for Pain***		
Drug	**Starting Dose (Oral)**	**Description**	**Comments**
Morphine (Roxanol, MSIR)	30 mg (q4h dosing)	Short-intermediate half-life; older people are more sensitive than younger people to side effects	Titrate to comfort; continuous use for continuous pain; intermittent use for episodic pain; anticipate and prevent side effects
Sustained-release morphine (MS Contin, Oramorph, Avinza)	MS Contin - 30-60 mg (q 12 h dosing) Oramorph - 30-60 mg (q 12 h dosing) Avinza - 30-60 mg (q 24 h dosing)	Morphine sulfate in a wax matrix tablet or sprinkles; MS Contin and Oramorph should not be broken or crushed; Avinza capsules can be opened and sprinkled on food, but should not be crushed	Titrate dose slowly because of drug accumulation; rarely requires more frequent dosing than recommended on package insert; immediate release opioid analgesic often necessary for breakthrough pain
Codeine (plain codeine, Tylenol #3, other combinations with acetaminophen or NSAIDs)	30-60 mg (q 4-6 h dosing)	Acetaminophen or NSAIDs limit dose; constipation is a major issue	Begin bowel program early; do not exceed maximum dose for acetaminophen or NSAIDs
Hydrocodone (Vicodin, Lortab, others)	5-10 mg (q 3-4 h dosing)	Toxicity similar to morphine; acetaminophen or NSAID combinations limit maximum dose	Same as codeine
Oxycodone (Roxicodone, OxyIR; or in combinations with acetaminophen or NSAIDs such as Percocet, Tylox, Percodan, others)	20-30 mg (q 3-4 h dosing)	Toxicity similar to morphine; acetaminophen or NSAID combinations limit maximum dose; oxycodone is available generically as a single agent	Same as morphine
Sustained-release oxycodone (OxyContin)	15-30 mg (q 12 h dosing)	Similar to sustained-release morphine	Similar to sustained-release morphine
Hydromorphone (Dilaudid)	4 mg (q 3-4 h dosing)	Half-life may be shorter than morphine; toxicity similar to morphine	Similar to morphine
Methadone (Dolophine)	Equal analgesic potency is dose-dependent and difficult to predict; significant overdose risk when switching from other opioids	Serum half-life 18 hr; analgesic half-life 8-12 hr. Highly lipid soluble; metabolism by oxidation and dependent on liver cytochrome enzyme activity.	Black box warning: Significant risk of drug accumulation.
Oxymorphone IR (Opana) Oxymorphone ER (Opana ER)	10-20 mg (q 4 h) 5 mg (q 12 h) in opioid naive	Slightly more potent than morphine, not as potent as hydromorphone	Same as morphine
Transdermal fentanyl (Duragesic)	25 µg patch (q 72 h dosing)	Reservoir for drug is in the skin, not in the patch; equivalent dose compared to other opioids is not very predictable (see package insert); effective activity may exceed 72 hrs in older patients	Drug reservoir is in skin, not patch. Titrate slowly using immediate release analgesics for breakthrough pain; peak effect of first dose may take 18-24 h; not recommended for opioid-naive patients
Fentanyl lozenge on an applicator stick	Rub on buccal mucosa until analgesia occurs, then discard	Short half-life; useful for acute and breakthrough pain when oral route is not possible	Absorbed via buccal mucosa, not effective orally

*A limited number of examples is provided. For comprehensive lists of other available opioids, clinicians should consult other sources.

elderly people may achieve pain relief from smaller doses of opiate drugs than younger people.

Opioid drugs have the potential to cause cognitive disturbances, respiratory depression, constipation, and habituation in older people. Drowsiness, performance-based measures of cognitive impairment, and respiratory depression associated with opioids should be anticipated when opioids are initiated and doses are escalated rapidly. Drowsiness, cognitive impairment, and respiratory depression occur in a dose-dependent fashion and can be used to judge dose escalations. If patients have unrelieved pain with little drowsiness or cognitive impairment, doses may be escalated. Tolerance usually develops in a few days to these side effects, at which time, patients usually return to a fully alert status and baseline cognitive function. Until tolerance develops, patients should be instructed not to drive and to take precautions against falls or other accidents. But once tolerance to these effects has developed, patients can return to normal activities including driving and other demanding tasks despite high doses of opioid drugs. In fact, cancer patients are often observed to improve physical function once pain is adequately relieved on opioid analgesics.

Constipation is a side effect of opioid drugs to which older patients do not develop tolerance. The management of constipation usually includes increasing fluid intake, maintaining mobility, and use of cathartic medications. Some patients find relief with remedies like prune juice or other natural laxatives. Other patients may require more potent osmotic laxatives such as milk of magnesia, lactulose, or sorbitol. But for many patients opioid-induced constipation may require potent stimulant laxatives such as senna or biscodyl. It should be remembered that stimulants should not be used until impactions have been removed and obstruction has been ruled out. Finally, some patients require regular enemas to ensure bowel evacuation during high-dose opioid administration for severe pain.

Nausea also occasionally complicates opioid therapy. Nausea from opioid medications may result from several mechanisms and may wane as tolerance develops. Traditionally, antiemetics such as prochlorperazine, chlorpromazine, and antihistamines have been the mainstay of treatment for nausea in younger patients. Recently low-dose haloperidol has been used, with anecdotally noting of a lower side effect profile compared to other neuroleptic drugs. It should be remembered that all of these agents have high side-effect profiles in elderly patients including movement disorders, delirium, and anticholinergic effects. Thus clinicians should choose antiemetic medications with the lowest side effects, and continue to monitor patients frequently.

It is important for clinicians who prescribe opioid analgesics to understand issues of tolerance, dependency, and addiction. Tolerance is a pharmacologic phenomenon that occurs with many drugs. Tolerance is defined by diminished effect of a drug associated with constant exposure to the drug over time. For opioid drugs, tolerance is difficult to predict. In general, tolerance to drowsiness and respiratory depression occur much faster than tolerance to analgesic properties of the drug. Previous reports that described tolerance among cancer patients resulting in the need for massive doses of morphine to achieve adequate analgesia were probably misinterpreted because those patients also had rapidly advancing cancer. More recent studies of opioid-managed arthritis pain have noted that tolerance was not often significant. In fact some patients have been noted to remain on stable doses of opioids for many years without demonstrating significant tolerance to the analgesic effects.

Dependency is also a pharmacologic phenomenon associated with many drugs including, for example, corticosteroids and beta-blockers. Dependency is present when patients experience uncomfortable side effects when the drug is withheld abruptly. Fortunately, these symptoms can be ameliorated easily by tapering opioids over a few days. It is important to remember that physiologic effects of opioid withdrawal are usually not life-threatening compared to the serious syndromes common with alcohol, benzodiazepine, or barbiturate withdrawal.

Addiction is a behavioral problem and is defined in such terms. Addictive behavior is defined by compulsive drug use despite negative physical and social consequences and the craving for effects other than pain relief. Addicted patients often have erratic behavior that can be observed in a clinical setting in the form of selling, buying, and procuring drugs on the street, and the use of medication by bizarre means such as dissolving tablets for intravenous self-administration. It is now clear that drug use alone is not the major factor in the development of addiction. Other medical, social, and economic factors play immense roles in addictive behavior. It is also important to not construe certain behaviors as necessarily addictive behaviors. Hoarding of medications, persistent or worsening pain complaints, frequent office visits, requests for dose escalations, and other behaviors associated with unrelieved pain have coined the term "pseudoaddiction". Laws, regulations, and unintentional behavior by prescribing clinicians may require patients to hoard medication and seek other physicians for additional help. In fact, true addiction is rare among patients taking opioid analgesic medications for medical reasons. This is not meant to imply that opioid drugs can be used indiscriminately, only that fear of addiction and side effects do not justify failure to treat pain in elderly patients, especially those near the end of life.

Other Nonopioid Medications for Pain

A variety of other medications not formally classified as analgesics have been found to be helpful in certain specific pain problems. The term "adjuvant analgesic drugs," although frequently used, is a misnomer in that some of these nonopioid drugs may, in certain cases, be the primary pain-relieving pharmacologic intervention. Table 16-2 provides some examples of nonopioid drugs that may help certain kinds of pain. The largest body of evidence available relates to the use of these drugs for neuropathic pain, such as diabetic neuropathies, postherpetic neuralgia, and trigeminal neuralgia. Tricyclic antidepressants, anticonvulsants, and local anesthetics are the most frequently used nonopioid analgesics for neuropathic conditions. In general, these drugs have had limited success in pain syndromes that are not associated with neuropathic mechanisms. Typically about 50% to 70% of patients have a measurable response and of those most only experience partial relief. Thus these drugs are not often panaceas and are rarely totally successful as single agents. Usually these agents work better in combination with other traditional drug and nondrug strategies in an effort to improve pain and keep other drug doses to a minimum. Failure of response to one

TABLE 16-2	Selected Nonopioid Medications for Pain*	
Drug	**Description**	**Comments**
Acetaminophen (paracetamol)	Mechanism of action not known (probably central-acting)	Drug of choice for mild to moderate musculo-skeletal pain; maximum dose = 4 gm/24 hrs; reduce dose by half in patients with severe hepatic insufficency
Nonsteroidal anti-inflammatory drugs (NSAIDs) Nonspecific COX inhibitors: Ibuprofen, naproxen, diclofenac	Effective for mild to moderate pain and inflammatory conditions; high side-effect profile in older persons including gastrointestinal bleeding, drug-drug and drug-disease interactions	Should not be used at high dose for long periods of time; proton pump inhibitors or misoprostol may reduce GI toxicity by 50%
Nonsteroidal anti-inflammatory drugs (NSAIDs) Specific COX-2 inhibitors Celecoxib (Celebrex), valdecoxib (Bextra)	No advantage over other NSAIDs in terms of pain efficacy or anti-inflammatory activity; GI toxicity compared to other NSAIDs is 50% less	Use has been controversial because of increased risk of myocardial infarction; one product (rofecoxib [Vioxx]) removed from the market in U.S.; continue aspirin in those with cardiovascular risk
Tricyclic antidepressants: (Amitriptyline, desipramine, nortriptyline, others)	Older people are more sensitive to side effects, especially anticholinergic effects; desipramine or nortriptyline is better choice than amitriptyline	Complete relief unusual; used best as adjunct to other strategies; start low and increase slowly every 3-5 days; not recommended for first-line therapy because of anticholinergic side effects
Norepinephrine modulating antidepressants: Duloxetine (Cymbalta), venlafaxine (Effexor)	Efficacy has been established, but studies are small and generally weak	Best in combination with other management strategies
Serotonin reuptake inhibitors (SSRI) Sertraline (Zoloft), paroxetine (Paxil)	Little or no effect on pain	Not recommended for pain
Anticonvulsants Clonazepam, carbamazepine	Carbamazepine may cause leukopenia, thrombocytopenia, and rarely aplastic anemia; clonazepine side effects may be similar to other benzodiazepines in the elderly	Start low and increase slowly; check blood counts on carbamazepine
Gabapentin (also an anticonvulsant) (Neurontin)	Less serious side effects than other anticonvulsants	Start with 100 mg and titrate up slowly; TID dosing; monitor for idiosyncratic side effects such as ankle swelling, ataxia, etc.; effective dose reported 100-800 mg q 8 h
Pregabalin (Lyrica)	Essentially identical to gabapentin	Start low and go slowly
Antiarrhythmics mexiletine (Mexitil)	Common side effects include tremor, dizziness, paresthesias; rarely may cause blood dyscrasias and hepatic damage	Avoid use in patients with preexisting heart disease; start low and titrate slowly; monitor EKGs; q 6-8 h dosing
Local anesthetics Lidocaine (intravenous) Lidocaine transdermal patch (Lidoderm) Capsaicin	IV lidocaine associated with delirium Transdermal patch has minimal systemic absorption. Capsaicin depletes nerve endings of Substance P.	IV lidocaine may predict response to anticonvulsants and antiarrhythmics May apply up to 3 patches alternating 12 h intervals to improve pain, reduce denervation hypersensitivity, and decrease systemic absorption May take 2 weeks to peak effect
Tramadol (Ultram)	Partial opioid and serotonin agonist; more of a norepinephrine antagonist; may cause drowsiness, nausea, vomiting, and constipation	Has ceiling effect; dose > 300 mg/24 h usually not tolerated because of nausea; q 4-6 h dosing
Muscle relaxants (baclofen, chlorzoxazone [Paraflex], cyclobenzaprine [Flexeril])	Sedation; anticholinergic effects; abrupt withdrawal of baclofen may cause CNS irritability	Mechanism of action not precisely known; monitor for sedation and anticholinergic effects; taper baclofen on discontinuation
Substance P inhibitors (capsaicin) Available OTC; for topical use only	Burning pain during depletion of substance P may be intolerable by as many as 30% of patients; may take 14 days for maximum response; avoid eye contamination	Start with small doses; can be partially removed with vegetable oil
NMDA Inhibitors Ketamine Dextromethorphan	N-Methyl-D-aspartate antagonists (NMDA) Ketamine: potent anesthetic Dextromethorphan: common cough suppressant	Ketamine only available IV Both may cause delirium

*A limited number of examples is provided. For comprehensive lists of other available pain medications, clinicians should consult other sources.

TABLE 16-2	Selected Nonopioid Medications for Pain—cont'd	
Drug	**Description**	**Comments**

Drugs for osteoporosis
  Calcitonin
  Bisphosphonates
	Pain-relief mechanisms unknown	Not effective on pain other than osteoporosis

Corticosteroids
  Prednisone
  Dexamethasone
	Decrease inflammation in many tissues.	Classic corticosteroid side effects limit overall usefulness in chronic pain.

particular class of drugs does not necessarily predict failure of another class of agents. In general, nonopioid medications for neuropathic pain should be chosen according to lowest side effects. Treatment should usually start with lower doses than recommended for younger patients and doses should be escalated slowly on the basis of known pharmacokinetics of individual drugs and appropriate knowledge of disease-specific treatment strategies. Unfortunately, most of the nonopioid medications for pain management have high side-effect profiles in elderly people. Thus these medications often have to be monitored carefully.

Tricyclic antidepressants have been the most widely studied class of nonopioid medications for pain. The mechanism of action for these drugs is not entirely known, but probably has to do with interruption of norepinephrine- and serotonin-mediated mechanisms in the brain. Because of the high level of anticholinergic side effects, most tricyclic antidepressants are no longer considered first-line therapy for neuopathic pain. Other studies of the serotonin reuptake inhibitors, which may have lower side-effect profiles for elderly people, have had mixed reviews and most have not been shown effective for pain management. Newer norepinephrine-modulating drugs such as duloxetine (Cymbalta) and venlafaxine (Effexor) may be more effective.

It has been known for many years that some medications with antiepileptic activity may relieve the pain of trigeminal neuralgia (tic douloureux). Among these drugs, gabapentin and pregabalin have become the drugs of choice for most neuropathic pain. Clinical observations suggest that these agents have a significant analgesic effect on many neuropathic pains with a much lower side-effect profile compared to other antiepileptic drugs and most antidepressants as well.

Muscle relaxant drugs include cyclobenzaprine, carisoprodol, chlorzoxazone, methocarbamol and others. It is important to know that cyclobenzaprine is essentially identical to amitriptyline with similar side effects, and carisoprodol has been removed from the European market because of concerns about drug abuse. Although these drugs may relieve skeletal muscle pain, their effects are nonspecific and not related to muscle relaxation. Therefore they should not be prescribed with the mistaken belief that they relieve muscle spasm. If muscle spasm is suspected to be at the root of the patient's pain, it is probably justified to consider another drug with known effects on muscle spasm (e.g., benzodiazepines, baclofen). Baclofen is an agonist of gamma butyric acid. It has been used as a second-line drug for severe spasticity related to central nervous system injury, demyelinating conditions, and other neuromuscular disorders. Discontinuation after prolonged use requires slow tapering because of potential for delirium and seizure.

Current information does not support a direct analgesic effect of benzodiazepines. Although they may be justified for management of anxiety or in a trial for the relief of muscle spasm, the high risk-profile of these drugs in elderly persons usually obviates the potential benefit as an analgesic.

Calcitonin may be helpful in various cases of bone pain and as a second-line treatment for some neuropathic conditions, particularly postosteoporotic vertebral fractures, pelvic fractures, and bony metastasis. The mechanism by which calcitonin relieves pain is unknown. Apart from hypersensitivity reactions, the main side effects include nausea and altered serum levels of calcium and phosphorus. Bisphosphonates may also provide analgesia in patients with cancer metastasis, particularly of breast, prostate, and multiple myeloma. Data are more promising for pamidronate and clodronate.

Topical analgesics may be helpful for certain regional pain syndromes. Placebo-controlled trials of lidocaine 5% patch have been largely limited to neuropathic pain. It has been shown to be helpful in cases of postherpetic neuralgia, but the benefit does not usually compare to that of systemic gabapentin or tricyclic antidepressants. Nonetheless, the patch has found widespread "off-label" use for a variety of conditions such as osteoarthritis and wound care. The patch is contraindicated in advanced liver failure because of decreased lidocaine clearance; however, among other patients, pharmacokinetic studies have suggested safe systemic lidocaine levels even with doses as high as four patches in 24 hrs. Adverse reactions are rare, mild, and mostly related to skin rash.

Eutectic mixture of lidocaine and prilocaine (EMLA) is a local anesthetic capable of penetrating the skin to produce cutaneous anesthesia. However, there is significant risk of systemic toxicity if used repeatedly or near mucous membranes or open wounds.

Topical capsaicin cream has been shown to provide some benefit in the reduction of both neuropathic and nonneuropathic pain, although as many as 30% of subjects may not be able to tolerate the burning sensation associated with treatment initiation. Depletion of substance P with resulting anesthesia may require several days or weeks of exposure. Newer formulations with NSAIDs, local anesthetics, or tricyclic antidepressants may help ameliorate the burning sensation and reduce premature treatment cessation.

Topical NSAIDs have shown some efficacy in a few studies of neuropathic and nonneuropathic pain. Studies of topical aspirin, indomethacin, diclofenac, piroxicam, and ketoprofen have been reported. The biology of these agents is not fully understood, although the reported toxicity seems to be low.

Antinociceptive effects have been observed with the use of cannabinoids in animal models and a few controlled human trials. In older patients, the therapeutic window for cannabinoids appears to be narrow because of the dysphoric response that older patients and those using higher doses may experience.

ANESTHETIC AND NEUROSURGICAL APPROACHES TO PAIN MANAGEMENT

A wide variety of anesthetic and neurosurgical approaches to pain are available and some require highly specialized skills. Although it is beyond the scope of this chapter to review details of all of these techniques, a few deserve mention.

Trigger-point injections have been used extensively for the treatment of myofascial pain syndromes. Myofascial pain with trigger points was first recognized more than 50 years ago. In a relatively high percentage of cases, trigger points may initiate a reflex mechanism that produces referred pain, tenderness, and muscle spasm. With local injection of the trigger point followed by stretching and reconditioning of the muscles, the myofascial pain syndrome usually subsides. More recently, similar results have been obtained using ice massage or vapocoolant spray applied topically, followed by specific muscle stretching and physical therapy techniques. Nonetheless, trigger-point injection with dilute local anesthetics may be highly effective when combined with specific physical therapy for many myofascial pain syndromes.

Continuous drug infusions are highly effective for providing steady-state analgesic drug levels. Continuous infusions can be maintained by implantable pumps or external devices to deliver intravenous, subcutaneous, intrathecal, or epidural medications. Continuous infusions of opioid drugs have found widespread use in severe chronic cancer pain, especially among those near the end of life. Other uses have included continuous infusion of muscle relaxants for patients with severe muscle spasm from spinal injury, multiple sclerosis, or end-stage Parkinson disease. Whether these invasive high-tech strategies are appropriate for patients with all kinds of chronic pain remains controversial. These techniques are very expensive, but they are often reimbursed by third-party payers. These issues have raised ethical issues about the application of high-tech strategies for patients who might be equally well managed using oral medications that are not reimbursable. In general, these methods should be used only when oral medications become ineffective or the oral route of administration is no longer viable. More work needs to be done to justify these risky and expensive techniques that need to be carefully monitored in nursing homes, home care, and other low-tech long-term care settings.

NONDRUG STRATEGIES FOR PAIN MANAGEMENT

Nondrug strategies, used alone or in combination with appropriate analgesic medications, should be an integral part of the care plan for most elderly patients with cancer pain. Nondrug strategies for pain management encompass a broad range of treatments and physical modalities, many of which carry low risks for adverse effects. Used in combination with appropriate drug regimens, these interventions often enhance therapeutic effects while allowing medication doses to be kept low to prevent adverse drug effects.

Physical exercise is important for most patients with pain. A program of exercise can be tailored to most patients' needs and is extremely important for rehabilitation and the maintenance of strength and endurance. There is no evidence that one form of exercise is better than another, so programs can be tailored for the individual's needs, lifestyle, and preference. The intensity of exercise along with frequency and duration must be adjusted to avoid exacerbation of the underlying condition while gradually increasing and later maintaining overall conditioning. It is important to remember that feeling better often gives rise to a false impression that the discipline of regular exercise is not necessary. Continued encouragement and reinforcement is often required. Unless complications arise, the program of exercise should be maintained indefinitely to prevent deconditioning and deterioration.

Psychological strategies have also been shown to be helpful for some with significant pain. Cognitive therapies are strategies aimed at altering belief systems and attitudes about pain and suffering. Cognitive therapies include various forms of distraction, relaxation, biofeedback, and hypnosis. Behavioral therapies are strategies aimed at enhancing healthy behaviors and discouraging abnormal behavior that is unpredictable and self-defeating. Cognitive therapy can be combined with behavioral approaches, and together they are known as cognitive-behavioral therapy. Cognitive-behavioral therapy in its purest form includes a structured approach to teaching coping skills that might be used alone or in combination with analgesic medications and other nondrug strategies for pain control. Effective programs can be conducted by trained professionals with individual patients or in groups and there is some evidence that the effect is enhanced with caregiver involvement. Although it may not be appropriate for those with significant cognitive impairment, there is evidence from randomized trials to support the use of cognitive-behavioral therapy for many patients with significant chronic pain.

Finally, a variety of alternative therapies are also used by many patients. Many patients seek alternative medicine approaches with and without the knowledge or recommendation of their physician or other primary care provider. Alternative medicine approaches to chronic pain may include homeopathy, spiritual healing, or the growing market of vitamin, herbal, and natural remedies. Although there is little scientific evidence to support these strategies for pain control, it is important that health care providers not abandon patients or leave them with a sense of hopelessness.

SUGGESTED READINGS

1. American Geriatrics Society Panel on Pharmacological Management of Persistent Pain in Older Persons: Pharmacological management of persistent pain in older persons, *Journal of the American Geriatrics Society* 57(8):1331–1346, 2009.
2. Paice JA: Pain at the end of life. In Ferrell BR, Coyle N, editors: *Oxford Textbook of Palliative Nursing*, ed 3, NY, 2010, Oxford Press, pp 161–885.
3. AGS Panel on Persistent Pain in Older Persons: The management of persistent pain in older persons, *Journal of the American Geriatrics Society* 50:S205–S224, 2002.
4. American Pain Society. Principles of Analgesic Use in the Treatment of Acute Pain and Chronic Cancer Pain. ed 5, Glenview, IL, 2003
5. Miaskowski C, Cleary J, Burney R, et al: *Guideline for the Management of Cancer Pain in Adults and Children*, Glenview, Il, 2005, American Pain Society.
6. Portenoy RK: Adjuvant analgesics in pain management. In Doyle D, Hanks GW, Mac Donald N, editors: *Oxford Textbook of Palliative Medicine*, ed 2, New York, 1998, Oxford Press, pp 361–390.
7. Hadjistavropoulos T, Herr K, Turk DC, et al: An interdisciplinary expert consensus statement on assessment of pain in older persons, *Clinical Journal of Pain* 23:s1–s43, 2007.
8. Weiner D, Herr K: Comprehensive interdisciplinary assessment and treatment planning: An integrative overview. In Weiner D, Herr K, Rudy T, editors: *Persistent Pain in Older Adults*, New York, 2002, Springer Publishing, pp 18–57.

with analgesic medications and other nondrug strategies for pain control. Effective programs can be conducted by trained professionals with individual patients or in groups, and there is some evidence that the effect is enhanced with caregiver involvement. Although it may not be appropriate for those with significant cognitive impairment, there is evidence from randomized trials to support the use of cognitive behavioral therapy for many patients with significant chronic pain.

Finally, a variety of alternative therapies are also used by many patients. Many patient seek alternative medical approaches without the knowledge or recommendation of their physician or other primary care provider. Alternative medicine approaches to chronic pain may include homeopathy, spiritual healing, or the consumption of vitamins, herbals and natural remedies. Although there is little scientific evidence to support these strategies for pain control, it is important that health care providers not abandon patients or leave them with a sense of hopelessness.

SUGGESTED READINGS

1. American Geriatrics Society Panel on Pharmacological Management of Persistent Pain in Older Persons. Pharmacological management of persistent pain in older persons. Journal of the American Geriatrics Society 57(8):1331-1346, 2009.
2. Pace JA. Pain at the end of life. In Ferrell BR, Coyle N, eds. Oxford Textbook of Palliative Nursing, ed 3, NY, 2010, Oxford Press, pp 161-185.

Cancer-Related Fatigue in the Older Patient

Betty Ferrell and Virginia Sun

CASE 17-1 **CASE STUDY**

Mr. D is an 80-year-old man who has been diagnosed with stage IV prostate cancer, with metastatic disease to the bones. He has a history of chronic arthritis and diabetes. His blood sugar is not optimally controlled, and he has had two recent visits to the emergency department for uncontrolled blood glucose. Over the years, as a result of his uncontrolled diabetes, Mr. D gradually developed diabetic peripheral neuropathy, and he uses a walker to help with ambulation. The neuropathy has interfered significantly with his functional status, and he relies on a niece who lives close by to shop for food and everyday essentials. His wife died six months ago, and he admits that he is still mourning his loss. He also reports that he is "exhausted," "tired to the bone," and is just "worn out." Mr. D has agreed to participate in a clinical trial testing a new chemotherapy to treat his prostate cancer.

This case study illustrates the multiple factors influencing cancer fatigue in the elderly. Cancer is a disease affecting predominantly older persons, with incidence and prevalence increasing with age.[1-4] In addition to cancer, many older persons have comorbid medical conditions (e.g., cardiomyopathies, diabetes, depression) rendering them more susceptible to illness and treatment and limiting their functional capacities.[5] Fatigue from cancer and/or its treatment is the most commonly reported symptom by older cancer patients and affects 70% to 100% of those receiving treatment for cancer.[3,6,7] The National Comprehensive Cancer Network (NCCN) defines cancer-related fatigue (CRF) as a distressing, persistent, subjective sense of physical, emotional, and/or cognitive tiredness or exhaustion related to cancer or cancer treatment that is not proportional to recent activity and interferes with usual functioning.[8] This chapter discusses the current evidence regarding cancer-related fatigue in the elderly and provides recommendations for the assessment and management of this distressing symptom in the elderly cancer population.

ETIOLOGY OF CANCER-RELATED FATIGUE

To date, the mechanisms and pathophysiology of CRF are largely unknown, although many studies have attempted to describe possible etiology and mechanisms related to its manifestation in cancer patients. Possible CRF mechanisms include cytokine production (i.e., IL-6), abnormal serotonin regulation, neuromuscular dysfunction, and abnormal levels of muscle metabolites.[9-12] CRF may also be caused by treatments such as chemotherapy, radiation therapy, bone marrow transplantation, biological response modifiers, or contributing factors such as pain, emotional distress, anemia, altered nutritional status, sleep disturbance, decreased activity, and comorbidities.[8] CRF is thought to have peripheral as well as central components as its biologic basis. Peripheral components are those factors that cause negative energy balance that result in fatigue. Factors that contribute to this negative energy balance include cancer, cancer treatments, systemic infections, hypothyroidism, anemia, malnutrition, metabolic abnormalities, sleep disorders, and psychological factors (depression, anxiety).[12,13] Central components include hypothalamic-pituitary-adrenal (HPA) axis hyperactivity, and increases in immunologic factors and cytokines (T lymphocytes, IL-1 antagonists, tumor necrosis factor receptor II).[12,14-18] All of these potential components of CRF are important in elderly cancer patients, and may contribute to the etiology of CRF in this older population.

CANCER-RELATED FATIGUE ACROSS THE DOMAINS OF QUALITY OF LIFE

CRF affects all aspects of the patient's quality of life (QOL) and can persist 5 to 10 years after completion of treatment.[19,20] The impact on the patient's physical functioning is exceptionally distressing and has been reported as being more distressing than pain or nausea.[21-23]

CRF affects physical functioning and can be very debilitating.[24-26] For the general geriatric population, the need for assistance with activities of daily living (ADLs) and instrumental activities of daily living (IADLs) is an independent predictor of morbidity and mortality. The older cancer patient is more likely to have functional limitations in ADLs than the general elderly population.[27] For many patients, physical activity levels decrease during and after treatment, with some patients not returning to prior treatment levels. This can lead to a cycle of declining physical activity leading to increased fatigue, which leads to further decreased conditioning, and increased weakness and fatigue during any physical activity.[4]

Luciani and colleagues conducted a retrospective cross-sectional study of 214 patients aged 70 or older, seen over the course of 3 months in their Senior Adult Oncology Program.[28] Patients were screened with a questionnaire assessing ADLs, IADLs, performance status (PS), cognitive impairment, depression, and malnutrition. In addition, each patient was assessed for fatigue using the Fatigue Symptom Inventory that measures four aspects of fatigue: severity, frequency, daily patterns of fatigue, and interference with daily activities; complete blood counts and chemical panels were also obtained. Eighty-one percent of the patients reported fatigue and the interference score of fatigue was a probable mediator for dependencies in ADLs ($p < 0.001$) and IADLs ($p < 0.001$), and poorer PS ($p < 0.001$). Data revealed a correlation between severity, interference, and frequency of fatigue and depression, but only hemoglobin level partially correlated with fatigue. Anemia correlated with decreased functional status. All fatigue dimensions were significantly associated with ADL and IADL dependencies and with the Geriatric Depression Scale. The authors concluded that fatigue in the elderly could represent a long-term complication of cancer and cancer treatment that may accelerate functional decline.[28]

Comorbid conditions in the older cancer patient are also causes of morbidity and mortality, affecting life expectancy, tolerance to treatment, and quality of life.[29,30] Those older than 65 years have an average of three comorbidities, with the most common being cardiovascular disease, hypertension, COPD, arthritis, and depression.[31] Comorbidities were found to be a prevailing issue among 867 elderly patients with newly diagnosed breast, prostate, lung, or colorectal cancer. Kozachik and Bandeen-Roche conducted a secondary analysis on this population and followed the patients at four points in time (6 to 8 weeks, 12 to 16 weeks, 24 weeks, and 52 weeks) during the year after their diagnosis.[2] The patients also completed a demographic questionnaire, the Comorbidity Index, and the Patient Symptom Experience. The researchers sought to determine whether the patient's sex, age, comorbidity status, cancer site, stage of disease, or treatment regimen predicted patterns of pain, fatigue, and insomnia over time. The mean patient age was 72.6 years, 54% were

men, and reported a mean of more than two comorbidities. Twenty-seven percent reported four or more comorbidities. The top four comorbid conditions reported were heart problems (31%), arthritis (20%), high blood pressure (50%), and chronic lung disease (16%). Results revealed that advanced age was not significantly associated with increased patterns of pain, fatigue, and insomnia. Comorbidities were correlated with pain, fatigue, and insomnia only at wave 1 and 4 observation times. Sex was associated with significant risks of reporting fatigue and insomnia or fatigue and pain, with women reporting the most fatigue and sleep disturbance. Treatment modality was associated with significantly increased risks of pain, fatigue, and insomnia. Having late-stage lung cancer and reporting pain, fatigue, and insomnia at wave 2, 3, and 4 observation times were significantly associated with death.[2]

The psychological impact of CRF in older cancer patients can greatly diminish their quality of life. CRF affects the patient's social activities, leisure time, and responsibilities.[32] There is debate as to whether a correlation exists between fatigue and depression. However, depression occurs in approximately 20% to 50% of patients with cancer.[33-41] It is the most common psychiatric disorder among cancer patients and yet is frequently undiagnosed because of the oftentimes coexistent symptoms from cancer and/or cancer treatment, such as fatigue, pain, and appetite loss.[42-44] As in the aforementioned case study, depression and grief for this elderly patient are important considerations in a plan of care.

Hwang, Chang, Rue, and Kasimis assessed multidimensional independent predictors of cancer-related fatigue and found that dyspnea, pain, lack of appetite, feeling drowsy, feeling sad, and feeling irritable predicted fatigue independently.[45] Physical and psychological symptoms predict fatigue independently in the multidimensional model and superseded laboratory data.[45] Liao and Ferrell assessed fatigue in the elderly and found a significant relationship between fatigue and depression, pain, number of medications, and physical function.[46] Respini and colleagues found that fatigue correlated with depression in older cancer patients to a degree comparable to that in younger patients.[7] This study assessed the prevalence and correlates of fatigue in 77 cancer patients aged 60 or older during outpatient treatment with chemotherapy or pamidronate. An older study conducted by Hickie and colleagues examined the prevalence and sociodemographic and psychiatric correlates of prolonged fatigue syndromes of 1593 patients attending four general primary care practice settings.[47] Twenty-five percent reported prolonged fatigue and 37% had a psychological disorder. Of the 25% with fatigue, 70% had both fatigue and psychological disorder, while 30% had fatigue only. Data revealed that patients with fatigue were more likely to also have a depressive disorder.[47] The literature clearly shows the interrelationship between fatigue and psychological disorders.

FATIGUE ASSESSMENT

CASE 17-1	CASE UPDATE

Mr. D comes to the clinic today for his third course of treatment and reports that he has been "very tired" for the past week, and that he is unable to perform some activities of daily living, such as buying groceries and cooking. When asked to rate his fatigue intensity over the past 7 days, he reports that it is a 6 out of 10. According to Mr. D's subjective rating, he is currently suffering from moderate fatigue. His oncologist initiated a more focused fatigue history and examination in addition to a comprehensive geriatric assessment. Mr. D was queried about the onset, pattern, and duration of his fatigue over the past 7 days. While conducting a thorough assessment of treatable contributing factors, his oncologist focused on Mr. D's two comorbidities: chronic arthritis and diabetes, as well as bereavement from his wife's recent death. On the basis of this medical history, the oncologist focused his queries around factors related to the comorbidities that may be contributing or exacerbating Mr. D's CRF: uncontrolled pain from his chronic arthritis and neuropathy, his activity level, his nutritional status, possible depression secondary to complicated bereavement, and possible anemia secondary to three courses of clinical trial treatment. Mr. D admits that the pain related to his chronic arthritis has been flaring recently, and that his activity level has been low. He also reports that he has been unable to sleep at night because of the arthritis flare-ups.

An essential component of managing CRF in the elderly is a thorough assessment. First, comorbidities need to be assessed and addressed to determine other factors that may be contributing to fatigue related to cancer treatments. Elderly patients with a history of diabetes or other comorbidities may be at higher risk for experiencing debilitating fatigue if treatment is planned. After assessing for comorbidities, patients should be asked to rate their fatigue level on a numerical analog scale (0-10). The NCCN guidelines recommend the following cut-offs for fatigue severity: 0 to 3 for "none to mild," 4 to 6 for "moderate," and 7 to 10 for "severe."[8] The guidelines recommend that all patients with a reported fatigue severity of moderate to severe intensity should be assessed using a focused history and examination to pinpoint treatable causes. Treatable causes include anemia, pain, insomnia, malnutrition, and emotional distress.[8] Finally, any referrals made to supportive care experts such as a dietician, rehabilitation, social work, psychology/psychiatry, or support groups should be documented. The NCCN guidelines recommend using an interdisciplinary model for managing CRF.[8]

FATIGUE MANAGEMENT

CASE 17-1	CASE UPDATE

On the basis of Mr. D's CRF assessment, referrals to supportive care experts such as a dietician, physical therapist, psychologist, social worker, and pain specialist were considered in order to manage the treatable causes. An endocrinologist was also consulted to assess whether Mr. D's diabetes continues to be poorly controlled. Mr. D was given patient education materials that included information about CRF and its management. His nurse discussed the education material, including strategies of fatigue management such as energy conservation and physical activity. His oncologist also discussed the use of medications such as Ritalin to manage his CRF, but Mr. D declines because he doesn't want to have to take another "pill."

Pharmacologic

A number of pharmacologic agents have been evaluated for the treatment of cancer-related fatigue. The class of pharmacologic agents that shows the most promise in managing cancer-related fatigue is psychostimulants, which are known to increase level of alertness and motivation. Methylphenidate has been evaluated in HIV patients and advanced cancer patients.[48,49] In a pilot study by Bruera and colleagues, an improvement was shown in general well-being and depression, as well as in fatigue scores as measured by the FACIT-F.[50] Because of the rapid onset of action and short half-life of methylphenidate, a subsequent double-blind, randomized, placebo-controlled trial by Bruera and colleagues tested a patient-controlled methylphenidate protocol for patients with a self-reported fatigue intensity of 4 or more as measured by the Functional Assessment of Chronic Illness Therapy – Fatigue (FACIT-F).[51] The dosage tested in this study was methylphenidate 5 mg or placebo every 2 hours as needed, up to four tablets per day, with fatigue assessment at day 8, 15, and 36. Fatigue intensity decreased significantly at day 8 in both groups, but there was no significant difference in fatigue improvement.[51] However, in the open-label phase, a significant improvement in fatigue was found between groups, and was sustained through days 15 and 36.[51] It was unclear whether the extended improvement during the open-label phase was an independent result or due to placebo effect. Although there is evidence on a preliminary level to support the effectiveness of psychostimulants for the treatment of cancer-related fatigue, some caution needs to be taken, particularly for geriatric oncology patients. Because of the rapid onset of these agents, as well as their behavioral effects and tolerance issues, there is an increased risk for side effects. The most common side effects of psychostimulants include agitation and insomnia, which may cause more harm than benefit for elderly cancer patients.[48] Cardiovascular side effects such as hypertension, palpitations, arrhythmias, as well as confusion, psychosis, and tremors are rare side effects, but again may be potentially dangerous for elderly cancer patients. These common and potential side effects limit the use of this class of agents for elderly cancer patients because of contraindications for cardiovascular and other comorbid conditions.

Modafinil has been tested as a fatigue treatment option. In a study of breast cancer survivors, Morrow and colleagues reported an 86% reduction of fatigue intensity with a modafinil dosage of 200 mg per day.[52] Donepezil, an agent used in the treatment of Alzheimer dementia, was evaluated by Bruera and colleagues in a double-blind placebo-controlled trial of donepezil 5 mg per day compared to placebo.[53] The study results were negative, with no statistically significant difference shown between groups. Toxicities are also a problem for this drug including nausea, vomiting, diarrhea, muscle and abdominal cramps, and anorexia, which may limit its use in the geriatric oncology setting.[48,54] Studies exploring the use of antidepressants as a possible mechanism for managing fatigue demonstrated no differences in fatigue scores.[12]

Nonpharmacologic

A number of systematic reviews and one Cochrane review have been undertaken to examine the efficacy of nonpharmacologic strategies, such as exercise, in fatigue management.[55-57] A detailed assessment by a rehabilitation expert such as a physical therapist should be accessed, if available, in order to prescribe a comprehensive and safe exercise regimen. The prescribed exercise regimen should be initiated gradually and at a pace based on the individual's capabilities. Table 17-1 provides an outline of key concepts to be included in patient education for CRF. The outline includes education points on what fatigue is, common causes of fatigue, common words used to describe fatigue, what patients should tell their clinicians about

fatigue, energy conservation principles, and the principles of exercise.

There are several treatable causes that have an impact on CRF. Nutrition is one that is of particular importance for the elderly cancer patient. Geriatric patients in general may also be at higher risk for malnutrition. Potential reasons include more difficulty accessing healthy food items, poorly fitted dentures, or inability to prepare healthy meals secondary to functional limits. Geriatric oncology patients may be particularly at risk because of gastrointestinal side effects (nausea, diarrhea) and poor appetite secondary to cancer treatment.[58] It is important in oncology to stress the importance of optimizing nutrition, particularly in relation to fatigue management. Patients should be provided with adequate information on potential side effects so they are aware of what to expect during treatment. If unable to eat regularly, patients can be advised to switch their eating habits from three large meals per day to six smaller meals spread throughout the day. The importance of maintaining adequate fluid intake should be emphasized, unless contraindicated. Finally, if available, referrals to nutrition experts such as dieticians should be initiated to aid elderly patients with optimizing their nutrition as a strategy for fatigue management.

Another treatable cause that may aggravate CRF is sleep deprivation. As a result of the natural course of aging, the length and quality of REM sleep decreases as the aging process continues.[5] Elderly cancer patients may be at higher risk for greater sleep disturbance. Patients can be instructed on the principles of sleep hygiene. These principles include the avoidance of caffeinated drinks or intense exercises before going to bed. Maintaining a dark, cool, and quiet sleep environment may help with inducing and enhancing sleep.[59] If possible, patients should be strongly encouraged to limit their daily nap times to no more than two 60-minute naps per day. This strategy will help in maintaining the quality of nighttime sleep. Relaxation or sleep-inducing strategies, such as warm baths, milk, or soothing music, can be used.

Stress-management strategies, such as meditation, massage, or muscle relaxation, may also be used to manage cancer-related fatigue.[60-62] Any contributing factors, such as anxiety, should be addressed by supportive care experts and assessed as a possible contributor to sleep disturbance. Patients should be assessed for any other symptoms, such as uncontrolled pain, that may be interfering with the quality of sleep. Maintaining physical activity during the day may help with promoting sleep at night, and patients should be encouraged to remain as active as possible. Finally, if pharmacologic intervention is warranted, clinicians can discuss the various options available either over the counter or prescribed and, together with the patient, a pharmacologic agent should be chosen that will provide the greatest benefit without debilitating side effects.

TABLE 17-1	Key Concepts for Patient Education on CRF

1. Definition of cancer-related fatigue (CRF)
2. Common causes of CRF
3. Common words used to describe cancer-related fatigue (i.e., feeling tired, weak, worn out, not being able to concentrate)
4. What to tell your clinician
5. Energy conservation principles (prioritize activities, ask for help, establish structured routine, balance rest and activities, establish regular bedtime)
6. Other management strategies (physical activity, sleep hygiene, maintaining adequate nutrition)

Adapted from Borneman T, Piper BF, Sun VC, et al: Implementing the Fatigue Guidelines at one NCCN member institution: process and outcomes. J Natl Compr Canc Netw 2007;5:1092-101.

THE NCCN CLINICAL PRACTICE GUIDELINES FOR CRF

The NCCN guidelines include several standards of care for the assessment and management of CRF. First, the NCCN recognizes that fatigue is a subjective experience that should be assessed using patient-reported outcomes.[8] Second, fatigue should be screened, assessed, and managed for all patients. Patients and families should be informed that fatigue management is an integral part of comprehensive oncology care.[8] Finally, fatigue should be included as an important component of all clinical outcomes research, and should be routinely assessed in all oncology research settings.[8]

Fatigue management within the NCCN guidelines is categorized on the basis of the subjective rating of the symptom on a 0 to 10 scale. It is recommended that all patients be screened for the presence or absence of fatigue. Management for patients who report absent or mild levels of fatigue (0 to 3) includes the provision of education about fatigue and common strategies for managing the symptom.[8] Periodic rescreening is recommended, daily for inpatient settings and during subsequent follow-up visits for outpatient settings.[8] It is also helpful for clinicians to understand the common barriers to optimal fatigue assessment and management. Table 17-2 provides a list of common patient- and professional-related barriers to fatigue management. Understanding and recognizing these potential barriers will aid the clinician in devising individualized fatigue management plan for elderly cancer patients.

As discussed previously in the case study, patients who report moderate to severe fatigue (4 to 10) should undergo a focused history and physical examination to determine the potential causes of fatigue. Table 17-3 provides a list of the essential components of this thorough evaluation. The NCCN guidelines identify seven treatable contributing factors of fatigue. These factors include pain, emotional distress, sleep disturbance, anemia, nutrition, activity level, medication side effects, and other comorbidities.[8] For elderly cancer patients, emphasis should be placed on potential medication side effects due to polypharmacy and comorbidities. Finally, because fatigue may be a problem at several different points throughout the disease trajectory, ongoing reassessment should be continued at all follow-up visits.

RESEARCH IN CRF MANAGEMENT

There are several important areas of research that are needed to further understand fatigue in elderly cancer patients and to further enhance assessment and management. First, CRF research should be designed specifically to target the elderly population. By doing so, the specific needs of elderly cancer patients can be better elucidated. Armed with more descriptive studies to explore the needs, attitudes, knowledge, and experience of CRF in the elderly, tailored patient education for the assessment and management of fatigue can be developed. Patient education for elderly cancer patients must acknowledge the fact that fatigue is common in cancer, and that elderly patients should be encouraged to discuss the symptom with their clinicians. Functional status should be assessed in detail for the elderly cancer patient, since a limitation in function may lead to inactivity or malnutrition, which can aggravate fatigue. Loss of functional independence has been associated with reduced survival, diminished quality of life, depression, and financial burden for patients, and fatigue is a primary cause of functional dependence for elderly cancer patients.[28] It has been reported that fatigue may accelerate the functional decline of elderly cancer patients.[28] Although evidence-based clinical guidelines are available for managing CRF, it is unclear whether these guidelines are generalizable to elderly cancer patients, because most of the evidence has not been tested specifically in an elderly sample population. While most recommendations can be applied to the elderly population, there may be issues that are specific

TABLE 17-2	Barriers to Effective Fatigue Management
Patient-Related Barriers	**Professional-Related Barriers**
1. Don't want to bother clinicians	1. Failure to initiate discussion regarding CRF
2. Concern that treatment may be altered	2. Assume that fatigue is related to the normal process of aging
3. Don't want to be perceived as complaining	3. Failure to recognize that fatigue is a problem
4. Assume that they just have to live with it	4. Not aware that there are effective treatments for fatigue
5. Belief that there are no treatments for CRF	5. Lack of knowledge in principles of fatigue assessment and management

See references 8, 65.

TABLE 17-3	Components of a Comprehensive Fatigue Assessment[8]

1. Current disease status
2. Type and length of treatment
3. Fatigue onset, pattern, duration, change over time
4. Associated or alleviating factors
5. Interference with function
6. Patient's perception of the causes of fatigue
7. Assessment of treatable contributing factors
   - Pain
   - Emotional distress
   - Sleep disturbance
   - Anemia
   - Nutrition
   - Activity level
   - Medication side effects (polypharmacy)
   - Comorbidities

to the elderly that are not thoroughly addressed in the guidelines.

Over the last decade, exercise and physical activity has emerged as a potentially effective strategy for managing CRF. The abundance of evidence can be recognized by the publication of numerous systematic reviews and a Cochrane review to determine the scientific evidence behind the efficacy of exercise. However, many limitations still exist in the current evidence on exercise. The quality of studies published thus far is widely variable.[55] There are issues with statistical power because many studies were limited by a small sample size.[55,63] In randomized controlled trials conducted on activity-based interventions, a variety of regimens were used. This variation makes it difficult to determine the most effective type of exercise for fatigue management. Future research is necessary to determine which parameters of exercise are most effective in managing fatigue. These parameters include type of exercise (aerobic or resistance), mode of exercise, length and frequency of sessions, and the amount of intensity that is required..[23,55,64] These parameters should also apply for developing activity-based interventions for the elderly cancer patient. Because comorbidities and functional dependence are common in the elderly population, it is crucial to develop modes of activities that are realistically feasible for this understudied population. Although experts are calling for research that produces more long-term follow-up outcomes of activity-based interventions, it may be equally important to focus on short-term outcomes in the elderly population. Finally, outcome measures used to assess fatigue in research should be psychometrically tested in elderly populations to establish reliability and validity, as perceptions of fatigue may be different.

Chapter Summary

 Cancer is primarily a disease of the older population. As the geriatric population of the United States increases, it is expected that more elderly individuals will be treated with cancer. Fatigue continues to be recognized as the most common and distressing chronic complication of cancer and its treatments. Fatigue affects all aspects of quality of life, and can lead to reduced social interactions and functional independence for the elderly. Clinicians should be aware of evidence-based strategies to assess and manage cancer-related fatigue. An interdisciplinary, comprehensive model of fatigue management incorporating focused assessment and patient education can be helpful in supporting elderly patients and families who are experiencing fatigue. Future research in fatigue should focus on describing the unique aspect of fatigue in the elderly cancer population and develop tailored interventions that are specific and realistic for this understudied population.

 See expertconsult.com for a complete list of references and web resources for this chapter

SUGGESTED READINGS

1. Rao AV, Cohen HJ: Fatigue in older cancer patients: etiology, assessment, and treatment, *Semin Oncol* 35:633–642, 2008.
2. Minton O, Richardson A, Sharpe M, et al: A systematic review and meta-analysis of the pharmacological treatment of cancer-related fatigue, *J Natl Cancer Inst* 100:1155–1166, 2008.
3. Kangas M, Bovbjerg DH, Montgomery GH: Cancer-related fatigue: a systematic and meta-analytic review of non-pharmacological therapies for cancer patients, *Psychol Bull* 134:700–741, 2008.
4. Dy SM, Lorenz KA, Naeim A, et al: Evidence-based recommendations for cancer fatigue, anorexia, depression, and dyspnea, *J Clin Oncol* 26:3886–3895, 2008.
5. Cramp F, Daniel J: Exercise for the management of cancer-related fatigue in adults, *Cochrane Database Syst Rev* CD006145, 2008.
6. Luctkar-Flude MF, Groll DL, Tranmer JE, et al: Fatigue and physical activity in older adults with cancer: a systematic review of the literature, *Cancer Nurs* 30:E35–E45, 2007.
7. Jacobsen PB, Donovan KA, Vadaparampil ST, et al: Systematic review and meta-analysis of psychological and activity-based interventions for cancer-related fatigue, *Health Psychol* 26:660–667, 2007.

Nausea and Vomiting

Roxana S. Dronca and Charles Loprinzi

CASE 18-1 **CASE PRESENTATION**

J.J., a 69-year-old woman, is a former smoker of 60 pack-years who presents with a stage IIIA (T2N2M0) primary lung adenocarcinoma. She was not considered a surgical candidate. The final treatment recommendation was definitive chemoradiation therapy, with plans for two cycles of neoadjuvant chemotherapy prior to the start of radiation because of the large lung mass and inability to deliver safe radiation doses. The initial chemotherapy plan included a combination of cisplatin (75 mg/m^2) and pemetrexed (500 mg/m^2) every 21 days.

On further discussion of potential chemotherapy side effects, Mrs. J. expresses concern regarding the potential for severe nausea and vomiting associated with the treatment, as she suffers from severe motion sickness and remembers having had significant nausea with her two pregnancies. She asks whether anything can be done to prevent and treat chemotherapy-associated nausea and vomiting.

Nausea and vomiting are two of the most feared and most commonly reported symptoms[1] in patients with cancer, and can occur either as a result of the malignancy itself or from antineoplastic treatment. Over the last few decades, significant progress has been made in the development of more potent and effective chemotherapeutic agents. However, there is a significant cost in term of toxicity and the side effects of treatment, which often limit management options. Among the cancer treatment-related side effects, chemotherapy-induced nausea and vomiting (CINV) are, historically, two of the most common[2-4]; they can significantly affect patients' quality of life, functional ability, and adherence to potentially useful and curative anticancer therapy.[5,6]

PATHOPHYSIOLOGY OF NAUSEA AND VOMITING

The vomiting reflex is triggered by afferent impulses to the vomiting center from vagus nerve terminals in the wall of the small bowel, the chemoreceptor trigger zone, or the cerebral cortex; the act of vomiting occurs when efferent impulses are sent to a number of organs and tissues such as the abdominal muscles, salivary glands, cranial nerves, and respiratory center. It is now thought that the central site of the emetic reflex, previously referred to as the "vomiting center"[7] and most recently named the "central pattern generator,"[8] is not an isolated area within the central nervous system but rather a group of loosely organized neurons throughout the medulla that interact through various pathways to coordinate the sequence of behaviors during vomiting.[9,10] The primary sources of afferent input to the central pattern generator include the area postrema (commonly referred to as the "chemoreceptor trigger zone")[11] and the gastrointestinal tract through vagal and splanchnic afferents,[12] which terminate primarily in the nucleus tractus solitarius[9] and, to a lesser extent, the area postrema. These two central nervous system centers are collectively referred to as the dorsal vagal complex.[11,13] The area postrema is located at the caudal end of the fourth ventricle, on the dorsal surface of the medulla oblongata where the blood-brain barrier is relatively permeable, and is therefore positioned to detect emetic stimuli in either the blood or the cerebrospinal fluid.[11]

The main neurotransmitters implicated in the pathogenesis of acute and delayed CINV include serotonin (5-HT), substance P, and dopamine, which bind to 5-HT$_3$, neurokinin-1 (NK1), and dopamine D$_2$ receptors, respectively.

- The 5-HT$_3$ receptors are found on the terminal ends of the vagal afferent nerves,[14] as well as in key areas of the human brain stem, including the area postrema and the nucleus tractus solitarius.[15] Preliminary evidence suggests that the selective 5-HT$_3$ receptor antagonists exert their action mainly by antagonizing the action of serotonin at the 5-HT$_3$ receptors on the peripheral vagal afferent terminals.[16,17]
- The tachykinin NK1 receptors are widely distributed throughout the central and peripheral nervous system, as well as the respiratory, cardiovascular, genitourinary, and gastrointestinal tracts.[18] It is currently thought that the NK1 receptor antagonists exert their action at a central level and that penetration of the blood-brain barrier is essential for their ability to prevent cisplatin-induced emesis.[19]

TYPES OF CHEMOTHERAPY-INDUCED NAUSEA AND VOMITING SYNDROMES

Three distinct chemotherapy-induced nausea and/or vomiting syndromes have been described: acute, delayed, and anticipatory. Although the exact mechanism behind each syndrome is unclear, this classification has important implications for both prevention and management of CINV. Acute CINV occurs within 24 hours of chemotherapy administration; it may occur within 1 to 2 hours, with a peak incidence at 4 to 6 hours.

Delayed CINV is arbitrarily defined as occurring more than 24 hours after chemotherapy. Although it is most common after high-dose cisplatin, it has been associated with other agents as well, such as carboplatin, oxaliplatin, or the combination of cyclophosphamide with an anthracycline. For cisplatin, nausea and vomiting typically reach maximal intensity at 48 to 72 hours, and can last up to 5 or more days.[20]

Anticipatory CINV is a conditioned response that tends to occur when nausea and vomiting have been poorly controlled with previous cycles of chemotherapy.[21,22] Previous neutral stimuli become conditioned stimuli that elicit anticipatory nausea and/or vomiting, which can then be brought on by the smell of the hospital, the sight of the clinic, the treating physician, or the chemotherapy suite. Although usually associated with negative past experiences, anticipatory nausea and/or vomiting has also been described in patients who have a high expectancy of developing nausea despite never having received any cancer treatment.[23] The incidence of anticipatory CINV can be as high as 57%,[24] with nausea occurring more commonly than vomiting. Risk factors associated with the development of anticipatory nausea and/or vomiting include previous history of motion sickness,[22] age younger than 50 years,[25] past history of anxiety or depression,[24] uncontrolled acute or delayed CINV with previous cycles,[22] or chemotherapy extended over a prolonged period of time.

EMETOGENICITY OF CHEMOTHERAPEUTIC AGENTS

The most important factor in predicting CINV is the emetogenicity of the chemotherapeutic agent(s) used. Several classification schemes have been proposed[26-29] that reflect the likelihood of emesis with both single agents and combination chemotherapy. The development of such algorithms has been of great value in providing a framework for the management of CINV and for the development of antiemetic treatment guidelines. In 2004, the Antiemetic Subcommittee of the Multinational Association of Supportive Care in Cancer (MASCC) held a consensus conference whereby a modification of the original schema of Hesketh et al.[26] was proposed.[29] This classification, utilized by both MASCC and the American Society of Clinical Oncology updated guidelines,[30] divides intravenous chemotherapeutic agents into four categories on the basis of risk (incidence) of emesis in the absence of prophylaxis (Table 18-1):

- High: greater than 90% emetic risk
- Moderate: 30% to 90% emetic risk
- Low: 10% to 30% emetic risk
- Minimal: less than 10% emetic risk

A new problem with utilizing this classification system is the growing use of oral chemotherapeutic

TABLE 18-1	Emetic Risk of Intravenously Administered Antineoplastic Agents
Emetic Risk (incidence of emesis without antiemetics)	**Agent**
High (> 90%)	Cisplatin
	Mechlorethamine
	Streptozotocin
	Cyclophosphamide $\geq$ 1,500 mg/m^2
	Carmustine
	Dacarbazine
	Dactinomycin
Moderate (30% to 90%)	Oxaliplatin
	Cytarabine > 1 g/m^2
	Carboplatin
	Ifosfamide
	Cyclophosphamide < 1,500 mg/m^2
	Doxorubicin
	Daunorubicin
	Epirubicin
	Idarubicin
	Irinotecan
Low (10% to 30%)	Paclitaxel
	Docetaxel
	Mitoxantrone
	Topotecan
	Etoposide
	Pemetrexed
	Methotrexate
	Mitomycin
	Gemcitabine
	Cytarabine $\leq$ 1 g/m^2
	Fluorouracil
	Bortezomib
	Cetuximab
	Trastuzumab
Minimal (< 10%)	Bevacizumab
	Bleomycin
	Busulfan
	2-Chlorodeoxyadenosine
	Fludarabine
	Rituximab
	Vinblastine
	Vincristine
	Vinorelbine

Reproduced with permission from Kris et al.,[30] by permission of J Clin Oncol.

agents, which tend to be prescribed over a period of several days to weeks. This makes it difficult to assess the contribution of acute versus delayed CINV and, as a result, antiemetic regimes recommended for single-dose intravenous agents may not apply to oral cytotoxic or targeted agents. The 2004 MASCC updated guidelines include[29] a separate listing of the estimated emetic risk of the most commonly used oral antineoplastic agents.

IDENTIFYING PATIENTS AT INCREASED RISK FOR DEVELOPMENT OF CINV

In addition to the emetogenic potential of chemotherapy drugs, there are also well-described patient factors predisposing for more or less emetic trouble with specific regimes, which have been supported in multiple studies. The patient characteristics predicting development of more severe CINV include:

- Poor emetic control with prior chemotherapy[31]
- Younger age (less than 65 years)[32,33]; increasing evidence indicates that older patients tend to tolerate chemotherapy better than younger patients
- Female gender[32]; in addition, emesis during pregnancy seems to be associated with an increased risk of developing CINV[34]
- Low alcohol intake (10 or less alcoholic drinks per week in one study)[32,35]
- Low social functioning or high fatigue scores[32]
- Tumor burden[36] – in one ovarian cancer study, patients 55 years or older with large (greater than 2 cm) tumors had more acute and delayed CINV
- Poor control of acute CINV increases the risk of delayed nausea and vomiting
- Presence of other causes of nausea and vomiting including constipation, which may be more frequent in elderly patients

Increased use of medications (polypharmacy) resulting from the presence of various comorbid conditions in older individuals may result in an increased risk of side effects and nausea.[37]

DIFFERENTIAL DIAGNOSIS OF NAUSEA AND VOMITING IN PATIENTS WITH CANCER

In addition to chemotherapy and radiation therapy, many other factors can contribute to the development of nausea and vomiting in patients with advanced cancer. While it may be difficult to distinguish among the various causes, most patients will have additional signs, symptoms, or test abnormalities that can be helpful in pointing to the correct etiology. A thorough history and physical examination, as well as guided laboratory and imaging evaluation, may be critical steps in the assessment of nausea and vomiting in this patient population.

The list is comprehensive, but most patients will have one or more of the contributing factors:

- Medications (most importantly narcotics, nonsteroidal anti-inflammatory drugs, antibiotics); a careful medication history, including nonprescription drugs is essential
- Postoperative nausea and vomiting following general anesthesia
- Gastroesophageal reflux disease (GERD) or peptic ulcer disease; absence of typical reflux symptoms does not rule out GERD
- Gastric outlet obstruction from malignancy or peptic ulcer disease
- Gastroparesis resulting from tumor involvement of the vagus nerve or lower thoracic spinal sympathetic plexus, paraneoplastic gastrointestinal dysmotility (described with small cell lung cancer and rarely other malignancies, and associated with antineuronal nuclear [ANNA-1, anti-Hu] or other antibodies[38,39]), and medications (i.e., anticholinergic drugs); patients usually complain of vomiting food eaten several hours earlier, and a succussion splash may be detected on physical examination
- Pancreatitis
- Cholecystitis
- Constipation
- Bowel obstruction; feculent vomiting suggests advanced obstruction or a gastrocolic fistula
- Peritoneal metastases and malignant ascites
- Mesenteric ischemia
- Increased intracranial pressure; vomiting may be projectile, and is usually associated with other focal neurologic signs or symptoms
- Metabolic causes (hyponatremia or hypernatremia, hyperglycemia, renal or hepatic insufficiency)

TYPES OF ANTIEMETIC AGENTS

Serotonin (5-HT$_3$) Receptor Antagonists

The successful development of 5-HT$_3$-receptor antagonists, a drug class that has a high therapeutic index for prevention of CINV, was a major breakthrough in the management of this clinical problem. A large number of clinical trials have since been conducted, proving their efficacy and safety. As of this date, five such 5-HT$_3$-receptor–selective antagonists have found their way in clinical practice: four first-generation agents (granisetron, ondansetron, dolasetron, and tropisetron) and one second-generation agent (palonosetron).

First-Generation 5-HT$_3$ Receptor Antagonists

- Numerous clinical trials using various doses, routes, and schedules of administration have demonstrated that first-generation 5-HT$_3$ antagonists are equally effective in preventing acute CINV.[40-43] This was further supported by the results of two large meta-analyses.[44,45]

- 5-HT$_3$ first-generation agents share similar low side-effect profiles, which most often include headache, constipation, transient asymptomatic elevation in liver transaminases, and reversible clinically insignificant ECG changes (including prolongation of the QTc-interval).[43] ECG changes are most prominent 1 to 2 hours after the drug administration and return to baseline within 24 hours. Although clinically important adverse cardiovascular events associated with these changes are excitingly rare,[46] particular care should be taken in elderly patients who are more likely to use other cardiovascular medications, therefore increasing the risk of drug-drug interactions and side-effects.

- A single daily dose of a 5-HT$_3$ receptor antagonist prechemotherapy seems to be as effective as multiple daily doses or a continuous intravenous infusion, offering both convenience and potential cost savings.[47] In addition, each drug has a plateau in therapeutic efficacy at a definable dose level, above which further dose escalation does not improve symptom control.[47]

- Oral administration is equally efficacious as the intravenous route, even with highly emetogenic therapy.[47] An orally disintegrating ondansetron tablet is also available for patients with dysphagia or anorexia and provides equivalent treatment to the oral swallowed formulation.[48] In addition, a granisetron transdermal patch was recently approved by the Food and Drug Administration (FDA)[49] and has been proven to be no less effective than oral granisetron when applied 24 to 48 hours prior to the first dose of chemotherapy [50]

- Combining 5-HT$_3$ antagonists with dexamethasone further improves their efficacy.[51]

- The role of first-generation 5-HT$_3$ receptor antagonists in preventing delayed CINV is less clear. A meta-analysis found that adding a 5-HT$_3$ antagonist to dexamethasone does not improve its effectiveness in preventing delayed emesis.[52] Similarly, a recent randomized study found that first-generation agents were not better than prochlorperazine in controlling delayed doxorubicin-induced nausea and that the proportion of patients reporting delayed nausea exceeded 70% in both groups.[53]

A Second-Generation 5-HT$_3$ Receptor Antagonist (Palonosetron)

- Palonosetron has a significantly higher binding affinity for the 5-HT$_3$ receptor and a longer half-life (approximately 40 hours) compared to first-generation agents.[54]

- A single intravenous dose of palonosetron was shown to be as effective as a comparable dose of dolasetron in preventing acute CINV and superior in preventing delayed emesis.[55]

- The safety profile of palonosetron is similar to first-generation 5-HT$_3$ antagonists.[55]

- No dose adjustments or special monitoring are required for geriatric patients.[56]

- Intravenous palonosetron is FDA-approved[56] for prevention of acute and delayed nausea and vomiting associated with moderately and highly emetogenic cancer chemotherapy as a single dose on day 1; repeat dosing in the days after chemotherapy or in the setting of multiday regimens has not been well studied.

Neurokinin-1-Receptor Antagonists (Aprepitant)

The implication of substance P in the pathogenesis of acute and delayed CINV has led to the development of aprepitant, a novel neurokinin-1 antagonist; preliminary trials conducted in late 1990s demonstrated the high clinical efficacy of neurokinin receptor blockage for the prophylaxis of acute and delayed emesis associated with highly emetogenic chemotherapy.[57] Subsequently, the approval of aprepitant for general use significantly improved the ability to prevent CINV in patients receiving moderately and highly emetogenic chemotherapy.

- Two phase III clinical trials, including a total of 1,043 patients receiving chemotherapy of high emetic risk (cisplatin), demonstrated a significantly improved control of acute and delayed CINV with the three-drug regimen of oral aprepitant (125 mg on day 1; 80 mg on days 2 and 3), ondansetron (32 mg intravenously on day 1), and dexamethasone (12 mg orally on day 1; 8 mg/d on days 2-4) over the standard combination of ondansetron (32 mg intravenously on day 1) and dexamethasone (20 mg orally on day 1; 8 mg twice daily on days 2-4).[58]

- Similarly, aprepitant was shown to be more effective in preventing emesis when added to a standard regimen of ondansetron and dexamethasone versus the standard regimen of ondansetron and dexamethasone in 866 patients with breast cancer undergoing moderately emetogenic chemotherapy (cyclophosphamide alone or in combination with doxorubicin or epirubicin).[59]

- Aprepitant plus dexamethasone alone does not seem to be as effective as the three-drug combination regimen including a 5-HT$_3$ receptor antagonist.[60]

- Aprepitant is FDA-approved for use, in combination with other antiemetic agents, for prevention of acute and delayed nausea and vomiting associated with initial and repeat courses of highly and moderately emetogenic cancer chemotherapy.[61]

- Chronic continuous use of aprepitant for prevention of nausea and vomiting has not been studied and is not recommended.[61]

- An intravenous version of aprepitant (fosaprepitant dimeglumine) has been recently approved for use in the United States as a 115 mg infusion 30 minutes prior to chemotherapy on day 1, followed by standard dose oral aprepitant (80 mg) on days 2 and 3.[62] Efficacy is thought to be similar to the oral regimen, although data are limited.[62]

- Aprepitant is both a moderate inducer and moderate inhibitor of cytochrome P450 enzyme 3A4 (CYP3A4) and a moderate inducer of CYP2C9[63] and therefore can alter the metabolism of certain drugs. Aprepitant should be used with caution in patients receiving concomitant medications that are metabolized through CYP3A4, as it could result in elevated plasma levels of these medications. Induction of warfarin metabolism may lead to clinically significant decrease in the International Normalized Ratio (INR) of prothrombin time and therefore increased monitoring may be required in the 2-week period following administration of aprepitant with each chemotherapy cycle.[61]

- The oral dose of dexamethasone (a CYP3A4 substrate) should be reduced by approximately 50% when coadministered with aprepitant, in order to achieve exposures of dexamethasone similar to those obtained when it is used without aprepitant.[61] Nonetheless, these recommendations do not apply when corticosteroids are used as anticancer therapy (i.e., part of a combination chemotherapy regimen).[30]

Dopamine Receptor Antagonists

Benzamides. Metoclopramide is the most commonly used drug in this class. It blocks type 2 dopamine receptors and 5-HT$_3$ serotonin receptors (when used in higher doses used to prevent CINV) in the chemoreceptor trigger zone, increases lower esophageal sphincter tone, and enhances bowel and gastric motility. The usual recommended doses are 20 to 40 mg orally every 4 to 6 hours (conventional dose) or 2 to 3 mg/kg (high dose).[64] Metoclopramide crosses the blood-brain barrier, and side effects include extrapyramidal reactions such as acute dystonia, akathisia, and possible irreversible tardive dyskinesia, especially with prolonged use of high doses and in the elderly. Diphenhydramine or hydroxyzine can be used to antagonize the dopaminergic toxicity of metoclopramide. In addition, metoclopramide can lower the seizure threshold and increase the risk of convulsions in patients with epilepsy.[37] In the past, metoclopramide combined with dexamethasone was the antiemetic regimen of choice for preventing delayed CINV,[65,66] but it has largely been replaced by the use of 5-HT^3 antagonists and aprepitant.

Phenothiazines. Phenothiazines, such as prochlorperazine (Compazine), thiethylperazine (Torecan), promethazine (Phenergan), and chlorpromazine (Thorazine) act predominantly as dopamine receptor antagonists, but they also have anticholinergic and antihistaminic blocking effects. Phenothiazines are useful in the treatment of nausea and vomiting caused by various gastrointestinal disorders, but their role in prevention of highly-emetogenic CINV is limited.[64] However, they still play a role in the treatment of mild CINV, as well as breakthrough nausea and vomiting.[29,67] Phenothiazines can be given intravenously, intramuscularly, orally, or rectally, making them very useful in patients who have difficulties with intravenous access or are unable to tolerate oral intake. Side effects include extrapyramidal symptoms (acute dystonia, akathisia, tardive dyskinesia), anticholinergic effects (dry mouth, urinary retention, tachycardia, drowsiness), and sedation. Acute dystonia is more common in younger, than in older, patients and, as with metoclopramide, diphenhydramine or hydroxyzine can be used to antagonize extrapyramidal system receptors. Intravenous administration of prochlorperazine can cause marked hypotension, especially in the elderly and especially if administered too rapidly.

Butyrophenones. The two drugs in this class, droperidol (Inapsine) and haloperidol (Haldol) are type 2 dopamine receptor antagonists. Although they have stronger antiemetic effects than phenothiazines, the incidence of extrapyramidal side effects is higher. Other side effects include sedation, hypotension, and clinically significant QTc prolongation associated with an increased risk of sudden death. Droperidol is currently rarely, if ever, used for the prevention of CINV. Haloperidol can be administered intramuscularly, intravenously, or orally; however, its prolonged half-life (18 hours) often limits its use. Before the introduction of 5-HT$_3$ receptor antagonists, butyrophenones were used as an alternative to high-dose metoclopramide[68]; however, their utilization has markedly decreased in recent years.

Atypical Antipsychotics. Olanzapine is a new atypical antipsychotic drug which blocks dopaminergic, serotoninergic, antihistaminic, muscarinic, and dopaminergic receptors. Olanzapine was initially found to be effective in patients with advanced cancer who required opioid analgesics for pain.[69] In a recently published small phase I study, Passik and colleagues used olanzapine for prevention of moderate and highly-emetogenic CINV in a dose of 5 mg daily for 2 days prior to chemotherapy and 10 mg daily for the subsequent 8 days (days 0-7).[70] Four of six patients receiving highly emetogenic chemotherapy and nine of nine patients receiving moderately emetogenic regimens achieved complete control of delayed nausea, with the main side effect being grade 3 depressed level of consciousness in 3 of 15 patients treated. A similarly high complete response rate and an acceptable toxicity profile were achieved in two subsequent phase II trials when olanzapine and dexamethasone were combined with granisetron and palonosetron, respectively.[71,72] Olanzapine is available in oral and injectable (intramuscular) formulations. The main side effects are extrapyramidal and anticholinergic reactions, sedation, as well as weight gain and an associated risk of diabetes when used for a prolonged period of time.[73,74]

Corticosteroids

Corticosteroids are among the most commonly used antiemetics because of their low cost, efficacy, and wide availability. At equivalent doses, all corticosteroids appear to have comparable efficacy and can be used interchangeably.[30] Dexamethasone and methylprednisolone are the most thoroughly studied; dexamethasone is used most often because of its availability in generic forms and the variety of dosage formulations. The efficacy of oral and intravenous formulations appears to be equivalent; therefore oral formulations are usually recommended because of ease of administration and low cost. The mechanism of action has not been fully elucidated and there is no clear evidence to support central neurotransmitter blockade with corticosteroid use. The main side effects include insomnia, agitation, mood changes, indigestion/epigastric discomfort, increased appetite, weight gain, and hyperglycemia.[75] Therefore, patients with a prior history of diabetes or those receiving NSAIDs should be closely monitored when corticosteroids are administered. Adrenal insufficiency has not been described with the short courses of corticosteroids (2 to 4 days) used in the prevention or treatment of CINV.

Single-agent corticosteroid treatment, such as dexamethasone (8 mg), is currently recommended for the prophylaxis of acute emesis with low-emetogenic chemotherapy.[29] Corticosteroids are most useful, however, when used in combination with aprepitant and 5-HT₃ serotonin receptor antagonists in patients receiving chemotherapy of moderate or high emetogenic potential.[30] For prevention of acute CINV induced by highly emetogenic chemotherapy, a dose of 20 mg of dexamethasone is recommended before chemotherapy, when given in combination with a 5-HT₃ serotonin antagonist,[76] but the dose should be decreased to 12 mg when aprepitant is added to the regimen.[29,30,77] For patients receiving moderately emetogenic chemotherapy, a single dose of 8 mg of dexamethasone is currently recommended before chemotherapy.[29,30,78] The recommended dexamethasone dose for prevention of delayed nausea is 8 mg daily for 2 to 3 days following chemotherapy.

Other Agents

Benzodiazepines. Benzodiazepines are weak antiemetic agents and their use as single agents to prevent CINV is not recommended. Benzodiazepines are mainly used as adjunctive agents to reduce anxiety, anticipatory nausea and vomiting,[79,80] and refractory emesis occurring despite adequate prophylaxis regimens.[30] Lorazepam (Ativan) and alprazolam (Xanax) are the most commonly used drugs in this class. The main side effect of benzodiazepines is sedation; therefore elderly patients and patients receiving medications with additional central nervous system depressant activity (e.g., phenothiazines, opioids) should be carefully monitored.

Antihistamines. Antihistamines do not have significant antiemetic activity and should not be used as single agents in the prevention or treatment of CINV. Antihistamines are mainly used as adjunctive agents to prevent dystonic reactions with dopamine receptor blockers, or for treatment of nausea in patients with advanced cancer when the nausea is thought to be mediated by the vestibular system.[81]

Cannabinoids. Despite the controversy that surrounds the use of cannabinoids for CINV, several studies using delta-9-tetrahydrocannabinol (THC) have shown this agent to be an effective antiemetic, compared to placebo and even prochlorperazine.[82,83] Drugs in this class are available as plant extracts (dronabinol or tetrahydrocannabinol) and semisynthetic substances (nabilone, levonantradol). The most frequently used doses are 5 to 10 mg orally every 6 to 8 hours for dronabinol and 1 to 2 mg orally every 12 hours for nabilone. In a systematic review[84] of efficacy and adverse effects of cannabinoids in the prevention of CINV, it was found that they were more effective antiemetics than prochlorperazine, metoclopramide, chlorpromazine, thiethylperazine, haloperidol, domperidone, or alizapride. However, cannabinoids have not been proven to be more effective in patients receiving mildly or very highly emetogenic chemotherapy. Side effects occurred more frequently with cannabinoids and included dizziness, dysphoria, depression, hallucinations, paranoia, and hypotension. Some potentially "beneficial" side effects include euphoria and sedation. As with other agents having a lower therapeutic index, cannabinoids should be reserved for patients who are intolerant of or refractory to 5-HT₃ serotonin receptor antagonists, aprepitant, or dexamethasone.[30]

Treatment Recommendations General Principles Regarding Emesis Control in Patients Receiving Chemotherapy

- The main goal of antiemetic therapy in patients with cancer undergoing chemotherapy is prevention of nausea and/or vomiting. Patients who experience acute nausea or emesis are also much more likely to develop these complications 24 hours or more after treatment.[20]
- Therapy should start before the administration of chemotherapy and cover at least the first 3 days for agents with high emetic risk.[20][29]
- Oral administration of antiemetic agents is equally efficacious as the intravenous route, even with highly emetogenic therapy, and therefore the oral route is preferred unless the patient is unable to tolerate or swallow oral medications.
- The choice of the antiemetic regimen should be based upon the emetogenic potential of the chemotherapeutic agent(s) used, side-effect profiles, and patient-specific factors including previous experience with antiemetics.

- For multidrug chemotherapeutic regimens, the choice of antiemetics should be on the basis of the drug with the highest emetogenic potential, although adding low- or moderate-risk agents usually increases emetogenicity by one level.[26]
- For multiday chemotherapy regimens, it has been recommended that antiemetics appropriate for the emetogenic risk of chemotherapy should be administered during each day of treatment. Nonetheless, there is a lack of formal guidelines for this situation.
- The best management of anticipatory nausea and/or vomiting is adequate control of acute and delayed CINV,[29] use of anxiolytics (although the response is usually not maintained as chemotherapy treatment continues),[29,85] and use of behavioral therapies involving desensitization.[29,86]
- Other potential causes of nausea and vomiting should be excluded and treated, if possible.

PREVENTION OF CHEMOTHERAPY-INDUCED NAUSEA AND VOMITING (CINV)

High-Emetic-Risk Chemotherapy

Acute CINV

- A three-drug antiemetic regimen is currently recommended to prevent acute nausea and vomiting in patients who receive highly emetogenic chemotherapy. The regimen includes a single dose of a 5-HT_3 receptor antagonist on day 1, along with aprepitant and dexamethasone.[29,30,87] (Table 18-2.)
- Other antiemetic agents, such as metoclopramide, butyrophenones, phenothiazines, or cannabinoids, are not appropriate first-choice agents in this patient population, unless they are intolerant or refractory to 5-HT_3 antagonists, NK1 receptor antagonists, and dexamethasone.[30,87]

TABLE 18-2	Dose and Schedule of Antiemetics to Prevent Emesis Induced by Antineoplastic Therapy, by Emetic Category Risk		
Emetic risk category	**Antiemetic regimen**	**Dose**	**Schedule**
High (>90%)	**5-HT_3 serotonin receptor antagonist**		
	• Ondansetron (Zofran)	Oral: 24 mg	Day 1 prechemotherapy
		IV: 8 mg or 0.15 mg/kg	
	• Granisetron (Kytril)	Oral: 2 mg	
		IV: 1 mg or 0.01 mg/kg	
	• Dolasetron (Anzemet)	Oral: 100 mg	
		IV: 100 mg or 1.8 mg/kg	
	• Palonosetron (Aloxi)	IV: 0.25 mg	
	• Tropisetron (Navoban)	Oral or IV: 5 mg	
	Dexamethasone	Oral: 12 mg	Day 1 prechemotherapy
		Oral: 8 mg	Days 2-4
	NK1 receptor antagonist		
	• Aprepitant (Emend)	Oral: 125 mg	Day 1 prechemotherapy
		Oral: 80 mg	Days 2,3
	• Fosaprepitant	IV: 115 mg	Day 1 prechemotherapy
Moderate (30% -90%)	**5-HT_3 serotonin receptor antagonist**		
	• Ondansetron (Zofran)	Oral: 16 mg	Day 1 prechemotherapy
		IV: 8 mg or 0.15 mg/kg	
	• Granisetron (Kytril)	Oral: 2 mg	
		IV: 1 mg or 0.01 mg/kg	
	• Dolasetron (Anzemet)	Oral: 100 mg	
		IV: 100 mg or 1.8 mg/kg	
	• Palonosetron (Aloxi)	IV: 0.25 mg	
	• Tropisetron (Navoban)	Oral or IV: 5 mg	
	Dexamethasone*		Day 1 prechemotherapy
	• without aprepitant	IV: 20 mg	Days 2,3[†]
		Oral: 12 mg	
	• with aprepitant	Oral: 8 mg	
Low (10%-30%)	Dexamethasone	Oral: 8 mg	Day 1 prechemotherapy
Minimal (< 10%)	Routine prophylaxis not recommended		

*The use of the three-drug antiemetic regimen is recommended for chemotherapeutic regimens incorporating a combination of anthracycline and cyclophosphamide.

[†]The value of administering dexamethasone beyond day 1 in patient receiving the three-drug antiemetic regimen has not been studied; in patients who do not receive aprepitant, oral dexamethasone on days 2 and 3 is recommended for prevention of delayed CINV induced by chemotherapy of moderate emetogenic risk.

- Lorazepam, diphenhydramine, H$_2$ blockers, or proton pump inhibitors may be useful adjuncts to antiemetic drugs, but they should not be used as single agents.[87]

Delayed CINV

- In all patients receiving cisplatin and all other chemotherapeutic agents of high emetic risk, the combination of aprepitant and dexamethasone is recommended to prevent delayed nausea and vomiting, on the basis of its superiority to dexamethasone alone (See Table 18-2).[29,30]
- The combination of dexamethasone and a 5-HT$_3$ antagonist to prevent delayed emesis is no longer recommended, as data have failed to demonstrate that the combination is superior to dexamethasone alone in this setting.[88,89] In addition, a recent trial has found that the combination of aprepitant and dexamethasone is superior to ondansetron and dexamethasone in the prevention of cisplatin-induced delayed emesis.[90]

Moderate-Emetic-Risk Chemotherapy

Acute CINV

- The standard antiemetic regimen to prevent acute nausea and vomiting in patients who receive moderately emetogenic chemotherapy is a combination of 5-HT$_3$ antagonist plus dexamethasone (See Table 18-2).[29,30] No clinically significant differences have been sufficiently clarified between the five different 5-HT$_3$ receptor antagonists for prevention of acute nausea in this setting and there is no difference in efficacy between oral versus intravenous administration.
- The MASCC and ASCO guidelines currently recommend the use of an aprepitant-based antiemetic regimen for any chemotherapeutic regimen that includes the combination of cyclophosphamide and anthracycline (which is technically classified as a moderately emetogenic regimen, but actually treated as a highly emetogenic regimen), on the basis of a recent trial in breast cancer patients.[59] This antiemetic regimen has not yet been tested specifically in patients receiving the CHOP (cyclophosphamide, doxorubicin, vincristine, prednisone) regimen.
- NCCN guidelines suggest that aprepitant be added for patients undergoing treatment with selected agents, such as carboplatin, doxorubicin, epirubicin, ifosfamide, irinotecan, and methotrexate, as these agents seem to be more emetogenic than the other moderate-risk agents.[87] However, no studies so far have investigated the use of the three-drug antiemetic regimen in patients receiving moderately emetogenic chemotherapeutic agents other than the combination of cyclophosphamide and an anthracycline.
- The recommended dose of dexamethasone for prevention of acute CINV is 8 mg on day 1 when used in combination with a 5-HT$_3$ antagonist.[29,30]

Delayed CINV

- In patients receiving a doxorubicin and cyclophosphamide (AC) regimen, aprepitant and dexamethasone is recommended for prevention of delayed nausea and vomiting.[30,91]
- Patients who receive chemotherapies of moderately emetogenic risk other than AC should receive antiemetic prophylaxis with oral dexamethasone (preferred) 8 mg daily on days 2 and 3[30] or a 5-HT$_3$ receptor antagonist (See Table 18-2).[29]
- Palonosetron is FDA-approved for the prevention of delayed nausea and vomiting with moderately emetogenic chemotherapies. In some randomized trials, palonosetron appears to be superior to other short-acting 5-HT$_3$ antagonists, particularly regarding delayed CINV. In these trials, about 5% to 10% of fewer patients vomited with palonosetron than with shorter-acting 5-HT$_3$ antagonists. The 2006 ASCO guidelines do not endorse the use of this drug over other 5-HT$_3$ antagonists, as the trials comparing this agent with other drugs in this class were designed as equivalency trials and did not include dexamethasone; also influencing this is the availability of aprepitant. Of note, the cost for palonosetron is significantly higher than for other oral 5HT$_3$ antagonists.

Low- or Minimal-Emetic-Risk Chemotherapy

- For patients administered low or minimal emetogenic risk chemotherapy there is little evidence from clinical trials to identify patients at risk for developing CINV.[29]

Acute CINV

- Single-agent dexamethasone (8 mg) is recommended for prophylaxis of acute emesis when low (10% to 30%) emetogenic risk chemotherapy agents are administered (See Table 18-2).[29,30]
- No routine prophylaxis is recommended for patients receiving minimal (<10%) emetogenic risk chemotherapy.[29,30]

> **CASE 18-1   CASE UPDATE**
>
> Mrs. J. has completed two cycles of neoadjuvant chemotherapy with a good response in the size of the lung mass. Her nausea and vomiting have been well controlled with the combination of granisetron, aprepitant, and dexamethasone, and she only required infrequent use of rescue prochlorperazine between treatments. She is now scheduled to start concurrent chemoradiation therapy with a planned radiation dose of 6000 cGy in 30 fractions along with cisplatin (50 mg/m^2) days 1 and 8, and etoposide (50 mg/m^2) days 1 through 5, both at a 15% dose reduction, administered every 4 weeks. She is asking about the side effects of daily radiation therapy and whether anything can be done to prevent nausea and vomiting related to this therapy.

Delayed CINV

- No routine prophylaxis is needed for prevention of delayed CINV in patients receiving low or minimal emetogenic risk chemotherapy.[29,30]

RADIATION-INDUCED NAUSEA AND VOMITING

The exact mechanism of radiation-induced nausea and vomiting has not been fully elucidated, but it is thought to result from the combination of direct mucosal injury and serotonin release.[92] In patients receiving radiation therapy (RT), nausea and vomiting is in general less problematic, but also less predictable than with CINV. It is therefore important to identify the populations at risk in whom antiemetic therapy should be administered routinely on a preventive basis, versus those in whom it may be administered as needed. The major risk factors associated with an increased risk of emetogenicity in context of RT include irradiated site and radiation field size (> 400 cm^2).[93] Other important considerations include dose of radiotherapy administered per fraction, total dose, and pattern of fractionation,[94] as well as patient-related factors, such as previous chemotherapy.[93]

The new MASCC guidelines[95] define four risk level categories on the basis of irradiated site:

- High risk (> 90% risk): total body irradiation
- Moderate (60% to 90% risk): upper abdomen irradiation
- Low (30% to 59% risk): thorax and pelvis irradiation
- Minimal (< 30% risk): head and neck/extremities/cranium/breast irradiation

PREVENTION OF RADIATION-INDUCED NAUSEA AND VOMITING

High Emetic Risk: Total Body Irradiation

- Recommended prophylaxis is with a 5-HT$_3$ receptor antagonist with or without a corticosteroid before each fraction and for at least 24 hours after.[30,95]
- Complete control of nausea and vomiting with 5-HT$_3$ receptor antagonists varies between 50% and 90%.[96-98]
- No randomized trial has evaluated the addition of dexamethasone, but the recommendation is made on the basis of the additive effect found in CINV control.

Moderate Emetic Risk: Upper Abdomen

- Recommended prophylaxis is with a 5-HT$_3$ receptor antagonist before each fraction for the entire duration of the cycle.[30,95]

- Published trials have demonstrated that 5-HT$_3$ receptor antagonists are more effective than phenothiazines, metoclopramide, or placebo in this patient population.[99-101]

Low Emetic Risk: Thorax, Pelvis, Craniospinal, and Cranial Radiosurgery

- Recommended prophylaxis is with a 5-HT$_3$ receptor antagonist before each fraction for the entire duration of the cycle.[30,95]
- No randomized trials have evaluated the effectiveness of different antiemetics in this patient population, but one trial suggested superiority of a 5-HT$_3$ receptor antagonist to placebo.[102]
- The incidence of emesis in patients undergoing craniospinal irradiation and cranial radiosurgery is not entirely known; therefore these patients are empirically judged as low risk and similar prophylaxis with a 5-HT$_3$ receptor antagonist is recommended.

Minimal Emetic Risk[30,95]

- Treatment should be administered on an as-needed basis for patients experiencing radiation-induced nausea and/or vomiting.[30,95]
- Recommended rescue treatment is with a 5-HT$_3$ or dopamine receptor antagonist.
- For patients experiencing nausea and/or vomiting, prophylactic treatment should then be continued for each remaining radiation day.

MANAGEMENT OF BREAKTHROUGH EMESIS

Breakthrough emesis is defined as vomiting that occurs on any day of treatment despite administration of optimal antiemetic prophylaxis.[29] Breakthrough emesis represents a challenging situation for the practicing physician, as it is difficult to reverse CINV when it has occurred despite round-the-clock administration of prophylactic medications. There are no randomized trials investigating the use of rescue antiemetics for breakthrough emesis and no clear guidelines for treatment of patients with breakthrough nausea and/or vomiting. General principles of therapy include:

- Rescue antiemetics should be administered on demand when breakthrough emesis occurs during chemotherapy.
- Rectal or intravenous administration may be necessary in patients unable to take oral medications.
- An additional antiemetic from a different drug class should be considered, although switching to a different 5-HT$_3$ receptor antagonist has also been proposed.[103]

- It is not known whether substituting to a second generation 5-HT$_3$ receptor antagonist (i.e., palonosetron) would be more beneficial in controlling breakthrough nausea occurring despite prophylactic use of first-generation agents.[29]
- Multiple concurrent agents in alternating schedules may be necessary,[87] such as adding dopamine receptor antagonists (e.g., phenothiazines, or high-dose metoclopramide[30]), neuroleptic agents (haloperidol, olanzapine), benzodiazepine (lorazepam), or cannabinoids (dronabinol, nabilone).
- Patients should be carefully evaluated for chemotherapy risk and prophylactic antiemetic regimen used, concurrent comorbidities (such as electrolyte abnormalities, presence of brain metastases, bowel obstruction, or other gastrointestinal abnormalities), and tumor burden/progression.
- Antacid therapy should be considered for patients with GERD or dyspepsia.[87]

CASE 18-1   CASE UPDATE

Mrs. J. has completed her therapy and did well for 12 months. Unfortunately, she suffered a relapse, with prominent liver metastases. She made an informed decision not to undergo any additional chemotherapy. She has, rather, opted for hospice care. Currently, her biggest symptoms are anorexia, nausea, and vomiting.

MANAGEMENT OF NAUSEA AND VOMITING IN PATIENTS WITH ADVANCED CANCER

Nausea and vomiting are common and distressing symptoms in patients with advanced incurable cancer and often pose significant challenges to treating medical oncologists and primary care physicians. Nevertheless, in the palliative care setting, there is a paucity of data regarding effective treatments for nausea and vomiting that occur independently of chemotherapy or radiation therapy. The following points are worth considering when treating nausea and vomiting in advanced cancer:

- The main goal is to treat and correct reversible underlying causes, if possible, such as treatment of brain metastases, metabolic abnormalities, constipation, or bowel obstruction. Nonetheless, in terminally ill patients, the etiology is frequently multifactorial and reversal of the underlying cause is oftentimes not very feasible.
- Dietary suggestions can be provided, such as intake of frequent small meals, or avoidance of food odors, although these have not been properly studied and likely have limited efficacy overall.

- Pharmacological therapies are the mainstay of treatment in most patients, although a recent systematic review of antiemetics in patients with advanced cancer[104] found that the available evidence is sparse and only a limited number of randomized controlled trials have been conducted. On the basis of the available data, the following conclusions can be made:
  - Metoclopramide seemed to be more effective than placebo for the treatment of cancer-associated dyspepsia[105]; dexamethasone may potentiate its antiemetic effect in patients in whom nausea persists.[106]
  - Data regarding the efficacy of 5-HT$_3$ receptor antagonists in this setting are conflicting,[104] although they probably do provide some benefit.
  - The evidence for other commonly used antiemetics in patients with terminal cancer (prochlorperazine, haloperidol, cyclizine, olanzapine) is weak or nonexistent.[104,107]
  - Megestrol acetate is helpful for appetite enhancement and control of nausea and vomiting in this patient population; the main adverse effects include venous thromboembolism[108] and edema.[109]
  - It is sometimes necessary to use a combination of drugs (added sequentially) that attack different receptors associated with nausea and vomiting:
    - Antidopaminergic (e.g., metoclopramide, prochlorperazine, or haloperidol)
    - Hormonal (e.g., dexamethasone or megestrol acetate)
    - Antihistaminic (e.g., diphenhydramine)
    - 5HT$_3$ receptor antagonist (e.g., ondansetron or granisetron)

The treatment of inoperable bowel obstruction in patients with terminal cancer is aimed mainly at symptom control. The goal of pharmacologic approaches is to preserve the patients' quality of life and to enable them to die comfortably "without tubes."[107] Clinical-practice recommendations for the management of bowel obstruction in patients with advanced cancer exist and have been published in 2001 by the European Association for Palliative Care (EAPC).[110]

- Dexamethasone is a standard recommendation for treatment of malignant bowel obstruction[104] given its anti-inflammatory effects and reduction of fluid influx into the bowel lumen, which could result in temporary reversal of the obstruction.[111]
- The prokinetic agents metoclopramide and domperidone are contraindicated in patients with complete obstruction, although they can sometimes still be considered for those with partial obstructions or ileus.[107]

- Antisecretory drugs such as anticholinergics, antihistaminics, proton-pump inhibitors, or octreotide may also help to control nausea and vomiting; a recent systematic review found octreotide to be superior to hyoscine butylbromide in the medical management of inoperable malignant bowel obstruction.[112]

Summary

In closing, the management of chemotherapy-induced nausea and vomiting (CINV) is a prominent clinical problem. Inadequately controlled nausea and vomiting can significantly affect patients' quality of life and functional ability and is a source of severe emotional distress for both patients and their families. While major advances have been made in recent years, nausea and vomiting in cancer patients remain problematic issues and continue to pose significant challenges to practicing oncologists and primary care providers. Over the past two decades, multiple treatment options have become available for treating nausea and vomiting in patients with cancer. However, the vast number of ways to intervene upon this problem may seem overwhelming to the busy practitioner whose patient is in the examination room waiting for a solution. Clinical guidelines are systematically being developed to assist physicians in delivering evidence-based care[30,113-115]; however, for numerous clinical situations there is no high-level clinical evidence or complete consensus among the experts. This chapter presents options for the prevention and treatment of CNIV on the basis of data and clinical experience gathered over the past several decades.

See expertconsult.com for a complete list of references and web resources for this chapter

SUGGESTED READINGS

1. Hesketh PJ: Chemotherapy-induced nausea and vomiting, *N Engl J Med* 358:2482–2494, 2008.
2. Hesketh PJ, Kris MG, Grunberg SM, et al: Proposal for classifying the acute emetogenicity of cancer chemotherapy, *J Clin Oncol* 15:103–109, 1997.
3. Grunberg SM, Osoba D, Hesketh PJ, et al: Evaluation of new antiemetic agents and definition of antineoplastic agent emetogenicity–an update, *Support Care Cancer* 13:80–84, 2005.
4. Roila F, Hesketh PJ, Herrstedt J: Prevention of chemotherapy- and radiotherapy-induced emesis: results of the 2004 Perugia International Antiemetic Consensus Conference, *Ann Oncol* 17:20–28, 2006.
5. Kris MG, Hesketh PJ, Somerfield MR, et al: American Society of Clinical Oncology guideline for antiemetics in oncology: update 2006, *J Clin Oncol* 24:2932–2947, 2006.
6. Kris MG, Gralla RJ, Clark RA, et al: Incidence, course, and severity of delayed nausea and vomiting following the administration of high-dose cisplatin, *J Clin Oncol* 3:1379–1384, 1985.
7. Osoba D, Zee B, Pater J, et al: Determinants of postchemotherapy nausea and vomiting in patients with cancer. Quality of Life and Symptom Control Committees of the National Cancer Institute of Canada Clinical Trials Group, *J Clin Oncol* 15:116–123, 1997.
8. Jordan K, Hinke A, Grothey A, et al: A meta-analysis comparing the efficacy of four 5-HT3-receptor antagonists for acute chemotherapy-induced emesis, *Support Care Cancer* 15:1023–1033, 2007.
9. Campos D, Pereira JR, Reinhardt RR, et al: Prevention of cisplatin-induced emesis by the oral neurokinin-1 antagonist, MK-869, in combination with granisetron and dexamethasone or with dexamethasone alone, *J Clin Oncol* 19:1759–1767, 2001.
10. Warr DG, Grunberg SM, Gralla RJ, et al: The oral NK(1) antagonist aprepitant for the prevention of acute and delayed chemotherapy-induced nausea and vomiting: Pooled data from 2 randomised, double-blind, placebo controlled trials, *Eur J Cancer* 41:1278–1285, 2005.
11. Hesketh PJ, Grunberg SM, Gralla RJ, et al: The oral neurokinin-1 antagonist aprepitant for the prevention of chemotherapy-induced nausea and vomiting: a multinational, randomized, double-blind, placebo-controlled trial in patients receiving high-dose cisplatin–the Aprepitant Protocol 052 Study Group, *J Clin Oncol* 21:4112–4119, 2003.
12. Randomized, double-blind, dose-finding study of dexamethasone in preventing acute emesis induced by anthracyclines, carboplatin, or cyclophosphamide, *J Clin Oncol* 22:725–729, 2004.
13. Warr DG, Hesketh PJ, Gralla RJ, et al: Efficacy and tolerability of aprepitant for the prevention of chemotherapy-induced nausea and vomiting in patients with breast cancer after moderately emetogenic chemotherapy, *J Clin Oncol* 23:2822–2830, 2005.
14. Aapro MS, Molassiotis A, Olver I: Anticipatory nausea and vomiting, *Support Care Cancer* 13:117–121, 2005.
15. Tramer MR, Carroll D, Campbell FA, et al: Cannabinoids for control of chemotherapy induced nausea and vomiting: quantitative systematic review, *BMJ* 323:16–21, 2001.
16. Razavi D, Delvaux N, Farvacques C, et al: Prevention of adjustment disorders and anticipatory nausea secondary to adjuvant chemotherapy: a double-blind, placebo-controlled study assessing the usefulness of alprazolam, *J Clin Oncol* 11:1384–1390, 1993.
17. Morrow GR, Morrell C: Behavioral treatment for the anticipatory nausea and vomiting induced by cancer chemotherapy, *N Engl J Med* 307:1476–1480, 1982.
18. Maranzano E, Feyer P, Molassiotis A, et al: Evidence-based recommendations for the use of antiemetics in radiotherapy, *Radiother Oncol* 76:227–233, 2005.
19. Glare P, Pereira G, Kristjanson LJ, et al: Systematic review of the efficacy of antiemetics in the treatment of nausea in patients with far-advanced cancer, *Support Care Cancer* 12:432–440, 2004.
20. Mercadante S, Casuccio A, Mangione S: Medical treatment for inoperable malignant bowel obstruction: a qualitative systematic review, *J Pain Symptom Manage* 33:217–223, 2007.
21. Herrstedt J, Roila F: Chemotherapy-induced nausea and vomiting: ESMO clinical recommendations for prophylaxis, *Ann Oncol* 19(Suppl 2):ii110–ii112, 2008.

Insomnia in Aging

Octavio Choi and Michael R. Irwin

This chapter will provide a broad overview of insomnia in aging, divided into three sections. The first section will review the epidemiologic literature as it relates to insomnia and aging. As will be discussed, older people suffer from higher rates of insomnia, and much of this increase appears to be related to the development of medical comorbidities, including cancer diagnosis and treatment, that interfere with sleep. The second section will provide a conceptual approach to the diagnostic assessment of insomnia in the elderly. Many of the most common insomnia-related conditions in the aged population will be reviewed. As most cases of insomnia in this population are associated with comorbid psychiatric and medical illness, a thorough evaluation of insomnia in older adults requires a systematic consideration of related comorbidities. Finally, the third and last section will discuss the health and quality-of-life consequences of insomnia in the older adult. The presence of insomnia is thought to exacerbate numerous health conditions including psychiatric illness, obesity, and pain syndromes, which together emphasize the clinical importance of diagnostic ascertainment and treatment of insomnia in older adults.

EPIDEMIOLOGY AND CLASSIFICATION

CASE 19-1

Ms. S is a 70-year-old woman with breast cancer, recently started on adjuvant hormone therapy, who is being seen by her physician for a routine examination. During the examination, she says she is tired and not sleeping well. What questions should her doctor ask to determine whether she might have insomnia?

Insomnia Prevalence in the General Population

In epidemiologic studies, the prevalence of insomnia in the general population is reported to vary widely, with estimates ranging from 6% to 48%,[1] with variation due in part to differing definitions of insomnia. More recent studies have increasingly used more precise and stringent definitions of insomnia, which has resulted in lower calculated prevalence rates. Epidemiologic studies of insomnia can be conceptualized as belonging to one of four

different categories, in a sense reflecting the evolution of insomnia definitions over time[1]:

1. Insomnia defined by the presence of insomnia symptoms, such as difficulty initiating or maintaining sleep, results in prevalence rates at 30% to 48% in the general population;
2. Insomnia defined by the presence of insomnia symptoms and daytime consequences, results in prevalence rates of 9% to15%;
3. Insomnia defined by subjective dissatisfaction with sleep quality, results in prevalence rates of 8% to 18%;
4. Insomnia defined by diagnosis using a formal classification system such as the Diagnostic and Statistical Manual of Mental Disorders, Fifth edition (DSM-V), results in prevalence rates of 4.4% to 6.4%.

The first group primarily includes older epidemiologic studies that detected insomnia simply by the presence of various symptoms, such as difficulty initiating sleep (DIS), difficulty in maintaining sleep (DMS), or early morning awakening (EMA). A representative study of this era is a 1979 study of 1006 adults, which reported an insomnia prevalence rate of 32.2% in the general Los Angeles population.[2] Subjects were simply asked whether they had trouble falling asleep, woke up during the night, or woke up too early in the morning; endorsement of any these insomnia symptoms was used to indicate insomnia. However, such a broad approach leads to an overestimation of the prevalence of clinically significant insomnia, as it includes people who may suffer from insomnia symptoms only occasionally, or experience only mild symptoms. To address this limitation, subsequent studies have refined the diagnosis of insomnia to include frequency and severity criteria. For example, when frequency criteria of insomnia symptoms of 3 or more times per week are included, prevalence rates drop to 16% to 21%. Similarly, if insomnia is defined as "great or very great difficulty" in initiating or maintaining sleep, prevalence rates drop to 10% to 28%.[1]

The second diagnostic approach restricts the definition of insomnia to require the presence of insomnia symptoms (such as DIS, DMS, or EMA), as well as daytime functional impairment, such as daytime sleepiness, irritability, and trouble concentrating. Using this more refined definition, prevalence rates range from 9% to 15% and average around 10% in the general population.[1] As will be discussed later in more detail, the presence of clinically-significant daytime impairment is a key criterion in establishing a diagnosis of insomnia in all modern sleep disorders classification systems.

The third diagnostic approach focuses on an alternative definition of insomnia, requiring only the report of a subjective sense of dissatisfaction with sleep quality, with the consequence of feeling unrested upon awakening. This definition yields prevalence rates similar to the second group, 8% to 18%. Importantly, this approach is a relatively recent definition, and there is still some controversy amongst sleep experts over whether individuals with this complaint share similar pathophysiologic mechanisms with insomniacs as defined in the first two groups.[3] For example, patients with obstructive sleep apnea may have severely disrupted sleep as a result of multiple apneic episodes throughout the night; however, they are often unaware of this and thus tend to answer "no" when asked whether they have difficulty falling or staying asleep at night. These subjects would thus not be categorized as insomniacs in the first two groups. However, they would tend to be included in the third group, as most patients suffering from this condition report waking up feeling unrested.[4] Despite this controversy, however, there is a general consensus that a subjective sense of sleep dissatisfaction is a useful marker of insomnia, and it is included in the diagnostic criteria for insomnia under the DSM-IV classification system as the criterion of "nonrestorative sleep."

The fourth approach ascertains insomnia using formal diagnostic classification systems, which together reflect the evolving understanding that insomnia is a constellation of symptoms that may be part of a larger disease process or a diagnosis in its own right, according to specific inclusion and exclusion criteria. Increasingly, insomnia is recognized to occur within the context of comorbid mental and physical illnesses, a point that will be discussed in more detail later in this chapter.

CASE 19-1 | **CONTINUED**

After hearing that Ms. S has been having trouble sleeping, the physician should inquire about the severity and frequency of the sleep problems by asking whether she has been having trouble going to sleep, waking up in the middle of night, or waking up too early and having difficulty going back to sleep—or all three symptoms. Ms. S reports that she only occasionally has difficulty going to sleep, but often wakes up and cannot resume her rest, reporting episodes of lying in bed where she is not sure whether she is sleeping or not for "hours on end" and "sometimes she gets up and begins her day even though she has not slept." Upon further questioning, it appears that these episodes of waking occur nearly every night during the week, and that she feels "exhausted" during the day and sometimes sad and depressed. She dismisses the notion that she snores, and says that her husband never complains of her snoring either at night or during her naps during the day.

Risk Factors for Insomnia

There are numerous risk factors for insomnia, including female gender, advancing age, social isolation (divorced/widowed/separated), low socioeconomic status, unemployment, drug use (alcohol or illicit substances), medication use, and medical and psychiatric comorbidities. Whereas many of these risk factors have been extensively reviewed elsewhere,[1] several of these risk factors deserve further discussion in this chapter. As most cases of insomnia in older adults occur within the context of comorbid illnesses, it is essential for the clinician concerned with insomnia to be aware of these comorbidities so they can be diagnosed and treated, with consequent impact on insomnia symptoms. Associated physical illness is especially prevalent in the elderly, and is a major contributing factor to insomnia in this age group; this will also be discussed later in this chapter.

Insomnia Comorbidities

Most of those with insomnia suffer from comorbid physical and mental illnesses, which are presumed to contribute to the onset and perpetuation of insomnia symptoms.[1,3,5] Indeed, one study showed that 53% of respondents with insomnia symptoms reported suffering from a "recurring health problem," and 33% reported "needing help for emotional problems" in the previous year, both significantly higher than noninsomniacs.[2] Subsequent studies have consistently reported that insomniacs suffer from rates of physical and mental illnesses that are higher than for persons without insomnia.[6-8]

However, when discussing medical and psychiatric conditions contributing to insomnia, sleep specialists are increasingly moving away from the term "secondary," preferring instead the term "comorbid." This change reflects an appreciation for the fact that with most diseases associated with sleep disorders, especially mental illness, causality is unclear and complex. For example, insomnia may be an antecedent of major depressive disorder, or may develop after depressive symptoms.[9,10] In addition, insomnia may persist after all other depressive symptoms remit, suggesting that once established, other factors, such as psychological conditioning, may perpetuate it. In such cases, it would be inaccurate to label the insomnia as "secondary" to the major depression, and treatment of major depression alone (for example with an antidepressant) would not be adequate for alleviation of insomnia. This is an important clinical issue, for the presence of insomnia alone is a major risk factor for future depressive relapse especially in older adults or older cancer patients. Hence, amongst clinicians, the term "insomnia secondary to" may focus treatment efforts on the comorbid illness, with a resulting potential to lead ultimately to undertreatment of the insomnia itself.

Insomnia and Psychiatric Illnesses

Cross-sectional surveys of insomnia and mental health symptoms have reported that 30% to 60% of those with insomnia symptoms have an associated mental disorder, compared with approximately 15% for persons without insomnia.[7,10] Major depressive disorder is most frequently associated with insomnia, followed by generalized anxiety disorder. Alternatively, over 80% of those with major depression, and over 90% of those with anxiety disorders, suffer from insomnia.[1] Indeed, the single most common comorbid disorders related to chronic insomnia are major depression and anxiety disorders,[11] with multivariate logistical regression models indicating that the presence of depression is the strongest single factor predicting insomnia.[6] Insomnia is more strongly associated with major depression than with any other medical disorder, with relative risk two to three times greater than all other medical conditions surveyed.

Longitudinal studies have established that insomnia in the absence of psychiatric symptoms is a risk factor for the later development of major depression, in both young[12] and aged populations[9,13,14] with odds ratios ranging from 3 to 4. Furthermore, when insomnia is chronic, the risk for developing major depression is significantly higher; one study reported that when insomnia was present for over 1 year, there was a four-fold increased risk for developing a major depressive episode in that year.[10] Interestingly, time sequence analyses have shown that insomnia symptoms precede the onset of depressive symptoms in most cases.[7]

Taken as a whole, it is of critical clinical importance to evaluate the presence of psychiatric comorbidity in patients presenting with insomnia. Clinicians should be especially vigilant for depression, as older persons are subject to psychosocial factors that increase the risk for depression, including retirement, social isolation, bereavement, and widowhood.[8] Furthermore, these data also suggest the potential for targeted treatment of insomnia, even in the absence of psychiatric symptoms, to reduce the risk of developing future depressive episodes.[15]

Insomnia and Cancer Survivorship

Poor sleep is one of the most common complaints in cancer patients. In breast cancer survivors, chronic diagnostic insomnia shows a prevalence of 19%, which is three to five times higher than rates of diagnostic insomnia diagnosis found in the general population.[16,17] Insomnia symptoms are also elevated in breast cancer survivors, with a prevalence of 51%, two to five times higher than the general population.[16,17] Finally, in heterogeneous samples of cancer survivors, a two-to-threefold increase in the prevalence of insomnia symptoms is found as compared to rates in healthy adults.[18,19]

In survivors of breast cancer, impairments of sleep are primarily characterized as problems falling asleep,[20] with difficulties of sleep maintenance[21] and duration also reported. Indeed, in women who have received a diagnosis of breast cancer and undergone treatments, over 45% continue to complain of sleep problems, with 25% of all breast survivors reporting use of sleep medications on a routine basis.[16] As noted earlier, 19% fulfill diagnostic criteria for chronic insomnia including prolonged (>30 minutes) difficulty initiating sleep or returning to sleep after nighttime awakening, which together are associated with distress and clinical impairments in daytime functioning. Moreover, high rates of sleep complaints are found several years after initiation of adjuvant therapy for cancer, suggesting that insomnia develops a chronic course in a substantial proportion,[16,22] contributing to continued impairment in quality of life.

Less is known about the clinical factors that precipitate and/or perpetuate insomnia in breast cancer survivors. While it is generally assumed that insomnia is secondary to psychological distress and anxiety of cancer diagnosis and treatment, sleep problems are frequent even in those patients who report low levels of anxiety.[23] Likewise in cancer survivors with insomnia, less than 20% are comorbid for depression and/or anxiety disorders,[24] consistent with comorbidity rates in the general population.[1,25] Nocturnal awakenings are also often attributed to symptoms of pain in cancer patients,[26] although pain is less likely to be a factor in breast cancer survivors who show no indication of residual or recurrent disease.[27,28] In contrast, among breast cancer survivors, social factors may be relevant; highly educated and single women have a fourfold increased risk of insomnia.[16] Moreover, older age also increases the vulnerability for insomnia in cancer survivors.

Other clinical factors, such as treatment variables, should also be considered. For example, women undergoing chemotherapy showed a progressive increase

---

CASE 19-1 | CONTINUED

Because Ms. S reports sleep problems and feeling depressed, her physician follows up and asks whether her sadness lasts all day long. She says that some days when she has not slept that she feels depressed all day, but then remembers that whenever she can get a nap or has a good night that she is her usual self, enjoying gardening and cooking for her family. However, further questioning reveals that there was a time after the death of her sister, who also had breast cancer, that she felt very sad and depressed, and that these feelings lasted nearly every day for nearly 6 months before she saw her previous physician who gave her an antidepressant medication. In fact, in recounting this episode, she notes that it was during the time that she was caring for her sister in the terminal stages of breast cancer that she became anxious about her own health and first began having trouble sleeping. Even after her mood returned to normal, she continued to have more nights than not in which she had problems sleeping. However, whenever she goes on a vacation or sleeps somewhere other than her bedroom, that her sleep is restful. She feels like her "bed is filled with worry."

in the number of awakenings, in which the number of awakenings increased with the number of treatment cycles, which was in turn related to increases in numbers of menopausal symptoms.[29] However, other studies report that the prevalence of insomnia was not related to time since diagnosis nor to treatment type,[16,30] and that the incidence of insomnia is similar across groups who receive different treatment (e.g., surgery, chemotherapy, radiation).[31] Among breast cancer survivors, hormone therapy (i.e., tamoxifen) is often used as an adjunct to radiation or chemotherapy, induces estrogen insufficiency, and is implicated in the onset of trouble sleeping because of menopausal symptom side effects. Although several studies have not consistently related tamoxifen treatment to either the onset or maintenance of insomnia symptoms,[32,33] nocturnal vasomotor symptoms are associated with less efficient and more disrupted sleep in healthy menopausal women.[34-37]

CASE 19-1 **CONTINUED**

After the diagnosis and treatment of her breast cancer, Ms. S further reported that her worrying about her health seemed to be about the same as it had been since her sister's death. However, now not only was she having trouble getting to sleep, but the problems waking up were more problematic. Sometimes, after the tamoxifen treatment, she had severe night sweats that woke her, but then again the main problem was getting back to sleep after she had woken. To help her with her sleep, she had started taking a sleeping pill to get through the night. Although she was able to sleep, she awoke feeling "fuzzy" in her thinking and had trouble even reading the newspaper. Finally, she stopped taking the sleeping pill after she had woken in the middle of the night and fallen as she was walking to the bathroom. Her physician completed her assessment, and found no other medical issues. On the basis of the severity and chronicity of her sleep complaints, the diagnosis of chronic insomnia was made and she was referred to a clinical psychologist for treatment with cognitive behavioral therapy for insomnia.

Insomnia and Aging

Numerous studies have documented a positive correlation between insomnia symptoms and advancing age, with prevalence rates reaching close to 50% in elderly individuals (defined as older than 65 years), depending on the definition of insomnia used. In one representative study, the incidence of insomnia symptoms (difficulty falling asleep, staying asleep, or early morning awakening) increased with age: 23% for 18 to 30 year-olds, 37% for 31 to 50 year-olds, and 40% for those older than 51 years,[2] with a composite rate for all age groups at 32.2%. Women had higher prevalence rates of insomnia at all age points studied, with an average ratio of 1.4:1.

Although the prevalence of insomnia *symptoms* increases with advancing age, the relationship between age and insomnia *diagnoses* is less clear, with some studies reporting a stable prevalence with age and others reporting

an increasing prevalence with age.[1] Taken as a whole, the rate of insomnia diagnoses appear to be stable between ages 15 and 45, increases from age 45 to 65, and remains stable after age 65. Interestingly, this correlates well with polysomnography studies, which indicate that sleep architecture in healthy subjects begins to change starting in early adulthood and become relatively constant after the age of 60. Age-related changes include decreases in sleep efficiency, decreases in percentage of slow-wave and rapid eye movement (REM) sleep, decreases in REM latency, and increases in percentage of stage 1 and 2 sleep.[38]

There are several factors that might account for the discrepancy between insomnia symptoms and insomnia diagnoses in terms of prevalence rates with age. For example, older people often report more sleep complaints, such as nighttime awakenings, but these complaints are often not associated with daytime functional impairment, a necessary criterion for an insomnia diagnosis. Hence many of these older adults receive a diagnosis of "dyssomnia not otherwise specified" rather than insomnia. In addition, older adults often suffer from a higher prevalence of nocturia, which may result in multiple nighttime awakenings. However, without difficulty falling back asleep, daytime functional consequences are minimal.[39] Finally, many elderly suffer from insomnia symptoms resulting from so called "primary sleep disorders" that are conceptualized as noninsomnia diagnoses within the DSM-IV classification system, such as circadian rhythm shift disorder, breathing-related sleep disorder, and limb movement disorders, and the prevalence rates of all these conditions increases sharply with age.[40]

Whereas it is not fully known what accounts for the rise in insomnia symptoms with age, the increasing prevalence of medical comorbidities is likely to play a key role. In 2004, a survey was conducted of 1506 older adults (aged 55 to 84 years) in the general United States population as part of the National Sleep Foundation's 2003 "Sleep in America" poll.[39] When comparing the 55- through 64-year-old to the 65 years and older groups, the older group reported significantly more heart disease, hypertension, arthritis, cancer, stroke, and enlarged prostates. Whereas 25% of the 55 to 64 year olds reported no medical conditions, only 12.8% of those older than 65 years reported no medical conditions, a statistically significant difference between the two age groups. In addition, this study demonstrated a significant inverse relationship between the number of medical conditions and self-perceived quality of sleep. Amongst subjects with no medical conditions, 54% reported an "excellent" quality of sleep, and only 10% reported a "fair/poor" quality of sleep. For those with one to three medical conditions, 42% reported excellent sleep, and 22% fair/poor sleep. For those with four or more medical conditions, only 32% reported excellent sleep and 41% fair/poor sleep. Interestingly in another study,[41] insomnia rates were not correlated with age amongst the elderly (those older than 65 years), after controlling for health status. In other words, age was not a significant independent variable in predicting sleep complaints in the elderly; rather, declines in physical and mental health predicted insomnia.

Taken as a whole, the data indicate that the elderly suffer from higher rates of insomnia symptoms compared with younger subjects, and much of this appears to be due to increasing medical comorbidities with age. Indeed, despite the normal age-related changes in sleep architecture mentioned earlier, healthy elderly appear to sleep as well as young adults. The prevalence of primary insomnia diagnoses (that is, insomnia without medical, psychiatric, or neurological comorbidities) is the same in elderly and young adults. Thus, when insomnia is detected in the elderly, it is incumbent upon the clinician to diagnose thoroughly and treat medical, psychiatric, and neurological comorbidities that may be interfering with sleep.

DIAGNOSIS AND EVALUATION

In this section, a systematic approach to the diagnosis and evaluation of insomnia in the elderly will be presented, taking into account the fact that most insomnia symptoms in the elderly occur in the context of comorbid health conditions. Often it will be important to interview not only the patient, but his or her caregiver, who may be more aware than the patient of sleep disturbances during the night, as well as symptoms such as snoring of which the patient may be unaware.

The clinician must ascertain if the patient has a complaint of difficulty initiating or maintaining sleep, or has a complaint of nonrestorative sleep, lasting for at least 1 month (the **First Criterion**). Moreover, the sleep disturbance must cause "clinically significant distress or impairment" during the day (the **Second Criterion**).

Useful screening questions are:

- Do you have trouble falling asleep or staying asleep at night?
- Does this cause problems for you during the day?
- Do you feel extremely sleepy during the day or have trouble staying awake?

The **Third Criterion** requires the clinician to rule out primary sleep disorders (which include narcolepsy, breathing-related sleep disorders, and circadian rhythm sleep disorders) and parasomnias. If there is a strong suspicion of a primary sleep disorder, a referral to a sleep specialist may be appropriate; additional testing including polysomnographic studies (Table 19-1) can be useful in establishing a definitive diagnosis.

The **Fourth Criterion** requires ruling out psychiatric comorbidities, especially major depression, which is the most common single diagnosis in individuals with insomnia. Clinicians should inquire whether their patients have been feeling sad or anxious, and whether they have risk factors for depression such as retirement, social isolation and bereavement. As mentioned earlier, because of the complex causal relationship between insomnia and mood disorders, treatment often involves treating both the mood disorder (i.e., with antidepressants) and insomnia symptoms (i.e., with hypnotics). Insomnia that persists after remission of depression substantially increases the risk of depressive relapse.[9]

The **Fifth Criterion** requires that the clinician rule out general medical conditions (Table 19-2), medications, and drugs of abuse (Table 19-3) as contributing factors to insomnia. As discussed earlier, medical conditions are frequently associated with insomnia symptoms

TABLE 19-1

Disorder	Description	Helpful Diagnostics	Treatment
Narcolepsy	Excessive sleepiness associated with sleep paralysis and hypnogogic hallucinations	Polysomnographic studies; caregiver interview	Sleep hygiene; lifestyle changes; medication
Obstructive sleep apnea	Distinctive snoring pattern (loud snores and brief gasps lasting 20-30 seconds)	Polysomnographic studies; caregiver interview	Treat underlying breathing disorder
Advanced sleep phase syndrome	Advancement of sleep/wake cycle such that they tend to fall asleep earlier and wake earlier	Sleep diary; caregiver interview	If needed, exposure to bright light later in the day to shift circadian rhythms
Restless leg syndrome	Disagreeable leg sensations ("tingling," "crawling," or "aching") that occur at bedtime and interfere with onset of sleep and are temporarily relieved by moving the legs	Caregiver interview	Sleep hygiene; lifestyle changes; medication
Periodic limb movement disorder	Clusters of repeated limb jerks that lead to brief awakenings	Polysomnographic studies; caregiver interview	Sleep hygiene; lifestyle changes; medication
Parasomnias	Behavioral or physiologic events during sleep-wake transitions (i.e., sleep terror, sleep walking, or REM behavior sleep disorder, which is an intermittent failure of sleep paralysis)	Polysomnographic studies	Psychiatric evaluation; neurologic evaluation; medication

TABLE 19-2	Common Drugs That Cause Insomnia

- Alcohol
- Caffeine
- Marijuana
- Chocolate
- Nicotine (including nicotine patch)
- Oral contraceptives
- Decongestants/cold medicines
- Antidepressants (e.g., SSRIs)
- Dopamine agonists
- Thyroid hormones
- Bronchodilators
- Anticonvulsants
- Antineoplastic agents
- Corticosteroids
- Beta-agonists
- Theophylline
- Antihypertensive agents
- Antilipid agents
- Diuretics
- Appetite suppressants
- Psychostimulants and amphetamines

TABLE 19-3	Common Conditions That Can Cause Insomnia

- Hyperthyroidism
- Arthritis or other painful condition, such as bone metastasis
- Chronic kidney disease
- Cardiovascular disease
- Chronic obstructive pulmonary disease
- Gastroesophageal reflux disease
- Brain tumors or metastasis
- Stroke
- Headaches
- Alzheimer disease
- Seizures
- Parkinson disease
- Diabetes
- Menopause

and in many cases are thought to play a role in causing or aggravating insomnia. Thus, it is imperative that the clinician first identify and treat medical comorbidities. Conceptually, they may be categorized as illnesses that give rise to respiratory distress (asthma, chronic obstructive pulmonary disease, pulmonary edema secondary to heart failure), pain (malignancy, arthritis, rheumatic disease, musculoskeletal pain, chronic pain, heart disease, GERD, diabetes), and neurodegenerative conditions (dementia, Parkinson disease, stroke). Hypertension has also been linked to insomnia in the elderly, perhaps as a marker for autonomic hyperarousal, or as a consequence of activating antihypertensive medications. In older men especially, nocturia secondary to prostate conditions may be a prominent cause of difficulty maintaining sleep; reduced fluid intake before sleep may be helpful in these cases. Older women may be prone to postmenopausal hot flashes that may interfere with sleep. Despite optimal management of medical conditions, separate treatment for insomnia symptoms may also be necessary, a topic that is discussed in detail elsewhere in this book.

Medications and Sleep

Numerous medications are thought to interfere with sleep (see Table 19-3). Activating medications include central nervous system stimulants, beta-blockers, bronchodilators, calcium-channel blockers, corticosteroids, decongestants, diuretics, stimulating antidepressants, and thyroid hormones.[40] Changing the timing of administration of stimulating medications to earlier in the day will often improve sleep at night. The clinician should also assess for substance use. Caffeine and cigarette use

both interfere with sleep and their use should be minimized. As caffeine has a half-life that ranges from 3 to 10 hours (averaging 5 hours), caffeine intake should be restricted to earlier in the day. It may be important to remind patients that caffeine is found not only in coffee, but in decaffeinated coffee, teas, and sodas.

The clinician should be aware that many people suffering from insomnia will use alcohol at night to help them sleep. Alcohol is a central nervous system depressant that does accelerate sleep onset. However, because of its short half-life, blood levels rapidly drop, causing awakening from sleep later in the night. In addition, there is rapid tolerance, such that prolonged use of alcohol at bedtime loses its effects on sleep onset, but sleep disruption remains. Patients should be counseled that the use of alcohol at night is counterproductive to good sleep and should be given other, more effective, treatment options.

TREATMENT

For patients suspected of having poor sleep hygiene and/or psychophysiologic insomnia, cognitive behavioral therapy (CBT) for insomnia may be especially helpful. CBT for insomnia, which combines stimulus control, sleep restriction, sleep hygiene (Table 19-4), and cognitive restructuring, has been found to be at least as effective as prescription medications for the treatment of chronic insomnia, with an efficacy in older adults comparable to the benefits reported in middle-aged adults.[42] For example, when temazepam was compared with CBT for the management of chronic primary insomnia in the elderly, both treatments were found effective when measured at 8 weeks. However, only the CBT groups (CBT alone, or CBT in combination with temazepam) maintained their clinical gains at 3, 12, and 24-month follow-ups.[43] The NIH noted in its "state of the science" consensus statement that while prescription hypnotics were found to be efficacious in the short-term management of insomnia, little data existed supporting long-term benefits.[3]

TABLE 19-4	Sleep Hygiene
Avoid alcohol, nicotine, caffeine, and chocolate several hours prior to bedtime.	
Reduce nonsleeping time in bed.	
Avoid a visible bedroom clock.	
Avoid trying to make yourself sleep.	
Establish a regular sleep schedule.	
Exercise every day.	
Deal with worries before bedtime.	
Adjust your environment.	
Make sure room is not too warm.	
Minimize light.	
Minimize sound.	
Make sure bed and pillow are comfortable.	

In addition, prescription hypnotics are associated with numerous side effects, including residual daytime sedation, cognitive impairment, and motor incoordination. As CBT does not appear to produce adverse effects, clinicians may wish to consider this as a more effective and potentially less harmful intervention for primary insomnia.

HEALTH AND QUALITY-OF-LIFE CONSEQUENCES OF INSOMNIA IN THE OLDER CANCER PATIENT

One of the challenges in determining the contribution of insomnia to health conditions is disentangling the role of insomnia per se from the comorbidities that usually accompany it. As reviewed earlier, chronic insomniacs as a population are sicker than noninsomniacs, because insomnia usually occurs in the context of medical or psychiatric illness. Most of the studies that will be discussed here are cross-sectional epidemiologic studies that are subject to this potential underestimation bias. In addition, these studies are not specifically focused on the older cancer patient. As a field, there is a strong need for more long-term prospective studies in older cancer patients, which would be less susceptible to this bias, as well as for interventional laboratory studies, which can more directly support causality.

Public Health Burden

Numerous studies have established that insomniacs utilize the health care system at higher rates than noninsomniacs. In a survey of 1,100 managed care enrollees in the United States, individuals reporting insomnia had significantly more emergency room visits, more calls to the doctor, and more use of over-the-counter drugs than those without insomnia.[44] Another survey of primary care clinic patients demonstrated that insomniacs had greater health care utilization, more days of disability due to health problems, and greater functional impairment as measured by self-reported physical and social disability.[45] In both of these studies, the associations persisted after controlling for medical and psychiatric comorbidities.

A 1995 study estimated the annual direct costs for insomnia in 1995 to be $13.93 billion.[46] This included costs for medications ($1.97 billion) and health care services related to insomnia ($11.96 billion). Somewhat surprisingly, the biggest expense in this analysis was nursing home costs, which totaled $10.9 billion, or 78% of total insomnia-related direct costs. Although this figure is seemingly high, 70% of caregivers cite sleep disturbances in their decision to institutionalize, often because their own sleep was affected, with 20% specifying sleep disturbance as their primary reason.[47] Estimates of total (direct and indirect) insomnia-related costs in the US alone range from $30 billion[48] to $107.5 billion annually.[49]

DAYTIME FUNCTIONAL IMPAIRMENT IN INSOMNIA

One of the most robust findings in the literature is that people with insomnia feel that their insomnia impairs their ability to function in a variety of domains. Compared with noninsomniacs, they report feeling more fatigued during the day,[50] and feel sleepier when driving a car.[51] Interestingly, one finding[49] was that in the 2-year period studied, insomniacs were involved in twice as many serious car accidents as noninsomniacs, although this result did not quite reach statistical significance. Amongst elderly insomniacs, sleeping difficulties contribute to slowed reaction times[52] and impaired balance leading to a greater risk of falls in this population.[53]

Insomniacs also complain that they have trouble remembering things,[51] have trouble concentrating, and more often feel confused than noninsomniacs, which may be why they report significantly lower levels of self-esteem, job satisfaction, and efficiency at work. A study in the elderly population[1] reported that the presence of excessive daytime sleepiness was a significant risk factor for cognitive impairment including attentional deficits, delayed recall, difficulties in orientation, and memory. These symptoms are of particular concern in older people, because they may be misinterpreted as symptoms of dementia or mild cognitive impairment.

INSOMNIA AND MORTALITY

If insomnia worsens medical and psychiatric conditions and increases the chances of falls and accidents, one may expect that insomniacs would be at higher risk for premature death. What is the evidence for this? A prospective study[54] of over one million people in the general population concluded that sleep durations of less than 6 hours and more than 8 hours were associated with a significantly increased risk of all-cause mortality over a 6-year period. The best survival was found among those who slept 7 hours a night, resulting in a U-shaped survival curve that has been replicated in other studies in the United States[55] and Japan.[56] This study also reported that severity of insomnia was associated with shorter survival in a dose-dependent fashion, although this effect went away after controlling for comorbidities. This result suggests that insomnia per se does not affect mortality; rather, it affects mortality exclusively by worsening other health conditions. However, a significant limitation of this study was that insomnia was not well-defined (participants were simply asked, "How many times a month do you have insomnia?" without providing criteria for what constituted insomnia), limiting the conclusions that may be drawn about insomnia in this study.

A more recent prospective study amongst healthy community-dwelling elderly provides strong evidence that insomnia is associated with increased mortality, by providing an objective assessment of sleep disturbance using polysomnography.[57] After controlling for age, gender, and medical burden, individuals with baseline sleep latencies of greater than 30 minutes were found to have 2.14 times greater risk of death over a mean follow-up of 12.8 years. Poor sleep efficiency and disturbed REM sleep were also found to be significantly correlated with greater risk of death. This study is remarkable in part due to the fact that sleep parameters were objectively measured with polysomnography for all 185 subjects, differentiating it from earlier studies that used subjective self-reports to measure sleep disturbance, with similar results.

Taken as a whole, the epidemiologic data support the hypothesis that insomniacs are at greater risk for premature death than noninsomniacs, even after controlling for medical and psychiatric morbidity, and that this is in part due to increased incidence of cardiovascular disease. Associational studies do not prove causality, however. Insomnia could either be a sensitive early marker of physical decline due to other causes, or it could play a more active role in contributing to a dysregulation of physiology that ultimately leads to disease.

Summary

Insomnia is a complex phenomenon. It is a sensitive marker for both medical and psychiatric illness, and also appears to be an active participant in causing disease.

Insomnia sits at the crossroads of multiple fundamental biologic mechanisms, through which it affects a dauntingly large array of illnesses including some of the most urgent health epidemics of our time such as cancer, cardiovascular disease, obesity, and diabetes. A note of hope for the clinician is that because insomnia is tied to so many fundamental disease processes, the application of effective treatments for insomnia may serve to have salutary effects on many of the conditions that are affected by it. The restoration of good sleep may prove to be a keystone in improving the health of older adults in general, older cancer patients undergoing treatment, and older cancer survivors.

See expertconsult.com for a complete list of references and web resources for this chapter

SUGGESTED READINGS

1. Morin CM, Hauri PJ, Espie CA, et al: Nonpharmacologic treatment of chronic insomnia. An American Academy of Sleep Medicine review, *Sleep* 22(8):1134–1156, Dec 15 1999.
2. Fiorentino L, Ancoli-Israel S: Insomnia and its treatment in women with breast cancer, *Sleep Med Rev* 10(6):419–429, Dec 2006.
3. Ancoli-Israel S, Moore PJ, Jones V: The relationship between fatigue and sleep in cancer patients: a review, *Eur J Cancer Care (Engl)* 10(4):245–255, Dec 2001.
4. Quesnel C, Savard J, Simard S, et al: Efficacy of congitive behavioral therapy for insomnia in women treated for nonmetastatic breast cancer, *J Consult Clin Psychol* 71:189–200, 2003.
5. Savard J, Morin CM: Insomnia in the context of cancer: a review of a neglected problem, *J Clin Oncol* 19(3):895–908, Feb 1 2001.
6. Savard J, Simard S, Blanchet J, et al: Prevalence, clinical characteristics, and risk factors for insomnia in the context of breast cancer, *Sleep* 24(5):583–590, Aug 1 2001.
7. Savard J, Simard S, Ivers H, Morin CM: Randomized study on the efficacy of cognitive-behavioral therapy for insomnia secondary to breast cancer, part II: Immunologic effects, *J Clin Oncol* 23(25):6097–6106, Sep 1 2005.
8. Savard J, Simard S, Ivers H, Morin CM: Randomized study on the efficacy of cognitive-behavioral therapy for insomnia secondary to breast cancer, part I: Sleep and psychological effects, *J Clin Oncol* 23(25):6083–6096, Sep 1 2005.

Nutritional Support for the Older Cancer Patient

David B. Reuben

Nutritional support for the older cancer patient varies at different points during the course of a malignancy (Table 20-1). At the earliest stage, nutritional support (e.g., supplementation with vitamin D) may be used to attempt to prevent cancer. A recent meta-analysis of cohort and case-control studies on the effects of vitamin D supplementation and blood-circulating 25-hydroxy vitamin D levels suggests a protective effective effect on the risk of developing breast cancer.[1] However, these observational data findings await confirmation in clinical trains and this approach is too preliminary to be recommended.

The second stage is at the time of diagnosis. If a tumor has been detected by screening, older cancer patients may have no symptoms; the main concern is whether they have any nutritional deficiencies that would interfere with primary treatment of the malignancy. In contrast, weight loss may be a presenting symptom for many malignancies, especially colorectal cancer and lymphomas.

During the course of cancer treatment, weight loss and nutritional complications may be the result of tumor progression causing anorexia, structural or functional disturbances of dentition or the gastrointestinal tract, depression that commonly accompanies cancer, or due to side effects of treatment (e.g., mucositis).

The cancer-related anorexia/cachexia syndrome is a hypercatabolic state (increased resting energy expenditure) with high levels of tumor-activated or host-produced immune responses (e.g., proinflammatory cytokines) to the tumor. Clinical manifestations include loss of appetite and weight, especially lean body mass; tissue wasting; metabolic alterations; fatigue; and reduced functional status.

Nutritional supplementation may be needed to allow the patient to continue to receive treatment or to maintain functional status. Sometimes older cancer patients may become so sick that they cannot tolerate oral feeding and more aggressive enteral or parenteral nutritional support may be considered. An emerging concept is the use of nutritional therapy (e.g., dietary modifications to reduce energy from fat and increased intake of vegetables, fruits, and fiber) to prevent recurrence of malignancies, especially breast cancer.

Finally, there is a stage of advanced cancer when nutritional support may be palliative (e.g., feeding the patient for comfort or pleasure in spite of risks of aspiration).

The knowledge base for nutritional support of the older cancer patient is limited, in part because of the difficulty in studying this population. The sickest, most malnourished patients are often excluded from clinical trials of nutritional support.[2] Even when eligible for clinical trials, sick older cancer patients may be reluctant to participate. Moreover, the published trials on nutritional support focus on older populations or cancer populations rather than older patients who have cancer. Hence, much of what can be gathered from the literature are extrapolations from studies conducted on one population or the other. Most of the clinical trials have focused on survival and cancer recurrence rather than functional status or quality of life. Many more published studies have relied on retrospective analysis of patients who did or did not receive a treatment. Because these patients were not randomly assigned to treatment, no conclusions can be reached about the effectiveness of these interventions; these studies are not considered in this chapter.

The approach to nutritional support of the older cancer patient is further complicated by general approaches and

TABLE 20-1	Nutritional Support by Stage of Cancer in Older Persons	
Stage	**Nutritional Support**	**Evidence**
Primary prevention	• Vitamin D	• Observational (cohort and case-control)
Early after detection	• Nutritional counseling	• Small clinical trials
	• VNS if malnourished	• Meta-analysis but not confined to cancer patients
	• PN if malnourished pre-operatively for head and neck cancer	• Small clinical trial
	• Treat depression	• Clinical trials but not confined to cancer patients
Tumor progression/ treatment side effects	• Disease treatment to relieve structural abnormalities	Anecdotal
	• Treat mucositis	
Cancer-related anorexia/ cachexia	• Megestrol acetate	• Clinical trials
	• Corticosteroids	• Small clinical trial
Prevention of recurrence	• Reduce energy from fat and increased intake of vegetables, fruits, and fiber	• Clinical trials (inconclusive)
Advanced cancer	• Palliative care	• Anecdotal

VNS, volitional nutritional support; PN, parenteral nutrition

some tumor-specific approaches. In particular, the role of nutritional support has been the focus of considerable research on head and neck and gastrointestinal malignancies. The findings of these studies may or may not be applicable to older persons with other malignancies.

In this chapter, approaches to nutritional assessment and monitoring, general approaches to nutritional support, pharmacologic appetite stimulants, and nutritional support of the patient with advanced cancer will be described, concluding with a summary of recommended care.

NUTRITIONAL ASSESSMENT AND MONITORING

Weight and Body Mass Index

Weighing the patient is easy and provides a general indication of whether the patient is getting adequate nutritional intake. Weight loss and low body mass index (BMI) have been associated with adverse outcomes in older persons. In a 4-year cohort study, the annual incidence of involuntary weight loss (defined as loss of more than 4% of body weight) among community-dwelling veterans was 13.1%. Over a 2-year follow-up period, involuntary weight losers had an increased risk of mortality (RR = 2.4, 95% CI = 1.3 to 4.4) that was 28% among weight losers and 11% among those who did not lose weight. Voluntary weight losers had a 36% mortality rate during this time.[3] Weight loss also has prognostic value among cancer patients independent of disease stage, tumor histology, and patient performance status.[4] Among community-dwelling old persons, body mass index (BMI) demonstrates a "U" shaped relation with functional impairment, with increased risk among those at the lowest and highest BMIs.[5]

In older persons, involuntary weight loss may be the presenting symptom of cancer. A case series of 306 patients with unexplained weight loss who were followed for at least 1 year reported that 38% had cancer; it also reported on blood tests (complete blood count, erythrocyte sedimentation rate, and biochemical profile) that were useful, particularly in excluding patients who had cancer. If none of these were abnormal, the likelihood ratio for a diagnosis of cancer was 0.2 (95% confidence interval 0.1-0.4).[6]

Nevertheless, the interpretation of weight as a nutritional indicator is complicated. Weight may remain stable or even increase among those who are progressively malnourished, because of other factors contributing to weight such as edema, ascites, and pleural effusions.

Depression Screening

Depression in cancer patients is a cause of anorexia and weight loss that may respond to antidepressant treatment or psychotherapy. A simple screen such as the Patient Health Questionnaire-9 (PHQ-9) (or its shorter version, the PHQ-2[7]) can be used to detect depressive symptoms.

Biochemical Measures

Serum albumin is the best-studied serum protein and has prognostic value for subsequent mortality and morbidity in community-dwelling older persons.[8,9,10,11] Because serum albumin does not fall quickly (half-life 18-21 days) in protein deprivation, it may be quite a useful indicator for chronic moderate to severe undernutrition. In contrast, proteins with shorter half-lives such as prealbumin (half-life 2-3 days) and transferrin (half-life 8-9 days) may respond to nutritional interventions more quickly and may be better for monitoring treatment.

Other Measures

Anthropometric measures such as midarm muscle circumference and skin-fold thickness tend to be less reliable in older persons.[12] Lymphocyte count, which is low (<1500 cells/mm^3) in protein-energy malnutrition, is also sometimes used as a measure but may not have independent prognostic value beyond albumin.[13]

GENERAL APPROACHES TO NUTRITIONAL SUPPORT

Nutrition Counseling

Nutrition counseling (NC) on the use of regular foods has resulted in less anorexia and better quality of life compared to nutritional supplements or ad libitum feeding in patients with colorectal cancer[14] or head and neck malignancies[15] receiving radiotherapy.

Volitional Nutritional Support

Volitional nutritional support (VNS) is defined as a "liquid formulation containing at least a nonprotein source of calories and nitrogen that is taken orally by the patient with specific instructions regarding its consumption on a scheduled basis."[2] These formulations are often used as supplements to oral diets and differ from supplements or snacks containing real food. A review of data from meta-analyses of 16 randomized clinical trials of mostly malnourished older persons (most of whom did not have cancer) indicated better survival among those receiving VNS.[2] The effects on functional status were more variable. In contrast, VNS has not been shown to have beneficial effects on mortality among patients undergoing chemotherapy or radiation therapy.

Enteral Nutrition

Enteral nutrition (EN) is defined as "the infusion of a putative complete nutrient formulation through a tube placed in the upper gastrointestinal tract."[2] In studies of patients receiving chemotherapy, surgical treatment, or radiation therapy, EN has not been beneficial. Gastrostomy tubes are associated with complications such as dislodgement, leakage with peritonitis, and aspiration.

Parenteral Nutrition

Parenteral nutrition (PN) is defined as "the intravenous provision of nitrogen and 10 kcal/kg/day of nonnitrogenous calories via either a central or peripheral venous catheter."[2] An American Gastroenterological Association technical review concluded that among cancer patients undergoing chemotherapy or radiation therapy, PN causes net harm.[16] In part, this poor risk-benefit ratio is because of parenteral nutrition's common complications of sepsis and catheter occlusions. Nevertheless, in both the United States and Europe, cancer is the most common diagnosis for which home parenteral nutrition is prescribed.

One situation in which parenteral nutrition may be beneficial is in malnourished (weight loss ≥ 10% of usual body weight) gastrointestinal cancer patients who are undergoing surgery. A randomized clinical trial indicated fewer overall complications rates among a group receiving preoperative PN for 10 days and 9 days postoperatively compared to a control group (37% versus 57%, p=0.03). Among the 40 patients aged 65 to 80 years, the trend was similar except there was no benefit on the rate of infectious complications, which occurred in 45% of treated elderly patients.[17]

When replenishing older cancer patients by means of any route, clinicians need to be alert to the possibility of precipitating the refeeding syndrome. This typically occurs in malnourished cancer patients who have had poor oral intake and then receive intravenous glucose-containing fluids, or enteral or parenteral nutrition. Symptoms occur most commonly within 2 to 4 days of refeeding and are caused by the glucose-induced acute transcellular shift of phosphate resulting in hypophosphatemia, hyperglycemia and hyperinsulinemia, which may be accompanied by hypokalemia, hypomagnesemia, and fluid retention. When serum phosphate levels drop below 0.5 mm/L, patients are at higher risk for cardiac arrhythmias, heart failure, respiratory failure, and neurologic complications such as paresthesias, delirium, muscle weakness, paralysis, and seizures. Supplementing intravenous fluids with potassium phosphate or oral phosphate and potassium may help prevent this syndrome.[18]

Pharmacologic Appetite Stimulants

Megestrol Acetate. Megestrol acetate is the most commonly used and best-studied appetite stimulant in cancer patients. A 2008 meta-analysis of patients with the cancer anorexia-cachexia syndrome concluded that megestrol acetate resulted in appetite improvement (RR 3.0, 95% CI 1.86-4.84) and weight gain (RR=1.71, 95% CI 1.24-2.36). Higher doses, 400 mg to 800 mg, were more effective than lower dosages. Slightly more than half of treated patients responded with increased appetite. However, less than one-third of patients responded with weight gain, and the effect was not statistically significant when outcomes of weight gain of at least 5% or 10% were considered.[19] The drug had no effect on survival or functional status. Megestrol (or medroxyprogesterone acetate) has also been combined with other agents including EPA, L-carnitine, and thalidomide. In a preliminary analysis of a five-arm trial treating the cancer-related anorexia/cachexia syndrome,[20] megestrol or medroxyprogesterone acetate was demonstrated to be superior to pharmacological support including eicosapentaenoic acid on outcomes of appetite, fatigue as measured by the Multidimensional Fatigue Symptom Inventory-Short Form, and quality of life as measured by the EuroQol (EQ-5D). Any potential benefit of megestrol must be weighed against potential adverse effects including thromboembolic events (e.g., deep venous thrombosis and pulmonary emboli) and adrenal suppression, which is of unknown clinical significance.

Cannabinoids. Cannabinoids have been reported to stimulate appetite. There are a variety of cannabinoids (single-extract and whole or partially purified extracts of

Cannibis sativa L.), as well as routes of their administration (oral and inhaled). In the United States, dronabinol, a synthetic delta-9-tetrahydrocannabinol (THC), and nabilone, a dronabinol analogue, are available by prescription. In a trial comparing oral THC, whole-plant cannabis extract, and placebo in treating the cancer-related anorexia/cachexia syndrome, there were no differences in appetite or quality of life among the three groups.[21] In a head-to-head comparison, megestrol was superior to dronabinol in improving appetite (75% versus 49%, p=.0001) and producing weight gain of at least 10% (11% versus 3%, p=.02); the combination of the two dugs provided no additional benefit.[22]

Corticosteroids. Corticosteroids are effective in reducing nausea and increasing appetite for a short time. However, these agents have not been demonstrated to increase weight.

Other approaches to treating cancer-related anorexia/cachexia include eicosapentaenoic acid (EPA), which is an omega-3 fatty acid that reduces lipolysis by attenuation of the stimulation of adenylate cyclase, and tumor necrosis factor-α (TNF-α) inhibitors. Neither approach has been demonstrated to improve appetite, weight, or clinical outcomes.

NUTRITIONAL SUPPORT OF ADVANCED CANCER

There is little evidence that nutritional support affects survival or quality of life in patients with advanced cancer. Nevertheless, two professional organizations have recommended nutritional support in certain circumstances. The French National Federation of Cancer Centers states that enteral or parenteral nutrition may be beneficial for patients with bowel obstruction or other sources of food intolerance but are not recommended in patients with a prognosis of less than 3 months or with a Karnofsky score of less than 50%. The Capital Health Home Parenteral Nutrition Program, in Edmonton, Canada, has established the following criteria for home parenteral nutrition: for a potential survival benefit, the duration of treatment is expected to be longer than 6 weeks, the Karnofsky score should be over 50%, and there must be a supportive home environment. In the United States, patients with advanced or terminal cancer are rarely given enteral or parenteral therapy and such treatment would not be covered under the Medicare hospice benefit.[23] Rather, management focuses on palliating symptoms in advanced cancer patients. For those who have dysphagia, approaches include:

- feedings that rely on small, frequent amounts of pureed or soft foods;
- avoiding spicy, salty, acidic, sticky, and extremely hot or cold foods;
- keeping the head of the bed elevated for 30 minutes after eating;
- treating painful mucositis, when present, with a 1:2:8 mixture of diphenhydramine elixir: 2%-4% lidocaine:

magnesium-aluminum hydroxide as a swish-and-swallow suspension before meals. If the cause is candidiasis, then clotrimazole troches or oral fluconazole would be appropriate.

For advanced-cancer patients who have anorexia, patient and family education on the effects of disease progression that result in lack of appetite and weight loss may be the most important intervention. Liberalizing the patient's diet to include calorically dense foods (e.g., sweets, ice cream, alcoholic beverages) may be helpful. Symptoms of dry mouth can sometimes be alleviated by ice chips, popsicles, moist compresses, or artificial saliva.

Summary

In summary, despite the importance of nutritional status in the older cancer patient, there is scant research that nutritional support is of value, except in certain instances. The best evidence supports the following:

- Patient weights are probably the most valuable method of detecting and monitoring nutritional status in older cancer patients.
- Nutrition counseling during treatment may be valuable in patients with gastrointestinal or head and neck cancers.
- Depression is a treatable cause of weight loss in cancer patients.
- Parenteral nutrition may be beneficial in malnourished (weight loss ≥ 10% of usual body weight) gastrointestinal cancer patients who are undergoing surgery.
- In higher doses, megestrol acetate provides a modest amount of benefit toward reducing weight loss in a minority of patients with the cancer anorexia-cachexia syndrome.
- Corticosteroids may reduce nausea and provide short-term appetite stimulation but have no benefit on weight.
- Use of volitional nutritional support (oral supplements), enteral nutrition, and parenteral nutrition is not supported by current scientific data.
- For older patients with advanced cancer, the care should focus on palliating symptoms and educating the patient and family about the disease progression and prognosis.

Further research will be necessary to identify optimal nutritional support for older cancer patients and for those with specific tumors (e.g., head and neck, gastrointestinal) that particularly affect nutritional status. Nutritional approaches to prevent cancer and its recurrence are exciting but unproven strategies. For those with more advanced cancer, providing adequate nutrition in the face of tumor-related effects on appetite and loss of lean body mass remains a challenge.

 See expertconsult.com for a complete list of references and web resources for this chapter

Complementary and Alternative Medicine in the Older Cancer Patient

Lisa M. Schwartz

J.D. is a 76-year-old woman with a history of breast cancer. She was diagnosed a little over 3 years ago with a 2.3 cm poorly differentiated infiltrating ductal carcinoma of the upper outer quadrant of the right breast. She elected to undergo a lumpectomy and sentinel lymph node biopsy. The tumor was estrogen and progesterone receptor-negative (ER/PR−) and HER-2/neu negative, the sentinel lymph node was negative, and there was some lymphovascular space invasion. She met with a medical oncologist who strongly recommended that she receive chemotherapy. The potential side effects of chemotherapy frightened her, and several months of chemotherapy would definitely interfere with her plans to cruise the Mediterranean with her newly retired husband. Her husband had worked very hard running the family business all the years that they had been married, and had promised to hand the business over to their children when he turned 75. The cruise was a fortieth wedding anniversary trip, and she was looking forward to finally spending some quality time with her husband. She declined any adjuvant therapy other than radiation and even compromised with her radiation oncologist to receive a shortened course of therapy with slightly larger doses of radiation each day, which was still an accepted course of treatment. She took a variety of "natural" remedies recommended by friends and family, which she used to maintain her general good health and boost her immune system. On her 3-year follow-up visit, her radiation oncologist appreciated a mass in the right axilla. A biopsy confirmed the presence of an ER/PR− infiltrating ductal carcinoma in an axillary lymph node. J.D. was told she needed surgery and chemotherapy or she would soon die of her breast cancer. Her feeling about the matter was that the recommended therapies would incapacitate her and she would much rather spend the time that she had left enjoying her 6-month-old and 2-year-old grandchildren. She presented to an integrative physician requesting alternative therapies for her recurrent breast cancer.

The use of complementary and alternative medicine (CAM) among the general population has grown tremendously in the last couple of decades. Eisenberg's initial report in 1993 and follow-up survey in 1997 shed light upon the number of American patients who sought out "unconventional care" (defined as therapies neither taught widely in medical schools nor generally available in most hospitals).[1-2] Those survey results revealed that in 1990, one in three patients (34%) reported using an unconventional therapy in the previous year, and by 1997, that number had increased to 42%, resulting in an estimated 629 million visits to CAM providers, which exceeded the number of visits to all U.S. primary care physicians during the same time period. According to the National Center for Health Statistics, Americans spent a staggering $33.9 billion out of pocket on CAM visits and products in 2007.[3] (Figure 21-1.)

This chapter reviews the incidence of CAM use among cancer patients, the pitfalls that may be associated with its use, and the evidence to support certain therapies during cancer treatment.

WHY DOCTORS NEED TO ASK

Primary care physicians and oncologists are very likely to have cancer patients using complementary therapies either during their active treatment or as survivors. A survey of 453 outpatients seen in the MD Anderson Cancer Center clinics between December 1997 and June 1998 showed that 83.3% had used some form of CAM.[4] A recent review of the literature revealed that between 64% and 81% of cancer survivors use vitamin or mineral supplements.[5] Gansler et al. examined the use of "complementary methods" in survivors of ten different cancer types using data from the American Cancer Society's Study of Cancer Survivors-I (SCS-I).[6] Among these 4139 cancer survivors the most commonly used therapies were as follows: prayer/spiritual practice (61%), relaxation (44%), faith/spiritual healing (42%), nutritional supplements/vitamins (40%), meditation (15%), religious counseling (11%), massage (11%), and support groups (10%).

Because women are more likely to use CAM,[7-8] it is not surprising that among cancer patients, breast or ovarian

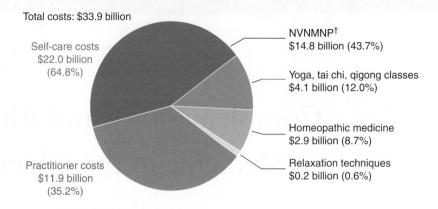

FIGURE 21-1 Out-of-pocket costs for complementary and alternative medicine. Americans spent a total of $33.9 billion out-of-pocket for complementary and alternative medicine in 2007. There were also more visits to complementary medicine providers than there were to primary care physicians.[3] *(Adapted from Nahin, RL, Barnes PM, Stussman BJ, Bloom B. Costs of Complementary and Alternative Medicine (CAM) and Frequency of Visits to CAM Practitioners: United States, 2007. National health statistics reports; no 18. Hyattsville, MD: National Center for Health Statistics. 2009.)*

TABLE 21-1	Reasons Patients Use CAM
Richardson[4] (cancer patients)	• A desire to feel hopeful • A belief that the therapies were nontoxic • A desire for more control in medical decision making
Barnes[7] (all patients)	• Conventional medical treatments would not help (67%) • Conventional medical treatments were too expensive (46%) • Therapy combined with conventional medical treatment would help (78%) • Suggested by a conventional medical professional (66%)
Astin[10] (all patients)	• More congruent with their own values, beliefs and philosophical orientations toward health and life
Verhoef[11] (cancer patients)	• Belief that it would work • Desire to gain some control over medical decision making • A feeling of hope in a last resort effort

cancer survivors are the most likely to use complementary therapies.[6] Between 63% and 83% of breast cancer patients use some form of complementary therapy.[9] The reasons patients give for trying CAM therapies are listed in Table 21-1.

In spite of the high proportion of patients using CAM, only a minority of them discuss it with their physicians. According to the Eisenberg surveys, 72% of patients who were using CAM did not discuss it with their physicians. A review of the literature revealed that between 31% and 68% of cancer patients do not discuss their supplement use with their physicians.[5] There are clearly barriers to communication between patients and their physicians regarding CAM therapies. Interviews with cancer patients have revealed three common themes describing these barriers: physicians' indifference or opposition to CAM use, physicians' emphasis on scientific evidence, and patients' anticipation of a negative response from their physician.[12]

COMPLEMENTARY, ALTERNATIVE, AND INTEGRATIVE: WHAT'S IN A NAME?

There is an important distinction to make between "complementary" and "alternative" medicine. The National Center for Complementary and Alternative Medicine (NCCAM) defines "complementary" therapies as those that are used in addition to conventional therapies and "alternative" therapies as those that are used instead of conventional therapies. The major categories of CAM therapies as defined by NCCAM are given in Table 21-2.

The term "integrative medicine" applies to a practice that incorporates evidence-based complementary therapies with conventional care; considers patients' beliefs about health, illness, and treatment when making recommendations; and empowers patients to participate in their health care decision-making process.[13]

One of the reasons physicians give for being reticent to use or recommend CAM is the paucity of well-conducted clinical trials involving CAM therapies. NCCAM is the branch of the National Institutes of Health (NIH) responsible for conducting research into CAM therapies and disseminating reliable information on CAM to the public. NCCAM started out in 1991 as the Office of Alternative Medicine (OAM) and its budget has grown from an initial $2 million to $128.8 million in 2010. Over $295 million was spent on CAM research at the NIH in 2009. This,

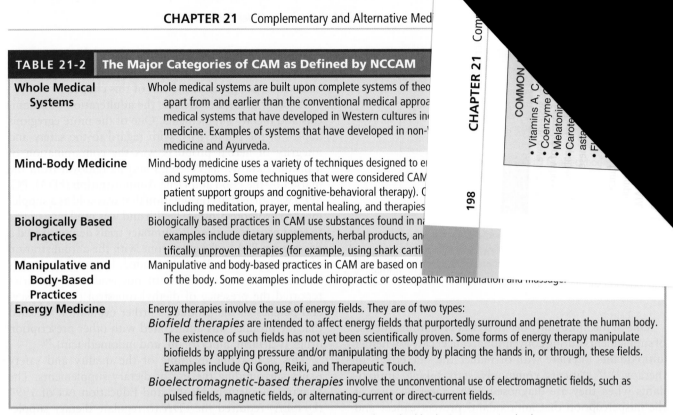

TABLE 21-2	The Major Categories of CAM as Defined by NCCAM
Whole Medical Systems	Whole medical systems are built upon complete systems of theo apart from and earlier than the conventional medical approa medical systems that have developed in Western cultures inc medicine. Examples of systems that have developed in non-' medicine and Ayurveda.
Mind-Body Medicine	Mind-body medicine uses a variety of techniques designed to e and symptoms. Some techniques that were considered CAM patient support groups and cognitive-behavioral therapy). C including meditation, prayer, mental healing, and therapies
Biologically Based Practices	Biologically based practices in CAM use substances found in n examples include dietary supplements, herbal products, an tifically unproven therapies (for example, using shark carti
Manipulative and Body-Based Practices	Manipulative and body-based practices in CAM are based on of the body. Some examples include chiropractic or osteopathic manipulation and massage.
Energy Medicine	Energy therapies involve the use of energy fields. They are of two types: *Biofield therapies* are intended to affect energy fields that purportedly surround and penetrate the human body. The existence of such fields has not yet been scientifically proven. Some forms of energy therapy manipulate biofields by applying pressure and/or manipulating the body by placing the hands in, or through, these fields. Examples include Qi Gong, Reiki, and Therapeutic Touch. *Bioelectromagnetic-based therapies* involve the unconventional use of electromagnetic fields, such as pulsed fields, magnetic fields, or alternating-current or direct-current fields.

From the National Center for Complementary and Alternative Medicine (http://nccam.nih.gov/health/whatiscam/overview.htm)

CASE 21-1	CASE HISTORY CONTINUED

J.D. met with an integrative physician and explained her reservations about receiving conventional care for the axillary recurrence of her breast cancer. She felt guilty about not taking the medical oncologist's advice but did not feel that he had listened to her concerns about therapy. She was anxious, depressed, and not sleeping. She was looking for a natural way to treat her cancer that she could control and which wouldn't have side effects that could interrupt her time with her grandchildren. After all, if she got chemotherapy now, she wouldn't be allowed to be around her grandchildren. Her niece had already recommended several supplements and dietary changes that she read about online and, although J.D. was heeding her niece's advice, she had doubts about the effectiveness of these interventions and her ability to continue to afford them. She also had noticed that the mass under her arm had gotten a little larger and was beginning to hurt. The integrative physician reviewed J.D.'s regimen with her including the evidence (or lack of evidence) to support each supplement's use. Ultimately, they decided that she would incorporate more soy, fruits, and vegetables in her diet; go for a 30 minute walk with her husband every day; and attend yoga and guided imagery classes at the cancer center. Her concerns and misconceptions about surgery and chemotherapy were addressed, as well as the impact these treatments would have on the time she spends with her family. She agreed to the surgery, and was encouraged to use acupuncture to manage the postoperative nausea that had been so debilitating after her first surgery.

---

however, pales in comparison to the amount spent on biomedical research, which, in 2003, was an estimated $94.3 billion.[14] Determining research methodologies pertinent to CAM therapies presents some obstacles as well. The challenges in conducting research on CAM therapies range from finding appropriate placebos for nonpharmacologic interventions to dismantling a whole systems practice like traditional Chinese medicine down to one well-defined intervention. The reductionist method is the standard in conventional medical research but may not be applicable to practices combining many treatment modalities as components of a comprehensive therapy. Nonetheless, there is a growing body of literature on the usefulness of some CAM therapies in the treatment of cancer patients, especially with regard to symptom management.

BOTANICALS AND NUTRITIONAL SUPPLEMENTS

Cancer patients commonly use dietary supplements, most often without the guidance or expertise of a knowledgeable practitioner. Well-intended oncologists sometimes resort to asking patients to discontinue all supplements during treatment, further diminishing a patient's sense of control over his or her own health care and promoting an attitude of nondisclosure. This lack of discourse can lead to harmful drug interactions, potentially decreasing the efficacy of some chemotherapeutic agents and radiation therapy. Opening a dialogue with patients about their supplement use helps to protect them, allows them to participate in their care, and promotes a sense of mutual respect between patient and physician. This section includes some general precautions about the use of dietary supplements; the remainder of the chapter will address some supplements and other interventions that are effective in treating common symptoms and side effects related to therapy.

ANTIOXIDANTS
and E
Q10 (ubiquinone)
noids (alpha and beta carotene,
xanthin, zeaxanthin, lutein, lycopene)
avonoids
Isoflavones
• Resveratrol
• Curcumin
• N-acetylcysteine
• Alpha lipoic acid
• Selenium
• Zinc

FIGURE 21-2 List of Common Antioxidants. These are some of the more common antioxidants that patients receiving chemotherapy and radiation should probably avoid.

One of the more hotly debated issues regarding the use of supplements during conventional cancer care is whether antioxidants interfere with or reduce the side effects of therapy.[15-19] Patients commonly start taking antioxidants when they are diagnosed with cancer because of the misperception that antioxidants prevent cancer and the assumption that what prevents cancer must also be good for treating cancer (Figure 21-2). In fact, there have been no large randomized controlled trials showing that antioxidants prevent cancer or reduce overall mortality.[20-21] In addition, the process of oxidation that results in the creation of free radicals is critical to the antineoplastic effects of radiation and many chemotherapeutic agents. Proponents of the use of antioxidants typically cite experimental and clinical data on tumoricidal effects, induction of apoptosis, and reduction in side effects from chemotherapy or radiation.[15] The obvious concern is that the administration of antioxidants leads to the protection of tumor cells, as well as normal cells, from oxidative damage. To illustrate this point, consider the largest randomized placebo-controlled clinical trial done examining the use of antioxidants during radiation in a group of head and neck cancer patients. In this study 540 patients were randomly assigned to receive α-tocopherol (a component of vitamin E) and β-carotene (a component of vitamin A) or placebo during radiation therapy. The patients in the α-tocopherol and β-carotene group had fewer adverse acute reactions (although no difference in quality-of-life measures), but local recurrence was 37% more likely in this group.[22] While future research may reveal antioxidants that help to mitigate treatment side effects without decreasing the efficacy of chemotherapy and radiation, the safest recommendation at present is to avoid antioxidants during treatment.[19]

Interactions with chemotherapy drugs and radiation are not the only concern in this population. The most common dietary supplement-drug interactions are with anticoagulants, cardiovascular drugs, oral hypoglycemics, and antiretrovirals.[23] These are all frequently used drugs in an aging population. Some of the more

common dietary supplement-drug interactions are listed in Table 21-3, and resources for evaluating a potential interaction are given at the end of this chapter.

Another area of concern is the adulteration of botanicals and dietary supplements. One of the more egregious abuses of the public trust with regard to the safety and integrity of herbal products was the contamination of a product known as PC-SPES and its removal from the market by the Food and Drug Administration (FDA). PC-SPES was an herbal combination that was sold as a supplement to promote prostate health and was used by patients to treat prostate cancer. Preliminary trials demonstrated a decrease in PSA and testosterone with the administration of this supplement. Publicly funded, larger clinical trials were planned for PC-SPES until independent laboratories reported the presence of diethylstilbestrol (DES) in several batches of the product. Further evaluation revealed that the product was adulterated with other prescription drugs (warfarin, alprazolam, and indomethacin).[26]

This is just one example of the quality and safety issues surrounding the use of dietary supplements. The Dietary Supplement Health and Education Act of 1994 (DHSEA) required the FDA to regulate dietary supplements as foods rather than as drugs, which means that supplements do not need approval from the FDA prior to entering the market. While this ensures the availability of these products to consumers, it comes with the consequence of a lack of regulatory oversight. The FDA does have the responsibility of regulating the manufacture of dietary supplements, and as of June, 2010, all manufacturers must be in compliance with current good manufacturing practices (cGMP). Given the large number of dietary supplement manufacturers, enforcement of these regulations may be difficult.

The industry is not completely without quality control, however. Many companies undergo voluntary independent testing of their products by the United States Pharmacopeia (USP) and ConsumerLab.com. Products displaying the USP verified seal or the ConsumerLab.com mark have completed this testing and been found to be of good quality.

While many physicians may not agree with the notions of patient self-diagnosis and self-treatment that are facilitated by the availability of dietary supplements, the fact remains that the practice exists. Hence the onus is on physicians to learn at least the basic essentials of indications, side effects, and potential drug interactions of dietary supplements.

CANCER-RELATED PROBLEMS AND CAM INTERVENTIONS

The remainder of this chapter provides recommendations that any physician can utilize to help cancer patients navigate the maze of treatment, side effects, and survivorship. The recommendations that follow are evidence-based. The evidence is not always from randomized,

TABLE 21-3	Common Herb-Drug Interactions and Precautions in Oncology[24-25]	
Botanical Product	**Common Uses**	**Potential Drug Interactions and Precautions**
Ginseng, American or Asian	To improve cognition, immune function, and energy; promotes blood sugar metabolism	None known but diabetics may need to monitor blood sugars due to a potential hypoglycemic effect
Black Cohosh	Menopausal symptoms	None known
Echinacea	Prevention of colds; used for immune support in cancer patients	None known; no documented interactions with immunosuppressive drugs
Garlic	Hyperlipidemia and atherosclerosis Prevention of colds	May enhance the effect of antiplatelet therapy and warfarin
Ginkgo	To improve cognition; to improve blood flow to the brain and extremities	Contraindicated in bleeding disorders; may enhance the effect of anti-platelet therapy and warfarin
Green tea	Reduce risk of cardiovascular disease and cancer	Can diminish the effect of dipyridamole; possible synergistic effects with sulindac and tamoxifen Large amounts of caffeine may increase the side effects of theophylline Antagonizes the tumorcidal effect of bortezomib (Golden 2009)
Ginger	Nausea	None known; anecdotal reports of interaction with warfarin but not proven
Kava	Anxiety and sleep	Should not be taken with alcohol, barbiturates, and other drugs with significant CNS effects Large doses may cause scaly ichthyosis
Milk thistle	Liver diseases and "cleansing"	An antioxidant; no known drug interactions
St. John's Wort	Depression	Should not be taken with prescription antidepressants; may interact with oral contraceptives, warfarin, theophylline, Indinavir, cyclosporine, digoxin Avoid alcohol Induces CYP3A4
Saw Palmetto	Prostate health, urinary outlet obstructive symptoms	None known; may cause mild nausea when taken without food

controlled trials, but it is enough to open doors to further exploration.

Nausea and Cachexia

Even with significant advances in pharmaceutical options for the treatment of chemotherapy-induced nausea, over 70% of cancer patients still report it as a problem.[27] Postoperative nausea may also be an unpleasant part of many cancer patients' experiences. Acupuncture (or a similar variation) has been shown in several studies to be useful for chemotherapy-induced and postoperative nausea. In fact, the 1997 NIH Consensus Conference on Acupuncture found that there was ample scientific evidence to support a recommendation of acupuncture for the treatment of postoperative and chemotherapy-induced nausea and vomiting.[28]

A more recent review of the literature examining trials of acupuncture point stimulation in preventing chemotherapy-induced nausea and vomiting found that acupuncture and electroacupuncture (applying an electrical current to the acupuncture needle while inserted) were significantly more effective than placebo or noninvasive forms of acupuncture point stimulation.[29]

Investigators at Duke University Medical Center examined the use of electroacupoint stimulation (slight electrical current applied through an electrode placed on an acupuncture point) in the treatment of postoperative nausea

and vomiting.[30] The participants were selected from a group of patients undergoing major breast surgery and were randomized to electroacupoint stimulation, ondansetron, or sham control (electrodes placed but without stimulation). Both treatment interventions were more effective at controlling nausea and emesis than the sham control. In addition, patients in the electroacupoint stimulation group had lower pain scores. A meta-analysis of nonpharmacologic methods of treating postoperative nausea and vomiting (acupuncture, electroacupuncture, transcutaneous electrical nerve stimulation, acupoint stimulation, and acupressure) showed that these methods were as effective as antiemetics in preventing early and late vomiting.[31]

Ginger (*Zingiber officinale*) is commonly used as a home remedy for an upset stomach. Traditional Chinese medicine uses ginger to treat nausea; it has also been useful in treating pregnancy-associated nausea.[32] In a randomized controlled trial of 644 cancer patients receiving chemotherapy, ginger capsules were found to be effective at significantly reducing nausea, even in the setting of standard 5-HT$_3$ receptor antagonist antiemetics.[27]

Another nutritional problem commonly encountered in oncology practices is cancer cachexia. Cancer cachexia is a condition involving complex metabolic processes, as well as reduced nutritional intake. It leads to a significant reduction in lean body mass, extreme fatigue, and ultimately immobility. In part, the metabolic hyperactivity in this condition is attributed to the production of proinflammatory cytokines. For this reason, omega-3 fatty acids as inflammatory mediators have been explored for supportive care in this condition. Several studies in pancreatic cancer patients have shown positive effects of omega-3 supplementation (especially eicosapentaenoic acid or EPA) in terms of weight gain, performance status, and quality-of-life measures.[33] A recent review of the literature on omega-3 fatty acids in the treatment of cachexia in patients with advanced cancer of the pancreas and upper digestive tract showed that supplementation with 1.5 to 2.0 grams per day of EPA and docosahexaenoic acid (DHA) resulted in improvements in multiple measures; one study actually showed a significant improvement in survival.[34-35]

Diarrhea and Mucositis

The gastrointestinal tract is often an innocent victim when it comes to the efficacy of therapeutic agents in destroying rapidly dividing cells. The loss of cells in the GI tract and bone marrow is sometimes the dose-limiting factor in administering chemotherapy or abdominal/pelvic radiation. In addition to routine supportive measures for diarrhea (hydration, small meals, avoiding fiber, and antidiarrheal drugs), patients may benefit from taking glutamine. Glutamine helps to maintain the mucosal integrity of the gut epithelium. In a randomized controlled trial of 70 patients who were receiving 5-fluorouracil (5-FU) chemotherapy for treatment of advanced colon cancer, oral glutamine at a dose of 6 grams three times a day significantly improved intestinal absorption and permeability compared to placebo.[36] Another placebo-controlled trial was done in breast cancer patients receiving cyclophosphamide, epirubicin, and 5-FU chemotherapy, with 30 grams of glutamine per day.[37] These investigators showed that glutamine lessened intestinal permeability and did not interfere with chemotherapy; however, no clinical difference was seen in diarrhea and stomatitis scores. There are also case reports that glutamine has been effective in preventing late diarrhea associated with irinotecan.[38]

Mucositis can affect up to 40% of patients receiving chemotherapy at standard doses and as many as 75% of patients receiving high-dose chemotherapy.[39] Also, despite advances in radiation therapy, mucositis is an almost universal side effect of head and neck irradiation. Ulceration of the oropharyngeal mucosa is painful, creates difficulty swallowing and speaking, inhibits adequate nutritional intake, and can lead to delays in treatment that potentially affect tumor control. Glutamine is useful in this group of patients as well. A randomized controlled trial of 326 breast cancer patients receiving anthracycline-based chemotherapy showed that glutamine in a proprietary drug delivery system (Saforis) significantly reduced the incidence of oral mucositis.[39] A pilot study in 17 head and neck cancer patients receiving radiation showed a reduction in oral mucositis with administration of a glutamine solution as an oral rinse four times a day.[40]

Xerostomia

Xerostomia, or dry mouth, is primarily caused by radiation to the head and neck region. With the development of more precise radiation treatment planning systems, better patient immobilization, and real-time imaging techniques, the incidence of permanent xerostomia has been significantly reduced, but it remains a significant quality of life issue for many patients. Acupuncture has proven to be very useful in improving salivary flow rates in patients who have received radiation to the head and neck. In one retrospective review of 70 patients with xerostomia from radiation, Sjögren syndrome, or other causes, patients received 24 acupuncture treatments; statistically significant differences were found in stimulated and unstimulated salivary flow rates compared to baseline.[41] These results were independent of the etiology of the xerostomia. At 3 years follow-up, those who had continued to receive some acupuncture treatments had significantly more salivary flow than those who did not receive additional treatment. Johnstone et al. developed a xerostomia inventory (XI) as a validated tool to help objectively measure the effects of acupuncture, as subjective measures of xerostomia are not always consistent with objective salivary flow rates. In a report on 50 patients who had received 318 treatments, 70% of patients had a response to acupuncture as indicated by improvements in the XI. Most patients required treatment every 1 to 2 months for a lasting effect; however, in 26% of the patients, the effect lasted for 3 months or more.[42-43]

Fatigue

The National Comprehensive Cancer Network (NCCN) defines cancer-related fatigue as "a distressing persistent, subjective sense of physical, emotional, and/or cognitive tiredness or exhaustion related to cancer or cancer treatment that is not proportional to recent activity and interferes with usual functioning."[44] Fatigue can be the result of treatment (surgery, chemotherapy, or radiation) or an effect of the disease itself. It is the most prevalent symptom reported by cancer patients,[45] and they often need reassurance that this is a common and expected part of their cancer journey. Patients should be screened for fatigue and referred to medical professionals experienced in dealing with cancer-related fatigue. The exact etiology is not clearly understood, and there are many related conditions including anemia, nutritional deficiencies, sleep disturbances, and emotional distress that contribute to the sensation of fatigue (Figure 21-3).

Nonpharmacologic evidence-based recommendations for dealing with fatigue include exercise and other activity enhancement (preferably under the direction of physical and occupational therapists), massage, yoga, meditation, and psychoeducational therapies aimed at stress reduction (Figure 21-4).[46-47] A recent phase II

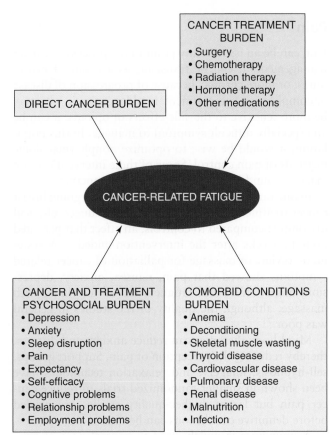

FIGURE 21-3 Related factors contributing to fatigue in the cancer patient. *(Reprinted with permission from Mustian KM, Morrow GR, Carroll JK, et al: Integrative nonpharmacologic behavioral interventions for the management of cancer-related fatigue. The Oncologist 12(suppl 1):52-67, 2007.)*

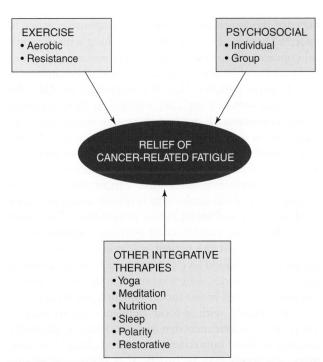

FIGURE 21-4 Nonpharmacologic interventions for cancer-related fatigue. *(Reprinted with permission from Mustian KM, Morrow GR, Carroll JK, et al: Integrative nonpharmacologic behavioral interventions for the management of cancer-related fatigue. The Oncologist 12(suppl 1):52-67, 2007.)*

study in cancer patients with persistent fatigue after chemotherapy showed that a short course (4 to 6 weeks) of acupuncture resulted in a mean improvement of 31% in the Brief Fatigue Inventory, a finding that met predefined criteria meriting it for further study. Perhaps what is most impressive about this finding is that the group of patients studied had completed their cytotoxic therapy an average of more than 2 years earlier and the fatigue had become chronic and persistent.[48]

Hot Flashes

Coping with menopausal symptoms is a fact of life for more than 50% of women and can interfere with quality of life for years after menopause.[49-50] Breast cancer patients are often faced with the symptoms of menopause around the time of their diagnosis and treatment either as a natural course of life or induced by chemotherapy and/or antiestrogen therapy. The difference in management for those who have or who are at risk for breast cancer is that hormone replacement therapy is an even less palatable treatment option than for the general population. An integrative approach to the management of menopausal symptoms in this group of patients involves advising patients about appropriate dietary, exercise,

and relaxation practices first, followed by advice about nutritional supplements and botanicals. Numerous studies have shown that a healthy diet is one that is largely plant based and includes lots of fresh fruits and vegetables, lean meats, whole grains, and olive oil.[51] There is evidence that lifestyle and dietary changes can positively influence hot flashes and mood changes.[52-53] Aerobic exercise has been shown to decrease hot flashes, improve sleep, elevate mood, and generally enhance quality of life in menopausal women.[54-55] Relaxation techniques may also be helpful in alleviating some of the symptoms of menopause. These include paced respiration (controlled diaphragmatic breathing), progressive muscle relaxation, and behavioral relaxation.[56] Anecdotally, relaxation practices such as meditation, yoga, or massage have been helpful.

Soy has long been of interest to women because of the association of a lower incidence of breast cancer in populations that tend to include more soy in their traditional diets. The evidence for the effectiveness of soy in the treatment of vasomotor symptoms of menopause is inconclusive.[57-59] There are some positive trials supporting the use of soy for the treatment of hot flashes.[59-61] Its effectiveness is presumably due to the fact that the isoflavones in soy have weak estrogenic activity. Because of this estrogenic activity, there is concern about the use of soy in breast cancer survivors or women at high risk for breast cancer. The soy isoflavone genistein can stimulate the growth of breast cancer cells,[62] interfere with the inhibitory effect of tamoxifen on breast cancer cells, and increase the expression of estrogen-responsive genes in mice.[63] These experimental findings, along with theoretical concerns, have resulted in anxiety among physicians and patients alike about the safety of soy consumption in breast cancer patients. Here it is important to make the distinction between soy consumption in food products versus concentrated soy isoflavones in nutritional supplements. In the Shanghai Breast Cancer Survival Study, 5042 female breast cancer survivors in China were followed for a median of 3.9 years, and information on various lifestyle exposures after cancer diagnosis was collected. Soy food intake was inversely associated with total mortality and breast cancer recurrence.[64] This effect was still evident regardless of estrogen receptor status or whether or not the patient was taking tamoxifen. In another study, blood levels of tamoxifen, its metabolites, and soy isoflavones were examined in an Asian-American population of breast cancer patients. Soy food intake was determined with a food frequency questionnaire. There was no evidence that soy food intake adversely affected levels of tamoxifen or its metabolites.[65] In summary, soy foods may be beneficial in breast cancer survivors with regard to total mortality and breast cancer recurrence; however, the data on the usefulness of soy foods in the treatment of hot flashes are inconclusive and further studies are warranted. Furthermore, concentrated soy isoflavones in the form of nutritional supplements should be avoided in breast cancer survivors given the potential for stimulation of breast cancer cell growth.

Black cohosh (*Actaea racemosa, Cimicifuga racemosa*) was once thought to have estrogenic properties but more recent evidence shows that it is actually not a phytoestrogen.[66] Numerous clinical trials have been conducted on the efficacy of black cohosh in the treatment of menopausal symptoms, with mixed results. Although these trials have varied significantly in methodologic quality, design, and type of herbal extract used, the preponderance of the evidence supports the use of black cohosh for the treatment of hot flashes,[56-57,66-67] with a recent meta-analysis showing a reduction in vasomotor symptoms by 26% with the use of black cohosh.[68]

Antiestrogen therapy is sometimes the cause of hot flashes and can lead to treatment compliance issues unless the symptoms are dealt with effectively. Although venlafaxine has been extensively used in this group of patients, it is not without its own side effects and antidepressant stigma. A recent randomized trial compared venlafaxine to acupuncture for control of vasomotor symptoms due to antiestrogen therapy. Both groups responded to treatment with a decrease in the number of hot flashes, fewer depressive symptoms, and general improvements in quality of life, with acupuncture being equivalent to venlafaxine. While the acupuncture group did not experience any adverse effects, the venlafaxine group reported 18 adverse events including nausea, dizziness, anxiety, and dry mouth. In addition, the acupuncture group reported improvement in energy, clarity of thought, and sense of well-being.[69]

Pain

Pain can be an issue at any point in the process of cancer management. It can be transient, as a result of procedures, or more chronic, because of progression of disease or complications of treatment. In older patients, who may be more sensitive to the side effects of opioids, it can be an especially difficult symptom to manage. In this population, it would be wise to optimize nonpharmacologic methods of pain control. Some of these interventions are massage, mind-body therapies, and acupuncture.

In one randomized study of women undergoing breast cancer treatment, massage significantly reduced physical discomfort compared to controls, an effect that persisted even 11 weeks after the intervention ended.[70] A systematic review of massage for palliation of cancer-related symptoms showed that pain, nausea, anxiety, depression, anger, stress and fatigue were all alleviated with massage, although the quality of the studies in general was poor.[71]

Mind-body therapies can reduce anxiety and distress, thereby reducing the perception of pain. Support groups, self-hypnosis, imagery, and relaxation techniques have been shown in smaller randomized trials to reduce cancer pain but larger, higher-quality studies are needed before definitive conclusions can be drawn.[72]

Acupuncture is widely used to control pain of various etiologies. The World Health Organization considers it effective for the treatment of cancer pain[73] and it is part of the National Comprehensive Cancer Network (NCCN) pain management guidelines as a recommended nonpharmacologic intervention.[74] A randomized controlled trial of auricular acupuncture for cancer pain was performed at a pain management clinic in a large comprehensive cancer center in France.[75] Ninety patients with chronic pain related to cancer were randomized to auricular acupuncture, placebo auricular acupuncture, or placebo auricular seeds. Auricular acupuncture resulted in a statistically significant decrease in pain compared to the two placebo groups (36% versus 2%). Acupuncture has also been examined in a randomized controlled fashion in patients who have pain and dysfunction after a neck dissection.[76] In this study, patients were randomized to acupuncture or usual care (physical therapy, analgesics, and/or anti-inflammatory drugs). Patients who received acupuncture rather than usual care had significantly better outcomes as measured by a composite score assessing pain, function, and activities of daily living. Acupuncture patients also fared significantly better with xerostomia, which was a secondary outcome measure.

In conjunction with the widespread use of aromatase inhibitors (AIs) in breast cancer, another painful scenario has emerged. A significant proportion of women taking AIs experience arthralgias that are serious enough to interfere with quality of life and medication compliance. A randomized, controlled, blinded study of true versus sham acupuncture was conducted in this group of patients. There was significant improvement in joint pain, stiffness, physical function, and physical well-being in women who received true acupuncture.[77]

Peripheral Neuropathy

The true incidence of chemotherapy-induced peripheral neuropathy (CIPN) is undetermined because of a lack of standards regarding symptom classification, measurement, and clinical evaluation.[78-80] For neurotoxic agents, CIPN is often the dose-limiting factor in administering the drug and can result in a dose reduction or a switch to a potentially less effective regimen. The most common offending agents are listed in Table 21-4. Standard pharmacologic interventions for symptom management are generally the same as those used for peripheral neuropathy due to other causes and include various antidepressants and anticonvulsants.

Several complementary therapies aimed at prevention of CIPN have been evaluated. A recent randomized, double-blinded, placebo-controlled trial examined the use of vitamin E in CIPN prevention and found that there was no effect of the vitamin E with regard to incidence of CIPN, time to onset of symptoms, or dose reductions in chemotherapy.[81] Glutamine has been effective in reducing the incidence of CIPN in breast cancer patients receiving paclitaxel.[82] In this nonrandomized trial, patients who received glutamine 10 mg tid for four days beginning 24 hours after the paclitaxel infusion had fewer symptoms and signs of CIPN, as well as less interference with activities of daily living. The authors of this study report that they did not find any alteration in the pharmacokinetics of paclitaxel with the administration of glutamine. Further study of this intervention in a larger, randomized controlled trial is warranted.

A meta-analysis of alpha lipoic acid in the treatment of diabetic polyneuropathy showed a 24% improvement in total symptom score with the administration of 600 mg of intravenous alpha lipoic acid each weekday for three weeks.[83] Unfortunately, as alpha lipoic acid is a potent antioxidant, it should probably not be administered concurrently with chemotherapy until there is evidence that it will not interfere with the chemotherapy's effectiveness. It may, however, be useful for patients with CIPN after therapy has been completed.

Although acupuncture for treatment of CIPN has only been reported in one small case series of five patients, these patients had significant relief of pain with treatment.[84] Acupuncture has been useful in the treatment of neuropathy related to diabetes and HIV.[85-88] One study also showed improvements in nerve conduction studies with acupuncture.[89]

LIFESTYLE CHANGES AND CANCER SURVIVAL

Many patients express an interest in adopting a healthier lifestyle after surviving cancer treatment.[90] Older cancer survivors are at increased risk for second malignancies, cardiovascular disease, obesity, and other comorbidities.[91] There is ample evidence that being physically active and eating a healthy diet are associated with an improved quality of life and lower risk of cancer recurrence. In a study of older long-term cancer survivors, greater amounts of exercise and better diet quality were associated with better physical quality of life outcomes and, in contrast, a greater body mass index was associated with reduced physical quality of life.[92] Breast cancer survivors with a high vegetable and fruit intake (≥5 servings per day) combined with a high physical activity level (≥9 MET-hrs/week or the equivalent of walking 30 minutes/day, 6 days/week) had a reduction in mortality of approximately 50% compared to survivors in the lowest quartiles for fruit and vegetable consumption and physical activity.[93] Holmes et al. found that the relative risk of death from breast cancer in women with hormone-sensitive breast cancer who exercised for 9 or more MET-hrs/week was half that of women who were less physically active.[94] Two separate prospective observational studies have also shown a decrease in risk of death in colon cancer survivors who exercise. The first involved 832 patients who were enrolled in a randomized adjuvant chemotherapy trial for stage III colon cancer.[95] The 3-year disease-free survival was 75% in patients who exercised for fewer than 18 MET-hrs/week compared to 84% in patients who exercised for more than 18 MET-hrs/week. The other observational group came from the Nurses' Health Study and involved 573 women with stage I-III colorectal cancer.[96] Cancer-specific and overall mortality were inversely related to physical activity levels.

In spite of this evidence, very few survivors actually meet the recommendations from the American Cancer Society regarding diet, exercise, and smoking cessation. A survey of over 9,000 survivors revealed that only 15% to 19% of patients meet dietary recommendations, 30% to 47% meet physical activity recommendations, and only 5% meet dietary, exercise, and smoking-cessation recommendations.[97] Clearly there is room for improvement in educating patients about the importance of lifestyle changes in cancer survivorship.

TABLE 21-4	Chemotherapies That Can Cause Peripheral Neuropathy
Drugs	**Malignancies for Which They Are Commonly Used**
Vincristine and vinblastine	Lymphoma and leukemia
Bortezomib and thalidomide	Multiple myeloma
Cisplatin, oxaliplatin, carboplatin	Ovarian, lung, colorectal, bladder, head and neck, cervical cancers
Paclitaxel and docetaxel	Ovarian, breast, lung cancers

Summary

The management of cancer patients is complex and that complexity only increases with age. A patient's utilization of therapies that are not a part of a physician's standard knowledge base presents additional challenges. The first step in addressing those challenges is to ask about the use of dietary supplements and complementary therapies. This chapter has reviewed some of the safety issues surrounding the use of CAM, as well as the evidence to support certain therapies. Equipped with even a modest understanding of these therapies, a physician should be able to engage his patients in a dialogue about CAM use, empower them to participate in their care, and guide their choices to keep them from potential harm.

See expertconsult.com for a complete list of references and web resources for this chapter

SUGGESTED READINGS

1. Eisenberg DM, Kessler RC, Foster C, et al: Unconventional medicine in the United States – prevalence, costs, and patterns of use, *NEJM* 328:246–252, 1993.
2. Eisenberg DM, Davis RB, Ettner SL, et al: Trends in alternative medicine use in the United States, 1990-1997 results of a follow-up national survey, *JAMA* 280:1569–1575, 1998.
3. Astin JA: Why patients use alternative medicine: results of a national study, *JAMA* 279:1548–1553, 1998.
4. Food, Nutrition, Physical Activity and the Prevention of Cancer: A Global Perspective: American Institute for Cancer Research Washington, DC, 2007, World Cancer Research Fund International, Last accessed May 27, 2010.
5. Bairati I, Meyer F, Gelinas M, et al: Randomized trial of antioxidant vitamins to prevent acute adverse effects of radiation therapy in head and neck cancer patients, *J Clin Oncol* 23:5805–5813, 2005.
6. Lawenda BD, Kelly KM, Ladas EJ, et al: Should supplemental antioxidant administration be avoided during chemotherapy and radiation therapy? *J Natl Cancer Inst* 100:773–783, 2008.

Rehabilitation/ Survivorship

The Role of Rehabilitation in the Older Patient with Cancer

Lucia Loredana Dattoma and Patricia A. Ganz

B.S. is a 77-year-old woman with a history of breast cancer, diagnosed at age 56 when she was found to have a right upper quadrant breast mass on screening mammogram, along with axillary lymphadenopathy on physical examination. She underwent right modified radical mastectomy and complete right axillary lymph node dissection. Pathologic examination confirmed right invasive cancer with lobular tubular features, well-differentiated, with six positive lymph nodes. The tumor was estrogen receptor and progesterone receptor-positive (ER/PR+). Imaging studies revealed no metastatic disease so the patient began radiation therapy and was placed on tamoxifen. She also developed right upper extremity lymphedema and arm dysfunction as a result of the surgery.

After remaining cancer-free for nearly 16 years, she presented to her physician complaining of radiating back pain, frequent falls, and increasing debilitation in the past 6 months from persistent right arm lymphedema and dysfunction. She was noted to have an elevated alkaline phosphatase and was found to have lumbar metastasis. Imaging studies revealed no further metastatic disease except for a new lesion in the left breast measuring 13 mm. She was treated with radiation to the lower back. While undergoing radiation she was offered subacute rehabilitation but refused it at first. Once she was educated on the benefits of "short-term" rehabilitation she agreed and was admitted to a skilled nursing facility (SNF), where she received physical and occupational therapy, pain management, and psychosocial therapy. Because B.S. was depressed and lacked adequate social support, she was adamant about not wanting to undergo another operation that would further debilitate her by also reducing her left arm function. After receiving radiation therapy, psychotherapy, and rehabilitation she agreed to undergo left modified radical mastectomy and modified lymph node dissection. Following her second operation, she returned to the SNF and received an additional 2 weeks of rehabilitation before she went home.

Rehabilitation services provide a multidisciplinary approach to preventive interventions that can enhance physical and psychosocial functioning; these interventions can be directed at limitations that may result from the diagnosis or treatment of cancer. The rehabilitation team begins by assessing and treating the whole patient and gaining an understanding of the individual's limitations and his or her disease process, along with an awareness of his or her leisure and vocational activities and desire to maintain a healthy and productive lifestyle, regardless of age or disease severity.

Rehabilitation plays an important role for the older adult patient with cancer. With the aging of the population, there will be an expansion of the number of older adults with cancer, as nearly 60% of all cancer diagnoses are made in patients 65 years old and older. As a result of older age, many of these patients already have multiple coexisting chronic conditions and functional limitations. Therefore it may be important to maximize overall quality of life and emphasize both mental and physical preparation prior to cancer treatment in the older adult. Anticipation of patient needs prior to treatment, as well as intervention with rehabilitation services during and after cancer treatment, may be particularly important in maintaining function and stable health when cancer co-occurs with other chronic health conditions.

As in the aforementioned case, patients who receive rehabilitation before and during aggressive cancer treatments have a higher likelihood of regaining premorbid functional status. Therefore rehabilitation promotes long-term health and wellness, whether as part of curative or palliative care.

REHABILITATION NEEDS OF THE OLDER PATIENT WITH CANCER

Treatment and technological advancements in medicine have led to prolonged survival rates in patients diagnosed with cancer. In fact, it is estimated that nearly two thirds of patients treated for a cancer will survive the initial phase. However, the sequelae of cancer treatment, whether it be surgery, hormones, chemotherapy or radiation, may lead to significant distress and hence make cancer a chronic disease. For example, B.S. developed right upper extremity lymphedema and arm dysfunction from her initial surgery nearly 20 years ago. This impairment was physically and emotionally debilitating, leading her initially to decline additional surgical intervention for her recurring cancer in the left breast.

Rehabilitation needs of the older adult with cancer vary according to the phase of the disease, with physical needs being greatest in advanced cancer. Cancer in all age groups, but particularly in older patients, is very heterogeneous in its manifestations, biology, responses to treatment, and time course. Being aware of the rehabilitation needs of the older adult with cancer as associated with disease phase, site-specific cancer, and treatment options and/or toxicities will empower the oncologic team and patient to initiate preventive interventions in a timely fashion.

Common Related Rehabilitation Issues The most common rehabilitative problem faced by an older patient with cancer is physical. The extent of dysfunction ranges from none to severe depending on the disease, time of diagnosis, and cancer severity. Ideally, all patients who receive a cancer diagnosis should have some degree of rehabilitation at some point during the course of the disease and its treatment. The key is to identify the problem and intervene early. In many cases, being proactive and getting a physical therapy consultation before the symptoms present may improve the long-term functional outcome. The goal in obtaining physical therapy is to maximize quality of life by maintaining mobility and stamina and retaining the ability to perform basic activities of daily living. Consultation with the hospital rehabilitation service before a patient's discharge from the hospital is invaluable, and maximizes the patient's chance of maintaining physical function and independence while at home.

The next most common rehabilitative problem in cancer patients is psychosocial issues including depression, anxiety, fear, sexual difficulties, and social and interpersonal problems. Psychosocial concerns are usually not acknowledged or understood by the older adult and are frequently missed by the treating physician. Hence they are often overlooked and may remain untreated until the later part of the disease course. A needs assessment should be done at the time of diagnosis, at the time of any recurrence, or whenever the prognosis has changed or is poor, as these are the periods when patients are most likely to develop psychosocial problems and may need professional intervention. Some patients may benefit from early consultation with a psychologist or psychiatrist. Psychosocial issues will be discussed further in a later chapter. (See Table 22-1.) Sexual difficulties are another area of rehabilitative need in some older patients with cancer. Depression, fatigue, distorted body image, hair loss, surgical scars, and weight loss can lead to decreased sexual desire and feelings of unattractiveness. Some surgical interventions and radiation therapies may lead to impairment in sexual function. Sexual problems

TABLE 22-1	Common Rehabilitative Issues

- Physical dysfunction – impaired mobility, stamina, and ADL
- Psychosocial problems – depression, anxiety and fear of recurrence
- Sexual difficulties – decreased sexual desire, sexual dysfunction
- Diet and nutrition – anorexia and malnutrition, obesity and decreased physical activity

are commonly overlooked by physicians and are frequently not discussed by the patient because of fears and embarrassment. It may help the patient and partner cope with posttreatment difficulties with sex and intimacy if the physician inquires about and discusses these issues with them. This may be particularly important for cancers that involve the pelvic organs, such as prostate cancer, rectal cancer, bladder cancer, and cervical cancer, especially when both surgery and radiation are used, and when stomas may be required. Sex therapy is warranted for some patients to help them recover.

A fourth area of rehabilitative need is diet and nutrition. Older adults with cancer are at very high risk for developing malnutrition, often because many of them also have comorbidities in addition to their cancer. Patients who have excessive weight loss due to early satiety and anorexia may derive benefit from a nutrition consultation to identify problems with the current dietary pattern and aid with a supplemental plan. A speech therapy consultation may be beneficial for patients with dysphagia or difficulties swallowing. Some patients may need an appetite stimulant such as megestrol acetate, which has been shown to have some benefit in preventing cachexia. However, megestrol acetate also has many adverse effects and is contraindicated in many older patients. Mirtazepine is an antidepressant that has been used successfully as an appetite stimulant and which has a lower side effect profile. This drug may benefit a depressed patient with anorexia who is also struggling with insomnia. Patients who become very malnourished, especially those requiring prolonged periods of radiation and/or chemotherapy, may benefit from a short period of intravenous hyperalimentation or gastrostomy tube placement for supplemental nutrition.

Obesity and lack of physical activity may be a problem for some cancer patients. Weight gain after cancer and/or obesity puts patients at higher risk for recurrence of breast, colon, and prostate cancers. Maintaining physical activity and a prudent diet can be an important focus for rehabilitation.

Cancer-Specific Rehabilitation Issues

Breast CancerAs with the patient described at the beginning of the chapter, many women suffer both physically and emotionally from the diagnosis and treatment of breast cancer. Breast cancer is the most common cancer in women in the United States. Surgical treatments for breast cancer have evolved over the past 30 years, so that modified radical mastectomies are done less frequently (about 35% of cases), and most women receive a segmental mastectomy with whole breast irradiation. Removal of the axillary lymph nodes and radiation to the axilla can lead to complications of arm swelling and difficulties with range of motion. Fortunately, these procedures are being done less frequently; the current strategy is biopsy of a "sentinel node" to determine whether the breast tumor has spread outside the breast. When this does not show spread, surgery to the axilla can be avoided. Nevertheless, there are many older women who have had mastectomies at an earlier time and who may experience problems with arm swelling and function. The most common problems that occur with the surgical treatment of breast cancer are upper extremity edema, limited mobility, pain, tingling, numbness and weakness, fatigue, difficulty lifting, and trouble following through with housework. For B.S., this significantly affected her quality of life and she nearly refused surgical intervention when her breast cancer recurred in the other breast. She underwent occupational therapy including an exercise program, elevation, and a supportive sleeve, which collectively improved her right arm function and decreased the edematous swelling. During this period, she also received psychotherapy, was started on an antidepressant, learned about the new conservative surgical options and therefore agreed to have surgery to remove the left breast cancer.

Surgical reconstruction of the breast should be offered to all women who undergo mastectomy. However, surgical reconstruction poses its own risks for the older adult and many patients either choose not to undergo this intervention or are not considered candidates for surgical reconstruction.

Other rehabilitative problems that occur with breast cancer are, as mentioned earlier, sexual and body image problems. This may be worse in patients who undergo concomitant radiation and chemotherapy, as these treatments may lead to decreased sexual desire and impaired vaginal lubrication. Sexual problems that continue or become psychologically debilitating should be addressed in sexual therapy with a qualified psychotherapist, to include the patient and her partner.

Prostate Cancer

Prostate cancer treatment can range from radical prostatectomy to pelvic irradiation or watchful waiting. Any or all of these can lead to sexual, urinary, and/or bowel dysfunction. Focus on quality of life during rehabilitation is important because patients with this disease may survive many years after their diagnosis. Sexual impairment such as erectile dysfunction or impotence occurs in the early stages of prostate cancer and is frequently caused by surgery such as radical prostatectomy or from body image distortion due to castration and/or pelvic irradiation. It remains controversial whether nerve-sparing surgeries

---

CASE 22-2

C.W. is a 76-year old man with a 10-year history of prostate cancer. At the time of diagnosis, his serum prostate-specific antigen level was 4.9 ng/mL and the tumor's Gleason score was 4+3. He was treated with external beam radiation therapy. He tolerated this therapy reasonably well except for some prominent urinary frequency and sexual dysfunction. This was emotionally distressing and he and his wife sought sexual therapy. His quality of life improved as a result and his PSA level dropped to 2.0 ng/mL (this suggests that the treatment did not eradicate his disease). However, his PSA level began to rise again, reaching 8.8 ng/mL about 3 years after treatment. A bone scan showed evidence of metastasis to a right seventh rib. He was placed on androgen deprivation therapy with a gonadotropin-releasing hormone analog and his PSA rapidly dropped to 3.0. He complained of worsening fatigue, urinary retention, and mid-to-lower back and right hip pain.

About 2 years later he had a third recurrence and received a series of endocrine therapies that eventually stabilized his PSA in the range of 3 ng/mL. However, he suffered a stroke with a left-sided hemiparesis about 2 years after the third recurrence and was hospitalized. As he recovered, he complained of fatigue, weakness, and depression. He was transferred to a skilled nursing facility where he underwent physical and occupational therapy and psychiatric evaluation and treatment. His prostate cancer symptoms of back and hip pain, urinary retention, and fatigue continued and his PSA rose to 9.1 ng/mL, so he was started on chemotherapy. However, after the first cycle of docetaxel chemotherapy he suffered considerable toxicity including diarrhea, stomatitis, and severe fatigue. It was at this time that he advised his oncologist that he did not wish to continue chemotherapy as it was impairing his quality of life. He agreed to undergo another course of rehabilitation before returning home to his family.

---

result in a lower incidence of sexual dysfunction. As in the patient discussed here, sexual therapy may be necessary for some patients, and should include both the patient and his partner.

The patient in Case 22-2 suffered from urinary incontinence; however, bowel incontinence is also a very common problem following radical prostatectomies or pelvic irradiation, while urinary retention is common when watchful waiting is practiced. Bladder and bowel training programs can be helpful in coping with these impairments. Pain control, through use of sustained-release narcotic analgesics, nonsteroidal anti-inflammatory agents, and palliative radiation therapy, should be a focus in patients with advanced disease. Maintaining physical function through pain control can prolong independence and improve quality of life.

Colorectal Cancer

The rehabilitative needs of patients who undergo treatment for colon cancer often relate to bowel changes and, in the case of advanced disease, obstructing lesions. For patients with a stoma, consultation with an enterostomal therapist is critical for education and for the management of the ostomy. Unfortunately, because of the urgency of this patient's need for surgery, he did not

F. H. is a 74-year-old man with end-stage colorectal cancer who was admitted to the hospital for nausea, vomiting, and abdominal pain. He was found to have colonic obstruction from a 5 cm cecal mass and two other lesions in the distal transverse and sigmoid colon. Review of systems revealed poorly controlled low back pain that began 3 months ago; poor sleep, which he attributed to pain; and several months of impaired concentration and anorexia, with a 40-pound weight loss.

F.H. underwent complete cecal excision and colectomy with subsequent right-sided colostomy. His hospitalization was complicated by prolonged intubation because of respiratory failure and hospital-acquired pneumonia, *Clostridium difficile colitis,* and deep vein thrombosis in the left leg. Anticoagulation had to be discontinued because of retroperitoneal bleeding; an inferior vena cava filter was placed. He was eventually extubated, but required placement of a gastrostomy tube because of severe dysphagia. Because of his debilitated state, he was deemed a poor candidate for chemotherapy; he was thus transferred to a skilled nursing facility for occupational and physical therapy.

The patient's SNF course was marked by frustration that resulted from persistent pain and alternating constipation and diarrhea. Both palliative care and psychiatric services were consulted to help manage his pain and to evaluate his cognitive difficulties. His back pain was caused by a metastatic lesion at L3 and was treated with escalating doses of controlled-release oxycodone and as-needed doses of short-acting oxycodone. His psychiatric history was unremarkable. On mental status examination, F.H. was awake and amiable, but uncomfortable. He denied feeling depressed or guilty. However, he said that he was embarrassed by having colostomy and would no longer enjoy his hobbies or spending time with family or friends.

As his SNF stay progressed, he appeared more withdrawn, had no interest in learning ostomy care, refused therapy, and became less hopeful that his pain, his difficulty maintaining attention, and his bowel problems would resolve. He was started on an antidepressant and psychotherapy and eventually began cooperating with physical and occupational therapy, became receptive to ostomy education, and experienced a reduction in pain to a tolerable level.

undergo excision of localized bowel tumors, hemicolectomies, or irradiation therapy. These may be improved by bowel training programs and, in seriously debilitating cases, a referral to a proctologist or gastroenterologist may be warranted.

Lung Cancer

Lung cancer is the single most common cause of cancer mortality in the United States today. This is especially true in the older adult population. The lung cancer survival rate is low, perhaps because the disease is usually at an advanced stage when diagnosed, as was true for the aforementioned patient. The significant toxicities of both chemotherapy and radiation therapy may also contribute to morbidity and mortality.

L.D. is a 71-year-old woman, formerly a heavy smoker, who was hospitalized after a 2-month history of worsening dyspnea, anorexia, and an unintended weight loss of 40 pounds. A chest x-ray revealed a left hilar mass, and ultrasound of the abdomen showed liver lesions indicating metastatic disease. Bronchoscopy was diagnostic for small cell lung cancer. She received a protocol of combination chemotherapy on a 4-week schedule. Subsequently, she suffered significant side effects of worsening anorexia, nausea, vomiting, and extreme fatigue. She spent all of her waking time in bed. She was thus referred for outpatient rehabilitation and received 1 hour of physical therapy three times per week.

At 3-month follow-up, she was found to be in complete remission. However, she presented 5 months later with worsening low back pain, dyspnea, and new-onset seizure disorder. Second-line chemotherapy and steroid therapy were initiated. She suffered significant toxicities from the chemotherapy without much clinical improvement. She became severely debilitated and developed cognitive impairment as a result of the brain metastasis. According to the patient's wishes, terminal supportive care was provided under the direction of her son who represented her interests with a durable power of attorney for health care.

receive ostomy information preoperatively; as a result, he suffered significant distress in the following months. His emotional difficulties adjusting to the stoma impaired his ability to learn ostomy care. It is important to encourage a patient who has an ostomy to view and touch it, so as to give him enough self-confidence and independence to provide ostomy care for himself.

Some patients also experience sexual dysfunction due to bodily distortion and function of elimination; erectile dysfunction is not uncommon in men who undergo invasive abdominorectal surgery. A patient's partner may have some difficulties adjusting to the bodily changes; this may lead to discord, feelings of lack of support, and sexual impairment. Some patients and their partners may benefit from sexual therapy.

Rectal dysfunction including constipation, diarrhea, and incontinence frequently occurs in patients who

Older adults with lung cancer commonly have serious pulmonary symptoms such as cough, dyspnea, fatigue and poor endurance. Addressing the issue of smoking cessation in these patients is often complex; cessation of smoking is advised to improve symptoms, but if the patient has advanced disease it may be psychologically challenging to address a lifelong addiction. In addition, chemotherapy and radiation treatments may compromise lung and cardiac function, leading to further exacerbation of symptoms. There may also be underlying coronary artery disease that preexisted the cancer diagnosis and which may be exacerbated by cancer therapy. Some patients will require supplemental oxygen for poor oxygenation and/or anxiety-related disorders. As described in Case 22-4, quality of life is often compromised by rapidly worsening disease and from the toxicities of chemotherapy. Patients with lung cancer experience greater severity of symptoms, physical distress, and emotional

TABLE 22-2	Cancer-Specific Rehabilitation Issues

- Breast cancer – Lymphedema, arm dysfunction, fatigue, therapy toxicities, sexual difficulties, body image problems, psychosocial
- Prostate cancer – Sexual, urinary, and bowel dysfunction; therapy toxicities; compromised quality of life; psychosocial.
- Colorectal cancer – Ostomy care, body image problems, sexual dysfunction, therapy toxicities, psychosocial
- Lung cancer – respiratory dysfunction, cardiovascular compromise, fatigue, therapy toxicities, psychosocial

distress than other cancer types. Low physical reserve prior to treatment is common. Often these patients are of lower socioeconomic status and may not have the supportive resources of more affluent patients. Subacute and outpatient physical and occupational therapy may be necessary in these patients and, for better results, should be initiated prior to the first cycle of chemotherapy and continued throughout the treatment course. It is advisable that psychotherapy and pharmacotherapy be initiated early in the diagnosis and treatment process given the aggressive nature and course of lung cancer. It is also wise to get pulmonary and cardiology consultants to work with the patient and his or her physicians; they can aid with the cardiopulmonary deterioration that accompanies lung cancer and its treatment course. (See Table 22-2.)

LATE EFFECTS AND REHABILITATION

The older adult with cancer is less likely to survive cancer than the younger adult. This is perhaps due to age and comorbidities. However, the few older adults that can be considered cancer survivors are at risk for suffering many different late effects. The late effects are usually a result of cancer treatments such as surgery, chemotherapy, and irradiation therapy.

To provide some examples: surgery for abdominal or pelvic cancers may lead to small bowel obstruction years later from surgical adhesions; chemotherapy agents such as doxorubicin can lead to cardiac problems; irradiation can lead to injury of soft tissue organs such as the bladder, causing a secondary cancer or bladder dysfunction.

Medical problems that develop secondary to a primary therapy can be treated with rehabilitation. Older patients with a history of cancer who develop cardiopulmonary dysfunction caused by chemotherapeutic agents benefit from physical therapy either in an outpatient or subacute setting, depending on the severity of the disease and its acute exacerbations. In addition, bladder dysfunction can be treated with a bladder training program and pelvic exercises.

Rehabilitation can play an important role in preventing and treating most late effects caused by cancer treatment. Rehabilitation for secondary cancers for older patients should be treated in the same way as rehabilitations for primary cancers, as discussed in this chapter.

BARRIERS AND POTENTIAL INTERVENTIONS FOR SUCCESSFUL REHABILITATION

Like all treatments, rehabilitation also faces its own barriers. Like the patient described in Case 22-1, if an older patient receives a new diagnosis of cancer during a hospitalization, when she is offered subacute rehabilitation while undergoing treatment such as irradiation therapy, she refuses because of the new found fears that surround her diagnosis and its current treatment. She is unaware of the debilitating effects of radiation and chemotherapy and therefore is unable to foresee her immediate need for physical and psychological rehabilitation. Her rehabilitation treatment leads to a stay in a skilled nursing facility, heightening her anxiety. When patients learn that SNF is a glorified name for a nursing home, they may adamantly refuse to go, because of the notion that nursing homes are for old, demented, and neglected patients. In addition, many perceive nursing homes as providing poor care. It may be beneficial to let patients know that nursing homes have two kinds of patients: the rehabilitation patient and the long-term care patient. The focus for the rehabilitation patient is short-term physical and occupational therapy, while the focus for the long-term care patient is making the SNF a safe home. It can also be helpful and empowering to encourage a patient to do his or her own research on local nursing homes and to check their rates. Lastly, encourage patients and families to tour potential SNFs so as to find the place where they will feel most at home.

Other barriers to rehabilitation options are adjustment and depression. Adjusting to the diagnosis of cancer at an advanced age leads to feelings of denial. Denial is one of the stages of grief and, if rehabilitation is offered during this stage, the patient is likely to decline. Low motivation and depression leads to poor participation with any type of rehabilitation; this can prove detrimental and lead to a downward spiral.

WHERE REHABILITATION CAN OCCUR

While many people think of substance abuse when they hear the word "rehab," rehabilitation therapy can take many forms. Rehabilitation can occur in several different settings depending on disease severity, duration of necessary therapy, insurance benefits, and patient preference. However, what is common among all forms of rehabilitation is that they include a multidisciplinary team consisting of a doctor, a nurse, and a therapist. There may be multiple therapists involved in the care of a single patient as the patient may require occupational, physical, speech, and/or psychosocial therapy.

Outpatient rehabilitation is less structured than inpatient or residential facilities. It indicates that a patient is well enough to leave the hospital and offers more continuity with daily living. The patient's physician is also confident that the patient is likely to complete a rehabilitation program on an outpatient basis. The number of sessions depends on the situation. Some patients attend rehabilitation once a day or multiple times per day, while others may attend outpatient rehabilitation once to three times per week. Outpatient rehabilitation is effective for cancer patients who would like to maintain their premorbid function while undergoing cancer therapy.

Inpatient rehabilitation takes two forms: subacute and acute rehabilitation. The difference between the two is the ability of the patient to participate in intensive physical or occupational therapy. Acute rehabilitation requires a patient to work 3 hours per day, 7 days a week. Usually these patients are medically stable, for example a premorbidly high-functioning stroke patient with minimal residual weakness. Generally, acute rehabilitation is not effective for cancer patients as they can be significantly debilitated and many are unable to sustain an intensive therapy program.

Subacute rehabilitation requires inpatient care for 1 to 2 hours of physical and/or occupational therapy per day 5 to 6 days a week. These therapy sessions may be divided for improved patient participation. Subacute rehabilitation is generally offered by skilled nursing facilities, better known as nursing homes. Patients in this setting may also benefit from speech and psychosocial therapy, and may be able to obtain additional treatments such as dental, optometric, and podiatric care.

Patients who qualify for subacute rehabilitation are those who need short-term rehabilitation, are motivated, and have a reasonable potential to meet their rehabilitative goals. The older adult cancer patient is at very high risk of developing debility during the course and treatment of the disease. Therefore, this patient would benefit from subacute rehabilitation either before initiating aggressive cancer therapy or throughout the treatment course to prevent a severe debilitating event. In addition, older cancer patients who become severely debilitated and deconditioned from a prolonged hospital course or surgical intervention are also good candidates for subacute rehabilitation.

Summary

Rehabilitation plays an important role in the care of the older adult with cancer. Rehabilitation needs of the older adult with cancer vary according to the phase of the disease. These needs vary from physical dysfunction to malnutrition to sexual impairment to psychosocial issues. Ultimately, the importance of rehabilitation of an older patient with cancer is its potential to minimize treatment exacerbations, improve overall quality of life, and maintain physical function. Hence, whatever a patient's diagnosis or course of treatment, it is important for his or her physician to consider rehabilitation as a preventive and/or concomitant treatment to maximize the patient's quality of life.

SUGGESTED READINGS

1. Lash TL, Silliman RA: Patient characteristics and treatments associated with a decline in upper-body function following breast cancer therapy, *J Clin Epidemiol* 53:615–622, 2000.
2. Pinto BM, Maruyama NC: Exercise in the rehabilitation of breast cancer survivors, *Psychooncology* 8:191–206, 1999.
3. Schover LR: The impact of breast cancer on sexuality, body image, and intimate relationships, *CA Cancer J Clin* 41:112–120, 1991.
4. Smoot B, Wong J, Cooper B, et al. Upper extremity impairments in women with or without lymphedema following breast cancer treatment, *Journal of Cancer Survivorship.*
5. Mulhall JP, Bella AJ, Briganti A, et al: Erectile function rehabilitation in the radical prostatectomy patient, *The journal of sexual medicine* 7(4):1687–1698, 2010.
6. Schmitz KH, Speck RM: Risks and benefits of physical activity among breast cancer survivors who have completed treatment, *Women's Health* 6(2):221–238, 2010.

Surveillance

Janet Pregler

As defined by the Institute of Medicine, surveillance in the context of the treatment of cancer survivors encompasses three elements: surveillance for cancer recurrence, surveillance for second cancers, and surveillance for medical and psychosocial late effects of cancer treatment.[1] In the care of the elderly, the approach to surveillance should be considered in the overall context of the health of the patient. As an example, active surveillance for cancer recurrence and second cancers may not be appropriate in patients whose comorbidities (e.g., moderate to severe dementia, end-stage chronic obstructive pulmonary disease) make further cancer treatment impossible or inadvisable. For these patients, the emphasis should be on initiating timely and appropriate palliative treatment if symptoms of cancer recurrence develop.

This chapter will discuss surveillance in the context of the treatment of cancer survivors who are considered to be in remission or cured, with an emphasis on cancers commonly encountered among the elderly. The strategies discussed presume that the overall health of the patient is such that active surveillance for cancer recurrence and second cancers is of potential benefit. Specific strategies and guidelines are reviewed for survivors of common cancers among the elderly, including breast, prostate, and colon cancer.

CASE 23-1

A 66-year-old woman presents for preventive care. Her past medical history is significant for stage 1 breast cancer diagnosed by mammography 2 years previously. The tumor was estrogen and progesterone receptor-positive and HER-2/Neu negative. She was treated with lumpectomy with sentinel node evaluation and radiation therapy. Her current medications include an aromatase inhibitor. She asks the following questions: (1) What follow-up tests do I need? (2) Should I have an annual breast MRI? (3) Should I be tested for the BRCA gene?

CASE 23-2

A 72-year-old man presents for preventive care. He underwent radical prostatectomy at age 60 for prostate cancer. His PSA is now undetectable. He asks: (1) How often do I need PSA testing? (2) Do I need to see a urologist on a regular basis?

GENERAL PRINCIPLES OF SURVEILLANCE

Surveillance strategies should be guided by available evidence, when possible. Although randomized trials have addressed many important surveillance issues for common cancers, published surveillance strategies are based partly on expert opinion.[2,3,4] An important element of performing surveillance in cancer patients who are free of disease is ensuring that other, unrelated medical issues or problems, as well as non–cancer-related preventive measures, are not overlooked. This is particularly relevant in the elderly, who frequently suffer from comorbidities that are unrelated to cancer.

Asymptomatic cancer survivors are often followed clinically on a regular basis for indefinite periods by medical, surgical, and/or radiation oncologists In recent years, there has been recognition that a "one size fits all" approach to selecting the appropriate clinician to perform follow-up of cancer survivors is not appropriate. Important issues to consider in determining which clinicians should provide surveillance for disease-free survivors include balancing access to appropriate expertise with overall accessibility, affordability, and coordination of care. Although more research is needed, available evidence suggests that well-trained generalists are as capable as oncologists of performing surveillance, and that nurses working with oncologists also provide high quality surveillance care.[3,4]

Because all elderly patients have significant preventive health needs, elderly cancer patients who are cancer-free should have a primary care clinician as part of their health care team. For many patients, once treatment is completed, surveillance may be effectively performed by the primary care clinician, with consultation with the oncologist on an as-needed basis. Elderly patients at high risk of recurrence may be best served by co-management by an oncologist and a generalist or geriatrician. Co–management may also be indicated for elderly patients who have a high likelihood of complications from therapy, particularly early in their posttreatment course. Co–management should also be available should the patient, the generalist or geriatrician, or the oncologist feel it is in the patient's best interest. Specialized survivorship clinics may be appropriate for some patients. Guidelines tools (described later) exist to assist physicians in performing evidence-based surveillance for patients who have been treated for common cancers.

Testing for recurrent disease should be performed proactively if recurrence can be treated for cure. Examples include serial PSA testing in prostate cancer patients, examination and mammography of preserved breasts in breast cancer patients, and computed tomography (CT) scanning to detect liver metastases in high-risk colon cancer patients. Randomized trials have not shown either survival or quality-of-life benefit for strategies that test for incurable disease before patients are symptomatic, even though such strategies may identify disease before it is clinically apparent.[2,4] For this reason, performing laboratory or radiological tests to detect asymptomatic metastatic disease that is incurable is not recommended. As an example, performing "routine" bone scans and liver-associated enzyme tests in asymptomatic breast and prostate cancer survivors is not recommended.[3,4]

Surveillance for second primary cancers is performed when such cancers are frequent. As an example, the absolute incidence of contralateral breast cancer in breast cancer survivors is 0.5% to 1% per year. Annual screening mammography is therefore recommended.[5] Appropriate genetic testing is indicated to identify cancer syndromes where enhanced screening and/or other preventive measures to prevent second cancers are available. Research suggests that screening and interventions are beneficial for such patients.[2,3] Because genetic testing has only recently been widely performed, it is important to ascertain the family history of all cancer survivors, including those whose treatment was remote, to identify those who may benefit from genetic testing.

Surveillance for medical and psychosocial aftereffects of treatment is often overlooked after the initial treatment is completed. All cancer survivors should have regular contact with a physician who accepts responsibility for this aspect of care. Long-term medical effects are treatment-specific; the physician responsible for identifying complications of treatment must therefore be informed of the treatment the patient received.

Patient education is an important element of surveillance. Patients should be informed of current recommendations for surveillance, as well as signs and symptoms of recurrence and late treatment effects. Physicians performing surveillance of medical and psychosocial effects should be aware of community and peer resources for their patients.

Recently, the Institute of Medicine has promoted the concept of a "survivorship care plan." A survivorship care plan provides a comprehensive summary of care and recommended follow-up in written (and, ideally, electronic) form, is clearly and effectively explained to the patient at the completion of active therapy, and is communicated to all members of the patient's health care team.[1]

SURVEILLANCE ISSUES FOR CANCERS WHERE SURVIVORS ARE COMMON AMONG THE ELDERLY

Breast Cancer

There are over two million breast cancer survivors in the United States.[6] Most of these women will die of causes unrelated to their breast cancer diagnosis. The risk of breast cancer increases with age, making breast cancer a common diagnosis among elderly women. Treatment usually consists of surgical resection of the cancer by lumpectomy or mastectomy and sentinal lymph node biopsy. Patients with positive lymph node biopsy may undergo lymph node dissection. Adjuvant therapy includes radiation therapy of the affected breast for patients treated with lumpectomy, and chemotherapy and/or hormonal therapy depending on the characteristics of the tumor. Commonly used chemotherapeutic agents include cyclophosphamide, methotrexate, fluorouracil, doxorubicin, and paclitaxel in various combinations, and trastuzumab. Hormonal agents include aromatase inhibitors (anastrozole, letrozole, and exemestane), and selective estrogen receptor modulators (tamoxifen).[7]

Surveillance for Cancer Recurrence. Recommendations for surveillance for recurrence among breast cancer survivors are mainly based on the results of large clinical trials performed in the late 1980s and early 1990s that randomized women to either intensive or conservative follow-up strategies. Both groups underwent periodic history and physical examination and mammography. The intensive follow-up groups in addition underwent periodic laboratory testing including both blood and radiological tests. Although women followed with batteries of tests had recurrences detected, on average, 3 months earlier, there was no difference in survival between groups after 10 years of follow-up, and satisfaction with care was identical in the two groups.[8,9,10] Although additional methods of early detection of distant recurrence, such as positron emission tomography/computed tomography (PET/CT) scanning and serological tumor marker testing, have become more widely used since the 1990s, the availability of these tests has not changed expert opinion that such testing is not beneficial.[3]

Surveillance for breast cancer recurrence focuses on the use of physical examination and mammography in preserved breasts to detect local recurrences, which are potentially curable, at an early stage. Surveillance for distant recurrence, which is incurable, is accomplished by history and physical examination, with additional testing as indicated. It is important that women be informed of the signs and symptoms of recurrence, because palliative treatment may be delayed if symptoms such as musculoskeletal pain or cough are not recognized as cancer-related. American Society of Clinical Oncology guidelines for surveillance in breast cancer are summarized in Table 23-1.

TABLE 23-1	**Summary of Frequently Cited Recommendations for Follow-up for Common Cancers** *(Assumes Patient is a Candidate for Further Therapy)*

Type of Cancer	Organization	Summary Recommendations
Breast	ASCO	History and physical examination every 3-6 months for 3 years, every 6-12 months for 2 years, then annually[*] Mammography 6 months after radiation therapy (if breast preserved), then annually Genetic (BRCA) testing when indicated (Table 23-2) Specifically NOT recommended in asymptomatic patients who lack other indications: CBC, chemistry panels, tumor markers (CEA, CA 15-3, CA 27.29), bone scans, liver ultrasounds, CXR, CT scans with or without PET, breast MRIs
Colon	ASCO	Colonoscopy 3 years after operative treatment, and then every 5 years if normal; flexible proctosigmoidoscopy every 6 months for 5 years for rectal cancer patients who have not been treated with pelvic radiation History and physical examination every 3-6 months for 3 years, every 6-12 months for 2 years, then at discretion of the physician for patients diagnosed with stage II or III colorectal cancer CEA measurement every 3 months for 3 years for patients diagnosed with stage II or III colorectal cancer CT of the chest and abdomen annually for 3 years for patients at high risk of recurrence[†] Specifically NOT recommended in asymptomatic patients who lack other indications: CXR, CBC, liver function tests
Prostate	National Comprehensive Care Network	PSA measurement every 6-12 months for 5 years, then annually Digital rectal exam annually[‡]

See references 2, 3, 23.
ASCO, American Society of Clinical Oncology; CBC, complete blood count; CXR, chest x-ray; CEA, carcinoembryonic antigen; PSA, prostate-specific antigen
[*]Includes patient education regarding symptoms of recurrence and "regular gynecological follow-up"
[†]Not rigorously defined. Includes stage III patients, some stage II patients with adverse risk factors
[‡]History and physical examination is recommended for patients at high risk of recurrence

Surveillance for Second Cancers. Compared to women who have not had breast cancer, breast cancer survivors have a two to six times greater risk of developing breast cancer in the contralateral breast. Physical examination and mammography are recommended to detect second cancers at an early stage. Unfortunately, studies have shown that many elderly breast cancer survivors do not receive appropriate mammographic screening. In one recent national study, over 30% of elderly breast cancer survivors did not receive recommended screening, despite being enrolled in integrated health care systems.[11]

Magnetic resonance imaging (MRI) with gadolinium has been shown to have increased sensitivity compared to mammography in women at highest risk for breast cancer, including women with BRCA mutation or equivalent risk. However, screening MRI is not currently recommended for women who, like most breast cancer survivors, do not have a lifetime risk of primary or recurrent cancer of 20% or greater[12] Lack of specificity of screening MRI continues to be a problem, with 25% or more of subjects in studies of screening MRI requiring additional imaging to further define abnormalities, the vast majority of which are benign.[13] The role of screening MRI continues to be studied.

Recently, increasing emphasis has been placed on identifying breast cancer survivors whose family history identifies them as being at high risk for carrying a BRCA gene. American Society of Clinical Oncology recommendations for selecting breast cancer survivors for BRCA testing are summarized in Table 23-2. Breast cancer survivors with the BRCA gene have a risk of developing ovarian cancer of 1.4% per year, which is ten times the rate observed in breast cancer survivors without the BRCA mutation. They also have a risk of developing contralateral breast cancer of over 5% per year.[14] These risks accrue over the patient's entire life, so otherwise healthy elderly women should be considered for testing as part of a strategy to prevent future cancers. For elderly women for whom genetic testing might not be indicated because of comorbidities, testing may still be indicated if the patient wishes to obtain genetic information to inform family members of the potential for genetic risk. In case-control cohort studies, prophylactic salpingo-oophorectomy reduces subsequent ovarian cancer risk by 90%.[15] Many women also choose prophylactic mastectomy. For BRCA-positive women who do not elect prophylactic mastectomy, annual screening MRI of the breasts with gadolinium is recommended.[12] The costs of genetic testing, prophylactic surgery, and screening MRI are generally included in insurance coverage for patients who meet published indications.

Late Medical and Psychosocial Effects in the Elderly. Fortunately, advances in surgical treatment have reduced the number of breast cancer survivors with severe lymphedema. However, a significant number of

TABLE 23-2	**Criteria for Referral of Breast Cancer Survivors for Genetic Counseling for BRCA Gene Testing**

Ashkenazi Jewish heritage
Personal history of bilateral breast cancer
Personal history of ovarian cancer
First- or second-degree relative with ovarian cancer at any age
First-degree relative with a history of breast cancer diagnosed
    before age 50
Two or more first- or second-degree relatives with breast cancer
    diagnosed at any age
Relative diagnosed with bilateral breast cancer
Male relative diagnosed with breast cancer

Adapted from Khatcheressian JL, Wolff AC, Smith TJ, et al. American Society of Clinical Oncology 2006 update of the breast cancer follow-up and management guidelines in the adjuvant setting. J Clin Oncol. 2006 Nov 1;24(31):5091-7. Epub 2006 Oct 10.

women still undergo lymph node dissection, and late presentation of lymphedema continues to occur. Patients are generally advised to avoid compression, venipuncture, and trauma to the arm ipsilateral to lymph node dissection. All patients who have undergone axillary lymph node dissection should be aware that they should report swelling to their clinician. Elevation and the use of a lymphedema sleeve are the usual treatments. Although patients have often been counseled to avoid weight lifting with the affected arm, a recent study suggests that exercise, including moderate weight lifting, may be beneficial in preventing or ameliorating lymphedema.[7,16]

Elderly women who were taking estrogen prior to their breast cancer diagnosis may develop hot flashes when estrogen is stopped. Treatment with aromatase inhibitors and tamoxifen are also associated with hot flashes. Selective serotonin reuptake inhibitors (SSRIs), selective serotonin and norepinephrine reuptake inhibitors (SNRIs), and gabapentin are effective interventions to treat vasomotor symptoms. SSRIs are generally avoided in patients taking tamoxifen because SSRIs may alter tamoxifen metabolism in some women, rendering it less effective. Vaginal dryness and dyspareunia may be treated with nonhormonal vaginal moisturizers or low-dose intravaginal estradiol (some experts recommend using intravaginal estradiol with caution).[5,7]

Women treated with aromatase inhibitors are at risk for treatment-associated arthralgias and musculoskeletal pain. Musculoskeletal symptoms also occur with tamoxifen treatment but less frequently. Imaging should be considered to evaluate for possible metastatic disease. Medical management with acetaminophen or other pain medications may be considered. Nonsteroidal anti-inflammatory drugs are avoided in the elderly, when possible, because of an enhanced risk of bleeding complications. Consideration of change or cessation of adjuvant treatment is sometimes unavoidable.[5]

Breast cancer survivors are at high risk of osteoporotic fracture. All breast cancer survivors should have adequate intake of calcium (1200-1500 mg daily) and Vitamin D (1000-2000 IU daily), and have bone densitometry performed at age 65 and each 5 years thereafter, or more frequently if indicated by low bone mineral density or other risk factors. Adjuvant treatment with aromatase inhibitors places patients at very high risk of fracture. For this reason, patients treated with aromatase inhibitors should have bone densitometry performed at initiation of therapy, and annually while receiving therapy. Bisphosphonate therapy is the preferred treatment of osteoporosis in breast cancer survivors.[17]

Patients who undergo radiation of the left chest wall are at increased risk of cardiovascular disease. The usual strategies to reduce cardiovascular risk, including screening and treatment of hypertension, diabetes, and hypercholesterolemia, as well as promotion of a healthy lifestyle including exercise, weight maintenance, and healthy diet, are recommended. Patients who receive treatment with anthracyclines or trastuzumab are at risk of congestive heart failure. No effective prophylaxis is known. Patients should be monitored and, if congestive heart failure develops, they should be treated according to the standard medical protocols.[7]

Patients treated with tamoxifen are at increased risk of uterine cancer, venous thrombosis, and cerebrovascular disease. Vaginal bleeding should be promptly evaluated by endometrial biopsy.

Cognitive dysfunction, depression, fatigue, and weight gain are all commonly reported in breast cancer survivors and they should be diagnosed and treated as per the usual strategies. Symptoms of cognitive dysfunction and fatigue should be fully evaluated in the elderly to ensure that they do not represent unrelated comorbid processes (such as Alzheimer disease, hypothyroidism, or other systemic disease).[5]

Prostate Cancer

Prostate cancer is the most common cancer in American men. Of the 10 million cancer survivors in the United States, 18% are survivors of prostate cancer. Treatment modalities include radical prostatectomy, external beam radiotherapy, and permanent (low-dose) brachytherapy. Active surveillance (close monitoring of men with prostate cancer with curative treatment offered only to those who fit certain criteria) and watchful waiting (management of men medically unsuitable for curative treatment consisting of initiation of palliative treatment for symptoms) are also strategies for management of prostate cancer. Patients with disease that is at very high risk of recurrence may be treated with androgen-deprivation therapy in addition to other modalities. These strategies will not be discussed further in this chapter. Recurrence (defined by elevated serum prostate-specific antigen [PSA] after initial treatment) is relatively common, ranging from 10% in those with low-risk cancers to over 60% in high-risk patients. Within 10 years of initial treatment,

10% to 20% of men with high-risk clinically localized prostate cancer die of the disease.[18]

Surveillance for Cancer Recurrence. The cornerstone of monitoring for cancer recurrence is serial PSA measurement. There is marked variation among various guidelines groups as to the recommended frequency of PSA measurement, which reflects the lack of randomized, controlled trial data on this topic. In general, testing is advised no more frequently than every 3 months, with many groups endorsing longer intervals after patients have been disease-free for a specified length of time. The role of digital rectal examination (DRE) is controversial. Some groups recommend it only if the PSA is judged to be abnormal. Others recommend annual examination. Guidelines from the National Comprehensive Cancer Network are summarized in Table 23-1.

Late Medical and Psychosocial Effects in the Elderly. Erectile dysfunction is reported by up to 80% of prostate cancer survivors. Erectile function may improve with time after prostate cancer surgery, but generally declines with time after radiation treatment. Phosphodiesterase inhibitors are effective in improving erectile dysfunction in up to 75% of men who have undergone nerve-sparing radical prostatectomy, as well as men who have undergone radiation therapy. Elderly men are less responsive to phosphodiesterase inhibitor treatment compared to younger men. Intraurethral and intracorporeal alpostadil is offered to men who do not respond to phosphodiesterase inhibitors, and is useful for men who have received all types of treatment, including those who had non–nerve-sparing treatment. In studies, about half of men show benefit.[19,20]

Urinary incontinence is reported by 10% to 20% of prostate cancer survivors. Urinary continence improves for up to a year after surgery. Urinary incontinence is treated with pelvic floor exercises, behavioral modification, and weight loss. Electrical stimulation for bladder retraining, periurethral collagen injection, and surgery to place an artificial sphincter or bulbourethral sling are sometimes recommended.[20]

Additional side effects in men treated with radiation therapy and brachytherapy include hematuria, cystitis, bladder contracture, urethral stricture, rectal bleeding, rectal ulceration, rectal/anal stricture, and chronic diarrhea. All are uncommon. Patients should be specifically asked about these complications, and treated or referred to specialists for treatment. Because these side effects are often associated with psychosocial distress, screening for depression is recommended by some experts.[4,20]

Colon Cancer

Colorectal cancer is a disease of the elderly. Two thirds of invasive colorectal cancers are diagnosed in persons older than 65 years. In persons older than 75 years, colorectal cancer is the most common cancer diagnosis. There are over 1 million survivors of colorectal cancer

in the United States.[1] Treatment generally consists of surgical resection, followed by adjuvant 5-fluorouracil, leucovorin, capecitabine, oxaliplatin, or irinotecan in various combinations for patients with high-risk stage II or stage III disease.[21]

Surveillance for Cancer Recurrence. According to current guidelines from the American Society for Clinical Oncology (Table 23-1), surveillance should include a history and physical examination, serial colonoscopy, and, for patients with rectal cancer who have not been treated with pelvic radiation, flexible proctosigmoidoscopy at frequent intervals. Serial carcinoembryonic antigen (CEA) testing is recommended for patients who are candidates for surgery or chemotherapy. Because several studies have shown survival advantage for colorectal cancer survivors with resectable metastases in the liver and lung, computed tomography of the chest and abdomen is recommended annually for three years for patients at high risk of recurrence, usually defined as those with node-positive malignancies, if the patient would otherwise be a candidate for resection. Chest x-rays, complete blood counts, liver-associated enzyme tests, and other molecular or cellular marker tests are not recommended at present.[2]

Surveillance for Second Cancers. In addition to serial colonoscopy as recommended for surveillance for cancer recurrence, colon cancer survivors should be assessed to determine whether testing for Lynch Syndrome (hereditary nonpolyposis colon cancer) is indicated. Experts recommend patients with Lynch Syndrome undergo colonoscopy every 1 to 2 years.

Patients with Lynch syndrome are also at risk for uterine, urological, and additional gastrointestinal malignancies. For women, prophylactic total abdominal hysterectomy and bilateral salpingo-oophorectomy may be of benefit. Enhanced surveillance for urological and upper gastrointestinal malignancies is also recommended by some experts.[22] Criteria for Lynch Syndrome testing in patients with colon cancer are listed in Table 23-3.

Late Medical and Psychosocial Effects in the Elderly. Long-term colorectal cancer survivors do not differ from healthy controls in terms of physical functioning. Advanced age and lower income are associated with lower levels of function. Long-term effects include fatigue, pain, and diarrhea. Bowel symptoms are more frequent among rectal cancer survivors. Although negative body image is more common among survivors with ostomies, as are symptoms of diarrhea and cramping, overall quality of life, social functioning, and activities of daily living do not appear to be permanently affected. Depression, however, is relatively frequently reported. Some experts recommend screening for depression in colon cancer survivors.[21]

Over 90% of patients treated with adjuvant oxaliplatin develop peripheral neuropathy during active therapy. However, only about one in 10 patients reports persistent symptoms after completion of treatment. Such

TABLE 23-3	Recommendations for Testing to Identify Patients Who May Have Lynch Syndrome (Hereditary Nonpolyposis Colon Cancer)

1. Patients should be offered genetic counseling and tumors should be tested for microsatellite instability when one or more of the following exist:
    - Colorectal cancer in patients younger than 50 years.
    - Colorectal cancer with suggestive histology including tumor-infiltrating lymphocytes, Crohn-disease–like lymphocytic reaction, mucinous or signet-ring differentiation, or medullary growth pattern in patients younger than 60 years.
    - Multiple colorectal cancer tumors, or colorectal cancer diagnosed in patients with a history of another tumor associated with Lynch syndrome (endometrial, stomach, ovarian, pancreatic, uterine, renal pelvic, biliary tract, brain, or small bowel cancer, or sebaceous adenomas or keratoacanthomas) in patients of any age.
    - Colorectal cancer or tumor associated with Lynch syndrome (endometrial, stomach, ovarian, pancreatic, uterine, renal pelvic, biliary tract, brain, or small bowel cancer, or sebaceous adenomas or keratoacanthomas) diagnosed before age 50 years in at least one first-degree relative.
    - Colorectal cancer or tumor associated with Lynch syndrome (endometrial, stomach, ovarian, pancreatic, uterine, renal pelvic, biliary tract, brain, or small bowel cancer, or sebaceous adenomas or keratoacanthomas) diagnosed at any age in two first- or second degree relatives.
2. Patients who fulfill above criteria and have high microsatellite inability and/or loss of DNA mismatch repair gene expression should be offered germline testing for Lynch syndrome genes.
3. When tumor testing is not feasible, testing for germline mutations may be considered for patients with a family history suggestive of Lynch syndrome.

Adapted from Lindor NM, Peterson GM, Hadley DW, et al. Recommendations for the care of individuals with an inherited predisposition to Lynch syndrome. JAMA 2006; 296:1507-17.

patients may benefit from pharmacological treatments for neuropathy, as well as specialty referral for pain management. Chronic diarrhea is generally managed with antidiarrheal regimens and the use of incontinence garments. Patients may not volunteer symptoms, so physicians should actively ask about bowel problems during follow-up. Patients who have undergone pelvic radiation for rectal cancer are at increased risk for pelvic fracture; thus all survivors with a history of pelvic radiation should undergo bone-mineral density testing, and medical treatment of osteopenia and osteoporosis should be considered. Survivors of pelvic radiation also commonly suffer from urinary and sexual dysfunction including urinary incontinence, erectile dysfunction in men, and vaginal dryness in women. Phosphodiesterase inhibitors have shown benefit for erectile dysfunction in men after pelvic radiation. Vaginal dilators may be of benefit for women with vaginal stenosis after pelvic radiation.[21]

REVIEW OF INTRODUCTORY CASES

CASE 23-1	CASE CONTINUED

A 66-year-old woman presents for preventive care. Her past medical history is significant for stage 1 breast cancer diagnosed by mammography 2 years previously. The tumor was estrogen and progesterone receptor-positive and HER-2/Neu negative. She was treated with lumpectomy with sentinel node evaluation and radiation therapy. Her current medications include an aromatase inhibitor. She asks the following questions: (1) What follow-up tests do I need? (2) Should I have an annual breast MRI? (3) Should I be tested for the BRCA gene?

ASCO guidelines recommend this patient be followed by serial history and physical examination and annual mammography, with further testing only for symptoms or physical findings. Because the patient is on an aromatase inhibitor, annual bone densitometry is recommended, with bisphosphonate treatment if osteoporosis is diagnosed. Annual breast MRI is recommended for patients with a lifetime risk of primary or recurrent breast cancer of 20% or greater. Women who carry the BRCA gene or who underwent chest wall radiation for Hodgkin disease between the ages of 10 and 30 years fit these criteria regardless of other factors. For other women, to determine whether MRI is indicated, one of several validated models that take into account family and personal historical factors to determine lifetime risk of breast cancer can be used (e.g., Gail, Claus, and Tyrer-Cusik models). These can be accessed electronically.[12] If the patient is of Ashkenazi Jewish descent, or fits family history criteria documented in Table 23-2, testing for the BRCA gene should be considered.

CASE 23-2	CASE CONTINUED

A 72-year-old man presents for preventive care. He underwent radical prostatectomy at age 60 for prostate cancer. His PSA is now undetectable. He asks: (1) How often do I need PSA testing? (2) Do I need to see a urologist on a regular basis?

Annual PSA testing is recommended for men who are disease-free 5 or more years after treatment for prostate cancer. Whether or not the patient sees a urologist should be determined by patient and physician preferences. However, if the patient elects not to be seen by a urologist, the primary physician should specifically inquire about erectile dysfunction and urinary incontinence and treat and/or refer if appropriate.

Chapter Summary

Surveillance in disease-free cancer survivors includes three elements: surveillance for cancer recurrence, surveillance for second cancers (including genetic testing to guide preventive and surveillance strategies, when appropriate), and surveillance for late medical and psychosocial effects. Surveillance strategies should take into account the patient's overall health status and treatment preferences. Although active surveillance for cancer recurrence and second cancers is appropriate for many elderly patients, some patients with significant comorbidities are not candidates for further curative treatment. For all patients, there should be strong emphasis on initiating timely and appropriate palliative treatment if symptoms of incurable cancer recurrence develop. Available evidence suggests that well-trained generalists can provide surveillance care equivalent to specialists for some common cancers. Co-management or specialized survivorship clinics with or without the involvement of specifically trained nurses may be indicated for some patients.

Guidelines are available to help determine surveillance strategies for survivors of common cancers. These are summarized in Table 23-1. Surveillance is an area of active research. More and better evidence-based information on how to best provide surveillance will likely be available in the near future.

 See expertconsult.com for a complete list of references and web resources for this chapter

Long Term Effects and Cancer Survivorship in the Older Patient

Mary E. Sehl, Erin E. Hahn, Amy A. Edgington, and Patricia A. Ganz

---

CASE 24-1 CASE 1: OLDER BREAST CANCER SURVIVOR PRESENTATION

M.H. is an 87-year-old woman who has been a breast cancer survivor for several years. She had been diagnosed 6 years earlier with a 2.3 cm, node-positive, estrogen receptor-positive, infiltrating ductal carcinoma. She was originally treated with lumpectomy, followed by chemotherapy and radiation therapy, which she tolerated well. She has since completed almost 5 years of endocrine therapy with an aromatase inhibitor. Her coexisting illnesses include osteopenia, gastroesophageal reflux disease, and glaucoma. The patient is a retired pianist who continues to perform as an entertainer locally. She has a very supportive social network of friends in the area and two sons who live out-of-state. She is also active with swimming and bridge.

CASE 24-2 CASE 2: OLDER PROSTATE CANCER SURVIVOR PRESENTATION

S.W. is a 79-year-old prostate cancer survivor. Eight years prior, he was referred for a prostate biopsy after his prostate specific antigen (PSA) level had risen to 5.4 ng/mL. The pathology revealed a Gleason 3+4=7 prostate cancer involving both the right and left lobes of the prostate with no capsular extension of disease. He underwent radical prostatectomy at that time and was followed with PSA measurements. Because of a rise in PSA level 3 years later, he was treated with external beam radiation. He is currently followed with yearly PSA measurements, which have been undetectable. The patient also has hypercholesterolemia, hypertension, aortic stenosis, congestive heart failure, multinodular goiter, osteoarthritis, and memory loss. The patient ambulates with a cane. He lives in an assisted living facility and has a caregiver during the day. He has a supportive family and they live close by.

With long-term survival from cancer rising, the number of cancer survivors is growing, and the majority (61%) of cancer survivors are aged 65 and older. According to a 2003 report of the National Cancer Institute (NCI) Office of Cancer Survivorship, there are over 10 million cancer survivors in the United States, representing 3.6% of the population. These numbers are expected to rise, given the increasing incidence of cancer and the aging of the population. Currently, an estimated one in every six people older than 65 years is a cancer survivor, highlighting the need to increase awareness and emphasize how to best care for this growing population in the oncology and geriatrics communities.

Because of improvements in cancer therapies, the 5-year and extended disease-free survival rates for early-stage breast, colorectal, and prostate cancer are over 90%. Likewise, early-stage melanoma, Hodgkin lymphoma, and cancers of the bladder, uterine cervix, and testes are associated with excellent survival outcomes. As a result, for most cancer survivors, death is more likely to occur from competing illnesses. However, cancer treatment modalities including surgery, radiotherapy, node evaluation, chemotherapy, and endocrine therapy have been shown to be associated with late effects that may persist for up to 20 years after initial treatment, including cognitive effects, physical effects, psychosocial adjustments, and functional decline. Many of these late effects overlap with physiological changes that occur with advancing age and with medical conditions associated with advancing age, making them an important focus in the care of the older cancer patient.

DEFINITION OF CANCER SURVIVOR

According to a broad definition developed in 1986 by the National Coalition for Cancer Survivorship, any cancer patient or close family member of a cancer patient, from the time of diagnosis until death, may be considered a cancer survivor. More recently, the term survivor has been used to denote a more focused period of time beginning after the completion of initial treatment with curative intent, when the patient is being seen posttreatment and in follow-up (Ganz 2005). It is this period of time that will be the focus of this chapter. Important issues that arise in this period of time with respect to managing symptoms and late effects, as well as health care maintenance and screening in this population, will be addressed.

HETEROGENEITY OF AGING CANCER SURVIVORS

Cancer in patients older than 65 years is a heterogeneous process in a heterogeneous population. Heterogeneity arises in the number and severity of coexisting illnesses, cognitive function, physical activity and performance status, and social connectedness. (Balducci 2008) While one patient aged 95 may be skiing, another aged 67 may be bed-bound. Surviving and thriving while experiencing the impacts of cancer and its therapy is a personal and individualized process, especially in the older patient. The two cases described earlier highlight the dramatic individual differences that can be seen in the older population.

PALLIATION, PREVENTION AND HEALTH PROMOTION

The goals of care for survivors have been well summarized as the 3 Ps of survivorship: palliation, prevention, and health promotion. (Ganz) With palliation, the intention is to improve quality of life. This goal is especially important in older people with complex and chronic illness. Concentration is placed on reducing the severity of prolonged disease symptoms where there is no curative medical treatment. These symptoms include pain, fatigue, depression, physical limitations, cognitive changes, lymphedema, sexual dysfunction, and menopause-related symptoms.

The main focus of the second P, prevention, is providing systematic follow-up required to screen for late-onset complications of cancer and its treatment. Complications that can arise as a result of treatment, such as osteoporosis, heart disease, and cataracts, are often conditions that are also associated with aging. The goal of this screening is early detection and early intervention for these complications. Another goal of prevention is to screen for second malignancies, and to counsel patients on chemoprevention and lifestyle modification that may decrease risk of a second malignancy.

Finally, the goal of health promotion is to endorse risk reduction for common health problems. In the older patient, these problems include other chronic diseases, such as diabetes and heart disease, as well as functional decline. Therefore, the focus of this third P is on educating patients about the importance of increasing physical activity, avoiding weight gain, and avoiding exposures that are harmful. For example, one harmful exposure, alcohol consumption, in older adults is associated not only with risk of malignancy, but also with increased risk of falls, medication interaction, and depression.

COMPREHENSIVE CARE FOR SURVIVORS

A clinical program designed to meet the special health needs of cancer survivors should be multidisciplinary in nature. Under this concerted approach, the patient undergoes a nutritional evaluation, psychological evaluation, social work assessment, and evaluation by physical therapy and occupational therapy. Recommendations are discussed as a team and an integrated care plan is formulated together with the primary care physician. This comprehensive model has already been proven to be effective in geriatric medicine and is likely to be of great benefit for older cancer survivors. The shared care model that has been recently developed for survivor care will be discussed later in the chapter.

LATE EFFECTS OF CANCER TREATMENT

Late effects have been attributed to chemotherapy, surgery, radiotherapy, and endocrine therapy; these effects can persist for decades. There is a great deal of overlap between late effects of cancer therapy and the physiological changes that occur with advancing age. Table 24-1 highlights this overlap and lists by system the late effects of therapy that commonly occur in cancer survivors alongside the potentially interacting age-related changes in that physiological system.

Functional decline is another important late effect that can occur in cancer survivors, and is a significant concern in the older patient. Cancer survivors are twice as likely as persons without a history of cancer to report limitation in an activity of daily living. Disability is an important concern in the older patient, highlighting the need for functional assessment in older cancer survivors.

CASE 24-1	**CASE CONTINUED CONCERNS RAISED**

M.H. describes feelings of anxiety regarding cancer recurrence. She also has been concerned about making commitments to piano performances that she may not be able to keep. Lately she has been suffering nocturnal leg cramps from her aromatase inhibitor therapy and, as a result, has been experiencing insomnia. She also notes a decline in how many laps she can swim at the pool, sometimes with difficulty catching her breath, although she does not have any shortness of breath at rest.

CASE 24-2	**CASE CONTINUED CONCERNS RAISED**

S.W. presents with symptoms of fatigue, memory changes, shortness of breath, and depressed mood. He sometimes feels sad and isolated, and describes worries about cancer recurrence, as his brother recently passed away from oral cancer.

TABLE 24-1	Late Effects of Cancer Therapy and Age-Related Physiologic Changes				
System	Chemotherapy	Radiotherapy	Surgery	Endocrine Therapy	Age-Associated Physiologic Changes
Cardiovascular	Cardiomyopathy, congestive heart failure	Scarring, inflammation, pericardial effusion, pericarditis, coronary artery disease	—	Venous thrombotic events	Decreased cardiac output, decreased maximum oxygen consumption, increased inflammatory cytokines
Pulmonary	Pulmonary fibrosis, inflammation interstitial pneumonitis	Pulmonary fibrosis, decreased lung function	Shortness of breath	—	Decreased FEV1, decreased D_LCO, decreased total lung capacity
Gastrointestinal	CASH, hepatic fibrosis, cirrhosis	Malabsorption, biliary stricture, liver failure	Intestinal obstruction, hernia, altered bowel function, nausea, vomiting	—	Impaired peristalsis, delayed gastric emptying time, impaired absorption, decreased liver blood flow
Genitourinary	Hemorrhagic cystitis	Bladder fibrosis, small bladder capacity	Incontinence	Vaginitis	Diminished bladder capacity, enlarged prostate
Renal	Decreased creatinine clearance, delayed-onset renal failure	Decreased creatinine clearance, hypertension	—	—	Increased blood pressure, decreased creatinine clearance
Hematologic	Myelodysplasia, acute leukemia	Myelodysplasia, cytopenias, acute leukemia	—	Anemia	Anemia
Musculoskeletal	Avascular necrosis	Osteonecrosis, fibrosis, atrophy, deformity	Accelerated arthritis	Osteopenia	Decreased bone density, decreased muscle strength and muscle volume
CNS	Problems with thinking, learning, memory; structural brain changes; paralysis, seizure; fatigue	Problems with thinking, learning, memory; structural brain changes; hemorrhage; fatigue	Impaired cognitive function, motor sensory function, vision, swallowing, language, bowel and bladder control, phantom pain (amputation), fatigue	Mood changes, fatigue, generalized weakness, hot flashes	Decreased brain weight, increased reaction times, diminished smell, decreased digit span and block span, impaired circadian rhythm and sleep
Peripheral nervous system	Peripheral neuropathy, hearing loss	—	Neuropathic pain	—	—
Pituitary	Diabetes	Growth hormone deficiency, other hormone deficiencies	—	—	Decreased growth hormone and DHEA, impaired insulin sensitivity
Thyroid	—	Hypothyroidism, thyroid nodules	—	—	Decreased thyroxine secretion
Gonadal	Sterility, early menopause	Sterility, ovarian failure, early menopause, Leydig cell dysfunction	Retrograde ejaculation, sexual dysfunction, testosterone deficiency	—	Decreased testosterone, decreased LH and FSH, decreased estradiol
Oral health	Tooth decay	Dry mouth, poor enamel, dental carries	—	—	Decrease in salivary flow rate

Continued

TABLE 24-1 | **Late Effects of Cancer Therapy and Age-Related Physiologic Changes—cont'd**

System	Chemotherapy	Radiotherapy	Surgery	Endocrine Therapy	Age-Associated Physiologic Changes
Ophthalmologic	Cataracts	Cataracts, dry eyes, visual impairment, retinopathy	—	Cataracts	Reduction in pupil size, loss of accommodation, impaired night vision
Skin	Rashes	Burn	Impaired wound healing, cosmetic effects	—	Epidermal atrophy, increased stiffness in dermal collagen, slower wound healing
Lymphatic	—	Lymphedema	Lymphedema	—	—
Immune	Impaired immune function, immune suppression	Impaired immune function, immune suppression	Impaired immunity and risk of sepsis (splenectomy)	—	Impaired cell-mediated immunity
All tissues	Second cancer	Second cancer	—	Endometrial cancer	Increased risk of cancer

FEV1, forced expiratory volume in 1 sec; D$_L$CO, lung diffusing capacity for carbon monoxide; CASH, chemotherapy-associated steatohepatitis; DHEA, dehydroepiandrosterone; LH, luteinizing hormone; FSH, follicle-stimulating hormone

NEED FOR SURVIVORSHIP CARE PLAN

On the basis of reviews of SEER Medicare claims data (Earle 2003, Earle 2006, Earle 2007, Snyder 2008), it has become apparent that a shared survivorship care plan is needed to ensure better preventive care for cancer survivors. In addition to the standard follow-up in oncology practice that focuses on surveillance for cancer recurrence and management of the adverse effects of treatment, the survivorship care plan needs to address the long-term effects of cancer and its treatment. (Earle 2006, Ganz 2008) The care plan should address the potential for late sequelae of treatment (Ganz 2006, Ganz 2008), particularly in an older population, who are at higher risk for organ dysfunction and second malignancies. In addition, there should be a focus on the ongoing psychosocial burden of a cancer diagnosis (Ganz 2008), which is an especially important concern in an older population that is at higher risk for depression and social isolation.

HOW TO FACILITATE SHARED CARE?

A very important component of the survivorship care plan is to facilitate the coordination of care with other physicians. (Ganz 2008) There has historically been some ambiguity about the responsibility for providing ongoing medical care for cancer survivors (Ganz 2005, Nekhlyudov 2009). According to a survey conducted by the ASCO Cancer Prevention Committee, when oncologists were asked the question, "To what extent do you provide ongoing medical care, including health maintenance, screening, and preventive services," 31% responded always, 48% sometimes, 15% rarely, and 5% not at all. (Ganz 2005) The majority (74%) felt that it was the role of the oncology specialist to provide this type of continuing care to cancer survivors and 66% felt

comfortable providing it. A recent study examining the attitudes of patients, oncologists, and primary care providers revealed that while patients expect their oncologists to be primarily responsible for cancer recurrence, they expected both their oncologists and primary care providers to be involved in surveillance for cancer recurrence and other cancer screening, and they preferred their primary care physicians to be solely involved in general preventive care and treatment of other coexisting illnesses. (Cheung 2009, Nekhlyudov 2009) Generally, primary providers and oncologists agreed with their patients. Although primary care providers expected most of the responsibility for preventive care, oncologists expressed interest in shared care for prevention. (Cheung 2009, Nekhlyudov 2009)

Under the shared care model, it will be important for both oncologists and primary care providers to take responsibility for incorporating interventions into routine care for cancer survivors. For example, at the beginning of adjuvant therapy for breast cancer, strategies of prevention for weight gain should be discussed. While many patients spontaneously initiate positive behaviors, such as diet and physical activity, many older patients do not. (Demark-Wahnefried 2005, Ganz 2005) It will be important to encourage modification of behaviors and initiate preventive exercise programs in this population at risk for decline in strength, functional activity, and independence.

CONTENTS OF TREATMENT SUMMARY AND SURVIVORSHIP CARE PLAN

Table 24-2 describes the contents of the treatment summary and survivorship care plan. In addition to a complete medical history, family history, and social history, the treatment summary should include both the history

TABLE 24-2	Treatment Summary and Survivorship Care Plan Contents

Treatment Summary

Provider contact information
   Medical oncologist
   Radiation oncologist
   Surgical oncologist
   Primary geriatrician
Surgical history
   Procedures and dates
   Complications
Pathology and stage
   Histopathology, TNM stage, biologic marker data
Chemotherapy history
   Treatments and dates
   List all agents and number of cycles received
   Total dose (e.g., anthracycline)
   Growth factors received, blood transfusions
   Complications
Endocrine therapy history
   Dates
   Side effects
Other therapies (e.g., biologically targeted therapy)
   Dates
   Side effects, adverse reaction
Radiation history
   Date started, date finished
   Fields radiated
   Total dose (Gy)

Survivorship Care Plan

Pertinent medical conditions
List of current medications, allergies
Family history, social history
Current symptom review
Current psychosocial assessment
Recent screening and diagnostic tests
Recommendations
   Cancer management and surveillance
   Late effects monitoring
   Psychosocial concerns
   Symptom management
   Health Promotion
   Prevention
      Bone health
      Weight management and physical activity
   ASCO guidelines for follow-up care for specific cancer

of cancer diagnosis, including detection, pathological findings, and staging; and a complete cancer treatment summary, including chemotherapy treatment summary, surgical history, and summary of radiation therapy and other oncologic medical therapies. The chemotherapy treatment summary should include the names and cumulative doses of each agent, and the radiation therapy summary should include the fields radiated as well as the total dose received.

The survivorship care plan should be comprehensive, should include psychosocial and supportive care needs, and should identify which providers will be responsible for specific aspects of continuing care. It should reflect the past and current toxicities experienced by the patient, and project long-term late effects that may potentially arise as a result of the treatment received. A current symptom review should be performed and included, as well as a current psychosocial assessment. The care plan should also contain pertinent recent screening and diagnostic tests for cancer recurrence and other medical conditions, such as mammography, bone density, lipid measurements, and other blood work (e.g., vitamin D level). The care plan should also include a complete list of providers, including primary geriatrician, surgeon, medical oncologist, radiation oncologist, and other specialists, such as pain specialist or pulmonologist, involved in the oncological care of the patient. Specific recommendations should be in the care plan, including cancer management and surveillance, late-effects monitoring, psychosocial concerns, symptom management, health promotion and prevention, and weight management and physical activity. Finally follow-up care and test recommendations regarding radiologic tests, self-examination, coordination of care, and genetic counseling referral should be included.

TIMING OF THE CARE PLAN

The treatment summary and survivorship care plan should first be delivered at the completion of surgery and adjuvant radiation and/or chemotherapy. Additional times to update the care plan include at the end of a course of adjuvant endocrine therapy, or after additional treatment decisions are made, such as after genetic testing that necessitates preventive surgery and other interventions.

WHO PREPARES THE CARE PLAN?

There is a great deal of variation in clinical settings and organization of care during the initial phase of cancer treatment. In some cases, the cancer patient is seen by several different cancer care providers, including a radiation oncologist, a medical oncologist, and a surgical oncologist. The medical oncologist will need to develop strategies to integrate survivorship care planning in the office practice. When patients receive surgery alone, the surgeon can serve as the designated clinician providing survivorship care planning. It is best to summarize the care plan in a report for the patient to keep. The report should also be placed in the chart, so that it can be accessed and updated by the primary care geriatrician and other specialists involved in the care of the patient.

Many times the physician is the sole practitioner in the office qualified to provide education and counseling regarding past cancer treatment and potential long-term and late effects of treatment, as well as advising the frequency and type of follow-up visits needed

CASE 24-1	**CASE 24-1: CONTINUED RECOMMENDATIONS**

Because this patient still has both breasts, her cancer surveillance recommendation included maintenance of regular breast exams and mammography. In addition, she was recommended to have cardiovascular surveillance with an echocardiogram, given her exposure to left-sided chest radiation and history of anthracycline. For her psychosocial concerns, she underwent a depression screen and discussion, which indicated that depression and anxiety may be contributing to her insomnia. It was recommended that she discuss pharmacological options with her primary care physician or be referred to a psychiatrist. For her insomnia, she was recommended to consider participating in a study on T'ai Chi and sleep seminars as nonpharmacologic treatment options for insomnia in breast cancer survivors.

CASE 24-2	**CASE 24-2: CONTINUED RECOMMENDATIONS**

Cancer surveillance was addressed for this patient with the recommendation to continue PSA monitoring with his primary care physician, with referral to a urologist if changes or symptoms were noted. For his fatigue and shortness of breath, he was referred to cardiology for complete evaluation of his cardiovascular health. For his cognitive changes, he was referred for cognitive rehabilitation services. A comprehensive geriatric assessment was recommended to evaluate both physical and emotional health and to discuss maintenance of a healthy nutritional status, increasing physical activity, and reducing the risk of falls. Finally, for his depressed mood, he was referred for individualized, short-term counseling.

TABLE 24-3	**Important Web Links/ Resources**

Resources for Survivors:

American Cancer Society Survivors Network: Available at www.cancer.org; csn.cancer.org

CancerCare: Available at www.cancercare.org

IOM report "From Cancer Patient to Cancer Survivor: Lost in Transition": Available at www.iom.edu/CMS/28312/4931/30869.aspx

Susan G. Komen for the Cure: Available at www.komen.org

Lance Armstrong Foundation: Available at www.livestrong.org

Living Beyond Breast Cancer: Available at www.lbbc.org

NCI Office of Cancer Survivorship: Available at http://cancercontrol.cancer.gov/ocs/

The Wellness Community: Available at www.thewellnesscommunity.org

The National Coalition for Cancer Survivors: Available at www.canceradvocacynow.org/

Cancer.Net: Available at www.cancer.net

People Living With Cancer: Available at www.cancer.net

Vita – Restoring Life after Cancer: Available at www.vita.mednet.ucla.edu

Resources on Preparing a Survivorship Care Plan:

ASCO treatment summary and care plan templates for breast and colon cancer: Available at www.asco.org/treatmentsummary

Haylock PJ, Mitchell SA, Cox T, et al: The cancer survivor's prescription for living, *Am J Nurs* 107:58-70, 2007.

Livestrong Care Plan from the OncoLink website: Available at http://www.livestrongcareplan.org/

Resources on Preparing a Survivorship Care Plan:

ASCO treatment summary and care plan templates, both generic and specific for breast, lung and colon cancer: Available at www.asco.org/treatmentsummary

Haylock PJ, Mitchell SA, Cox T, et al: The cancer survivor's prescription for living, *Am J Nurs* 107:58-70, 2007.

Livestrong Care Plan from the OncoLink website: Available at http://www.livestrongcareplan.org/

Journey Forward survivorship care plan builder: Available at http://www.journeyforward.org

to monitor for cancer recurrence. In larger practices, where oncology nurse specialists or advanced practice nurses participate in patient care, components of the survivorship care planning visit can be delegated to the nurse. Primary care physicians can also be involved in ensuring that components of the survivorship care plan are complete, and that comprehensive care has been addressed.

ACCESS AND IMPLEMENTATION OF CARE PLAN

Recommendations for monitoring for cancer recurrence and recommended strategies for health promotion and disease prevention are summarized in the treatment summary and survivorship care plan, which can be given to the patient and placed in the patient's chart so that it can be conveyed to the primary geriatrician. Ideally, enough time should be set aside at key transition points where care planning is indicated. Screening for depression and anxiety is vital at these times, with referral to a mental health specialist if there are any signs or symptoms of depression, along with referral to appropriate support

groups and community resources. Concerns regarding sexuality, intimacy, and vocation should also be addressed at the end of acute treatment, with resource referral when needed.

Establishing practice models in the community setting to improve the coordination of care for cancer patients in the posttreatment phase of the illness trajectory is vital to successful shared-care specialist/primary care collaboration. ASCO has developed templates for treatment summaries and care plans for breast and colon cancer. These and other resources on preparing a survivorship care plan are listed in Table 24-3. It is important for the oncologist and geriatrician to try to coordinate care with the patient's other physicians and to identify, with the patient, who will take care of ongoing health needs. Care of cancer patients is often subsumed by oncologists during the acute phase of their disease because of the complexity of the cancer and its treatment. However, especially in the older patient, it is important to attend to chronic care needs and health promotion during this time, as well as in follow-up; this is best done in the primary care setting. A clear and concise treatment summary and survivorship care plan can empower the older cancer survivor and the primary care physician to take charge of future care, with consultation of the medical oncologist and other specialists as necessary.

RESOURCES AVAILABLE TO CANCER SURVIVORS

The treatment summary and survivorship care plan can serve as both a communication vehicle and an educational resource for the cancer survivor. Table 24-3 lists additional resources available to cancer survivors. In the older patient, focus should be placed on establishing a social network for education and resources on wellness, and promotion of preventive strategies such as nutrition and physical activity. Patient empowerment is critical to ensuring successful implementation of the care plan.

SUGGESTED READINGS

1. Aziz NM: Cancer survivorship research: State of knowledge, challenges and opportunities, *Acta Oncologica* 46:417–432, 2007.
2. Cheung WY, Neville BA, Cameron DB, et al: Comparisons of patient and physician expectations for cancer survivorship care, *J Clin Oncol* 27:2489–2495, 2009.
3. Demark-Wahnefried W, Aziz NM, Rowland JH, et al: Riding the crest of the teachable moment: Promoting long-term health after the diagnosis of cancer, *J Clin Oncol* 23: 5813–5830, 2005.
4. Droz J, Aapro M, Balducci L: Overcoming challenges associated with chemotherapy treatment in the senior adult population, *Crit Rev Oncol Hematol* 68S:S1–S8, 2008.
5. Earle CC, Schrag D, Woolf SH, Ganz PA: The survivorship care plan: what, why, how and for whom. In Ganz PA, editor: *Cancer Survivorship*, New York, 2007, Springer, pp 525–531.
6. Earle CC: Failing to plan is planning to fail: Improving the quality of care with survivorship care plans, *J Clin Oncol* 24:5112–5116, 2006.
7. Earle CC, Burstein HJ, Winer EP, Weeks JC: Quality of non-breast cancer health maintenance among elderly breast cancer survivors, *J Clin Oncol* 21:1447–1451, 2003.
8. Ganz PA, Hahn E: Implementing a survivorship care plan for patients with breast cancer, *J Clin Oncol* 26:759–767, 2008.
9. Ganz PA, Casillas J, Hahn EE: Ensuring quality care for cancer survivors: implementing the survivorship care plan, *Semin Oncol Nurs* 24:208–217, 2008.
10. Ganz PA: Monitoring the physical health of cancer survivors: a survivorship-focused medical history, *J Clin Oncol* 24:5105–5111.
11. Ganz PA: A teachable moment for oncologists: cancer survivors, 10 million strong and growing! *J Clin Oncol* 23: 5458–5460, 2005.
12. Ganz PA: *Overview of cancer survivorship*. http://www.cancer.ucla.edu/Modules/ShowDocument.aspx?documentid=387.
13. Nekhlyudov L: "Doc, should I see you or my oncologist?" A primary care perspective on opportunities and challenges in providing comprehensive care for cancer survivors, *J Clin Oncol* 27:2424–2426, 2009.
15. Snyder CF, Earle CC, Herbert RJ, et al: Trends in follow-up and preventive care for colorectal cancer survivors, *J Gen Intern Med* 23:254–259, 2008.

SECTION VI

Special Issues

Managing the Older Cancer Patient at Home

Pattie Jakel and Joseph Albert Melocoton

It is estimated that by the year 2050, about 79 million individuals in the United States will be older than 65 years.[1] Older adults are the fastest growing segment in the U.S. population. Cancer incidence is projected to rise as the general population ages, and is a leading cause of mortality in the elderly.[2] Because of advances in modern medicine, life expectancy has increased significantly and cancer has become a chronic disease. Cancer is a major health concern in the United States, yet information about the services and programs for older adults with cancer are still limited.[3] The current health care system has undergone major changes regarding reimbursement. Inpatient lengths of stay have been significantly reduced under curtailed reimbursement, and the burden of care has shifted to outpatient and home care. The older adult population has unique needs that pose a tremendous challenge to health care professionals. Designing a comprehensive plan of care after hospital discharge should address the behavioral and functional issues prevalent among elderly patients with cancer, such as medication adherence and home safety. Furthermore, an understanding of specialized programs or geriatric resources (involving a multidisciplinary approach) is essential to optimizing health outcomes for this important patient population.

MEDICATION ADHERENCE AMONG ELDERLY CANCER PATIENTS

CASE 25-1

H.T. is a 65-year-old woman who has been newly diagnosed with chronic myelocytic leukemia (CML) in its chronic phase. Her medical history is significant for hypertension, diet-controlled diabetes, and depression. She received patient education on her diagnosis and the intended therapies. She does not yet fully comprehend her diagnosis and is overwhelmed at the prospect of cancer treatments. She lives alone in an apartment with no immediate family. She drives a long way to her medical appointments.

She started treatment with an oral antineoplastic agent, and experienced nausea with the medication despite antiemetic therapy. She returned to the clinic a week later complaining of nausea and vomiting; her serum potassium level was 3.

Scope of Problem

As the nature of cancer therapy shifts from acute to chronic care, medication adherence or compliance has become an increasingly important concern. Compliance or adherence refers to the ability to maintain health-promoting regimens, whether it involves taking a medication, performing an exercise program, or carrying out lifestyle changes.[4] Some experts assign a subtle difference to the meaning of compliance and adherence but they will be used interchangeably for the purpose of this chapter.

Because the elderly often have multiple comorbidities, an older adult takes, on average, three to twelve prescription drugs and one to four nonprescription drugs per year. However, it is estimated that only about 60% take their prescribed medications properly. There are currently more than 20 oral agents in the cancer armamentarium and dozens more in the pipeline. With the significant increase in the use of oral agents for treating cancer or otherwise, there is also a concurrent potential increase in the risk of nonadherence among the elderly. Nonadherence to oral medications is a barrier to optimal therapy and can impair health through delayed healing, promote disease recurrence, or even hasten death. Nonadherence is not only an impediment to the full therapeutic benefit of the regimen but is also associated with increased health care costs due to frequent physician visits and hospitalizations.[5, 6]

Factors Involved in Nonadherence

The financial impact of medication nonadherence to the U.S. health care industry is estimated to be $100 billion per year.[7] To ensure safety, quality of care, and improved treatment outcomes, it is imperative that patients adhere to a medication regimen. Nonadherence can have crucial implications to oncology. Nonadherence to a drug regimen is a multifaceted issue and involves three major variables: *patient, physician, and treatment.*[8]

Patient variables relate to individual factors that are associated with medication adherence such as physical and cognitive decline, intentional nonadherence, inadequate support system, lack of belief about treatment, and psychological illnesses, particularly depression. Memory deficits, poor visual acuity, and diminished manual dexterity can also contribute to medication nonadherence. The elderly may have challenges understanding complex regimens and therefore may have difficulty complying with the directions as instructed. Furthermore, nonadherence can be intentional; the reasons for this are complex. A study on chronically ill patients who were starting a new medication found that a third did not comply with the prescribed regimen; for 50% of these, the nonadherence was intentional because of medication side effects.[9] Knowledge and beliefs about health can also influence medication-taking behavior, although these variables have yet to be validated in research studies. Patients may adhere to the medication regimen if they believe that the medication will help and that the potential benefit outweighs the risk. In addition, mood disorders such as depression can also influence medication adherence. Depression is a common comorbid chronic illness in older adults that is underdiagnosed and undertreated. Compared to patients who are mentally stable, the medication nonadherence rate is 27% higher among depressed patients.[10] Physician factors refer to the patient-physician interaction. The relationship between the doctor and the patient, the communication skills involved, and the physician's cultural competence, as well as his or her comfort in dealing with older patients, all contribute to adherence to therapy. Poor patient-provider communication, inadequate discussion of side effects, and lack of patient understanding about the effectiveness of treatment may foster dissatisfaction and mistrust that can hamper effective medication adherence.[5] Another problem is the lack of awareness and recognition by health care providers of the existing problem of medication nonadherence.

Treatment variables refer to the medical and economic considerations that can affect medication adherence such as side effects, duration of treatment, medication costs, polypharmacy, and complexity of drug regimen. Because of chronic conditions, the elderly tend to be on multiple medications. Medication side effects are a major reason that older adults skip doses or stop taking their medications. A study on adjuvant therapy with tamoxifen revealed that women were four times more likely to be nonadherent to the regimen if they experienced side effects.[11] Thirty-five percent of older adults who took five or more medications were prone to adverse reactions.[12] Likewise, patients who are on therapy for an extended period have a high rate of discontinuation. The higher the number of medications, the less likely the elderly will adhere to therapy. The elderly take, on average, four to seven prescription medications, three over-the-counter medications and one herbal supplement.[13, 14] Polypharmacy and multiple medication doses required per day create a complex of medication regimen and increase the risk of drug reactions among the elderly.

Solutions to the Problem

Patient education is important to promoting medication adherence in the elderly. A specific set of educational methods should be tailored to their learning needs, and assessment should focus on their memory, attention, and executive functioning. There are several aids to medication planning and organization. Methods that were found to be beneficial in promoting medication adherence include utilization of a timed pill box, placing containers in a familiar location, taking medications in synchrony with meals/bedtime, getting reminders from others, and using a check-off list or written instructions.[15] Written instructions in large letters or bullet and list format seem beneficial. When discussing medications, it is likewise helpful to provide general information first, followed by how to take the medicine, the outcomes or side effects to watch for, and signs or symptoms of when to call the doctor. Memory-enhancing methods such as medication schedules, refrigerator medication charts, electronic reminders or alarms, or an electronic medication-dispensing device can also enhance patient medication adherence. Medication cards that list current medications can heighten drug compliance; this list can be shared with other prescribing providers who can update and review drug regimens at each clinic visits.

Refilling prescriptions can also be challenging for the older adults. A system to assist in procuring or refilling prescriptions such as a mail-order pharmacy, pharmacy automatic-refill service, or telephone reminder calls can be very beneficial. Modified medication containers or blister packs may make it easier for those who are physically challenged to open medication containers. The pharmacy can be a good resource when choosing alternatives for preparing medications for administration, such as utilizing tablets that are easier to break or providing correct medication dosages that don't require breaking. A comprehensive pharmacy medication adherence program or system that includes patient education, pharmacy consultation, and follow-up can enable elderly patients to adhere more closely to their medication regimens.[16] Pharmacy reviews to decrease polypharmacy, such as the Beers criteria[17] for potentially inappropriate medication use, can be a helpful guide when considering medications that should be avoided in patients age 65 and older and can identify adverse drug interactions.

The importance of engaging the help of family members or supportive caregivers can never be overemphasized. Family members and caregivers provide emotional and regimen-specific support. They provide important clues and information that are valuable when considering the functional status, cognitive capacity, health maintenance, and medication habits of the aging population.

Overall, there is no single best method to promote medication adherence in the older adult population. A multifaceted approach is warranted (Table 25-1 for a summary of practical recommendations to improve medication adherence in the elderly).

TABLE 25-1	Practical Strategies to Improve Medication Management for the Elderly	
Factors associated with nonadherence to oral medications	**Helpful recommendations for increasing adherence**
Patient-related variables	
Cognitive deficits	*Use of memory cues* (taking medications based on routine or synchrony with meals/bedtime); *Memory-enhancing methods or devices* (pre-poured or timed pill box; utilizing a medication dispensing service; automatic dispensers with voice-activated message; telephone call reminders; placing containers in a familiar location; medication calendar or charts; wristwatch with alarms; medication diary; dose-reminder cards)
Physical deficits	Use of blister packs, or easy-open containers/non-childproof containers; consult with pharmacy regarding medication modification (correct dose of medications, easy-to-break tablets)
Other: depression, intentional nonadherence, lack of belief about treatment, inadequate support system.	Assess and treat depression; explore health concerns for noncompliance; reinforce benefits of therapy; discuss the danger of missed medications; refer to social worker or discharge planner on community resources; enlist help of family members/caregivers; annual physical exams
Physician-related variables	
Poor patient-provider relationship or communication	Regular contact and consistent patient support (nonjudgmental attitude, active listening, reinforce adherent behaviors, cultural sensitivity, convenient follow-up schedules) Provide patient education and periodic drug review (medication side effects, benefits of therapy, asking for feedback, keeping messages simple, providing informational resources)
Treatment-related variables	
- Side effects	- Modify regimen to reduce adverse effects
- Complexity of regimen	- Simplify the regimen and dosing schedule: Review prescribed and nonprescribed medications; Enlist the help of other physicians involved.
- Medication costs	-Seek assistance with procuring medications; learn about insurance coverage; consult with other physicians about availability of drug samples; use of generic drugs; participate in drug company programs; refer to social worker regarding Medicare prescription coverage (www.medicare.gov/MedicareReform). Review if drug regimen is efficacious and economical.
- Polypharmacy	- Medication review semi-annually; check duplicate drug therapies; use combination drugs or alternative routes; screen for drug interactions; create an updated medication list to share to providers; apply Beers criteria on medication review.[17]

Health Care Providers' Role

The physician's role is central and key to successful medication adherence in the elderly. The physician should constantly assess personal characteristics (physical/cognitive/emotional skills), relationship orientation, and the way a patient absorbs and process information (self-efficacy), because all patients are unique. Listening to the patient is very important. It helps to have comfort in dealing with older patients. Enhanced patient-provider communication fosters adherence by creating trust and improves patient satisfaction with care.[5] It is essential to have regular contact and consistent patient support at all levels of care. During a patient clinic visit, it is important for providers to screen for potential adverse drug interactions and identify any medications of concern. It is necessary to have an updated list of all medications including dose frequency and to have the patient provide this list to other prescribing providers when necessary.[18]

Elderly patients require a substantial need for more information when starting a new medication. It is necessary keep the information simple and clear, both in verbal and written form. Start with what the patient already knows and discuss the names of the drugs being ordered and its effect. Always provide time for questions. Physicians should carefully explain information regarding treatments and should reinforce disease characteristics, risks and benefits of treatments, and the proper use of medication.[7] It is important to discuss medication side effects from the start of treatment so that patients may know what to expect and be better able to deal with adverse reactions to therapy. An understanding of how some medications might have different effects on people of various ethnicities, as well as a knowledge of age-related changes in metabolism and drug interactions are essential.

Also, it is imperative to identify barriers to adherence; questioning techniques about medication-taking behaviors should be nonjudgmental and may include statements such as "How do you take your medications?" "Do you stop taking medication when you feel better/when you feel worse?" and "Are you having difficulty taking your medications daily?" It is also helpful to inquire about situations that may have an impact on medication adherence such as missed doses and what the patient should do in the situation of a missed dose. Caregivers should be involved in the plan of care. They can reinforce adherent behaviors. Getting feedback at each clinic discussion can help to uncover and address issues that can have important implications to medication adherence and overall health. If the patient has difficulty understanding a particular medication at a previous clinic encounter, then reviewing the drug again at the next visit would be very helpful to encouraging adherence. It is also beneficial to discuss special instructions such as taking medication with food or the proper way to use an inhaler, as well as side effects to monitor or report.

Assistance Programs

It is a known fact that the more costly the medication, the less likely that older adults will procure the medication or adhere to a regimen that includes it. Lack of funds, especially at the end of the month, is a major factor in why older adults have difficulty filling their prescriptions.[19] The out-of-pocket costs, high copayment, or a lack of prescription drug coverage can create a tremendous financial burden for chronically ill adults and can be a major barrier to medication adherence.

Helpful suggestions to ease medication procurement for the elderly include the use of drug samples from prescribing physicians, participation in copayment assistance programs from pharmaceutical corporations, and pharmacy consultation on utilizing generic instead of brand name drugs. Patients can be referred to a social worker to navigate the system or to help them obtain Medicare or other insurance coverage.[20, 21] Several states have pharmacy assistance programs that help eligible persons pay for their prescription drugs.

CASE 25-1 | CONTINUED

H.T. had been unable to fill her antiemetic prescription because of a high copayment for drug regimens. She had thought of stopping therapy entirely, because of her limited income, but had reluctantly refilled only her oral antineoplastic agent and not the antiemetic medication. At this clinic visit, an antiemetic and replacement with intravenous potassium were ordered. The oncologist explored her economic challenges to filling her prescriptions, assessed her self-care skills and her current stressors or depression, and offered encouragement and support to maintain a proactive stance in her medical oncology care. During this clinic visit, the physician modified her antiemetic regimen; a cheaper alternative prescription to manage delayed nausea was ordered, and a drug sample was given. She was also referred to the nurse navigator and social worker regarding local/national cancer support groups or other resources that she might find helpful. She was also informed about psychosocial assistance when necessary. A copay assistance program was also explored and a pharmaceutical drug representative was contacted.

Specific information regarding expected side effects, adverse reactions of the medication regimen, and commonly encountered drug-drug interactions were reiterated. Her questions were answered and she feels satisfied to continue with her cancer therapy. The oncologist also collaborated with the patient's primary care doctor and discussed what they would do to comanage this patient's care effectively.

HOME SAFETY

Homecare Services

The older adult population's cancer illness experience and needs differ substantially from those of younger age groups because of multiple chronic medical conditions that often compound the oncologic diagnosis. The current health care system, typified by shorter hospital stays and an increased shift of cancer treatments from hospital to ambulatory settings, has concomitantly caused a great challenge for older adults by making it necessary for them to cope in the home setting with the physical and psychosocial difficulties associated with cancer. Homecare for older adults with cancer may necessitate a multidisciplinary approach, requiring integration, continuity of care, and coordination of a number of service disciplines such as social workers, pharmacists, physical therapy (PT), speech therapy (ST), or occupational therapy (OT). A description of these skilled and ancillary services can be found in Table 25-2. Several patient-safety issues that

TABLE 25-2	Skilled Home Care Services	
Services	**Indications**	**Example**
Physical Therapy	Functional limitations in mobility, strength, range of motion; wound debridement	Gait training and strengthening exercises
Speech-Language Pathology Services	Language, speech, and swallowing disorders	Assessment, evaluation, and therapy to regain or strengthen speaking and swallowing skills (also listening, reading, and memory skills)
Occupational Therapy	To improve activities of daily living and achieve independence through therapy; occupational therapists can also perform environmental assessments	Therapeutic activities, energy conservation methods, task simplification, use of adaptive equipment
Ancillary Services		
Social services	Psychosocial assessment and evaluation of patient and caregiver that affect treatment or recovery	Counseling, resource finding, referrals
Home health care aide	Support services for skilled nursing therapy (not covered by Medicare unless patient is receiving skilled nursing care).	Custodial care or assistance with activities of daily living (bathing, grooming, transportation, meal preparation, and light housekeeping tasks)

can affect health outcomes upon discharge relate to issues including but not limited to medication adherence, living situation, and physical and cognitive functioning. Much of the decision is left to clinicians' individual assessment and clinical judgment when it comes to identifying characteristics of patients needing homecare referral, as Medicare regulations only dictate that patients be homebound and have a need for skilled assistance.[22] In addition, situational variables that present special challenges to recovery, health maintenance, and safety for this high-risk population include transportation, social support, maintaining independence, and financial resources. To be eligible for Medicare reimbursement, home health services should be deemed medically necessary by a physician and should be provided on an intermittent or part-time basis. Medicare law prohibits reimbursement for ancillary services unless a skilled service is initially ordered and provided. Physicians can refer to home health services or services may be requested by a family member or patients themselves.

Homecare is significantly different compared to the hospital setting and, thus far, there is limited data and research on patient safety problems encountered at home.[23] Issues for patients who are receiving care at home may be its unregulated setting compared to the hospital setting, greater autonomy exercised at home, and the complex physical, social, emotional and functional dimensions involved. Quality care for the elderly should consider safety risks during discharge planning. Doran et al. in a 2009 study[24] identified the most prevalent safety risks in the older adult population; they were polypharmacy, physical decline, cognitive decline, living alone, and a history of two or more falls. For the elderly with cancer, impaired functional status is the most frequent predictor of the need for homecare referral, although cancer stage and plans for adjuvant therapy are important when making informed referral decisions.[25]

Discharge planning should take into account the identification of patients likely to suffer adverse health consequences. It should consider the patient's care needs, preferences, caregiver support, and financial responsibilities so as to promote safe transition across care settings. The discharge plan focuses on the medical and social resources of the patient and should address his or her physical and cognitive function, postacute living arrangements, and functional status in areas such as eating, dressing, toileting, and ambulation. Factors to include in determining discharge needs include goals of care (rehabilitation, palliation, hospice), skilled nursing needs (PT, OT, ST), functional capacity (before and during hospitalization), equipment and supportive needs, social support, medication lists, insurance, and prognosis.

Home Safety Evaluation

Problems with an older adult's environment can interfere with optimizing his or her health and with achieving goals of care; thus an environmental or home assessment

is warranted. Furthermore, unintentional falls are a growing public health concern and a common cause of nonfatal injuries for people older than 65 years.[26] The goal of a home safety evaluation is to develop and implement strategies to preserve a person's ability to function safely and independently at home and may include an assessment of the environment, residential observation of the elderly, and determination of the older adult's fall risk and health status.[27]

A home safety evaluation can be performed to assess for actual and potential safety problems in a patient's home environment. When doing a home safety evaluation, the physical infrastructure, bathroom facilities, storage layout, room features, accessibility, and even medical waste disposal and availability of resources or support persons are considered.

Some home safety assessment recommendations are covered by Medicare/Medicaid. Services can be paid out-of-pocket or by insurance. Home safety evaluation is necessary to identify factors that affect home safety (lighting, overall aesthetics, furnishings, clothing, rooms, electronic appliances, rooms, bathroom equipment, doors, handles, locks, stairs, light switches, remote controls, handrails, tub or faucet handles). Extrinsic factors are also considered (entryway, driveway, walkway). Safety hazards can be identified (clutter, electronic equipments, extension cords, pool, hot tubs, water temperature) and steps can be ensured to promote a safe environment for the elderly patient. Home hazard modifications can thus be recommended, which may include setting goals, enlisting social support, coordinating care, providing referrals, and planning with the patient, family, and health care professionals. A home safety evaluation can be performed by a registered nurse (RN), physical therapist, or occupational therapist. Performance of a safety evaluation involves a team approach. The physician, nurse practitioner, or physician assistant may order a home safety evaluation. Home safety evaluations are also available through community service programs, and a number of private agencies can do home safety evaluation.

If the individual has a history of safety "red flags" (history of falls, mobility/balance difficulties, cognitive impairments), a home safety evaluation by a trained health professional such as a nurse, physical therapist, or occupational therapist can be initiated for further assessment and a house visit can then be made (Table 25-3 for sample checklist). The need for assistive devices is also part of the assessment and a prescription can be obtained as indicated.

A typical scenario in a home safety evaluation consists of the physician recognizing a homebound patient needing skilled services. In conjunction with hospital discharge planners, a referral for home health care services will be made. A home hazard and safety assessment will be performed prior to patient discharge or can also be initiated upon discharge. If a home safety evaluation is performed during discharge, a physical therapist or occupational

TABLE 25-3	Sample Home Safety Evaluation Checklist
Floors	Clear pathway (no objects or clutter on the floor); no throw rugs or use of double-sided tape to prevent slipping; no exposed or frayed cords or electrical wires
Stairs and steps	No uneven or broken steps; adequate lighting; accessible light switches; no torn or loose carpets; available handrails (loose handrails are fixed and available on both sides of the stairs); marked steps for easy identification
Kitchen	Things are accessible or at waist level; steady step stool
Living room	Removing unsafe chairs (too low or no arms)
Bathrooms	Nonslip rubber mat; available grab bars or support inside tub or next to toilet; water temperature at 120° F
Bedroom	Easy-to-reach lamp; adequate distance of the side of the bed to the wall
Others	No toxic substances (should be properly stored if present); appropriate medication storage; first-aid kit availability; telephone access; waste disposal

therapist will transition the client from wheelchair to car. The therapists will follow the older adult at home, and the physical therapist can start a safety evaluation by, for example, measuring the height of the bed or the width of the door, while the occupational therapist assesses safety barriers as well. Safety deficits are identified after the evaluation and then modifications, adaptive techniques, and recommended safety devices are discussed with the patient, family, or caregivers, on the basis of the assessment. Environmental safety recommendations are advocated and family members or caregivers can be trained on other accommodations or adaptations to ensure an optimal level of daily performance and improve patient outcomes overall.

Other Homecare Issues

Other practical issues pertinent to a patient's plan of care relate to resources. Many community agencies offer senior programs and services. Several local cancer support groups, faith-based groups, and agencies on aging in the community can provide resources for transportation, chore services, adult day care, and a variety of senior activities. Local and national cancer agencies provide assistance with transportation, such as the Road to Recovery program of the American Cancer Society, and other public or private sector programs. Some transportation services are provided in the community on the basis of age and health insurance.

Preserving independence while maintaining safety should always be the goal, and physicians should always be alert and assess the cause when a deficit is noted. Long-term treatment and medical care for the older adult with cancer often involves periodic medical visits, lifestyle

modifications, and prolonged medication or equipment use to manage symptoms or side effects of cancer treatments. Unmanaged symptoms from cancer and its treatments expose the elderly patient to depression or psychological disabilities. Alternative living arrangements such as nursing home placement may be necessary when it is no longer safe or possible to keep the elderly patient functioning adequately at home. The home environment may not be the best place for maintaining health when someone has vision, hearing, or mobility deficits. Factors to consider when recommending long-term care placement include medical stability, orientation, activities of daily living (ADL), skilled therapy requirement, living condition, and resources. Potential issues of guilt or role-restructuring within a family or caregiver network should be addressed and caregiver support should be considered when long-term care placement is the best course of action for the patient.

A doctor's order for homecare should include and specify the type of skilled care and unskilled services required as well as the frequency of the services ordered. It should clearly explain to the payer why rendering the service is reasonable and necessary. If orders have to be amended, it should clearly specify and indicate what is to be changed and the reason for the changes. The frequency of the service incorporated in the care plan should be justified by the changes in the patient's medical condition.

LONG-TERM CARE OPTIONS FOR THE OLDER ADULT

The aging population in the United States has resulted in a large number of people with chronic illness and a declining ability to care for themselves in their homes. Many older patients do not suffer from a single life-threatening illness but rather a slow progression of illnesses with physical and psychosocial burdens that can elicit caregiver burnout. Studies have shown that elderly patients with comprehensive discharge plans by skilled professionals such as advanced practice nurses have much lower risk for discharge failures.[28-29] If these patients are followed up in their homes, they have decreased readmission rates and a longer time at home between hospitalizations. Comprehensive plans need to be prepared with the family to allow for successful transitions between hospital, home, and skilled nursing facility (SNF).

Locating services for the elderly can be a daunting task for the patient, the family, and the health care provider. It is critical to understand the Medicare system and what is covered for the patient older than 65 years. It is important to note that some patients may have Medicare supplement insurance plans, either from the American Association of Retired Persons (AARP) or as part of their retirement package.[30] These policies are usually purchased by a Medicare patient. This insurance usually covers only 20% copayment for Medicare benefits and does not cover long-term custodial care (Table 25-4).

TABLE 25-4	**Medicare**

Medicare Basics

- People age 65 or older
- People under 65 with certain disabilities
- People of any age with end-stage renal disease

The Different Parts of Medicare

Medicare Part A (Hospital Insurance)

- Helps cover inpatient care in hospitals
- Helps cover skilled nursing facility, hospice, and home health care

Medicare Part B (Medical Insurance)

- Helps cover physician services, outpatient care, and home health care
- Helps cover some preventive services

Medicare Part C (Medicare Advantage Plans – like HMO or PPO)

- A health coverage option run by private insurance companies approved by and under a contract with Medicare

Medicare Part D (Medicare Prescription Drug Coverage)

- Prescription drug option run by private insurance companies approved by and under contract with Medicare

Medicare Coverage Choices

Original Medicare

- Fee-for-service coverage
- Federal government management
- Provides Part A and B coverage
- Patient can see any doctor or hospital that accepts Medicare
- Patient can join a Prescription Drug Plan
- Patient can buy a Medigap (Medicare Supplement Insurance) policy sold by private insurance companies to fill the gaps in Part A and Part B

Medicare Advantage Plans (HMO or PPO)

- Run by private insurance approved by and under contract to Medicare
- Provides Part A and Part b coverage but can charge various amounts for certain services

TRICARE Coverage

- Coverage for active-duty military or retirees and their families.
- Retired military must enroll in Part B to keep TRICARE coverage

Other Medicare Health Plans

- Part of Medicare but not a Medicare advantage plan
- Most plans provide Part A and Part B coverage, and some also provide prescription drug coverage
- Include Medicare Cost Plans, Demonstration/Pilot Programs and Programs of All-Inclusive Care for the Elderly (PACE)*.
- Patients may choose a Homecare Agency from the participating Medicare-Certified Home Health Agencies in their area. Medicare Advantage Plan (HMO or PPO) or other Medicare Health Plans may require the patient to use a contracted agency. Medicare has a "Home Health Compare" tool on the web that compares agencies by location. Check www.medicare.gov- click "Resources" and then "Home Health Agencies." Please see Table 4 on options for elderly patients covered by Medicare.

Medicaid

- Joint Federal and state program that helps pay medical costs for those with low-income; programs vary from state to state
- Possible coverage for services that Medicare does not cover (nursing home, home health)

Note: Based on information from the U.S. Department of Health and Human Services- Centers for Medicare and Medicaid services.[30]
*PACE is a Medicare and Medicaid program that allows patients who would need a nursing home to remain at home. PACE provides all the care and services covered by Medicare and Medicaid as well as additional medically-necessary care and services not covered. There are limited service areas that provide PACE services. Check this website for covered areas: www.medicare.gov/Publications/Pubs/pfd/11341.pdf

DL is a 69-year-old widowed man with stage III colon cancer who completed 6 months of chemotherapy. Various family members stayed and offered assistance to the patient. The patient presented for follow-up with his primary physician approximately 6 months after chemotherapy, appearing unkempt. His son reported that the patient has not been eating, has not been taking his medications correctly, and has not been participating in activities at the senior center.

Possible warning signs that elderly patients are failing to care for themselves at home:

- *Personal hygiene changes, i.e., failure to bathe, wearing the same clothes all the time, or sleeping in the same clothes*
- *Responses such as, "Why should I bathe or change my clothes? I do not go out anymore."*
- *A dusty/dirty residence that was formerly neat*
- *A lack of food in the refrigerator or placing to-go orders on a regular basis may signal difficulty driving, or a physical problem with lifting groceries*
- *Tiredness and constant complaints may be a sign of depression*
- *Forgetting to pay bills, turn off stove, leaving water running, not taking medications, or leaving the phone off the hook*

The physician ordered a home safety evaluation and the physical therapist reported that the patient was struggling at home. Meals-on-wheels were provided for the patient and it was arranged that the senior access shuttle would provide transportation to the senior center once a week.

One month later, the patient was admitted for 3 days with uro-sepsis, and was confused and weak. To qualify for Medicare SNF coverage, the patient must be hospitalized for at least 3 days. The patient was sent to a subacute rehabilitation facility (acute rehabilitation requires performance of physical/occupational therapy for 3 hours per day) with a skilled need of IV antibiotics and daily physical therapy. He stayed 30 days, with Medicare paying 80% of the cost and the other 20% paid for by the patient's retirement health insurance plan with Blue Cross. His family arranged for the patient to sell his home and the patient was moved to an assisted living complex. The patient will receive services: shower help, daily dressing help, three meals per day, shuttle rides for appointments and shopping, and twice-daily medication administration. The cost for this patient is between $1,800-2,500 per month. If the patient's physical needs increase, assisted living will be able to care for the patient until he requires total care. If an elderly patient requires 24-hour care and does not have a skilled need, the patient must pay for custodial care (Medicare does not cover this type of care). If the patient qualifies for Medicaid, there are a limited number of beds in a SNF that can care for these patients.

Summary and Conclusions

Aging has become a worldwide phenomenon and United States demographics indicate an unprecedented growth of the older adult population. Geriatric care poses a unique challenge to health care providers and the health care system in general. Managing older adults with cancer and associated chronic conditions can be complex, as cancer management extends well beyond the initial diagnosis and treatment. This chapter has reviewed factors, such as medication adherence, that can have an impact on effective disease management for the older adult population. The elderly are the largest users of prescription medications and are at risk for problems in medication management. Since a drug's effectiveness is dependent on its therapeutic concentration, medication adherence has critical implications for older adults with cancer. Practical recommendations for increasing adherence were outlined. This chapter also discussed safety considerations for an older adult transitioning care from hospital to a home setting.

More people are surviving cancer as a result of breakthroughs in cancer screening, diagnosis, and treatment. The period following hospitalization may be one of the most challenging times for cancer symptom management. Discharge planning should consider a comprehensive geriatric assessment to guide individualized client service planning for a variety of home health and home care services. Also, home safety evaluation to identify safety risks (modifiable and amenable to interventions), should be considered when setting priorities for service provision upon discharge. Lastly, uncoordinated health care services can adversely affect health outcomes for the elderly. Health care providers are encouraged to keep abreast of state and federal regulations concerning health care. Use of community resources is highly advocated. Useful links and resources for supportive geriatric care are also provided.

In summary, interdisciplinary management is crucial to ensure a positive effect on the health outcomes of older adult patients with cancer. Systematic approaches are needed to determine resources available, to identify the type of health care assistance needed, and to refer to appropriate services as required. Comprehensive geriatric care is best provided by a team of health care professionals with the goal of preserving the elderly person's social, cognitive, and physical function, thereby reducing health care costs and maintaining quality of life.

TABLE 25-5	Long-term Care Options and Medicare Coverage

Types of Long-Term Care	Services

A. Home Health Care
• Medicare may pay if patient is elderly or disabled living in their own home.
• Patient must be home bound
• Covered under Part A & B
• Plan of care must be signed by MD and services provided by a Medicare certified agency
• Medicaid programs may pay for home health aides depending on the state
	• Skilled nursing care- services and care that can only be performed safely and correctly by a licensed registered nurse, e.g., IV medications, pain pumps, wound care, TPN, and tube feedings
	• Homemaker/Health Aides- 2-3x/week
	   - House Cleaning; laundry; bathe and dress
	   - Plan and shop for meals
	   - Move patient from bed
	   - Physical Therapy- 2x/week
	• Speech Language pathology
	• Occupational Therapy

	Durable Medical Equipment (DME) Patient pays 20% of Medicare- approved amount in Parts A & B • Oxygen Equipment • Wheelchairs (non-electric) • Walkers • Hospital Beds. Medicare Does Not Cover DME services such as: • 24 hour care at home • Meal delivery • Homemaker care (bathing, shopping, cleaning laundry, and mobility help) when there is no skilled nursing need. • Shower chairs and commodes
B. Hospice Care Medicare will cover hospice care if the physician certifies that the patient has less than 6 months to live.	
	• Hospice staff on call 24/7 • Manages patient's pain • Assists family to care for patient • Assist patient and family with emotional, psychosocial and spiritual aspects of dying • Provides medications supplies and all equipment
Four Levels of Medicare Coverage for Hospice • Routine Home- Nursing Care and Home Health Aide, Social Work and Chaplain • Continuous Home Care- allowed only in periods of crisis; can be at home or inpatient hospice. • Respite Care- 5 days of consecutive care. Inpatient Hospice, hospital of SNF. • General Inpatient Care- only for pain control and symptom management. Medicare does not cover the room and board in a SNF under hospice for reasons other than those listed here. Some states have "homes for the dying" in the community. These homes can be at no charge or just cost between 6,000-8,000 thousand dollars per month. The home usually is staffed by an RN, care partner and volunteers. Patients can also be seen by a hospice nursing agency with nursing support, chaplain, and aide visits. Check this informative website: www.compassionandsupport.org	

Continued

TABLE 25-5	Long-term Care Options and Medicare Coverage—cont'd	
Types of Long-Term Care		**Services**

C. Skilled Nursing Facility/Nursing Home

Patient responsibility with Medicare:
- **$0 for the 1st 20 days each benefit period**
- **$137.50 per day for days 21-100 each benefit period**
- **All cost for each day after day 100 in a benefit period.**

Admissions allowed only after a 3-day inpatient hospital stay for a related illness or injury or within 30 days of hospitalization.

- Semi-Private Room
- Meals
- Skilled Nursing Care (intravenous medications, wound care)
- Rehabilitative Services including physical therapy, occupational therapy and speech therapy
- To qualify the patient must have a skilled nursing need such as.
- SNF may specialize in short term or acute care nursing care, intermediate care or long-term care.

Medicare does not cover long-term or custodial care in this setting.
Web Links for Choosing SNF:
- www.medicare.gov/nhcompare
- www.aarp.org_promtions/text/life.nursinghomechecklist.pdf
- www.aarpmagazine.org
- www.nccnhr.org/public/50_156_455.cfm.

D. Assisted Living for Seniors
- **Non-medical aspects of daily living**
- **Medicare covers none of the cost**

Cost Range from $800-$ 4,000 or more per month depending on location

- Help with aspects of daily living- bathing, dressing, mobility, and eating
- Separate private living areas with a common dining room and social room
- Social activities
- Transportation
- Physical activities
- Some have specialized care for: cognitive disabilities, respite care, short term care, and hospice.
- Some states allow for medication distribution by a non-license medical assistant under the direction of an RN

E. Board and Care
- **Not covered by Medicare**
- **Can be senior subsidized housing, Housing and Urban Development (HUD), or Section 8 Housing**
- **Rent based on ability to pay**
- **Long waiting lists for limited income patients**

- Apartment setting for 100 residents
- Home setting for 6 residents or less
- Activities of daily living (ADL) assistance
- Communal meals
- Daily staff contact
- Usually with 24-hour non-medical supervision

Useful links:
www.helpguide.org/elderly/board_care_homes_seniors_residential.htm

F. Adult Day Care
- **No Medicare coverage**
- **Medicaid may pay for services provided in a state licensed facilities**
- **Some private long-term insurance may pay**

- Health monitoring
- Social activities
- Meals
- Safety and security
- Alzheimer's/dementia care
- Assistance with ADLs
- Exercise
- Mental stimulation
- Transportation

Note: Based on information from the U.S. Department of Health and Human Services- Centers for Medicare and Medicaid services.[30]
SNF, skilled nursing facility

See expertconsult.com for a complete list of references and web resources for this chapter

Caregiver Burden

Barbara A. Given, Charles W. Given, and Paula Sherwood

A cancer diagnosis is often acute in onset and sparks an abrupt need for diagnostic and treatment decisions for the patient and family. Family members find that the patient's cancer treatment trajectory poses physical, psychological, and social challenges, particularly for older patients. Shortened inpatient care and more complex outpatient treatment regimens require family members to become active partners in cancer care. This complex and changing care by family members challenges their knowledge and skills, as they do not know how to provide "cancer care."

Family members often take primary responsibility for symptom management, wound care, pumps and equipment, transportation, mental health, support, and medication administration, while maintaining their own daily responsibilities, as well as those of the person with cancer, and coping with their emotional responses to the patient's diagnosis and the uncertainty of the future.[1] Uncertainty is intensified by the disease, treatment responses or failures, the patient's emotional and physical responses, and how these demands and pressures bear upon family caregivers. In addition, cancer and cancer-related treatment may alter family functioning and communication patterns, family member occupational roles, and social roles.[2] Increasingly, the health care system demands that informal caregivers behave more like formal care providers to achieve optimal patient clinical outcomes. In turn, caregivers require support and training, as well as coordination and communication with health care providers, to carry out the tasks of care. Patients' outcomes depend on the partnerships among the patient and his or her family caregiver and oncology providers. Providers need to recognize that patients and family members react as a unit and thus both members of the dyad have a legitimate need for assistance and care.

The purpose of this chapter is to review caregiver burden: the needs, roles, and concerns of family caregivers (typically spouses or adult children) providing care to older cancer patients undergoing cancer treatment. Spouses of older patients will be the primary focus because they comprise the largest group of caregivers for the older adult. Implications and recommendations for improving practice suggest how providers can engage family caregivers to participate more effectively in patient care.

DEFINITION OF BURDEN

Family caregiving is defined as the provision of unpaid aid or assistance and care by one or more family members (defined broadly) to another family member with cancer. This care extends beyond the usual family activities, such as cooking or household chores that are a part of normal daily life; it also includes critical components of health care. Among them are symptom management, nutrition support, response to illness behaviors (e.g., anger), modification of usual roles, interpersonal care (e.g., communication), implementation of prescription regimens, acute episode management, use of community resources, and navigation of the health care system.[3-5] Caregivers make major decisions, adjust to change and challenges, access resources for care, provide direct care, and coordinate patient visits with the health care system. Coordinating care (such as scheduling appointments, requesting medical records, and arranging transportation) can add substantially to caregivers' responsibilities and may increase burden.[6,7]

Burden, a negative reaction, is a multidimensional concept that stems from the imbalance between the social, psychological, and economic consequences permeating a care situation and the caregivers' coping strategies to meet the demands of patient care.[4,5,8-12] Caregivers who are unable to apply effective coping strategies to care demands may develop burden, which, if sustained, may lead to depression (see Assessment).[13-19]

Caregiver depression is considered to be a secondary or long-term mood disturbance that may develop as a result of unrelieved stress or burden.[20-24] Depression may emerge as a consequence of sustained caregiver burden and may be manifested by feelings of loneliness, sadness, isolation, fearfulness, and irritability.[25] Caregiver depression may be less dependent on recent changes in the patient's status and more dependent on whether the caregiver is able to employ coping mechanisms to alleviate burden before it progresses to depression.[2,19,23-27] In order to stop the progression of caregiver burden into more serious psychological responses, it is imperative that health care providers communicate with patients and their families to define and prioritize appropriate care demands and care tasks. Defining expectations for family caregivers can be beneficial for patients and families, as well as for oncology providers. The establishment of clear instructions, along with education on what to expect in the way of possible side effects or complications and what can be done to manage care at home will engage family members in assisting the patient and will reduce their uncertainty. For providers, patients and families become allies in patient care management, as well as sentinels to detect and report problems and clinical complications. If these problems are identified early, they can help prevent interruptions or delays in treatment.[23,25,28] While providing care may result in negative emotional and physical consequences for caregivers, it is important to remember that care provision can also engender satisfaction and meaning. Positive consequences, such as rewards, self-esteem, support, uplifts, and satisfaction, may provide a buffer to the negative effects of caregiving.[29-31] More research is warranted to identify ways of expanding positive aspects of care in the face of increased and recurring care demands.

CASE 26-1

The patient is a 68-year-old woman who presented for evaluation of unusual behavior: she kept asking her 72-year-old husband whether he could smell the oranges. Computed tomography (CT) of the brain did not show a bleed, but magnetic resonance imaging (MRI) demonstrated a mass. Surgery and a biopsy were scheduled for the next day to have the tumor removed; the diagnosis confirmed glioblastoma multiforme.

The patient was experiencing left-sided weakness and extreme fatigue. She was unable to properly bathe and feed herself or use the bathroom unaided. Her husband had to quickly figure out the proper ways to take care of her. He set up a bed for her on the first floor of their house.

Every morning, the patient's husband had to take her to the hospital for treatment. After treatment, she usually experienced nausea, loss of appetite, and increased fatigue. Her husband also had to learn to take notes at all of her doctor's appointments so that he could effectively manage her care and help with symptom management.

As the patient's condition began to deteriorate, her personality changed and she became very demanding and irritable. Her husband began to feel alone and distressed and didn't know how to do deal with his situation. He appreciated the help that he received, but he began to lose sleep and felt physically and mentally exhausted. He wanted to take care of his wife, but he was having trouble coping and felt burdened with the required care.

CAREGIVER CARE DEMANDS

Care demands include dealing with patients' physical care, nutrition, spiritual support, symptom management, housekeeping, transportation, and financial needs. Regardless of the level or intensity of involvement, disruption of daily activities, competing demands, and unfamiliar physical care demands, those that produce anxiety or uncertainty have been shown to result in caregiver

burden.[31-33] Each type of caregiver task involvement demands different skills and knowledge, organizational capacities, and social and psychological strengths.[5,11] Unmet demands for care are a large source of burden for family caregivers and have been associated with poorer caregiver health, higher costs of care, and higher incidence of psychiatric diagnosis.[34,35] Caregivers also need information about their own self-care, the importance of networking with other caregivers, the importance of maintaining social support and contacts, and warning signs about their own levels of stress.[2,36]

Care demands stemming from the presence of neuropsychiatric and cognitive dysfunction (e.g., agitation, inappropriate behavior, and apathy) are particularly stressful for caregivers.[37-39] Management of cognitive and neuropsychiatric sequelae may produce higher levels of caregiver distress than assisting with impaired physical functioning.[31,39-41]

Moreover, as the caregiving situation evolves, there are additional opportunities for role ambiguity, role confusion, and role overload. Negative consequences for the caregiver, such as increased burden, can arise as caregivers seek to balance caregiving with work, family, and leisure activities.[42-45] The key to overcoming role ambiguity is to understand when new changes are likely to occur or when expectations shift as patient status changes.[46]

CASE 26-2

J., 64, taught children with learning disabilities, while her husband B., also 64, worked from home as a consultant.

When B. was diagnosed with a brain tumor, words that J. could not understand swirled through her mind: grade III, astrocytoma, malignant neoplasm, radical resection, biopsy, parietal, craniotomy.

She read journals, blogs, and Web sites and was overwhelmed with the diversity of the information she was reading. The thought of potential care demands competing with her work hours caused considerable stress.

Direct-Care Tasks

For caregivers of older cancer patients, direct-care activities occur at end of life or among patients who are disabled. These direct-care tasks include dressing changes, catheter care, wound care, and equipment and medication management. Medication management may be particularly burdensome for family caregivers. Older patients often have numerous comorbid conditions in addition to cancer. For the caregiver, the severity of patients' functional impairment and disability has been consistently shown to increase care demands on the caregiver and restrict other caregiver roles, thereby increasing caregiver distress.[40,47,48] Caregivers should be encouraged to facilitate the patients' return to normal physical functioning; however, this assistance may be problematic for older caregivers who have their own functional limitations. Providers can offer guidance and direction so caregivers can receive the assistance they need to provide care.

Cancer treatment can complicate preexisting medication regimens for other comorbidities, which means that caregivers must receive training, guidance, and access to comprehensive information to help them perform safe and effective medication administration. For example, oral-targeted therapies are especially complex; with oral agents, caregivers must rely on different sources for refilling prescriptions (specialty pharmacies, mail-order plans) and may rely on other mechanisms for reimbursement (e.g., private insurance and Veterans Administration benefits). Caregivers require education not only on how to administer medication but also on how to monitor for side effects and make critical decisions (e.g., dosing, withholding, and discontinuation).[49,50]

Symptom management often becomes a primary role for caregivers as a result of patient treatment, and successful management of symptoms is associated with lower caregiver burden. Patients experience multiple and severe symptoms from treatment, including pain, nausea, fatigue, shortness of breath, and anorexia.[15,29,51-57] Several researchers have demonstrated that patient depression is closely linked to caregivers' mental health.[58,59] This shared level of distress demonstrates that both the patient and caregiver need care consideration.[58] Patients and their family caregivers should be screened for depression throughout the care trajectory and receive treatment if they are clinically depressed.

Increased symptoms can occur in elderly patients with multiple comorbid conditions and may also accompany different cycles of treatment or certain protocols. Interventions designed to help the caregiver with patient symptom management may lower the negative reaction and burden.[60] Unfortunately, symptom resolution does not eliminate the caregiver role; caregivers report that they continue to provide assistance and are often on call for months after active treatment is over.[2,47]

Employment

Caregivers must adapt their employment obligations so as to manage and meet care demands,[8,61-63] which may result in missed days, work interruptions, leaves of absence, and reduced productivity. While vacation and personal time are always options, caregivers may also use the Family Medical Leave Act, which provides family members time to provide care. Generally, studies on employed caregivers report that 20% to 30% experience work-related challenges and distress.[64,65] When faced with employment demands, women appear particularly at risk for emotional distress and greater perceived care demands.[66] For some caregivers, however, employment provides respite and serves as a buffer to distress.[27,66-68]

CAREGIVER-RELATED ISSUES

Multiple caregiver characteristics have been linked with the degree to which a family member will perceive burden associated with providing care. Understanding these groups of caregivers is vital for identifying those at risk for burden. Gender, for example, has been established to be differentially related to caregiver distress. Overall, caregiving is reported to be more stressful for women (wives and daughters) than for men (husbands and sons), yet women have been shown to be more responsive to caregiver interventions.[2,47,69]

Older age presents challenges, especially for caregiver spouses who may be on fixed incomes, and who may be in poor physical health themselves. Low personal and household incomes, loss of income, out-of-pocket expenses, and limited financial resources all contribute to caregiver stress for these older caregivers.[45,47,68,70] However, studies have consistently revealed that adult children, especially daughters, exhibit higher levels of burden and lower well-being than older caregivers. This may be related to an increase in competing demands of family, work, leisure, and social obligations for younger caregivers.

CAREGIVER HEALTH CONDITIONS

Caregivers who are burdened consistently report lower levels of physical health. Although the sources of caregivers' lower levels of physical health are multifaceted and to some extent unexplored, caregivers report higher levels of chronic conditions, pain, sleep disturbance, fatigue, headaches, lower immune functioning, altered response to influenza immunizations, slower wound healing, higher blood pressure, and altered lipid profiles.[19,29,71-79] Caregivers have been shown to have marked changes in a broad array of neurohormonal and inflammatory parameters in the year after patient diagnosis. The most striking changes were in systemic inflammation and increased risk for coronary heart disease. Data suggest that caring for a family member with brain cancer may heighten vulnerability to coronary disease, as well as other metabolic, autoimmune, and psychiatric conditions sensitive to inflammation.[25] Older caregivers with higher levels of depression, fatigue, and pain reported lower physical functioning.[80]

In addition to burden, depression, and demands of the tasks of care, older caregivers may themselves have chronic diseases, which are often left unattended as a result of care demands. Caregivers may forgo personal health maintenance due to the pressures of providing care for others.[13,81] Primary care providers need to encourage caregivers to manage their own health problems to continue providing quality care. Studies have shown negative caregiver outcomes when spouses are hospitalized.[82,83] Providers must remain vigilant of caregivers' health and the potential impact this may have on their ability to provide patient care.

CASE 26-3

L.'s husband has colorectal cancer and is unable to provide basic self-care as a result of disease progression. An aide comes in daily for an hour to bathe him. He has a colostomy that needs vigilant attention. The skin surrounding his stoma looks normal and the stoma is pink and appears healthy. The room is filled with medical supplies.

L. confided that her symptoms of congestive heart failure have gotten worse in the past couple of weeks. She states that she gets winded very easily and she has occasional chest pain. She also has a history of atrial fibrillation and she can feel her heart fluttering. She does not want her health to keep her from caring for her husband. She is intentionally keeping her health problems from her husband's medical team. She states her diabetes is well controlled with insulin injections. She takes alprazolam for anxiety, which has gotten much worse since her husband's diagnosis.

Social Support

The availability and use of social networks and social interaction have been shown to alleviate and prevent caregiver burden.[84] Feelings of emotional connectedness and cohesion with one's social network protects caregivers from burden and distress. Support such as understanding, counseling, and acting as a confidant may help moderate their burden.[74,85,86] It is important for providers to communicate with caregivers on how to effectively monitor and manage their patients.

Relationship to the Patient

Wives, husbands, daughters, and sons approach the practice of caregiving in different ways.[31] Spousal caregivers of older cancer patients have been shown to be at high risk for caregiver burden because they live with the patient, provide the most extensive and comprehensive care, maintain their role longer, often assume other household tasks, and tolerate greater levels of patient disability.[29,87] Alternatively, spouses may have stronger established patterns of decision making with the patient, which can facilitate treatment and symptom management decisions. Other researchers report that adult children are at high risk for burden because of a larger disruption in lifestyle from competing demands (careers, children, their own spouse).[88] Providers should assess the patient/caregiver relationship from the beginning and observe changes over time to understand when mounting strain, tensions, and burden may occur.

Preexisting discord in family relationships may be aggravated by the care process, by decision making, and by how different family members respond to the challenges of cancer care.[89-91] Perceived family conflict, withdrawal, changes in family dynamics, and loss of intimate exchange with the cancer patient may be associated with a range of negative psychosocial patient outcomes, as well as with caregiver burden. Among caregivers in relationships that are less mutually satisfying, patient needs may restrict caregivers' usual activities, which in turn may increase caregiver resentment and burden.[15,47,90,92]

Socioeconomic Status and Insurance

Socioeconomic status poses unique challenges for caregivers of cancer patients. For most caregivers of spouses, Medicare provides basic coverage of health benefits, yet there are limits to coverage for ambulatory care services, some home care services, and limitations in payment for some drug protocols, particularly those that are newly approved by the FDA. The challenges for older cancer patients and their caregivers include copays and supplemental insurance for new expensive treatments. Medicare coverage is limited in what is covered and the amount covered. Out-of-pocket costs are often high. Concerns about financial status are pervasive; for example, oral agents may cost thousands of dollars per month, often with a copay.[63,70]

CASE 26-4

A. is a 68-year-old woman whose husband was recently diagnosed with lung cancer. A. reports a very weak family support system. She has two daughters who are married and live out-of-state.

A. has a great deal of concern about her finances; her husband was laid off around the same time as the diagnosis and is having trouble finding new employment because of his physical limitations. She has extremely large copayments for the medical care. She would like more financial assistance but there seems to be none available and she feels the pressure of financial costs. Above all, A. wants to take care of her husband, and feels burdened by the financial uncertainty and by her husband's future.

CAREGIVER TRAITS

Providers should assess caregiver traits and personal resources to help them alleviate distress. Dispositional optimism is a stable personality trait that can be thought of as a generalized expectancy of good outcomes, even in the face of adversity. Those with a sense of optimism feel they can better endure the negative effects of caregiving. Caregiver optimism has been associated with better quality of life, lower depression, less delay and anxiety in seeking care, and higher expectation of a positive outcome of medical care, making optimism a protective mechanism against burden. Optimists may be using different coping strategies than pessimists when confronted with stressful events.[93,94] Pessimism has been found to be a warning sign for compromised health in the caregiver. Caregiver optimism, for example, is directly related to how family members perceive the care situation and, in turn, relates to the degree of burden caregivers will perceive.[85,90,95,96] Another caregiver trait similar to optimism is mastery, which is the perception of their sense of worth as a caregiver and how they perceive their ability to meet the demands of providing care.[66,85,97] Interventions are recommended to strengthen optimistic attitudes and weaken the pessimistic view, without giving a false sense of optimism when a cure is not possible. Mastery has been shown to positively influence caregivers' level of burden, their depressive symptoms, and their response to care.[98,99] Caregivers with a high sense of mastery have reported using more problem-focused coping strategies to meet care demands[100-102] and ultimately have indicated a lower level of caregiver burden.[30,103,104] Health care practitioners can strive to improve caregivers' sense of mastery by enhancing their knowledge and skills and reducing their feelings of uncertainty, thus lowering the risk for emotional distress. Caregiver mastery can also be improved by implementing educational and cognitive behavioral interventions for meeting caregiver needs to provide care.[97]

RISK ASSESSMENT FOR CAREGIVER BURDEN

Risk assessments for caregivers are vital to identify individuals at risk for negative outcomes and to provide information on resources for patient and caregiver care, such as cancer-related community resources (e.g., major cancer support organizations), as well as sources of additional information (e.g., Internet Web sites). The assessment should address major areas of functioning including role, social, and family functioning and should identify any practical problems stemming from care demands, such as managing equipment, finances, household tasks, arranging appointments, and transportation).

A risk appraisal measure (RAM), a brief screen for caregivers, has been used for dementia. It assesses multiple dimensions of risk and adverse outcomes in six areas: depression, burden, self-care and health behaviors, social support, safety, and patient problem behaviors. The RAM (Table 26-1) appears to be an efficient and easily administered tool that could provide a "road map" of interventions for providers. Such a tool would increase the likelihood for a caregiver to receive assistance in the areas needed to prevent or relieve burden.[105] (See Table 26-1).

Another caregiver assessment form has been developed by the American Medical Association.[106] This assessment focuses on caregiver stress, depression, need for support, and need for decision making. Both assessment forms are brief and may be useful for screening caregivers for emotional and physical distress. A more in-depth multidimensional caregiver burden tool, such as the Caregiver Reaction Assessment,[9] is suggested for long-term monitoring and planning interventions.

Overall areas to be included in a comprehensive assessment include: relationships between members of the dyad; necessary role changes; patient care requirements (symptoms, ADL, IADL); information needs about diagnosing treatment and expectations; care coordination;

TABLE 26-1	Risk Appraisal Measure (RAM)
Domain	**RAM Items**
Self-care and healthy behaviors	Sleep
	Rating of physical health
Patient problem behaviors	Information symptoms
	Feels stress with trying to help patient with ADL
Burden	Stress trying to meet responsibilities
	Strain around patient
	Feels good as a result of caregiving
Depression	Felt depressed last week
Social support	Satisfaction with help from friends
	Satisfaction with support from others
Safety	Felt like yelling
	Felt like hitting
	Able to leave patient alone

ADL, activities of daily living.

hours of care; capacity of caregiver; caregiver's own health status and expected role in care and support; and resources available for care. (Table 26-2).

ASSESSMENT OF FAMILY CAREGIVER TO PLAN CARE

Cancer caregiver needs vary across experiences and thus providers must identify those needs and know they may change at key transition points, such as when the patient's care level goes from active treatment to palliative care. Reassessment is necessary and should be conducted regularly. Health care providers need to recognize that caregivers have varying levels of knowledge and skills and shoulder different levels of burden as they deal with constantly changing stages of patient demands. Providers must consider their approach on the basis of a given caregiver's skills and level of knowledge, and tailor their interventions to those needs. Personal and community resource referrals also depend on family caregiver needs.

CAREGIVER CHARACTERISTICS

Caregiver Self-Care

Caregivers involved with older cancer patients need to ensure that they consider their own self-care. Studies have shown that they discontinue vital health screenings and self-care such as exercise. Some studies have shown that increased health care use, increased total costs of care, and increased rates of psychiatric diagnosis may occur up to 2 years after caring for an older patient with cancer.[35]

Role of Primary Care Provider. With appropriate information and support in place, primary care physicians[107] appear willing to assist cancer patients and their family caregivers during treatment. Primary care physicians

TABLE 26-2	**Assessment of Family Caregiver to Plan Care**

Type and Quality of Prior Family Relationship (Prior to incident of care)
1. What was the quality of the relationship between the patient and family?
2. What is the usual decision-making and communication pattern about health care within the family?

Initiation and Maintenance of the Family Role
1. What is the duration of the "care" relationship expected to be with the formal system?
2. What are the expectations for patient and family involvement in care?

Patient Characteristics:
1. What are the care requirements?
2. What are the signs and symptoms of disease or treatment that require family assistance?
3. What are the emotional and supportive needs?

Care System and Involvement Required:
1. What are the care requirements?
2. What is the patient's functional level and what family involvement is needed?
3. What are the hours of care per week? Per day?
4. What components of home care cause the *family* difficulty or distress?
5. What are the skills and assistance needed from the formal system?

Factors Related to Diagnosis and Treatment:
1. What are the patient and family expectations and knowledge about the course of the disease and its treatment?
2. What is the expected length of the overall treatment?
3. What is the likely treatment outcome? (Is recovery expected?)

Family Member Characteristics:
1. What is the relationship of the patient to the family members assisting with care?
2. What other family, work, or social roles exist for those helping with care?
3. What roles have been given up by the family to maintain the care (work, family, social)?
4. What are family member/formal system interactions around care?
5. What emotional support do family members need, are they burdened? Do they express burden?

Patient's and Family's Role in Care:
1. What is the availability of family members to assist with care?
2. Do the family members feel they have adequate knowledge/skills needed to provide care?
3. Does the family feel "prepared" and competent to care?
4. In what areas do family members need assistance? Which treatments?
5. What skills do family members need?

Support and Resources for Care
1. What "other" family resources are available to assist with care?
2. Is there adequate perceived support available?
3. What other resources should be mobilized to assist the family?

Care Outcomes and Status:
1. What negative reactions or burdens from home care are evident from the family member?
2. What is the perceived impact of care on the family member's physical and mental health?
3. How does the family perceive that care affects their daily activities and role responsibilities? Do they express burden?

can regularly monitor caregivers for distress, particularly at critical time points in the patient's disease trajectory. Referrals for psychological counseling and support, caregiver education, and assistance toward improving communication are vital.

INTERVENTIONS TO SUPPORT CAREGIVERS

Family caregivers need to feel better prepared to handle care demands including decision making, symptom control, and medication administration. When caregiver needs are not addressed, their physical and mental health

is at risk, which may threaten the level of care the cancer patient receives. To ensure the appropriate and effective delivery of services, providers need to: (1) link patients and families to needed community and health care services; (2) coordinate care; (3) ensure that patients and families receive follow-up care; and (4) monitor the effectiveness of services upon patient referral. Often, family members do not take advantage of the available services. The capacity and ability of the caregiver also determines what resources are needed.

Caregivers develop a pattern of care, such as shared involvement, often within the first 6 to 8 weeks of care. They often describe their approach as trial and error.

Caregivers share care activities and respond together along with the patients to the demands of the illness and the patient's plan of care. Patients' preferences and abilities are the driving force in determining what the pattern of care is. Caregivers faced with unclear, incomplete, unknown, and changing role expectations may experience more role strain and burden and may not perform their duties as effectively as possible. Caregivers should be a major part of the plan of care developed for the older cancer patient. Providers need to assist caregivers to perform care tasks, coordinate resources, or find the support they need.

Interventions to help the patient with cancer require the caregiver to build skills, solve problems, and set priorities specific to the needs of the older patient. Interventions must help to alleviate caregiver distress, improve patient outcomes, and reduce health service utilization. Interventions should also be directed toward caregivers' emotional needs including assistance with stress reduction, time management, burden reduction, depression and anxiety management, and consideration of the caregiver's own health maintenance and self-care.[108] From the interventions used to help caregivers, only small to moderate effects have been found, but caregivers' burden can be reduced, their ability to cope can be improved, and their confidence in their ability to provide care can be increased. More-prepared, less-distressed caregivers will be better equipped to provide positive care for patients.

Educational and Informational Interventions

It is important that caregivers get education to help with problem solving and decisions, as well as information about the disease, its treatment, management of signs and symptoms, and prevention of adverse events. However, caregivers often become saturated and overwhelmed with too much information, which may not be tailored to their needs and which may be contradictory and irrelevant. Caregivers should be receiving information as they need it and when they can use it. A coach, mentor, or guide is found helpful by caregivers as they try to apply their new knowledge and skills.[4] In turn, caregivers can use that information to learn how to make care decisions.[109] When information alone is provided, it should give caregivers an opportunity to translate their new knowledge into action for patient care. There are numerous modes for information delivery, such as voice response systems, Web-based sites, and printed toolkits; all are readily available to aid patients and caregivers. Cancer centers can then provide recommendations about these informational resources to caregivers so that they will be directed to appropriate and credible sites. Caregivers need information in order to know and understand the patient's illness, his or her care needs, and their own role in that care. Information can improve caregivers'

self-efficacy and may increase their accuracy in determining which symptoms patients are experiencing.[110]

Social Support Interventions

Caregivers need support from their families, from their coworkers, and from health care providers,[2] and should identify a key support person in each of these areas. Social support may come in various forms; several Web-based social networks have shown promise in reducing burden. There is preliminary evidence that telephone counseling may also increase social problem-solving skills and provide social support.[111] Good relationships, contact with friends, and social support from family and friends contribute to positive caregiver responses.[112] Social networks have proven vital in determining caregivers' responses to providing care: Those with strong social networks can receive much-needed guidance and support.[95] Supportive interventions focus on building rapport and creating an opportunity and forum to discuss difficulties, successes, and feelings about caregiving. Social support interventions[113] allowed participants in group settings to provide mutual support to one another, provided opportunities to share methods of dealing with caregiving difficulties, and identified strategies to incorporate these ideas into care.

Problem-Solving Skills and Psychoeducational Interventions

Psychoeducational interventions that concomitantly focus on providing information, teaching problem-solving skills, and utilizing psychological support and counseling approaches to decrease caregiver distress have lent tremendous support to caregivers. Psychoeducational interventions often involve multiple components that address areas such as symptom management, monitoring of problems, coordination of resources, health care communication, cognitive reframing, and emotional support,[16,114,115] and have produced improvements in caregiver levels of emotional tension and confidence, as well as in positive problem-solving skills for the management of care demands.[59,116-121]

Providers can assist caregivers by encouraging them to challenge negative thoughts, engage in positive activities, and develop problem-solving abilities that focus on time management, emotional control, and incorporating these skills into day-to-day care demands.[122,123]

Home Health Care Interventions and Care Coordination

Few intervention studies have focused on how home care support for family caregivers enhances coordination of care, improves support, and benefits caregiver outcomes.[124] Unfortunately, home health care interventions are unlikely to be reimbursed unless skilled care is required. Although community services may provide assistance to family members, particularly older spouses, the need to arrange community resources contributes to the complexity of the care family members must provide. In addition, they may be reluctant to accept help for a variety of reasons. They often need help in finding the resources that are available in the community. Interventions that help family members mobilize resources such as chore services, homemaker services, or transportation should be considered. Assessing need and the care trajectory over time is crucial.

Summary

The duration and depth of care provided by family members and its impact on patient outcomes is under-recognized and often underappreciated. Concern for caregivers as partners in patient care and caregiver outcomes deserves careful attention by providers. A family plan of care should also be considered when an older person has a cancer diagnosis. Providers are challenged to recognize the value of the early and continued involvement of family members as care partners. Once this occurs, practitioners can more accurately identify situations that place caregivers at risk for burden and distress, which ultimately will decrease untoward hospitalizations and emergency department visits and improve patients' quality of life. Balancing the achievement of patient outcomes against the impact that providing this care has upon family members is the ultimate goal for family cancer care.

See expertconsult.com for a complete list of references and web resources for this chapter

SUGGESTED READINGS

1. Bradley CJ, Given B, Given C, et al: Physical, economic, and social issues confronting patients and families. In Yarbro C, Frogge M, Goodman M, editors: *Cancer Nursing: Principles and Practice*, ed 6, Boston, 2004, Jones and Bartlett Publishers.
2. Czaja S, Gitlin L, Schulz R, et al: Development of the risk appraisal measure: A brief screen to identify risk areas and guide interventions for dementia caregivers, *JAGS* 57:1064–1072, 2009.

3. Gallagher-Thompson D, Doon D: Evidence-based psychological treatments for distress in family caregivers of older adults, *Psychol Aging* 22:37–51, 2007.
4. Gaugler JE, Linder J, Given CW, et al: Family cancer caregiving and negative outcomes: The direct and meditational effects of psychosocial resources, *J Fam Nurs* 15:417–444, 2009.
5. Given B, Sherwood P, Given C: What knowledge and skills do caregivers need? *Am J Nurs* 108(Suppl 9):28–34, 2008.
6. Lobchuk M, McClement S, Daeninck PJ, et al: Asking the right question of informal caregivers about patient symptom experiences: Multiple proxy perspectives and reducing inter-rater gap, *J Pain & Symptom Manage* 33:130–145, 2007.
7. Lobchuk MM, Vorauer JD: Family caregiver perspective-taking and accuracy in estimating cancer patient symptom experiences, *Soc Sci Med* 57:2379–2384, 2003.
8. Reiss-Sherwood P, Given B, Given C: Who cares for the caregiver: Strategies to provide support, *Home Health Care Manage Prac* 14:110–121, 2002.
9. Robison J, Fortinsky R, Kleppiner A, et al: A broad view of family caregiving: Effects of caregiving and caregiver conditions on depressive symptoms, health, work, and social isolation, *J Gerontol B Psychol Sci Soc Sci* 64:788–798, 2009.
10. Rohleder N, Marin T, Ma R, et al: Biologic cost of caring for a cancer patient: Dysregulation of pro- and anti-inflammatory signaling pathways, *J Clin Oncol* 27:2909–2915, 2009.
11. Swore Fletcher BA, Dodd MJ, Schumacher KL, et al: Symptom experience of family caregivers of patients with cancer, *Oncol Nurs Forum* 35:E23–E44, 2008.
12. Toseland R, Naccarato T, Wray L: Telephone groups for older persons and family caregivers: Key implementation and process issues, *Clin Gerontol* 31:59–76, 2007.
13. Zarit S, Femia E: Behavioral and psychosocial interventions for family caregivers, *Am J Nurs* 108:47–53, 2008.

Communication and Coordination

Peter Ward and James W. Davis Jr.

Coordination of care between oncologists and geriatricians is essential in the care of patients with cancer. Geriatric patients with cancer often have multiple complex comorbidities, making their oncology care more complex as well. Studies have shown that shared care models, where primary care physicians (PCPs) and geriatricians have an active role in the management of geriatric oncology, may improve patient satisfaction. Good communication between geriatricians and oncologists is the key part of this shared care model, but many other disciplines may be involved as well. In this chapter, a case study is presented that illustrates potential pitfalls in communication between the oncologist and the geriatrician during the different stages of cancer care. The chapter will also demonstrate how a shared care model works, the preferred methods of communication in certain circumstances, and how good communication may improve outcomes.

CASE 27-1

A.G. is an 81-year-old woman with a history of hypertension; a widow, she lived alone and was independent in her daily activities. She had complained about declining memory and family members had become concerned about her ability to continue to live alone and drive a car. She was forgetful about taking medications but her score on the Folstein mini-mental state examination (MMSE) was 28/30 (within normal limits). She declined to have help at home and was considering a move to assisted living. Several months prior to diagnosis she began to lose weight. She later complained of a dry cough. Chest x-ray showed a large (9.5 cm) mass in the right upper lobe of the lung.

WORKUP

The geriatrician or PCP usually initiates the workup of most cancers. There can be many potential ways to conduct the workup and preliminary consultation with an oncologist at this time can be helpful. For example in the case described above, the PCP may not know whether the patient needs to see a pulmonologist to attempt a diagnosis via bronchoscopy or if it would be more

expedient to have an interventional radiologist perform a computed tomography (CT)-guided biopsy. It is preferable that these tests and procedures be ordered prior to the first consultation with the oncologist. There is often an urgency to make a diagnosis, especially if the patient is at a potentially curable stage. The fastest and most efficient way to communicate during this stage of cancer care is directly by phone or via email. Not only can this expedite the workup, but the PCP can also try to set up the initial consultation for the patient with the oncologist, assuming the workup will be completed in 1 to 2 weeks. This can be a critical time for the development of shared care, where the PCP and the oncologist begin to define their respective roles in communicating diagnosis, prognosis, and plans for future care. It is essential to give the patient and family clear information and to establish lines of communication so the family will know how to access care and address problems as they arise.

Often, these impromptu consults are termed "curbside" consults. Studies of "curbside" consultations have shown that advice by means of email, fax, and telephone has been shown to be very useful.[1] They can often be used to determine the need for a more formal consultation. This may be especially true in geriatric oncology. The geriatrician who has a high suspicion of cancer in a patient may be unsure whether to pursue a time-consuming, expensive, and potentially distressing workup for a patient with multiple comorbidities. A "curbside" consultation may help clarify whether or not the patient would be fit enough to tolerate treatment before embarking on the workup. "Curbside" consultations have also been shown to improve or maintain good relationships with other physicians. Interestingly, more subspecialists than primary care physicians felt that "curbside" consultations were important for maintaining good relationships among physicians.[2] However, these types of informal consultations have potential pitfalls. Studies have shown that the information conveyed may be incomplete or inaccurate. Also many physicians, especially subspecialists, may dislike "curbside" consultations because of the potential legal ramifications of giving such informal advice; also, there may be no reimbursement for time spent answering these types of consults.

Another barrier to communication is the preference of the oncologist to have a tissue diagnosis before getting involved in a case. This is more often a problem in the academic setting where physicians tend to be salaried than in community cancer centers where oncologists see patients on a fee-for-service basis and are competing for referrals. However, if the referring physician knows the oncologist and maintains open lines of communication, especially in the academic setting, there is usually more willingness to assist in the workup before the first formal consultation.

DIAGNOSIS AND REFERRAL

CASE 27-1	CONTINUED

A.G. failed to keep several appointments for interventional radiology and diagnostic studies. Social services were contacted and the family became more involved. She appeared weaker and more confused. She was brought to appointments by family members but did not always recall the purpose of the visits. With the help and encouragement of her family, she moved into an assisted-living facility. Her lung biopsy revealed well-differentiated squamous cell carcinoma. She and family members met with a geriatric oncologist.

The time between the diagnosis and referral can be crucial. Good communication between the oncologist and the PCP can reduce delays between diagnosis and treatment. The uncertainties of treating geriatric patients with cancer can sometimes exacerbate these delays. In a study of breast cancer patients, the main factors that were independently related to delays in care were older age, lack of Social Security, and advanced stage.[3] Other barriers that may prevent older patients from being referred to an oncologist have been identified. The most common issues cited by PCPs are long waiting lists, mandatory tissue diagnosis before referral, and the belief that oncologists seldom relate to PCPs. In this same study, 86% of PCPs said they would refer an older patient with early-stage, potentially curable cancers, but only 65% would refer those with advanced-stage, potentially incurable cancers. Factors that influence the PCP's decision to refer were a patient's desire to be referred, the type of cancer, the stage of the cancer, and the severity of the cancer symptoms. According to this study, age was not a factor in the primary's decision of whether or not to refer the patient.[4]

When the decision to refer the patient is made, what is the best way to refer? This depends on the urgency of the referral. Someone with life-threatening disease is usually hospitalized where multiple subspecialists can be consulted simultaneously and a treatment plan can be made together. In patients who have rapidly progressive disease but are medically stable, coordination of care usually occurs in the outpatient setting. These urgent

TABLE 27-1	When Should a Referral Be Communicated By Phone?

- When the consult is urgent
- When there is sensitive information to convey (i.e., patient dissatisfaction with previous consultants)
- If there are any psychosocial problems that may affect treatment
- If the case is too complex to convey in a written form

consults are best communicated by phone. As electronic medical records and resources become more frequently used, email may also be an effective way of communicating an urgent consult. A study of an email consultation service at the Walter Reed Army Medical Center showed that this could be a viable option. In a 20-month period, 3121 consultations were logged. The average time to response was approximately 12 hours. The implementation of the system required little extra training on the part of the users. In general, the use of this system mirrored the usual clinical practice of consultation and response. However, the study did identify potential barriers, such as a lack of secure communication and difficulty assigning workload credit for the participants, which may limit the use of this system in a broader setting.[5] Other reasons to refer by phone or email, as opposed to sending a letter, are to convey sensitive information, to relate any psychosocial problems that may affect treatment, or to convey information that may be too complex to communicate through a letter (Table 27-1).

Although telephone consultations seem to be the quickest and most direct way to initiate a consultation, some potential pitfalls of using this method of communication have been studied. A qualitative study of telephone consults between physicians identified five sources of tension: presentation, context, fragmented clinical process, reason for call, and responsibility. Consultants complained that the pace of conversation was too fast or too slow. Sometimes information was not conveyed because of the accent of the caller or because the caller was disorganized when describing the case. A case that may be extremely urgent from the perspective of the caller, may be just one of 10 phone consults that an oncologist receives during a day in which he is seeing 20 other patients in the office. The clinical process in phone consultations is fragmented and information passed from caller to consultant can be inaccurate or incomplete. A PCP may call a consultant for reassurance about a case; the consultant may view this as inappropriate, especially if his or her opinion is different from the caller's. Responsibility for a case may cause tensions in both directions. A caller may be trying to pass the responsibility of a complex case on to a consultant; alternatively, a consultant may find it easier to have a patient transferred to his or her hospital so as to see the patient in person, while the caller is reluctant to release the patient from his or her own care. All of these tensions tend to undermine the quality of care. (Table 27-2.)

TABLE 27-2	Five Sources of Tension during Telephone Consultations
Tension	**Examples**
Presentation	The pace, accent, organization, and tone of the caller or consultant may make it difficult for the other to understand or may create emotional tension.
Context	An urgent and important case to the caller may be just one of 10 telephone calls the consultant receives while rounding on other patients.
Fragmented Information	The consultant has to rely on observations and knowledge of the caller and information may be inaccurate or incomplete.
Responsibility	It may be easier for the consultant to take over the care of the patient, while the caller is only asking for advice and is not willing to give up the responsibility of the patient's care.
Reason for Call	The consultant may be asked to provide information that the caller could find in the medical literature, but may not have time to search for.

TABLE 27-3	Essential Information on Referral From PCP to the Oncologist

- Reason for consult
- Past medical history/chronic medical conditions that may affect oncology treatment
- Current medications
- Pertinent information on tests performed and the results
- Contact information of other consultants involved
- What the patient has been told about his or her diagnosis
- Concerns about any psychosocial problems that may affect treatment
- If there is a need for an interpreter and whether the patient is competent to make decisions

TABLE 27-4	Essential Information in the Consultation Reply Letter

- Restatement of the reason for consult
- Diagnosis and prognosis
- Details of the treatment plan
- Treatment goals and patient wishes/expectations
- Potential toxicities of the treatment and suggestions for management of these toxicities
- Concerns about psychosocial problems that may affect treatment
- What the patient has been told
- How to contact the oncologist

In the same study, the caller's and consultant's strategies for averting these tensions were reported. In some instances, the strategies used by the consultant to abate tension were seen by the caller as exacerbating tension. An example that was cited was a case where a consultant asked for the patient's laboratory results and the caller reported them as "all normal." The consultant then asked for the specific values of certain tests and the caller felt he was "being talked down to." Although they didn't offer specific strategies to avoid these circumstances, the authors of this study felt that it was important for both callers and consultants to recognize these tensions. They concluded that many physicians are poorly trained in professional communication skills and recommend that this be given greater importance in medical school curricula.[6]

In some circumstances, consults are made by means of a referral letter. A study of referral letters from PCPs to oncologists showed that the amount of information contained in the letters was quite variable. The key pieces of information for the PCP to convey to the oncologist are outlined in Table 27-3. As illustrated in the case above, the patient's "back story" can often be as important as the diagnosis and comorbidities. As pertains specifically to geriatric patients, a knowledge of geriatric syndromes such as cognitive impairment, history of falls, or other signs of frailty can strongly impact the oncologist's treatment plan. If this information has not been passed on from a physician who knows the patient well, it can sometimes be missed in an initial visit with the oncologist, who usually does not have the time to do a complete geriatric assessment.

In the initial consult note from the oncologist to the PCP, there are certain pieces of information that the

PCP regards as essential, as listed in Table 27-4. When patients first consult with an oncologist, they often find the amount of information they are given to be overwhelming. They then see their PCP and ask for information on things such as prognosis and potential toxicities. They may even ask the PCP whether or not to pursue treatment. If this information is conveyed in the oncologist's consult note, it can keep everyone "on the same page."[7]

TREATMENT

CASE 27-1	CONTINUED

After A.G.'s consultation with the geriatric oncologist, plans were made for her to begin chemotherapy treatment for her lung cancer. Before treatment began, the patient was seen in the emergency room for a fall and a lumbar spine compression fracture was found. She became less mobile and required increased assistance in her assisted-living facility.

Good communication leading up to the point when the patient starts treatment can make the comanagement easier. Many questions arise at this point, such as how care will be coordinated and how complications will be monitored and treated. If the patient is hospitalized, who will assume responsibility during hospitalization? The answers to these questions may depend on the setting.

In a small community hospital, patients may be under the care of a hospitalist or the primary physician, with oncology consulting, whereas most academic centers have oncology wards where patients are primarily cared for by oncologists. One may assume in most settings that the oncologist would make most treatment decisions at this point, but a recent study of patient preferences showed that greater involvement by the PCP was associated with better patient satisfaction. Patients often prefer having treatment options described by the oncologist, but they depend on their PCP to discuss goals of care. Oncologists also prefer the PCP's involvement in discussions regarding goals of care.[8]

Patients often turn to their PCP when they are faced with difficult medical decisions after visits to specialists. This can be very evident when a geriatric patient is offered enrollment in a clinical trial. Most frequently, the invitation to participate in a clinical trial is introduced by the oncologist. Patients may feel pressured and suspect that the oncologist may be biased towards having the patient participate in the trial. Before enrolling in the trial, the patient may consult with his or her PCP. This is the time when the communication between the PCP and the oncologist will be crucial in order to do what is best for the patient. During this interaction, the oncologist can stress that there is a lack of level I evidence for optimal treatment of geriatric oncology patients. If there is good trust between the patient and the PCP, the importance of clinical trials can be presented in an unbiased way.

During the patient's cancer treatment, there are many aspects of care that the PCP may have more experience with, such as diabetes, COPD, or other chronic conditions. In many circumstances, the PCP may be the first to recognize signs of depression in a patient during treatment. In the same regard, the PCP may have more experience with treatment of depression. Close collaboration with the oncologist can minimize potential drug interactions between chemotherapy and any new medications added to the patient's regimen during this phase. Other issues that may fall under the expertise of the PCP during treatment include sexual concerns, fertility, contraception, and general health and nutrition.[14] In the case described above, a geriatrician would likely have more experience and knowledge about what additional services the patient may need in the assisted-living facility to improve her performance status before she begins chemotherapy.

Many of the common cancers in geriatric patients have a prolonged course of treatment. Breast cancer and prostate cancer patients often survive for many years. What prevents good communication during the treatment phase? A survey of PCPs comanaging patients undergoing chemotherapy showed that one of the most valued aspects of communication is the accessibility of the oncologist.[9] Both the oncologist and the PCP are extremely busy, and trying to reach one another by phone can often interrupt other patients' visits. A solution to this problem is for the oncologist to provide an email address in the consult reply letter. The PCP often serves as the first contact for health concerns that arise either as a consequence of the cancer or for unrelated problems such as in the aforementioned case. The PCP can alert the oncologist of such events before the patient's next visit and adjustments can be made in the treatment plan, so that unnecessary visits may be avoided. In the case above, the PCP alerted the oncologist to the patient's change in performance status and her treatment was delayed.

TOXICITIES

CASE 27-1	CONTINUED

After physical therapy and increased support from her family, A.G. was able to improve her functional status and began treatment for her lung cancer. She received her first cycle of gemcitabine, which she tolerated without any immediate side effects. About 12 days later, she began to have nosebleeds and presented to her geriatrician's office. A complete blood count was checked and she was found to be thrombocytopenic.

Managing toxicities of chemotherapy can be challenging for PCPs. As the armamentarium of chemotherapy continues to expand, it is increasingly difficult for PCPs to keep up with potential side effects of newer agents. In the case above, the primary care physician may or may not recognize thrombocytopenia as a common side effect of gemcitabine. Even if the PCP does recognize it, he or she would most likely call the oncologist to discuss how to manage this toxicity. As mentioned before, it is important to explain potential toxicities and strategies for management of these side effects in the initial consult note sent from the oncologist to the PCP. A simple and effective way of doing this is to include in the reply letter a standard information sheet with data regarding the cancer type, potential side effects, and recommendations for their management. Less than 20% of oncologists' consult letters contain this information. A group of general practitioners (GPs) in Australia were randomized to receive either a fax of an information sheet regarding a patient's chemotherapy regimen in addition to a consult reply letter or to receive just the reply letter alone. The intervention group showed a significant increase in their confidence in being able to manage the side effects of chemotherapy. They also showed increased satisfaction with communication. When compared to the reply letter alone, the information sheet was shown to be significantly more instructive. In addition to these findings, it is notable that the study had a response rate of 84%, which speaks to the utility of this intervention. Interventions such as these not only help to inform the primary care physician, but they can potentially also help oncologists by decreasing the number of patients that are seen in their treatment centers for care of chemotherapy toxicities. This is a win-win situation, and one which can help maintain good lines of communication between oncologists and PCPs.[10]

FOLLOW-UP/SURVEILLANCE

CASE 27-1 CONTINUED

A.G. appeared to have a partial response after four cycles of therapy. She returned to her geriatrician with the understanding that her chemotherapy was finished and she did not require any further treatment. Her geriatrician and her oncologist had not spoken since the treatment had completed. The geriatrician was unsure of the follow-up plan and of whether she was in fact done with her treatment.

In the same way that it is important for the oncologist to inform the PCP about potential toxicities during the treatment phase, it is equally important for information on survivorship care to be communicated. As the number of long-term cancer survivors continues to grow and oncologists are forced to give preference to patients who are being actively treated, some of the burden of providing survivorship care will be carried by PCPs. During the surveillance period the PCP may not know how often the patient will need follow-up labs, CT scans, or other screening measures. In the case above, the PCP isn't sure if and when the patient may require more treatment. In addition, many chemotherapeutics may have long-term toxicities, such as heart failure with anthracyclines, which PCPs will need to follow as well. A study of PCPs who provide survivorship care showed that many of them feel undertrained to take on this burden. The study also showed that 82% of those surveyed believed that primary care guidelines for adult cancer survivors were not well defined.[11] Another study of breast cancer survivors looked at the patients' confidence in their PCP's ability to provide survivorship care. These women rated their PCP-related survivorship care at a level of 65 out of 100. They felt confident in the PCP's ability to provide general care, psychosocial support, and general health promotion, but expressed doubt about the PCP's knowledge of follow-up care, long-term toxicities of chemotherapy, or treatment of cancer-related symptoms. Unfortunately, only 28% of these patients felt that their PCPs and oncologists communicated well.[12]

In the geriatric population of cancer survivors, the issue of frailty is especially important. PCPs play an important role not only in screening and assessing for frailty in cancer survivors, but in managing frailty and keeping it from progressing. Cancer treatment can push a patient who is close to becoming frail past the threshold and into frailty. In these situations, it is best that the PCP take the lead in managing the patient, while the oncologist plays the role of advisor.

A study of collaboration between oncologists and PCPs in Canada showed that oncologists desire more involvement from PCPs in taking care of patients in remission. Both oncologists and PCPs expressed frustrations when trying to collaborate. The PCPs cited difficulty accessing oncologists and reluctance to contact oncologists because they were embarrassed by their own lack of knowledge. Oncologists surveyed in this study cited inadequate time, difficulty contacting, and unfamiliarity with most of the family physicians because there were so many of them. They noted that these PCPs varied in their interest in providing survivorship care. The oncologists also felt that PCPs sometimes gave patients preconceived ideas that exaggerated the toxicities of chemotherapy prior to the first consultations, thereby creating mistrust. Oncologists stressed the importance of passing information both ways between them and the PCPs. As much as they want to educate PCPs about potential toxicities, they also want to receive information from PCPs about when patients are admitted to the hospital, their tests, their surgery reports, and their incidental illnesses.

The oncologists expressed that they believed their role in survivorship care should be providing reassurance, managing toxicities, detecting recurrences, and gathering data for clinical trials. The authors noted that although oncologists treat patients with a multidisciplinary approach, they rarely include family physicians in these teams. They point out that there can often be an exclusive nature to cancer centers and they can be thought of by PCPs as a "black box." In the conclusion of the study, the authors identify several solutions to these problems. One proposal is for oncologists to identify a core group of PCPs who have a special interest in providing survivorship care. In order to provide survivorship care, it is important that the oncologist and the PCP discuss the patient at the beginning and the end of the cancer treatment. The authors also point out the importance of establishing follow-up guidelines that delineate who will be responsible for the patient in which circumstances. As a way of helping PCPs and oncologists get to know each other, the oncologists suggested holding informal seminars with case presentations to provide continuing medical education. They also suggested having an open house as a way of dispelling the idea of the cancer center as a black box.[13] (Table 27-5).

Although the roles of the PCP and the oncologist may be well defined during the surveillance period, it is less clear who is responsible for the patient at the end of life. At the end of life, whose responsibility is it to arrange for hospice care? This will to a great extent depend on patient preference. There may be other factors that influence this such as the stage at presentation to the oncologist, the length of treatment time, and the frequency of visits to the PCP during treatment. This is one of the most critical times for good communication between the

TABLE 27-5	System-Based Strategies for Improving Communication between Oncologists and PCPs

- Using templates when composing consult letters
- Including standardized educational materials with consult reply letters
- Including back-office phone numbers with consultation letters
- Giving patients discharge summaries to hand-deliver to the next provider after hospitalization
- Holding an open house at the cancer center
- Maintain a two-way flow of information

oncologist and the PCP. In cases where the PCP knows the patient well and has maintained contact during the treatment, it may be important to have a sense of closure with the patient and their family. In cases where the patient has progressed through multiple lines of therapy and it is unclear whether he or she would benefit from more treatment, the responsibility of introducing the concept of hospice clearly falls on the oncologist.

Summary

 Good communication between primary care physicians and oncologists from the workup to end-of-life care has been shown to improve patient satisfaction. This can be accomplished by the transfer of key pieces of information at the time of referral, after the initial consultation, and at times of transfers of care. The development of shared-care models during oncology treatment is increasingly important as patients navigate systems with multiple different specialties involved. PCPs often feel inadequately trained in their ability to comanage patients with cancer and they appreciate when oncologists share educational materials about treatment, toxicities, and surveillance. Most oncologists are not trained to recognize and manage geriatric syndromes and they rely on the referring geriatricians to point out signs and symptoms of frailty that may complicate cancer treatment. Methods to improve communication start with availability, outreach, and recognition of tensions during transmission of information. In the future, it will be important to study whether shared-care models have any impact on outcomes such as morbidity and mortality.

 See expertconsult.com for a complete list of references and web resources for this chapter

Palliative Care, Hospice and End of Life

Susan Charette and Elizabeth Whiteman

Cancer is a feared diagnosis at any age and, for the older patient, it can present a greater challenge and options for cure may be more limited. Traditional cancer care is typically focused on the disease process: reducing tumor burden and achieving remission. However, when patients are asked what kind of care they want if serious and life-threatening disease occurs, their preferences include pain and symptom control, avoidance of prolongation of the dying process, a sense of control, concern for the burden they may place on family, and an opportunity to strengthen relationships with loved ones.[1]

Palliative care addresses these issues and is an invaluable asset in the management of the older cancer patient. Much like the discipline of geriatric medicine, the palliative approach is interdisciplinary and addresses issues that arise in physical, psychological, social and spiritual domains. Unfortunately, many health care providers believe that palliative care and hospice are only indicated when the patient is in the final stage of their illness and near death. This limited view of palliative care and hospice is commonplace and does not address their potential usefulness and benefit in the care of the older cancer patient.

This chapter will provide an introduction to palliative care and hospice for the older cancer patient. Special attention will be paid to common issues that arise for these patients including pain and nonpain symptom management, as well as the Medicare Hospice Benefit, determining prognosis, and advance directives.

PALLIATIVE CARE AND HOSPICE

The terms palliative care and hospice are not synonymous but complementary. Palliative care is centered on the relief of suffering for patients with life-threatening or debilitating illness and the improvement of quality of life for patients and their families.[2] Palliative care focuses on the needs and goals of the patient and his or her family, in addition to the tumor and its treatment. Pain control, symptom management, psychosocial needs, goals of care, and quality of life are primary endpoints. Palliative

> **CASE 28-1**
>
> Mrs. T. is an 85-year-old woman with a history of rheumatoid arthritis and mild cognitive impairment. She is a widow who lives in her own apartment two blocks away from her only child, a daughter. She is independent in her activities of daily living and her instrumental activities of daily living. At a routine doctor's appointment, Mrs. T reports a persistent cough and mild dyspnea on exertion for the past 2 months. A chest x-ray demonstrates a mass with an associated postobstructive pneumonia. Further studies are obtained and Mrs. T. is diagnosed with stage 4 non-small cell carcinoma of the lung. Both the patient and her daughter are shocked by the diagnosis. Upon meeting the oncologist for the first time, the daughter asks, "What are my mother's options?"

care is interdisciplinary and incorporates medicine, nursing, social work, psychology, nutrition, and rehabilitation.[3] Treatments and interventions are used to control symptoms but not to advance or accelerate the death process.[4]

Mrs. T. has stage 4 non-small cell lung cancer and she will not be cured. She and her daughter need to be informed that while curative treatment is not available, there may be treatments that may decrease her tumor burden, reduce her symptoms, maintain her function, and improve her quality of life. By choosing a palliative chemotherapy or referring a patient for palliative radiation, the oncologist is doing palliative care. If the oncologist or primary medical doctor needs help controlling symptoms or discussing goals of care, an inpatient or outpatient palliative medicine consultation may be available to help address these issues. For older patients with cancer, especially those with advanced disease at the time of diagnosis, palliative care should start early in the course of care.

"Hospice" can represent a philosophy of practice as well as an agency or facility that provides care for patients with end-stage disease. Hospice utilizes a comprehensive, palliative approach to care that is interdisciplinary and symptom-focused. Most older patients in the

United States with advanced cancer will be eligible for the Medicare Hospice Benefit under Medicare Part A. Eligibility for Medicare Hospice benefit is determined by four criteria. First, the patient must be eligible for Medicare A. Next the patient must have a terminal condition and two physicians must certify that life expectancy is 6 months or less, given his or her prognosis. The patient must choose hospice care and the patient or agent must give informed consent. Finally, comprehensive care has to be provided by a Medicare-certified hospice. If these criteria are satisfied, all medicines, durable medical equipment, and care related to the terminal diagnosis are covered. Medicare Part B will still pay for covered benefits for any health problems that are not related to the terminal diagnosis.[5] Patients who meet criteria for hospice benefit have to be reviewed by the interdisciplinary team and certified by the medical director or hospice physician. Benefit periods consist of two 90-day periods, followed by an unlimited number of 60-day periods if life expectancy remains at 6 months or less.

Under the Medicare Hospice Benefit, the hospice team must include a physician, nurse, bath aide, social worker, chaplain, volunteers, and possibly therapists when appropriate.[6] Bereavement support for 1 year after a patient's death is also included in this benefit. All medical supplies and durable medical equipment and any medication related to the terminal diagnosis and for symptom control are covered by the benefit. Most patients receive hospice services in their private home or in the nursing home setting. Although not commonplace, freestanding hospice facilities provide room and board along with care by the hospice team when the patient qualifies under "Inpatient Status," which is typically for symptoms out of control. Most private insurance companies will also use Medicare-certified hospice criteria to enroll patients in hospice. Hospice care must provide comprehensive palliative care for terminally ill patients with a usual estimated life expectancy of 6 months or less. The care must include treatment of physical symptoms, social support, spiritual and emotional care, and bereavement care. Hospice benefits can play an important role when the patient and the physician agree that inpatient or other aggressive treatments are not in the patient's best interest. The patient care will focus on symptom management with a switch to full palliation of symptoms and care, usually outside the inpatient hospital setting.

Hospice care can take place in different settings and the Medicare benefit provides four levels of care: routine home care, continuous home care, general inpatient care, and respite care.[7] Routine home care is the most common level of care. Most patients receiving this level of care are in the home or nursing home setting. Patients have to be able to care for themselves at home or have appropriate caregiver support. The Medicare Hospice Benefit does not cover the cost of caregivers or nursing home room and board. All other services mentioned above are covered and the hospice must provide 24-hour on-call services. Continuous home care is for crises and for management of acute symptoms. This care can be provided in the home or in a long-term nursing home setting as well. Nursing care from 8 to 24 hours is arranged to provide intensive palliation of symptoms; such care may include titration of pain medications and the use of intravenous medications to gain control of symptoms. General inpatient care is for control of acute pain or symptoms that cannot be managed in the home or nursing home. This level of care can be provided in an inpatient hospital or freestanding hospice. Respite care is provided for caregivers that need relief or a break and is offered for up to 5 days at a time. Care can be provided 24 hours per day and includes custodial care at a hospice facility, intermediate care facility, or a hospital that contracts with the hospice.

EPIDEMIOLOGY

The need for palliative care among our older cancer patients will continue to grow in the coming years. There were nearly 1.5 million new cancer cases in the United States projected for 2009.[1] One in four Americans die from cancer, and 70% of these cancer-related deaths occur in persons older than 65 years.[1,8] These numbers are expected to increase dramatically with the aging of our population; also, older patients are more likely to have advanced or incurable disease at diagnosis and therefore are in greatest need of palliative care.[8]

An ongoing challenge will be how to meet the palliative care needs of these patients. While the number of hospitals with palliative care programs has doubled over the last 10 years, the 2008 American Hospital Association Annual Survey of U.S. Hospitals reported that only 31% of hospitals have such programs.[9] These hospitals tend to be the larger hospitals, often those affiliated with academic medical centers; large segments of the population are therefore left underserved.

Hospice agencies are more commonplace, yet referrals are often made late and their services are underutilized. Patients are dying in the hospital when they want to die at home. The median length of stay in a hospice during 2005 was 26 days; one third of patients enrolled during the last week of life and 10% on the last day of life.[10] Hospice admissions happen late for a wide range of reasons. Most notably, it is often difficult for patients, families, and the health care team to switch out of treatment mode, give up the hope for a cure, and discuss worsening prognosis and death.[3] In states where there is more access to palliative care services, patients are less likely to die in a hospital and are less likely to spend time in an intensive care unit or critical care unit during their last 6 months of life.[3]

Mrs. T. is found to be a poor candidate for surgical resection due to the extent of her disease. However, she is offered radiation treatment which she accepts. She and her daughter were informed of the risks of radiation, which may include fatigue in older patients. They also were told the radiation was palliative and would not cure the cancer at this stage. Now Mrs. T. spends most of her days in bed. She has little energy and needs help with dressing and bathing. She ambulates with a walker.

DETERMINING PROGNOSIS

(For a more comprehensive discussion on functional assessment, see Chapter 4 on "Functional Assessment.") Determining prognosis is a challenge for most physicians. Not only must a difficult prediction be made but also, the physician must often break bad news to the patient and his or her loved ones. Almost universally, patients and their families want to maintain hope for a cure, and if that is not possible, the hope that the cancer will not progress. Elderly cancer patients may have multiple medical problems, cognitive impairment, and functional limitations at baseline. These deficits may reduce their ability to tolerate cancer treatments, increase their risk of side effects, and adversely impact their prognosis. For older patients in whom cure is not possible, the goals of care should focus on controlling symptoms and maximizing function.

The best predictor of prognosis among cancer patients is performance or functional status. Functional status refers to one's ability to carry out his or her activities of daily living and instrumental activities of daily living. For older patients, functional status is often impaired at baseline and may decline following interventions such as surgery, chemotherapy, and radiation; it may not recover. This impaired functional status may limit cancer treatment options and contribute to physical and psychological distress. Cognitive impairment is more common in older patients and, depending on the degree of the deficit, may not only reduce available treatment options but also increase the risk of delirium and worsened cognitive impairment during the course of treatment.

There are a number of different tools that have been developed to assess function. Two well-known scales are the Karnofsky Performance Status Scale and the Eastern Cooperative Oncology Group (ECOG) scale. The Karnofsky Performance Status Scale rates function from 100% (normal) to 0 (dead). The ECOG rates function from 0 (normal) to 5 (dead). A median survival of 3 months roughly correlates with a Karnofsky score less than 40% or ECOG greater than 3.[11] Typically, if a patient spends more than 50% of his or her time in bed, with progressively worsening function and an increase in other symptoms, then a prognosis of less than 3 months is likely.[11] Newer tools are available and incorporate function, signs, and symptoms: the Palliative Prognostic Score (PaP) and

the Palliative Performance Scale.[12,13] These scales utilize more patient information and the added detail may help provide a more comprehensive and reliable assessment.

Discussing prognosis early in the course of care is ideal. It gives patients and their families the opportunity to consider their options and understand what to expect. Discussions should address how the patient's concomitant medical conditions may affect the cancer course, the treatment choices, and the overall prognosis. For older patients with multiple comorbidities, poor functional status, and moderate to advanced cognitive impairment, a palliative approach may be appropriate earlier in the course of care and, for some patients, it may be indicated at the time of diagnosis. These recommendations should be shared with patients and their families, and will likely evolve over the course of care.

Mrs. T. has been undergoing radiation therapy. She arrives in your office in a wheelchair, as her shortness of breath with exertion has worsened. She also states her appetite is low and that she is constipated. She feels anxious about what is going to happen next.

Laboratory studies reveal that she is hypercalcemic; an x-ray shows progressive growth of the tumor mass.

Her hypercalcemia is treated with IV fluids and she is placed on routine medication to prevent her constipation. Discussions about future goals of care reveal she would like to continue further palliative radiation if possible, but wishes to be more comfortable.

In a discussion about advance directives, Mrs. T. states that, if she had a reversible condition, she would want it to be treated with antibiotics or other short-term treatments. If she was not going to recover, or if the risk of treatment outweighed the benefit, she would not want her life to be prolonged on machines. She fills out an advance directive stating her wishes and lists her daughter as her power of attorney in the event she cannot make decisions on her own.

ADVANCE DIRECTIVES

An advance directive is a legal document by which patients specify their treatment preferences, goals of care, and an alternate decision maker or agent if they are unable to make their own decisions. A living will is a legal, written document that outlines a patient's treatment preferences if and when there is a time that he or she is unable to communicate them. A durable power of attorney (DPOA) is a commonly used document by which patients appoint an agent to be their decision maker or healthcare proxy if they lose the capacity to make decisions. A DPOA is useful in that it ensures a flexible form of decision making, since the agent can respond to unanticipated problems that a written document may not predict. Advance directives are state-specific and patients must complete the form from their own state to ensure that their wishes will be carried out. It is very important that an advance directive is completed for the older cancer patient. If a patient chooses to list a DPOA, it should be a person who will respect and follow the patient's wishes.

The Physician Orders for Life-Sustaining Treatment (POLST) Paradigm program is designed to improve the quality of care people receive at the end of life.[14] The POLST is a new form that has been implemented in some states, including California and Oregon (Figure 28-1). The POLST outlines the patient's treatment preferences and underlying medical condition and must be completed and signed by the patient or health care proxy and by his or her physician. The POLST specifically documents

HIPAA PERMITS DISCLOSURE OF POLST TO OTHER HEALTH CARE PROFESSIONALS AS NECESSARY

EMERGENCY MEDICAL SERVICES AUTHORITY · EMSA · CALIFORNIA

EMSA #111 B
(Effective 1/1/2009)

Physician Orders for Life-Sustaining Treatment (POLST)

First follow these orders, then contact physician. This is a Physician Order Sheet based on the person's current medical condition and wishes. Any section not completed implies full treatment for that section. Everyone shall be treated with dignity and respect.

Last Name	
First/Middle Name	
Date of Birth	Date Form Prepared

A *Check One*

CARDIOPULMONARY RESUSCITATION (CPR): ***Person has no pulse and is not breathing.***

☐ **Attempt Resuscitation/CPR** ☐ **Do Not Attempt Resuscitation/DNR** (Allow Natural Death)
(Section B: Full Treatment required)

When not in cardiopulmonary arrest, follow orders in **B** and **C**.

B *Check One*

MEDICAL INTERVENTIONS: ***Person has pulse and/or is breathing.***

☐ **Comfort Measures Only** Use medication by any route, positioning, wound care and other measures to relieve pain and suffering. Use oxygen, suction and manual treatment of airway obstruction as needed for comfort. Antibiotics only to promote comfort. ***Transfer*** *if comfort needs cannot be met in current location.*

☐ **Limited Additional Interventions** Includes care described above. Use medical treatment, antibiotics, and IV fluids as indicated. Do not intubate. May use non-invasive positive airway pressure. Generally avoid intensive care.

☐ ***Do Not Transfer to hospital for medical interventions. Transfer*** if comfort needs cannot be met in current location.

☐ **Full Treatment** Includes care described above. Use intubation, advanced airway interventions, mechanical ventilation, and defibrillation/cardioversion as indicated. ***Transfer*** *to hospital if indicated. Includes intensive care.*

Additional Orders: ____________________

C *Check One*

ARTIFICIALLY ADMINISTERED NUTRITION: ***Offer food by mouth if feasible and desired.***

☐ No artificial nutrition by tube. ☐ Defined trial period of artificial nutrition by tube.
☐ Long-term artificial nutrition by tube.

Additional Orders: ____________________

D

SIGNATURES AND SUMMARY OF MEDICAL CONDITION:

Discussed with:
☐ Patient ☐ Health Care Decisionmaker ☐ Parent of Minor ☐ Court Appointed Conservator ☐ Other:

Signature of Physician
My signature below indicates to the best of my knowledge that these orders are consistent with the person's medical condition and preferences.

Print Physician Name	Physician Phone Number	Date
Physician Signature (required)	Physician License #	

Signature of Patient, Decisionmaker, Parent of Minor or Conservator
By signing this form, the legally recognized decisionmaker acknowledges that this request regarding resuscitative measures is consistent with the known desires of, and with the best interest of, the individual who is the subject of the form.

Signature (required)	Name (print)	Relationship (write self if patient)
Summary of Medical Condition	Office Use Only	

SEND FORM WITH PERSON WHENEVER TRANSFERRED OR DISCHARGED

FIGURE 28-1 Example of the California POLST Form.

HIPAA PERMITS DISCLOSURE OF POLST TO OTHER HEALTH CARE PROFESSIONALS AS NECESSARY

Patient Name (last, first, middle)		Date of birth	Gender: M F
Patient Address			

Contact Information

Health Care Decisionmaker	Address		Phone Number
Health Care Professional Preparing Form	Preparer Title	Phone Number	Date Prepared

Directions for Health Care Professional

Completing POLST

- Must be completed by health care professional based on patient preferences and medical indications.
- POLST must be signed by a physician and the patient/decisionmaker to be valid. Verbal orders are acceptable with follow-up signature by physician in accordance with facility/community policy.
- Certain medical conditions or medical treatments may prohibit a person from residing in a residential care facility for the elderly.
- Use of original form is strongly encouraged. Photocopies and FAXes of signed POLST forms are legal and valid.

Using POLST

- Any incomplete section of POLST implies full treatment for that section.

Section A:

- No defibrillator (including automated external defibrillators) should be used on a person who has chosen "Do Not Attempt Resuscitation."

Section B:

- When comfort cannot be achieved in the current setting, the person, including someone with "Comfort Measures Only," should be transferred to a setting able to provide comfort (e.g., treatment of a hip fracture).
- IV medication to enhance comfort may be appropriate for a person who has chosen "Comfort Measures Only."
- Non-invasive positive airway pressure includes continuous positive airway pressure (CPAP), bi-level positive airway pressure (BiPAP), and bag valve mask (BVM) assisted respirations.
- Treatment of dehydration prolongs life. A person who desires IV fluids should indicate "Limited Interventions" or "Full Treatment."

Reviewing POLST

It is recommended that POLST be reviewed periodically. Review is recommended when:

- The person is transferred from one care setting or care level to another, or
- There is a substantial change in the person's health status, or
- The person's treatment preferences change.

Modifying and Voiding POLST

- A person with capacity can, at any time, void the POLST form of change his/her mind about his/her treatment preferences by executing a verbal or written advance directive or a new POLST form.
- To void POLST, draw a line through Sections A through D and write "VOID" in large letters. Sign and date this line.
- A health care decisionmaker may request to modify the orders based on the known desires of the individual or, if unknown, the individual's best interests.

This form is approved by the California Emergency Medical Services Authority in cooperation with the statewide POLST Task Force.

For more information or a copy of the form, visit **www.capolst.org**.

SEND FORM WITH PERSON WHENEVER TRANSFERRED OR DISCHARGED

FIGURE 28-1, cont'd

preferences regarding cardiopulmonary resuscitation, medical interventions, and artificial nutrition. The premise for the POLST is effective communication of patient wishes, documentation of medical orders on a brightly colored form, and a promise by health care professionals, including emergency medical personnel, to honor these wishes.[15]

SYMPTOM MANAGEMENT

Pain

(For a more detailed discussion of the evaluation and management of pain, see Chapter 17 entitled, "Pain.")

Pain is prevalent among older cancer patients, yet it often goes undiagnosed and undertreated. Research has shown that as many as 80% of older persons diagnosed with cancer experience pain during the course of their illness.[16] Pain control is critical, as uncontrolled pain may affect quality of life, diminish hope, increase depression, and contribute to disordered sleep, appetite disturbances, and cognitive dysfunction.[17,18]

There are numerous challenges to optimal pain evaluation and management in older cancer patients. Persistent pain is epidemic among older adults and is most commonly associated with musculoskeletal disorders such as degenerative spine conditions and arthritis.[19] Other prevalent pain conditions include peripheral neuropathy, postherpetic neuralgia, nighttime leg cramps, and claudication.[19] These conditions may cloud the picture of new or worsening cancer-related pain and impede its treatment. Patients and their families are often hesitant to use opioids due to the potential for adverse drug reactions and addiction.[20] Physicians and other health care practitioners have similar concerns and, typically, receive minimal training in pain management. These factors contribute to the reluctance among physicians to prescribe opioid medications to older patients.[18] These concerns have been augmented by increased attention in the media on the potential for abuse and overdose. While barriers exist, pain management is essential for optimizing function and improving quality of life.

The first step in pain management is assessment. Unfortunately, many older patients and health care professionals expect pain to be a normal part of aging. Patients do not think to report their pain, or they try to bear it and accept it. Other patients may think that their physician is too busy and do not want to be viewed as a "bad patient" with another complaint. Physicians may be focused on the management of the cancer and complaints of pain and other symptoms may get deferred. The best place to begin a pain assessment is to ask, "Are you in pain?" This question has been validated in patients who are cognitively intact as well as those with mild to moderate cognitive impairment. A variety of assessment tools are available including pain scales, the pain thermometer and the faces scale as well as more comprehensive tools.

Pain management is an integral part of palliative care. A wide range of pharmacologic agents are available to manage pain. Nonsteroidal anti-inflammatory drugs (NSAIDs) may be effective for bony pain from bone cancer and metastases; however, they must be used with discretion in older patients because of their potential side effects including elevated blood pressure, renal insufficiency, dyspepsia, and upper gastrointestinal bleeding. NSAIDs are best used for short periods of time, and the concomitant use of an antacid agent or proton pump inhibitor may reduce their risk for GI side effects. For mild pain in a patient with multiple comorbidities and no contraindications, acetaminophen may be useful, especially if dosed around the clock. For older patients with moderate to severe pain, stronger agents such as tramadol and opioid agents such as morphine, oxycodone,

or hydromorphone will be required, and dosing will likely need to be around the clock with as-needed dosing for breakthrough pain. Adjuvant agents offer synergy in pain control and address specific types of pain. Antidepressants and antiepileptics for neuropathic pain, corticosteroids for inflammation, and bisphosphonates for bone pain have been shown to be effective. Additionally nonpharmacologic approaches such as radiation treatment, acupuncture, massage, TENS units, and other types of therapy may be useful additions to a pain management plan. For pain that is difficult to control, a palliative medicine consult or pain management consult may be needed.

CASE 28-1 | **CONTINUED**

Mrs. T. is continuing with her radiation. She was placed on low-dose morphine for her shortness of breath and is using oxygen as needed. She feels she is able to be more active and get out of the house with assistance in her wheelchair. Her constipation is controlled with around-the-clock anticonstipation medication and her appetite is stable. Despite feeling better, her weight continues to drop and her CT scans show the cancer is progressing.

Constipation

Constipation is a common problem in the elderly and may be more severe near the end of life. Multiple factors contribute to this, such as opioid use, immobility, and dehydration due to poor oral intake. Patients need to be evaluated for treatable causes such as medications or electrolyte abnormalities. Associated abdominal pain may contribute to other problems such as anorexia, nausea, or vomiting. Constipation can be controlled and the goal is to keep stool moving and avoid impaction.

Table 28-1 lists some common laxatives that can be useful in treating constipation. Docusate sodium and other stool softeners often are not strong enough alone to treat cases of severe constipation. They need to be used in combination with stimulant laxatives. Fiber products may have to be discontinued, especially if a patient's fluid intake is poor, as these products may contribute to more impaction. When opioids are started, a laxative should always be given routinely to prevent constipation.[21] The patient needs to be monitored for worsening symptoms. Stimulant laxatives such as senna, cascara, and bisacodyl can be used on a routine basis to keep bowel movements regular and patients comfortable. Side effects, however, may be abdominal cramping, and bloating. Saline laxatives such as magnesium hydroxide and magnesium citrate often work faster; however, caution should be taken in patients at risk for electrolyte depletion and dehydration. These can be harsher on the gastrointestinal tract. Osmotic laxatives may be easier to tolerate but side effects can include pain and bloating. Polyethylene glycol can be used for constipation, mixed in water or juice. Methylnaltrexone is a newer agent approved for

TABLE 28-1	Treatment for Constipation		
Drug	**Mechanism**	**Dose**	**Comment**
Docusate sodium	Softener	100-250 mg bid	Often minimally effective used alone
Senna	Stimulants	187-1496 mg bid	Can cause cramps
Cascara		325 mg qd	
Bisacodyl		5-20 mg po or pr qd	
Magnesium hydroxide	Saline laxative	15-40 mL po qd-bid	Diarrhea, electrolyte abnormalities
Magnesium citrate		120-240 mg qd	
Sodium phosphate		20-30 mL po or pr	
Lactulose	Osmotic	5-40 mL po qd-bid	Pain and bloating, diarrhea, dehydration
Sorbitol		15-30 mL po qd-bid	
Polyethylene glycol		17-36 mg po qd-bid	
Psyllium	Bulk-forming	1-2 tablespoons qd	Need adequate fluid intake
Methylcellulose		1-2 mg qd	Need adequate fluid intake
Methylnaltrexone bromide	Selective mu-receptor blocker	8-12 mg SQ QOD	NOT for bowel obstruction

subcutaneous injection for opioid-induced constipation. It has been used in patients receiving palliative care who have been unresponsive to laxatives. It is a selective mu-receptor blocker.[22] It will not reverse the pain control of opioids and does not cross the blood-brain barrier. It is, however, contraindicated for patients in whom there is suspicion of gastrointestinal obstruction.[23] Also, it has only been tested for short-term use. Patients should always be assessed for fecal impaction. Suppositories or enemas must be used in patients who have poor rectal tone or who are too weak to assist in defecation. Also, in cases of severe fecal impaction, trained staff must manually disimpact the rectum prior to starting any laxative treatment. Patients should be routinely monitored and reassessed for symptoms, as adjustments in medication may need to be made.

Nausea and Vomiting

Nausea and vomiting is a common problem. Multiple etiologies such as underlying diseases other than cancer, the cancer itself, medications, or severe constipation can all add to the symptoms. First, the underlying cause must be determined so that the appropriate treatment can be provided. Causes of nausea can be broken down into four categories: central nervous system (CNS), gastric obstruction or ileus, medication side effect, or metabolic abnormalities. Patients may also have other contributing factors. Once the main cause is determined, appropriate treatment can begin. The oral route is preferred; however for those with intractable symptoms, rectal or parenteral routes are an option (Table 28-2). Dopaminergic agents such as prochlorperazine and promethazine can be used orally, rectally, or intramuscularly. These agents are often useful for treating drug-induced nausea and vomiting. The side effects of these antiemetics include drowsiness and extrapyramidal symptoms. Despite these potential side effects in the elderly, these medications can be very helpful and short-term use may benefit patients

by controlling symptoms and improving quality of life. For CNS causes of nausea and vomiting, haloperidol or droperidol can be helpful. Patients who are at risk for increased intracranial pressure may be started on corticosteroids and these may concomitantly improve their symptoms of nausea and vomiting. For patients with significant bowel disease, corticosteroids can relieve bowel edema and improve nausea. High doses of corticosteroids should be used with caution in the elderly as they can lead to gastric irritation, delirium, and fluid retention. Serotonin-receptor blockers are often helpful in cases of chemotherapy-induced nausea and vomiting. Anticholinergics and antihistamines can be useful, especially in cases of vestibular nausea and central nervous system disease. However, care should be taken with these agents, as anticholinergic side effects such as dry mouth, drowsiness, dizziness, blurry vision, and confusion can be difficult for elderly patients to tolerate. Benzodiazepines are often helpful and may help relieve nausea, especially if the nausea is related to anxiety. Patients must be continually reassessed for the underlying cause of nausea and vomiting; they should use these medications on an as-needed basis.

Dyspnea

Dyspnea can be a debilitating symptom for many patients. Causes may include the underlying cancer or progression of illness and terminal condition. Patients may have an uncomfortable awareness of breathing, rapid breathing, or air hunger.[24] Dyspnea can be significantly uncomfortable for patients, and their families may be distressed by the patient's fluctuating respiratory rate, by hearing increased secretions, and by the gurgling sound or "death rattle" that often is heard when a patient is nearing death. It is important to assure patients that the relief of these symptoms and overall comfort is the goal of care (Table 28-3). Often, other treatments must be reassessed for appropriateness; these should be discussed with the

TABLE 28-2	Treatment for Nausea and Vomiting			
Drug	**Mechanism**	**Dose**		**Comment**
Prochlorperazine	Dopamine antagonist	5-20 mg PO/IM/IV q4-6h, 25 mg PR q 8-12h		EPS side effects
Promethazine	Dopamine antagonist	25 mg PO/PR q4-6h		EPS side effects
Droperidol	Dopamine antagonist	2.5-5 mg IM/IV q4-6h		EPS side effects
Haloperidol	Dopamine antagonist	0.5-5 mg PO/IV/IM/SC q4-6h		EPS side effects
Metoclopramide	Dopamine antagonist	5-20 mg PO/IM/IV/SC q6h		EPS side effects
Ondansetron	Serotonin receptor blocker	8 mg PO/IV/SC q8h		Chemotherapy-induced nausea
Granisetron	Serotonin receptor blocker	0.5-1 mg PO/IV/SC q12h		Chemotherapy-induced nausea
Diphenhydramine	Antihistamines	25 mg PO/IV/IM q4h		For vestibular symptoms
Meclizine	Antihistamines	25-50 mg PO q4-6h		For vestibular symptoms
Dexamethasone	Corticosteroid	1-4 mg PO/IV q6h		For chemotherapy induced nausea, or increased intracranial pressure
Prednisone	Corticosteroid	5-20 PO q4h		For chemotherapy induced nausea, or increased intracranial pressure
Scopolamine	Anticholinergic	1.5 mg patch q72h		Delirium risk
Hyoscyamine	Anticholinergic	0.125 mg tid		Delirium risk
Dronabinol	Cannabinoid	2.5-7.5 mg PO bid-tid		Chemotherapy-induced nausea
Lorazepam	Benzodiazepine	0.5-2 mg PO/SC/IM q4h		For reducing anxiety, nausea
Diazepam	Benzodiazepine	5-10 mg q4h		For reducing anxiety, nausea

TABLE 28-3	Treatment for Shortness of Breath and Increased Secretions			
Class of Drug	**Examples**	**Dose**		**Comment**
Shortness of Breath				
Oxygen		2-10 L/min by nasal cannula		Use for patient comfort, shortness of breath
Opioids	Morphine	5-15 mL PO/SL/PR		Decrease patient perception of breathlessness; titrate up to patient comfort
	Methadone			
	Oxycodone			
Benzodiazepines	Lorazepam	1-2 mg PO/SL		Can help with anxiety and breathlessness
	Diazepam	2.5-10 mg PO/SL		
Secretions				
Scopolamine patch		1-3 patches q1-2 days		In alert patient, may cause dizziness and dry mouth
Hyoscyamine		0.125 mg PO q4-6h		Less sedation than scopolamine
Glycopyrrolate		0.2-1 mg PO q4-6h		Least sedation and fewer CNS side effects
Atropine drops		2-4 drops PO/SL q2-4h		Can be used when patient is unable to swallow and as needed

patient, the family and the physician. Interventions such as antibiotics for acute infection and diuretics for fluid overload can be considered based on the patient's preference and the stage of the disease process.[25]

As the body starts to shut down, renal function decreases, the circulatory system slows, and patients are at higher risk for fluid overload. Treatment with intravenous fluids may make symptoms of shortness of breath worse. Also, tube feedings may have to be slowed or discontinued, as the patient may be at higher risk of fluid overload and aspiration. Patients should be allowed to eat as they can tolerate; however, food consistency may have to be changed if they are having more difficulty chewing or swallowing. Patients who are too lethargic to eat should not be forced, as aspiration is a high risk and can make the breathing even more labored.

Oxygen is used to improve patient's symptoms and can be used easily. Patient's life expectancy will not be prolonged by the use of oxygen; however, the patient may have less air hunger and may have the sensation of breathing easier.[26] Opioids are the main pharmacologic agents for treating dyspnea. Morphine sulfate can be used orally, sublingually, intravenously or rectally. Doses can begin very low, starting at 5 to 10 mg every 2 to 4 hours. However, it should be titrated up at least by 30% to 50% until symptoms are controlled. Patients can be placed on continuous long-acting doses of the opioid preparation, but short-acting opioid formula should still be available for severe symptom control as needed. Titration should be based on the patient's symptoms, not on his or her respiratory rate. Studies on nebulized morphine and hydromorphone have shown variable results. The benefit over enteral narcotics is still unclear and more research is needed.[27,28]

Benzodiazepines can also be effective in treatment of dyspnea. Patient may feel symptomatic relief as well as less anxiety and air hunger when symptoms are more severe. Benzodiazepines may need to be used around the clock and may need to be titrated based on the patients symptoms. Nonpharmacologic methods to help reduce shortness of breath include placing the patient in a more open room, using air from a fan, keeping the patient in an upright position, relaxation techniques, and support for the patients spiritual or psychological needs.

Dyspnea at the end of life is often caused by secretions and difficulty with swallowing. Many patients have recurrent aspiration. If a patient is still eating, the benefit of quality of life versus the risk of aspiration must be considered. Many patients are willing to take some risk for the benefit of being able to enjoy food. Many patients may be more uncomfortable due to increased secretions from fluid overload, aspiration, infections, and inability to control secretions. Often medication to help dry secretions can be beneficial. Scopolamine patches can be used and are helpful in drying secretions. Side effects include dizziness, blurred vision, and oral dryness. Hyoscyamine is less sedating than scopolamine and can be used orally when the patient can still swallow. Glycopyrrolate has fewer CNS side effects and can be used orally and intravenously. It does not cause as much drowsiness compared to the others and the risk for delirium is low. This is often a safer alternative in the elderly patient who still is awake and at high risk for delirium. In patients who cannot swallow and who are mostly unconscious, atropine drops can be used orally or sublingually. These can be used to dry oral secretions and help reduce the gurgling from the throat often heard when a patient is nearing death and has no control over secretions, sometimes referred to as the "death rattle." Medications to help control secretions are listed in Table 28-3. Often, patients' caregivers can be trained to help clear secretions by using swabs to clear out the oropharynx, suctioning gently with a bulb syringe, and making postural changes to clear the airway.

Depression

(For more comprehensive discussion and treatments, see Chapter 16 on "Depression.")

Depression is a common problem among elderly cancer patients. A recent systematic review found that approximately 15% of palliative care inpatients suffer from major depression and that the prevalence of all depressive disorders including minor depression, dysthymia, and depressive adjustment disorders is likely to be twice this value.[29] Unfortunately, depression is often overshadowed by other physical complaints. Depression is reported less often than pain and fatigue when patients are asked about common symptoms.[29] It can be especially confusing with cancer patients, because many of the biological symptoms of depression are expected consequences of cancer and its treatment such as fatigue, sleeplessness, change in weight, and loss of appetite.[29]

Other indicators of depression in the terminally ill are suicidal ideation and feelings of hopelessness, helplessness, worthlessness, and guilt.[30] Anxiety often coexists with depression and may be an associated symptom. Older cancer patients facing death may experience a depressed mood; it can be difficult to differentiate when depressed mood or normal grief becomes clinical depression.[29] These distinctions are important, as depression significantly impacts functional status and quality of life.[29,30]

Given these complexities, what is the best way to identify depression in elderly cancer patients? The short answer is to ask the patient. Research has shown that patient interviews are superior to self-report and visual analogue scales for the identification of depression, and a diagnostic interview is the gold standard.[29,31] Certainly, the ideal tool in the clinical setting would be one that is quick, easy, and reliable. Chochinov et al. demonstrated that incorporating a single-item interview for depressed mood and asking "Are you depressed?" reliably and accurately diagnosed the presence of depressed mood.[31] The authors also suggested that inquiry regarding loss of interest and pleasure in activities may be additive.[31] Once identified, further questioning is required through thorough history taking and possibly the implementation of additional questionnaires such as the Geriatric Depression Scale (GDS) or the Patient Health Questionnaire-9 (PHQ-9). Other questionnaires ask more questions and have been found to be reliable; examples include the Hospital Anxiety and Depression Scale and the Beck Depression Inventory.[32,33] These may be useful and offer a more definitive diagnosis of depression rather than just the identification of depressed symptoms; however, their length and requirement for prolonged attention may make them hard to complete with frail elderly patients.[29] While self-report and visual analog scale measures are not reliable in making the diagnosis of depression, they may be useful to quantify the severity of a depressive syndrome, once it is identified, and in monitoring change over time.[31] Once depression is suspected in a patient, further history should be obtained and further information gathered to assess for a history of depression, its prior treatments, successes and failures; medical etiologies; or contributors such as thyroid disease, anemia, and electrolyte disturbances.

Treating depression may lead not only to an improvement in physical symptoms but also have a major impact on quality of life and, possibly, survival.[34] Treatment may be effective even in those who are terminally ill and it carries minimal risk. A consensus panel by the American College of Physicians/American Society of Internal Medicine reported that psychotherapeutic interventions have been shown to be effective in relieving depressive symptoms, improving quality of life, and prolonging life, while psychopharmacologic treatments may relieve depressive symptoms and alleviate psychological distress in a majority of patients.[30] Simultaneous symptom management, especially pain control, is essential, as poorly controlled pain is a risk factor for depression.[30] Additional nonpharmacologic interventions are also important including psychological support, spiritual support, and symptom management. Talking through concerns, answering questions, and reassuring the patient that his or her pain will be relieved are all important. This type of support can be provided in the context of an office visit or visit to the infusion center by staff and by the interdisciplinary team if hospice is involved. A palliative care approach will help ensure that comprehensive care is provided.

There are many available antidepressants; it may seem difficult to choose the right one for an older patient with advanced cancer. The risk/benefit ratio is low with treatment and there is little reason not to consider a trial of intervention. Important considerations include: good side effect profile, little or no interaction with other drugs used in palliative care, additional benefits (e.g., helpful with neuropathic pain or somnolence), quick onset of action, and safe in liver or renal failure.[34] Citalopram and sertraline are selective serotonin reuptake inhibitors that have been shown to be effective and well tolerated in palliative care patients.[34] These agents are preferred, as they have few active metabolites to accumulate and cause toxicity when compared with fluoxetine.[30] Mirtazepine, a noradrenaline and specific serotonin antagonist (NaSSA), is particularly useful in patients with insomnia, poor appetite, nausea, and anxiety.[34] Duloxetine may be a good choice in patients with concomitant neuropathic pain. Venlafaxine may be useful for patients not responsive to the SSRIs. Antidepressants typically require a 4-week trial period to determine effectiveness. If one agent has not been effective, then try switching to a different agent. If there is still no improvement, or if additional symptoms such as paranoia, delusions or active suicidal ideation are present, then the involvement of a psychiatrist is recommended.

Depression routinely goes unaddressed in the older cancer patient. Physicians may not recognize depression in their patients and often lack the knowledge and skills to identify depression.[29,30] Patients, their families, and health care providers believe that psychological distress is a normal feature of the dying process and fail to differentiate natural, existential distress from clinical depression.[30] Other barriers exist including the stigma of depression, a lack of time to address the issue during clinical encounters, the concern that talking about depression will cause further distress, and physician reluctance to prescribe psychotropic agents.[30] Optimal care for the older cancer patient requires that depression be looked for and treated.

Anxiety and Agitation

Anxiety and agitation are common near the end of life and may be more difficult to control than other symptoms. Terminal restlessness can be assessed and treated to improve the patient's life. Patients may have multiple factors adding to agitation such as disease process, electrolyte abnormalities, shortness of breath, uncontrolled pain, medication side effects, or psychological fear and depression. Intervention goals are to provide patients with comfort and the best-possible quality of life. Patients with advanced cancer who have anxiety are more likely to have difficulties in the physician-patient relationship.[35] In the elderly, depression, delirium and the possibility of cognitive dysfunction can make evaluation and treatment more complex.

As for depression, anxiety can present in many ways. Poor symptom management can add to more anxiety. Patients should be assessed for uncontrolled pain, shortness of breath, constipation, and nausea at every encounter. Poor sleep can also lead to anxiety. Patients may have depression with an anxiety component and appropriate medication should be started. Patients who are debilitated or who require more care may often feel anxious about becoming a burden on family or caregivers. Appropriate and early intervention to discuss care needs and possibilities for care facilities should come earlier in the course of illness. Social, spiritual, and cultural aspects also must be addressed. A patient whose death is impending may wish to reconcile with loved ones with whom he or she lost contact. Some patients may need religious or spiritual support. All these disciplines should be offered and considered in a patient who seems to be more anxious. Medication can often help in patients who are still undergoing active care and even for those on hospice care. SSRIs are common antidepressants that can help with anxiety, as well as with depression. Anxiolytics, such as benzodiazepines, can often be used in acute anxiety. Caution should be taken in the elderly, as the side effects of benzodiazepines can include confusion and agitation. They are not recommended for long-term use for chronic anxiety in the elderly.[36] For those who are near the end of life, they can be used more acutely. During the dying process, when some patients may suffer from terminal delirium and agitation, around-the-clock benzodiazepines and, often, antiseizure medications can be used for sedation. Antipsychotics, especially atypical antipsychotics, are often used and can be helpful in acute anxiety or agitated state, particularly in patients with underlying cognitive impairment. Mood disorders and underlying psychiatric disorders should be assessed and treated. Patients may also benefit from psychological support, spiritual support, and social support. Anxiety often stems from patient's fears of pain and suffering. There is a high association of depression and anxiety in patients with chronic medical problems, as is the case for many elderly. The addition of a cancer diagnosis will often exacerbate the condition. Use of interdisciplinary team members, spiritual support, family involvement, and psychiatric and psychological support should be instituted early.

Delirium

Delirium is also highly prevalent at the end of life and in acute illness. Delirium is defined as an acute state of disturbed consciousness. Usually, it is abrupt in onset and associated with fluctuating symptoms. Patients may be lucid at intervals then decline again. These symptoms can be treated and it is often reversible. Patients who are over 65 years old are at the highest risk for delirium. Delirium can increase length of hospital stay in older patients and can increase mortality.[37] Delirium in cancer can be a challenging diagnosis. It can represent a reversible condition, new disease in the brain, or an irreversible part of the evolution of the terminal disease.[38] Distinguishing delirium from dementia can often be difficult, especially in patients with a history of dementia. In delirium, confusion occurs acutely and is associated with altered consciousness. Dementia is usually a slow and progressive cognitive loss. When delirium is superimposed on a patient with dementia, diagnosis can be difficult.[39]

As delirium can be a reversible condition, it is important to evaluate the cause and to treat it if possible (Table 28-4). One of the main causes of delirium is drug toxicity. Medications to treat acute illness such as antibiotics, centrally acting antihypertensives, and steroids are common in the acute-care setting. In addition, medications used for palliation of symptoms including opioids, benzodiazepines, antipsychotics, anticholinergics, and antiseizure drugs can all cause delirium, especially in older patients. Metabolic abnormalities and endocrine disorders as well as acute fever, hypotension, and infection are all risks for confusion. Patients with cancer are highly susceptible to delirium from the disease itself or due to consequences of the cancer treatment. Hematologic abnormalities and neurologic causes including new cerebral vascular event, infection, head trauma, seizures, or bleeding should be considered. Toxic effects of antineoplastic treatments and new CNS tumor to the brain and meninges can cause acute changes in consciousness.[40] In elderly patients, underlying psychiatric disorders such as dementia can make delirium more pronounced and difficult to diagnose. Patients with depression, anxiety, or agitation can present with confusion as the main symptoms.[41] Alcohol, drug, or medication withdrawal can add to delirium. In an elderly patient, environmental changes such as sleep deprivation, inability to communicate because of hearing loss, vision loss, and change in environment can increase the confusional state.

After addressing the reversible causes, delirium is usually treated with antipsychotic agents. In an elderly patient, care must be used in dosing and the potential for oversedation is high. Often, older patients will better tolerate atypical antipsychotics. Side effects can be detrimental to patients; they should be monitored for extrapyramidal symptoms manifested by stiffness, tremor, and confusion. Benzodiazepines are also often used but should be used with caution as they can cause more

TABLE 28-4	Causes of Delirium

Drug toxicity
- Steroids, antibiotics, narcotics, benzodiazepines, antipsychotics, antihypertensives, anticholinergics, antiseizure drugs

Metabolic
- Electrolyte abnormalities: sodium, calcium
- Renal or liver failure
- Paraneoplastic syndrome

Endocrine abnormalities
- Glucose
- Thyroid disorder

Infections and fever

Hematologic abnormalities

Neurologic
- New CVA, infection, head trauma, seizures, bleed

Nutritional deficiencies: B12, thiamine, folic acid

Toxic effects of antineoplastic treatments
- Chemotherapy
- Radiation therapy

CNS tumor: brain metastasis, meningeal metastasis

Hypoxia
- Respiratory failure
- Cardiac failure
- Metabolic

Alcohol or drug withdrawal
- Chronic or acute alcohol
- Benzodiazepines
- Antipsychotics
- Antidepressants

Psychiatric illness
- Depression, psychosis
- Underlying dementia (higher risk)

Environmental
- Sleep deprivation, pain, unfamiliar surroundings
- Poor vision, hearing loss, immobility

CASE 28-1	CONTINUED

Mrs. T. is admitted to the hospital with increased confusion. A CT scan of the brain reveals a new brain lesion with edema. She is started on IV steroids; her oncology team requests a Palliative Care consult as she is not a candidate for any further radiation due to her severe decline and progression of the disease. At this time, Mrs. T. is unable to comprehend the medical situation and lacks the capacity to make decisions. Her daughter wants to know what her options are for care. She believes her mother would like to be at home.

Mrs. T. becomes hypotensive and is in respiratory distress. Her daughter understands that her mother's current condition is irreversible and that, if she is intubated, it is unlikely that she would return to her prior level of function. Based on previous discussion and her mother's advance directives, she decides to make her mother's status "Do not resuscitate" (DNR) and to make comfort the goal. Mrs. T. is placed on IV morphine and all blood draws are stopped. Her breathing becomes more comfortable and she dies in the hospital with her daughter and friends at her bedside.

confusion, especially in the elderly.[42] Patients may have a paradoxical reaction and become more acutely hyperactive and more confused.

The Last Hours

The end of life is never easy. It can be difficult for patients and families, as well as for the health care team. As a patient enters the last few days to hours of death, physical capabilities diminish and need for care increases. The goals of care need to be readdressed and treatments often must shift to assure patients comfort. Normal physiologic changes usually include weakness, decreased appetite, neurologic dysfunction, and decreased blood perfusion. Families and health care team should focus on a treatment plan with comfort as the goal. Routine use of artificial nutrition and IV fluids is not recommended during terminal care. Too much fluid can cause more discomfort and can add to breathlessness, cough, and secretions. Edema and skin breakdown can be more painful and intravenous lines can cause more discomfort.[43] As death approaches, there may be changes in respirations including Cheyne-Stokes breathing, accessory muscle use, and death rattle. Appropriate medication for comfort should be instituted. Patients are at risk for terminal delirium; medications for pain, agitation and confusion can be given routinely. Decreased perfusion will present as mottling of the skin; tachycardia and hypotension are part of the natural dying process. It is important to attend to skin care, repositioning of the patient, and control of increased secretions, as these will provide more comfort for the patient. Invasive and potentially uncomfortable treatments, such as suctioning, should be avoided. Swabbing the oral cavity, as well as applying moisture to the lips and moisture drops to the eyes can reduce discomfort.[44] During this time, any spiritual and cultural support should continue and family should be allowed to be with the patient and trained to assist in care if they wish.

IMPROVING END OF LIFE CARE FOR OLDER CANCER PATIENTS

Palliative medicine is gaining recognition as a valid and important field in medicine. Over the last 10 years, significant advances have been implemented to improve the palliative care that patients receive, including national guidelines for quality of care, multidisciplinary educational offerings, research opportunities, and resources for clinicians.[3] Through these efforts, palliative care knowledge and expertise is increasing among health care providers.[3]

"Hospice and Palliative Medicine" became a recognized subspecialty within the American Board of Medical Specialties (ABMS) in 2008. "Hospice and Palliative Medicine" is a subspecialty of ten participating boards including the American Boards of Internal Medicine, Anesthesiology, Family Medicine, Physical Medicine and Rehabilitation, Psychiatry and Neurology, Surgery, Pediatrics, Emergency Medicine, Radiology, and Obstetrics and Gynecology. The American Board of Internal Medicine (ABIM) is responsible for administering the certification examination on behalf of all 10 cosponsoring boards. Physicians who demonstrate the requisite experience in hospice and palliative care may sit for the examination during the grandfathering period from 2008 to 2012. After 2012, physicians will be required to complete a minimum of a 12-month or ACGME-accredited fellowship in Hospice and Palliative Medicine.

Multiple educational opportunities have been developed to improve the knowledge and skills in palliative care among health care practitioners. The End-of-Life Nursing Education Consortium (ELNEC) is a train-the-trainer model for nurses of all levels including faculty, ward nurses, and advanced care specialists in palliative and end-of-life care.[45] Over 5000 nurses in 50 states have received ELNEC training through these national courses and are sharing their new expertise in educational and clinical settings.[3] While this is a significant effort, this number reflects less than 0.2% of practicing nurses.[3] Utilizing a similar model, the Education for Physicians on End-of-Life Care (EPEC) is also a train-the-trainer program created to introduce physicians to the core competencies of palliative care.[46] The curriculum components include a comprehensive syllabus, trainer notes, recommended teaching approaches, slides, video trigger tapes, and an annotated reference list.[3] EPEC-Oncology (EPEC-O) was designed for practicing oncologists and the interdisciplinary team caring for persons and families with cancer and offers the same EPEC curriculum with a focus on patients with cancer.[3] These three curricula can be accessed at national courses and through Web-based learning. The End-Of-Life/Palliative Education Resource Center (EPERC) is an online resource for palliative care educational material supported by the Medical College of Wisconsin.[47] EPERC offers "Fast Facts," a collection of over 200 peer-reviewed and evidence-based summaries on key topics including pain, nonpain symptoms, communications skills, ethics, terminal care, and clinical interventions used near the end-of-life.[47] These "Fast Facts" are useful for self-learning as well as teaching students and trainees. Other EPERC offerings include suggested articles and links to other Web-based resources.

Additional resources offer guidance in the development and implementation of a palliative care program. The Center to Advance Palliative Care (CAPC) is a national organization whose mission is to provide "health care professionals with the tools, training, and technical assistance necessary to start and sustain successful palliative care programs in hospitals and other health care settings."[48] CAPC provides a large number of services including a comprehensive Web site, training and mentoring programs through their Palliative Care Leadership Centers™ (PCLC), online courses, discussion boards, and publications.[3,48]

Over the last 10 years, there have been increased research efforts in palliative medicine. Areas that continue to lack adequate data and need rigorous research include treatment decisions, family care, and advance directives.[3] Funding is becoming increasingly available for research in palliative care; two current options are include the National Palliative Care Research Center and the American Cancer Society (ACS) Initiatives for Palliative Care Research.[3] The doors are wide open for research pursuits in palliative medicine. Further high-quality research in hospice and palliative medicine is essential to develop a foundation for evidence-based practice.

| CASE 28-1 | **CASE REVIEW** |

In the case of Mrs. T., there are several important considerations that might have improved her end-of-life care. As an elderly patient with other comorbidities, with functional limitations, and who was diagnosed with an incurable cancer, she was at high risk for side effects and decline. Discussions on goals of care could have been held earlier with the patient and primary medical doctor. The patient would have preferred to be at home at the end of her life. But once her condition took an acute turn, she was too unstable to be moved. Initiating hospice earlier in the course of her care could have allowed her to complete palliative radiation, as well as allowing for improved symptom management and quality-of-life focus. The hospice would probably have provided more social support for the patient and her daughter and she might have been able to stay in her home, if that was her wish. In a case such as this, palliative care can be initiated at the time of diagnosis and follow-up can be in a palliative clinic, which can work in conjunction with the oncologist and primary physician.

CONCLUSION

Palliative care and hospice are invaluable resources in the care of the older cancer patient. In the United States, medical care for patients with advanced illness has been characterized by untreated physical symptoms, poor communication between providers and patients, and

treatment decisions in conflict with patient and family preferences.[3,49] With the aging of our population there will be more and more older patients diagnosed with cancer, many of whom may have advanced disease at the time of diagnosis, and the need for knowledge and clinical skills in palliative care by the oncologists and interdisciplinary team that care for them will only grow. National experts recommend a change in health care to include palliative care early in the course of cancer, in order to familiarize patients and their families with palliative care and hospice services, start communication about death earlier in the course of cancer treatment, and provide an opportunity for a discussion of goals of care among the physician, patient, and family.[3]

Palliative medicine offers health care professionals a holistic model of care and an approach to older cancer patients that addresses their physical and psychosocial needs. Essential components include a discussion of prognosis, as well as discussion of expected symptoms and how they will be managed. Such discussions should also clarify expectations, address fears, review goals of care, and determine treatment preferences, including intensity of care and code status. Improving the care of older cancer patients requires that the medical community have greater awareness of the importance of these issues and how they affect disease course, functional status, and quality of life. Physicians and other health professionals who care for older patients with advanced cancer need to be competent in the management of pain and nonpain symptoms and know when to ask for help. Educational, clinical, and research opportunities in palliative medicine are available; however, they must continue to be expanded and, most importantly, health care providers must access and utilize them. Palliative care consultation and referrals to hospice should be implemented earlier and ultimately should become standard-of-care in the management of the older cancer patient.

See expertconsult.com for a complete list of references and web resources for this chapter

Ethical Issues Related to Assessing Decision Making Capacity

Anne Walling and Neil S. Wenger

CASE 29-1 **CASE DESCRIPTION**

Ms. S. is a 74-year-old woman with colorectal cancer metastatic to liver and brain. Although she has told friends that she no longer wants aggressive therapy and would not want to be intubated or spend time in intensive care and would like to die at home "when it is my time," she has been hesitant to bring this up with her doctor as she knows that he was considering recommending her for a new clinical trial. She was an only child, her husband died 10 years ago, and she never had children. She does not have an advance directive and has not specified a durable power of attorney agent to make health care decisions. Her next door neighbor brings her to the emergency department one night for progressive confusion and fever. At presentation, her blood pressure is low and her cognitive status fluctuates. The emergency physician explains to the patient that she requires treatment in the intensive care unit (ICU). The patient states that she wants to go home. What should the emergency physician do?

Great importance is placed on the ethical principle of autonomy in medicine, as practiced in the United States today, and ensuring that a patient's medical care is guided by his or her preferences is central to upholding this ethical principle.[1] Ideally, patients would always actively participate in decisions about their own medical care. Unfortunately, the brain commonly becomes dysfunctional in the setting of organ failure and severe illness, and this is particularly true in the cancer patient. Patients with cancer can lose the ability to direct their care because of malignancy directly affecting the brain, as an effect of severe illness elsewhere in the body, and as a result of medication effects. Delirium is common in elderly patients and in patients with advanced cancer.[2,3,4] Delirium often presents just as patients are becoming more seriously ill (and often will need decisions to be made regarding aggressiveness of care) and right before death. For example, in the Study to Understand Prognoses and Preferences for Outcomes and Risks of Treatments (SUPPORT), 28% of patients with lung or colon cancer suffered from confusion in their

last 3 days of life.[5,6] However, such cognitive changes can be reversible and, in one study, 50% of episodes (often those precipitated by a change in opioid dose or by dehydration) in patients with advanced cancer were reversible.[2] In addition, elderly patients have increasing rates of impaired cognition as they age. Patients with cognitive impairment who retain the ability to make decisions at baseline are at greater risk of developing delirium under the stress of illness.[7]

Cognitive dysfunction has many implications for the elderly cancer patient. In general, cognitive dysfunction is a poor prognostic sign in older patients.[8] Patients with cognitive dysfunction are also particularly challenging to care for and require special attention to care planning above and beyond the average patient. For example, patients with cognitive dysfunction may have problems with adherence to treatments and may require the assistance of a caregiver. In addition, these patients may lack the capacity to make decisions about their own health care. Because of the prevalence of delirium and cognitive impairment among elderly patients with cancer, assessment of decision-making capacity will almost always be necessary in the trajectory of disease of an older cancer patient; for this reason, it is essential to understand what decision-making capacity is. Decision-making capacity is defined as the ability to participate in making medical decisions. To have this capacity, a patient must: (1) understand the relevant information needed to make an informed decision; (2) have the ability to appreciate the clinical situation and its consequences; (3) reason about treatment options; and, ultimately, (4) communicate a choice.[9,10]

For example, a man with myeloma who sustained a pathologic femur fracture and is refusing pinning of the fracture but cannot understand that surgery is needed or is unable to conceive of the risks and benefits of surgery lacks decision-making capacity because he does not understand the relevant information. If the man refused surgery but did not understand that without the procedure he will be unable to walk for months, if ever again, and that he would be likely to die if left to lie in bed for this time does not exhibit decision-making capacity because he cannot appreciate the clinical situation and its consequences. If the man refused surgery because "all operations are scary" and cannot even consider the option of surgery or the risks and benefits of surgery versus alternative treatments, then the case would be an example of a patient who lacks decision-making capacity because he cannot reason about treatment options. Lastly, a man who cannot or will not communicate a decision does not exhibit decision-making capacity. In nearly all cases, more than one aspect of capacity is compromised in a patient lacking decision-making capacity. Yet, teasing out the aspect of capacity that is lacking when a patient is deemed incapable can be a valuable exercise to ensure that a patient lacks capacity and also as a focus to attempt to enhance capacity.

Capacity is evaluated by a physician asking a series of questions. Table 29-1 shows specific questions and comments that can aid a physician in assessing capacity. For example, a physician can assess a patient's understanding by asking, "Please tell me in your own words the problem with your health now." "What is the recommended treatment?" A physician could then assess a patient's ability to appreciate the situation and its consequences by asking, "What is treatment likely to do for you?" or "What do you think will happen if you choose not to proceed with the treatment?" A patient's ability to reason through treatment options might be determined by asking, "Why do you prefer (or why do you not want) the treatment?" Lastly, asking, "Can you tell me your decision?" helps assess the patient's ability to communicate his or her decision. If a patient is able to answer these questions in a coherent fashion (that is the patient displays decision-making capacity), then he should be

TABLE 29-1	**Legally Relevant Criteria for Decision-Making Capacity and Approaches to Assessment of the Patient**			
Criterion	**Patient's Task**	**Physician's Assessment Approach**	**Questions for Clinical Assessment**	**Comments**
Communicate a choice.	Clearly indicate preferred treatment option.	Ask patient to indicate a treatment choice.	Have you decided whether to follow your doctor's [or my] recommendation for treatment? Can you tell me what that decision is? If no decision: What is making it hard for you to decide?	Frequent reversals of choice because of psychiatric or neurologic conditions may indicate lack of capacity.
Understand the relevant information.	Grasp the fundamental meaning of information communicated by physician.	Encourage patient to paraphrase disclosed information regarding medical condition and treatment.	Please tell me in your own words what your doctor [or I] told you about: the problem with your health now; the recommended treatment; the possible benefits and risks (or discomforts) of the treatment; any alternative treatments and their risks and benefits; the risks and benefits of no treatment.	Information to be understood includes nature of patient's condition, nature and purpose of proposed treatment, possible benefits and risks of that treatment, and alternative approaches (including no treatment) and their benefits and risks.
Appreciate the situation and its consequences.	Acknowledge medical condition and likely consequences of treatment options.	Ask patient to describe views of medical condition, proposed treatment, and likely outcomes.	What do you believe is wrong with your health now? Do you believe that you need some kind of treatment? What is treatment likely to do for you? What makes you believe it will have that effect? What do you believe will happen if you are not treated? Why do you think your doctor has [or I have] recommended this treatment?	Courts have recognized that patients who do not acknowledge their illnesses (often referred to as "lack of insight") cannot make valid decisions about treatment. Delusions or pathologic levels of distortion or denial are the most common causes of impairment.
Reason about treatment options.	Engage in a rational process of manipulating the relevant information.	Ask patient to compare treatment options and consequences and to offer reasons for selection of option.	How did you decide to accept or reject the recommended treatment? What makes [chosen option] better than [alternative option]?	This criterion focuses on the process by which a decision is reached, not the outcome of the patient's choice, since patients have the right to make "unreasonable" choices.

From Applebaum, PS. Assessment of Patients' Competence to Consent to Treatment. N Engl J Med 2007;357:1834-40.

able to accept or reject medical care, even if the physician disagrees with the patient's decision.[9]

It is important to note that decisions about a patient's capacity have to be made on an individual basis. It is often possible for patients with psychiatric disorders or dementia to make at least some decisions, if not all of them. Although a patient's past history can inform a capacity assessment, prior capacity determinations or prevalent diagnoses should not be assumed to deem a patient incapable of making future decisions. For example, a patient with a history of schizophrenia and a history of lacking decision-making capacity who is now receiving treatment that controls psychosis may be able to participate in his health care treatment decisions. In addition, a patient with a history of dementia, who had been actively participating in decision-making concerning breast cancer treatment, may suffer a decline in her cognitive abilities so that she is no longer able to meaningfully choose between treatment options.

When should a physician complete a capacity assessment of a patient? A good rule of thumb is that any time informed consent or refusal is required in medical care, it should be clear that a patient has decision-making capacity. In the above case, Ms. S. is refusing admission to the ICU and demanding to go home. However, she shows signs of a serious infection and is, at times, lethargic. In order to accept Ms. S.'s refusal of ICU admission, the emergency physician must assess her capacity to make that decision.

CASE 29-1 | CONTINUED

After explaining to the patient her current situation, the recommended treatment and why it is needed, the emergency physician asks Ms. S. to tell him in her own words what her health problem is and the recommended treatment. Ms. S. is unable to answer this question. She also does not respond meaningfully when the doctor asks her additional questions about what is happening to her. Although lethargic, she continues to demand that she go home. The emergency physician decides that Ms. S. does not have the capacity to make decisions, admits her to the intensive care unit (using implied consent), and attempts to identify a potential surrogate decision maker for the patient.

Although Ms. S. is able to communicate that she wants to go home, she is unable to articulate why and how she came to this decision. Therefore she does not have decision-making capacity to make the venue-of-care decision. Since Ms. S. does not have an advance directive or any prior medical record note regarding preferences for care, the emergency physician decides that the appropriate course of action is to treat the patient in the intensive care unit.

In practice, a formal evaluation of capacity is not completed for every patient who expresses preferences regarding the acceptance or refusal of a medical intervention.

However, some degree of judgment about the patient's ability to form and express preferences must occur every time a patient makes a decision.[11] For selected patients, it is important that a formal capacity assessment be performed and documented in the medical record. If a patient has an underlying cognitive impairment, if a patient is at high risk of delirium due to an underlying medical condition, or if a patient's expressed preferences fall outside of a range generally comprehensible to others, a more rigorous evaluation of capacity that covers all four of these elements is required, especially if the proposed procedure or clinical condition has serious clinical consequences to the patient.[1] It is important to recognize that some patients, especially those with slowly emerging dementia, are able to mask their cognitive impairment. Mini-mental status exams (MMSE) and other objective tests should be considered in all vulnerable elders to assess cognitive status when important decisions are being made.[12]

Ms. S., in the case above, is an elderly woman with metastatic brain disease and signs of acute infection, all of which put her at high risk of delirium; thus she deserves a formal evaluation of capacity. Documentation about decision-making capacity for a patient should cover all four areas that are assessed: understanding of relevant information, ability to appreciate the clinical situation and its consequences, ability to reason about treatment options, and ability to communicate a choice. In this case, a physician might document, "Ms. S. is expressing the desire to go home. Although comfort-oriented care at home may be a reasonable option given her metastatic disease, we have no evidence that she previously desired this course of treatment. Ms. S. is unable to describe or understand her current clinical situation, does not understand the implications of her situation, and cannot engage in reasoning about her treatment options. Therefore, despite the fact that Ms. S. is asking to go home, this cannot be considered a reasoned decision. Ms. S. lacks decision-making capacity at this time. Because she has a potentially life-threatening condition that needs emergent care, we will treat her using implied consent and search for an appropriate surrogate decision maker until she regains the ability to make decisions for herself." On the other hand, if Ms. S. had been able to express that she knew she had cancer and had decided that she never wanted to go to an ICU, was ready to die, and did not want to die in a hospital, she would have displayed that she had capacity to make this decision (even though she has risk factors for incapacity).

There are methods or tools available to assist in the assessment of decision-making capacity. Many of the tools available for clinical research are not adequate for assessing all four domains of decision-making capacity.[13] Some tools for clinical practice have been developed; however, these are often time-consuming. For example, the MacArthur Competence Assessment Tool (MacCAT-T) assesses the domains of decision-making capacity using a structured interview format. The Capacity to Consent to Treatment Instrument varies from the MacCAT-T in that it uses clinical vignettes to test a patient's understanding rather than using a structured interview format. The Hopemon Capacity Assessment Interview (HCAI) is also similar to the MacCAT-T but uses semistructured interviews and was initially designed to specifically assess medical and financial decision making in nursing home patients.[14]

THE PATIENT DOES NOT HAVE CAPACITY. WHAT NEXT?

Once a patient is deemed to lack capacity, a physician must decide how to proceed. Regarding Ms. S., the physician should make sure that there is not an advance directive or POLST (Physician Orders for Life Sustaining Treatments) form that states the patient would not want ICU care. If no such documentation exists, in an emergency situation the physician often must act without explicit informed consent from the patient. In a less emergent situation, the physician would look for an appropriate decision maker and ask the surrogate decision maker how to proceed. A surrogate decision maker should always be advised to make decisions based on a patient's previously expressed wishes and, if there had been no wishes expressed, to make a "substituted judgment" that considers a patient's values and prior behaviors to figure out what the patient would want.[15]

CASE 29-1   CONTINUED

Ms. S. is transferred to the ICU where she receives antibiotics and fluids. Mechanical ventilation is not required overnight. Upon examination in the morning by the ICU team, although Ms. S. is still somewhat lethargic, she seems less confused. Her capacity is reassessed. Although she still is unable to answer all questions about her treatment options and reason through a decision, she identifies her neighbor (at her bedside) by name as her dearest friend. She also says that her neighbor is like her sister and knows what she wants. Although the doctors don't think she has the capacity to make a treatment decision, they believe that she is capable of identifying a surrogate decision maker. Later, the physicians return to assess the consistency of her wishes and the patient is able to clearly confirm that she wants her neighbor to make medical decisions for her.

One must also take into account the practical aspects of care in designing treatment options for a patient. Issues of "practical" versus "best" treatment often arise in considering treatment options for a patient incapable of making a treatment decision. For example, if an incapable patient is refusing to ingest a particular medication, it may be impossible to force him or her to take the medication. Despite the fact that this medication might be the preferred treatment, it might not be a reasonable option for this patient; a different set of

potential treatments must be considered. The long-term consequences of a therapy also should be considered. For example, for a patient with severe chronic psychosis who develops leukemia, it may be feasible to sedate the patient to receive outpatient chemotherapy as an inpatient, but it may be infeasible to keep that patient hospitalized for the following weeks to monitor for fevers and neutropenia, especially if he or she is not cooperative with hospital staff. Treatments must be practical in order to be implemented.

There are two points about decision-making capacity raised in this part of the case. One is that decisional incapacity is not necessarily a permanent condition.[16] In fact, decision-making capacity often fluctuates. In this case, the patient initially presented with delirium and did not have the ability to make decisions. However, after receiving fluids and antibiotics, her delirium diminished and her ability to make decisions increased. As delirium can wax and wane, so can a patient's ability to make decisions. Patients who are found to lack capacity for a decision at one point should be continually assessed and, in particular, should be reassessed during treatment of the underlying condition. Patients who lack capacity due to psychotic and mood disorders may regain capacity with treatment. There are situations in which patients lack capacity because they lack trust in the information provided or the providers. In such circumstances, decision-making capacity may, at times, be enhanced by improved communication or even by changing providers.

As noted in the case continuation above, even if a patient lacks capacity to make one medical decision, this does not necessarily mean that she lacks capacity to make all decisions.[17,18,19] Drane suggests that a "sliding scale" exists in which increasingly more stringent standards of capacity are required as the consequences of the patient's decision embody more risk.[20] For example, it is generally accepted that the capacity requirements for a patient to name a surrogate decision maker are less stringent than for more complex medical decisions. Some suggest that even patients with severe dementia may be able to identify a surrogate decision maker if they can pass a careful screening process. A set of criteria that could be used to judge whether a nursing home resident has the ability to name a health care proxy showed reasonable reliability and validity when tested among 200 nursing home residents. Even among patients who had a MMSE score of less than 10, 50% were able to name a health care proxy.[17]

Who can assess decision-making capacity in a patient? Any able treating physician can evaluate decision-making capacity, and it is the responsibility of a physician proposing a treatment that requires consent or refusal to ensure that the patient making the choice has the capacity to do so. This responsibility can be fulfilled by the physician carrying out the capacity evaluation or by consulting another physician to perform the assessment. A common misunderstanding is that a psychiatric consult is necessary to perform a formal capacity evaluation.

Although a psychiatric consult can be useful in cases in which a patient is thought to lack decision-making capacity due to a psychiatric disorder, for most medical cases (where incapacity is due to dementia or delirium) any medical doctor with experience in capacity assessment can become qualified to carry out a formal capacity assessment.

How does one deal with uncertainty when assessing decision-making capacity? Test, retest, and retest. When possible, the best way to deal with uncertainty is reassessment. Usually, over time, a patient's mental capabilities will improve or worsen, making the decision less uncertain. Information garnered early in the effort often can inform later retesting and provide insight into a patient's beliefs and capabilities so as to solidify the assessment of each of the aspects of capacity. When prior information about values and behaviors is available, this can inform the capacity assessment as well. When practical aspects of a case make it impossible to take this approach, consider consulting a specialist with expertise in capacity assessment, such as a psychiatrist. An ethics consultation might also be considered. Refusal to participate in a psychiatric assessment—such as refusal to participate in decision making— can constitute incapacity if a patient's capability cannot otherwise be known.[21] The courts are another approach to capacity assessment; however, they are not usually available in a timely fashion and should be reserved for situations in which a decision maker will have to be appointed or for the rare circumstance in which there is uncertainty that requires a legal solution.

CASE 29-1 | **CONTINUED**

In a bedside discussion with the physicians and nurses, Ms. S.'s neighbor and surrogate decision maker is asked about her friend's overall goals for care. She is able to recall multiple conversations that she has had with Ms. S. in which Ms. S. indicated that when it was her time, she wanted to avoid aggressive measures such as mechanical ventilation, and that she wished to die peacefully at home. The neighbor also explained that Ms. S. had felt in recent weeks that her "time" was here. Ms. S.'s neighbor also said that she was willing to care for her friend at home. Based on these preferences, the physicians recommend transferring Ms. S. home with hospice care. Ms. S.'s neighbor strongly believes this is what Ms. S. would want and Ms. S. nods in agreement.

Although not legally appointed, Ms. S.'s neighbor is an acceptable surrogate decision maker. The goal of a surrogate decision maker is to make a decision that is consistent with what the patient would want. Ms. S.'s neighbor did not have difficulty with this because the patient and her neighbor had had clear, frequent, and recent discussions about the patient's preferences for care. In turn, Ms. S.'s neighbor was clear, consistent, and reasoned in her decision making.

Surrogate decision making is not always this easy. One challenge is that the identified surrogate decision maker must demonstrate decision-making capacity. If a surrogate decision maker is deemed incapable (applying the criteria discussed above) to make decisions, an alternate decision maker must be found. Most advance directives designate an alternate. Most states have laws that designate the closest available relative as an appropriate surrogate decision maker. As a last resort, a court-appointed decision maker may be necessary.

Another common challenge to surrogate decision making comes when the surrogate does not have a clear idea of what choices the patient would make. If the surrogate cannot explain the patient's previously stated wishes and a substituted judgment (based on the values and prior behaviors of the patient) is impossible, then the surrogate decision maker should be guided to make a "best interest" decision *from the patient's perspective*. A common pitfall is a surrogate deciding to pursue a plan that fits what he or she would personally want for the patient rather than placing himself in the patient's shoes. While some surrogate decision makers get this concept implicitly, with others considerable effort is needed to help them overcome the strong desire to make a self-serving choice.

A physician may be able to help guide decision making by stimulating conversation about the patient's personality, passions, and attitudes toward their disease and medical care. For the surrogate who is unable to relate the patient's preferences or to make a substituted judgment, we have found it valuable to have the surrogate recount "who this person is." What was this patient like? What were her goals and aspirations? What made him tick? If it cannot be known what this patient would want right now, what sorts of decisions would be most consistent with the essence of her being?

AVOIDING A COMMON MISTAKE

A common mistake made by physicians who care for elderly patients with complex medical issues is to not assess capacity until the patient disagrees with the physician's recommendations (Table 29-2). Patients with various levels of cognitive impairment may not have the capacity to make decisions, for example, about whether to initiate chemotherapy. This might not be obvious, especially if a patient is agreeing to recommended therapies. Testing for and documentation of decision-making capacity in older patients who are making important medical decisions should be routine.[16]

PLANNING FOR INCAPACITY

Even among critically ill cancer patients,[22] only a small proportion of individuals have completed an advance directive. In addition, studies suggest that patients with terminal illness often do not communicate their preferences for care either to their surrogate decision makers or their physicians.[23,24] Thus the high rate of incapacity anticipated among elderly cancer patients means

TABLE 29-2
Ten Myths About Decision-Making Capacity
1. Decision-making capacity and competency are the same.
2. Lack of decision-making capacity can be presumed when patients go against medical advice.
3. There is no need to assess decision-making capacity unless patients go against medical advice.
4. Decision-making capacity is an "all or nothing" phenomenon.
5. Cognitive impairment equals lack of decision-making capacity.
6. Lack of decision-making capacity is a permanent condition.
7. Patients who have not been given relevant and consistent information about their treatment lack decision-making capacity.
8. All patients with certain psychiatric disorders lack decision-making capacity.
9. Patients who have been involuntarily committed lack decision-making capacity.
10. Only mental health experts can assess decision-making capacity.

From Ganzini L, Volicer L, Nelson WA, Fox E, Derse AR. Ten myths about decision-making capacity. J Am Med Dir Assoc 2005;6(3 Suppl):S100-4.

that preserving autonomy in this vulnerable population requires primary care physicians, oncologists, and other clinicians caring for these patients to discuss the importance of surrogate decision makers and advance care planning early in the trajectory of illness, as well as at sentinel events, such as onset of metastatic brain disease, beginning of a palliative chemotherapeutic regimen, and admission to an ICU.[25] Discussing patient preferences for care and documenting a surrogate decision maker for cancer patients can improve the match of treatment with prognosis and preferences. If Ms. S. had been unable to name her neighbor as her surrogate decision maker, there would have been no way to ensure that medical decisions reflected what she would have wanted. Discussing these topics in advance, while sometimes difficult, will ultimately increase patient autonomy and make it more likely that the care patients receive is consistent with their goals.

INFORMED CONSENT AND CANCER CLINICAL TRIALS

This chapter uses a clinical case to display the importance of decision-making capacity in informed decision-making. It is important to note that assessment of and attention to decision-making capacity is also critical in research. Providing informed consent for participation in a cancer clinical trial requires a high level of understanding and the capacity to reason through complex trade-offs. For the older cancer patient, assessment of decision-making capacity prior to obtaining informed consent for research should be routine.[26]

FUTURE RESEARCH

Evidence suggests that physicians, even including psychiatrists, may inconsistently apply the standards for decision-making capacity.[27] There is still a great deal to learn about decision-making capacity and the best ways to care for patients who lack decision-making capacity. It is important to study how capacity is tested in practice, what errors are common, and the clinical implications of such errors. In addition, better standardized methods of measuring decisional capacity that are practical for the clinical setting are needed. Such tools should account for the magnitude of the decision and should have the capability to be used in a serial fashion to assess change over time. Moreover, we need to know more about how to enhance capacity among patients who are marginally capable of making decisions or whose capacity waxes and wanes. The better the set of tools available to assess and maximize decision-making capacity, the greater the likelihood that decision-making capacity will be appropriately used in clinical care.

Chapter Summary

Ideally, a patient would always actively participate in decisions about his or her own medical care. Unfortunately, delirium and cognitive impairment are common among elderly patients with cancer and therefore capacity assessment will almost always be necessary in the trajectory of disease of an older cancer patient. In most situations, capacity assessment can be performed by the physician obtaining consent from a patient for treatment; however, psychiatric or ethics consultation may be helpful in some cases. A strategy for assessing decision-making capacity has been suggested.

When a patient lacks decision-making capacity, an appropriate surrogate decision maker should be identified and counseled about making a substituted judgment on behalf of the patient. Advance care planning is recommended in the elderly cancer patient to ensure that treatment decisions are made in accordance with a patient's goals, even after the patient loses the capacity to actively participate in decision making.

ACKNOWLEDGMENT

Some of the concepts developed in this chapter were derived from UCLA Clinical Ethics Rounds that included James Hynds, PhD, and Katherine Brown-Saltzman, RN, MA.

See expertconsult.com for a complete list of references and web resources for this chapter

SUGGESTED READINGS

1. Appelbaum PS: Assessment of patients' competence to consent to treatment, *N Engl J Med* 357:1834–1840, 2007.
2. Appelbaum PS, Grisso T: Assessing patients' capacities to consent to treatment, *N Engl J Med* 319:1635–1638, 1988.
3. Ganzini L, Volicer L, Nelson WA, et al: Ten myths about decision-making capacity, *JAMDA* S100–S104, 2005.

Economic Burdens and Access to Care Barriers for the Older Cancer Patient

Scott D. Ramsey, John F. Scoggins, and Veena Shankaran

CASE 30-1 | **CASE DESCRIPTION**

A 75-year-old man with type 2 diabetes and hypertension presented to his physician with fatigue and constipation. His complete blood count showed a low hemoglobin level and evidence of iron deficiency; colonoscopy revealed a sigmoid colon mass. He had missed a routine screening colonoscopy appointment 3 years ago, but a prior colonoscopy approximately 15 years ago had been unremarkable. He subsequently underwent surgical resection of the mass, which was found to be a T3N1M0 adenocarcinoma of the sigmoid colon. His surgical course was complicated by a wound infection but he has been continuing to recover slowly from his hospitalization. His daughter has been helping with his wound care and dressing changes. His oncologist recommends adjuvant chemotherapy with a 6-month course of oral capecitabine, and he leaves the clinic with a prescription, along with instructions for proper use of the medication.

Up until now, he has been purchasing his antihypertensives and diabetes medications online from a Canadian pharmacy and has therefore not enrolled in a Medicare Part D prescription plan. His wife died 3 years ago from breast cancer, and he lives with his daughter and son-in-law. He does receive monthly Social Security checks. Although he has a small amount of savings left, much of it was depleted by expenses related to his wife's cancer.

After checking online, he discovers that a 1-month supply of capecitabine will cost approximately $2,000, which he knows he cannot afford. He decides not to mention this to his daughter, since she has been so worried after her husband lost his job a month ago. He calls the nurse at the oncologist's office to tell her that he is not interested in adjuvant chemotherapy, but that he will come back for routine checkups. A follow-up appointment is scheduled in 3 months.

About a year later, he develops pain on the right side of his abdomen. A computed tomography (CT) scan shows extensive metastases to the liver. Systemic chemotherapy is recommended, and he is now going to the oncologist's office every 2 weeks to receive FOLFOX + bevacizumab. He develops significant neuropathy and nausea from chemotherapy. He has been taking his nausea medications only when the nausea is severe, because the medication is quite expensive. Because his neuropathy has worsened, his daughter now has to drive him to all of his clinic appointments and chemotherapy appointments. Because of side effects from chemotherapy, he does not have the energy to play with his grandkids. He feels nauseated, tired, and sad most of the time. He feels guilty and wishes he could just "slip away."

Old age is typically a period of declining income and increasing health care expenditures. For example, Americans older than 85 who do not have cancer have household incomes 47% lower and out-of-pocket health expenditures 77% higher than those between 55 and 65 years of age. Between these two age groups, out-of-pocket health expenditures increase from 3% to 9% of household income (Table 30-1).[1]

The economic realities can be even harsher for those older Americans who suffer from cancer. Out-of-pocket health expenditures are 32% higher for cancer patients over age 65 than for people in this age group without cancer.[2] The Consumer Bankruptcy Project (CBP) found that 10% of families of all ages that filed for bankruptcy

due to medical reasons cited cancer as their main illness.[3] These higher economic burdens borne by elderly cancer patients persist in spite of a high percentage of health insurance coverage for this age group relative to younger people (99.6% vs. 86.4%).[4]

To understand the special economic problems encountered by older cancer patients, an examination of the patchwork system of insurance coverage in the United States is necessary. In addition, any discussion of the economic burdens of older cancer patients should include the costs incurred by relatives and other uncompensated caregivers. This chapter describes the coverage system under Medicare and Medicaid for the majority of older adults in the United States, focusing on potential sources

TABLE 30-1	Income, Out-of-Pocket, and Total Health Expenditures by Age Group and Cancer Diagnosis (1996-2006)					
	Income		Total Expenditures		Out-of-pocket	
Age	Not Cancer	Cancer	Not Cancer	Cancer	Not Cancer	Cancer
55 - 65	$33,065	$33,122	$4,264	$15,705	$894	$1,762
65 - 75	$24,045	$25,359	$5,396	$13,585	$1,037	$1,408
75 - 85	$19,551	$20,408	$7,047	$12,773	$1,296	$1,656
≥ 85	$17,522	$18,817	$7,741	$12,172	$1,586	$1,945

of high out-of-pocket expenses for patients with cancer. Average out-of-pocket expenditures for older patients with and without a cancer diagnosis are described using data from the Medical Expenditures Panel Survey (MEPS). MEPS is a nationally representative survey of medical expenditures by households and individuals that has been conducted by the Agency for Healthcare Research and Quality (AHRQ) every year since 1996.[5] Finally, the costs and burdens borne by family members of elderly patients with cancer are explored.

HEALTH INSURANCE BENEFITS AND COSTS

Medicare

Medicare covers 98.9% of all Americans age 65 and older. It is available to all those who qualify for Social Security benefits and is by far the largest health insurer in the U.S. There are four major parts of Medicare coverage. Part A covers hospitalization (excluding physician fees), home health, hospice, and a limited number of days of nursing home care. Part B covers physician fees and outpatient care. Part C is a managed care option operated by private companies and covers the same expenses (and sometimes more) that Parts A and B cover. Part D covers prescription drugs.[6]

Most Medicare enrollees do not pay any premiums for Part A coverage, but do pay a deductible ($1,068 in 2009) and coinsurance (from $0 to $534 per day in 2009, depending on the length of stay) for each hospital stay. The few who do pay premiums (i.e., people who do not qualify for Social Security, also known as *voluntary* Part A beneficiaries) are charged $443 per month for basic coverage.[7] Medicare also pays for part or all, up to the first 100 days (in a lifetime), of long-term hospitalization or nursing home care. Specifically, Medicare pays for all of the first 20 days and the enrollee must pay $133.5 per day for stays between 21 and 100 days.

Because of the limits to Part A coverage, the greatest exposure to high out-of-pocket expenses for Part A enrollees comes from hospital stays that last for more than 60 days and nursing home stays that last for more than 20 days. For example, a 120-day hospital stay would generate $25,000 of expenses not covered by Medicare and a 100-day nursing home stay will generate

$10,000 in noncovered expenses. Long nursing home stays are quite common. 8.5% of all nursing home residents over the age of 65 have a diagnosis of cancer and 72.6% of those cancer patients have stays that last longer than 100 days. With an average monthly charge of $4,290 in 2004, the out-of-pocket cost of a long nursing home stay can be financially devastating.[8]

Part B beneficiaries pay a monthly premium of $96.40—more if their individual income is over $85,000 per year. In addition to the monthly premium, Part B beneficiaries pay an annual deductible of $135 plus 20% of all Part B payments to providers. Medicare Part B facility payments are determined by prospective payment systems that dictate the payment for each type of patient visit. Physician fees paid by Medicare are determined by the resource-based relative value scale (RBRVS).

Part C (Medicare Advantage) is an optional type of insurance coverage that Medicare beneficiaries can substitute for Part A, Part B and Part D coverage. These plans are administered by private insurance companies, mainly health maintenance organizations (HMOs) and preferred provider organizations (PPOs). As of 2009, 23% of Medicare enrollees are covered by Medicare Advantage plans.[9] Medicare pays the plan administrators approximately 15% more per enrollee than it pays for fee-for-service enrollees. This relatively generous payment system is responsible for the increased participation in Medicare Advantage plans by private insurers in 2003. This increased competition has attracted many enrollees to Medicare Advantage plans, but is a source of controversy.

Part D, implemented in 2006, provides coverage for prescription drug costs. Enrollees pay a minimum monthly premium of $24.80, a $180 to $265 annual deductible and 25% of full drug costs up to $2,400. Once out-of-pocket expenses reach $3,850, the enrollee pays only 5% of additional drug costs.[10] The range of uncovered drug costs is known as the "donut hole", a gap in coverage. In 2008, the coverage gap was $3,216 for plans offering the standard Medicare Part D benefit; by 2019, it is projected to be nearly $6,000.[11]

Medicaid

Medicaid covers 8.7% of all Americans age 65 and older who are actively treated for cancer.[12] Each state determines its own terms of eligibility for Medicaid coverage

TABLE 30-2	Out-of-Pocket and Total Health Expenditures by Cancer Diagnosis and Expenditure Category, Age 65 and Older (1996-2006)					
	Expenditures					
	Without Cancer		With Cancer		Difference	
Category	Out-of-pocket	Total	Out-of-pocket	Total	Out-of-pocket	Total
Drugs	$738	$1,437	$895	$1,771	$157	$334
Office visits	$138	$1,247	$247	$3,232	$110	$1,985
Home health	$90	$569	$133	$867	$43	$298
Hospitalization	$33	$2,321	$67	$5,371	$34	$3,050
Outpatient	$20	$427	$41	$1,816	$21	$1,389
Other	$316	$1,002	$388	$1,755	$73	$753
Total	$1,335	$7,003	$1,772	$14,812	$437	$7,809

but, in general, Medicaid is intended to cover the indigent population. Consequently, Medicaid coverage does not normally require premiums, deductibles, or coinsurance payments. Indeed, Medicaid often pays the Medicare premiums, deductibles, and coinsurance payments for people who are enrolled in both Medicare and Medicaid.

In 2008, Medicaid physician fees were 72% of Medicare physician fees.[13] Consequently, Medicaid's fee payments are so low that some physicians claim to not accept new Medicaid patients. This could result in less access to health care for Medicaid patients; however, this access problem for Medicaid enrollees may be less acute for cancer patients than for other types of patients. In a 2006 survey of physicians who accepted new patients, only 4% of oncologists responded that they did not accept new Medicaid patients, while none responded that they did not accept new Medicare patients. Primary care physicians and other specialists responded that 18% did not accept new Medicaid patients and 12% did not accept new Medicare patients.[14]

Importantly, Medicaid covers nursing home expenses. Since Medicare coverage ends after 100 days, many long-term nursing home residents must deplete their life savings before becoming eligible for Medicaid. For nursing home residents over the age of 65 with a diagnosis of cancer, 34% are covered by Medicaid at the start of a stay that lasts for more than 100 days; however, the percentage jumps to 65% by the end of the stay.[1]

TOTAL AND OUT-OF-POCKET HEALTH EXPENDITURES

The costs of cancer care to Medicare are substantial and vary by tumor site, phase of care, stage at diagnosis, and survival. Costs are greatest in the initial year of treatment and in the final year of treatment and also increase with stage.[16,17,18] Older patients being treated for cancer—regardless of their insurance status—face significantly higher out-of-pocket and total health expenditures than patients without cancer.[19] From 1996 to 2006, annual total health expenditures for members of this age group being treated for cancer were more than double those

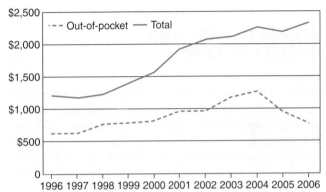

FIGURE 30-1 Annual per Capita Drug Expenditures by Cancer Patients Age 65 and Older, 1996-2006 (2006 dollars)

for members not being treated for cancer ($14,812 vs. $7,003). Out-of-pocket expenditures for these two groups averaged $1,772 and $1,335, respectively—a 33% increase from the noncancer group.[20] Although the difference in total health expenditures is due mainly to expenditures for office visits, hospitalization, and outpatient visits, the single largest component of the difference in out-of-pocket expenditures is for prescription drugs, $896 vs. $738. Over this time period, half of total drug expenditures for older cancer patients were paid out-of-pocket. Only 7% of other types of health expenditures are paid out-of-pocket.[20] Table 30-2 provides complete figures.

It was because of high out-of-pocket expenditures for prescription drugs that the Medicare Prescription Drug, Improvement, and Modernization Act (i.e., Medicare Part D and Medicare Advantage Plans) was enacted in 2003. Figure 30-1 shows the annual per capita drug expenditures for cancer patients age 65 and older from 1996 to 2006. Although total drug expenditures continued their upward trend over this time span, out-of-pocket drug expenditures have decreased from $1,269 to $777 (39%) since 2004.[20] This sizable decrease in out-of-pocket drug expenditures for the elderly cancer patient is likely due in part to Medicare Part D; however, since Part D did not become operational until 2006, it is also likely that some of the decrease, especially in 2005, was due to the enhancement of Medicare Advantage plans that began earlier than 2006. The decrease in some of these out-of-pocket prescription costs might have been offset by premiums and deductibles related to Medicare Part D and Medicare Advantage plans.

Despite the variable total expenditures by cancer type, cancer patients uniformly experience significant out-of-pocket costs (range $257-$1,620). Table 30-3 shows the geometric mean values for annual total and out-of-pocket expenditures by type of cancer.[20]

Patient time during treatment is a nonpecuniary cost that is usually not included in out-of-pocket costs. One 2007 study concluded that the value of patient time totaled $2.3 billion in 2005 and varied substantially by tumor site.[21]

ACCESS TO CARE AND QUALITY OF CARE

Some studies have concluded that access to care and quality of care for the older cancer patient are not all that they could be. Many clinicians may be influenced by ageist beliefs that are not supported by scientific evidence. For example, one study concluded that oncology health care professionals had negative attitudes towards elderly people with regards to their residential patterns, cognitive style, personal appearance, and personalities.[22] Another published report noted that mastectomy has been used as a standard treatment for older women, because it was believed that changes in body image would not bother them, although evidence shows that older women also suffer problems with body image after mastectomy.[23]

Inadequate local therapy is associated with reduced survival in elderly women treated with breast-conserving therapy.[24] Older adults being treated for cancer may not be provided appropriate palliative care[25] and may often experience diminished quality of life.[26] Some limits to care could be self-imposed. In a survey of elderly adults, respondents were more likely to recommend end-of-life treatment for a spouse when it was financed by Medicare than by the patient's own savings.[27]

Despite the near universality of health insurance coverage of the elderly, many cancer patients perceive problems in the quality of their care. Even when restricting the sample to those who have health insurance, cancer patients aged 65 and older are less likely than younger cancer patients to report that their doctors listen to them (odds ratio [OR] = 0.76, p < 0.01), explain their treatment to them so that they will understand (OR = 0.78, p < 0.01), and show them respect (OR = 0.74, p < 0.01). Also, older cancer patients are less likely to report that their doctors spend enough time with them (OR = 0.82, p = 0.04). Overall, older cancer patients are less likely than younger cancer patients to give their doctor a high overall ranking (OR = 0.79, p = 0.01).[28]

Older cancer patients' perceptions of their access to care are generally more favorable than their perceptions of their quality of care. Older cancer patients were nearly half as likely as younger cancer patients with health insurance to report any difficulties or delays in getting needed care (OR = 0.55, p < 0.01) and there was no statistically significant difference between older and younger patients in the percentage reporting that they were able to obtain health care when needed (OR = 0.92, p = 0.54).[31]

TABLE 30-3	Annual Total and Out-of-Pocket Expenditures by Type of Cancer, 1996-2006 (2006 Dollars)						
		Total Expenditures			Out-of-Pocket Expenditures		
			95% Conf. Int.			95% Conf. Int.	
Type of Cancer	n	Mean	LB	UB	Mean	LB	UB
Pancreas	14	$30,594	$13,635	$68,647	$928	$336	$2,559
Multiple Myeloma	15	$16,658	$8,208	$33,807	$1,620	$944	$2,779
Liver	33	$16,116	$8,941	$29,047	$1,246	$594	$2,612
Lung	140	$16,054	$13,411	$19,220	$1,023	$763	$1,371
Ovary	15	$15,936	$3,530	$71,948	$765	$307	$1,910
Thyroid	20	$15,627	$7,246	$33,699	$1,337	$854	$2,092
Colorectal	184	$11,707	$9,594	$14,286	$873	$775	$984
Cervix	10	$11,380	$6,597	$19,629	$588	$218	$1,586
Kidney	25	$10,595	$5,659	$19,834	$683	$166	$2,816
Bone	44	$10,523	$8,141	$13,602	$1,119	$887	$1,412
Non-Hodgkin	69	$9,375	$7,138	$12,314	$966	$684	$1,365
Bladder	85	$8,443	$7,182	$9,927	$1,098	$816	$1,476
Leukemia	90	$8,125	$6,229	$10,599	$937	$825	$1,065
Uterus	30	$7,511	$4,708	$11,981	$1,563	$924	$2,646
Breast	431	$6,723	$6,214	$7,275	$1,299	$1,177	$1,433
Prostate	562	$6,354	$5,935	$6,802	$826	$776	$879
Melanomas	63	$6,090	$4,706	$7,880	$890	$777	$1,020
Head and Neck	78	$5,687	$3,362	$9,621	$805	$600	$1,079
Stomach	24	$5,187	$1,650	$16,305	$257	$165	$401

CAREGIVER COSTS

Many costs of caring for older cancer patients are borne by their friends and relatives. These costs include financial and productivity losses and psychological and physical stressors. For all types of illnesses, one study in 1997 concluded that the cost of informal caregiving was more than six times as great as formal home health care.[29] Another study found that caregivers of elderly cancer patients sacrifice more than 3 hours per week more than caregivers for noncancer patients.[30] This loss in productivity surpassed a billion dollars for the United States in 2001. Yet another study found that when family labor is included in the cost calculations, average cancer home care costs for a 3-month period are not much lower than the costs of nursing home care.[31] Out-of-pocket and labor costs for family caregivers of breast cancer patients have been found to be equal to approximately half of the amount of costs borne directly by the patient.[32]

Several studies have found that caregivers of elderly cancer patients have higher depression scores or worse health than control subjects.[33-36] The mental health effects on the spouse of the elderly cancer patient can continue well beyond the death of the patient.[37] Providing care for older cancer patients can be especially stressful because such patients often have premorbid or comorbid conditions, such as dementia.[38] Caring for an elderly cancer patient can also have its rewards, since some caregivers report feelings of satisfaction and a greater sense of self-worth.[39]

CONCLUSION

The older cancer patient encounters many serious economic consequences. At a time in their lives when incomes are fixed and declining with every additional year of age, out-of-pocket costs are increasing. Time costs for older cancer patients and their informal caregivers are also quite burdensome. The physical and emotional effects on the friends and relatives are difficult to measure monetarily, but are very substantial nonetheless.

Although the out-of-pocket costs are significant, they are quite small in comparison with total monetary costs of care, because of the near universality of health insurance coverage for the elderly in the United States. In recent years, out-of-pocket prescription drug costs have declined significantly as a result of changes in Medicare coverage. Despite these changes, cancer patients, as compared with patients with other diseases, may be more vulnerable to high out-of-pocket costs related to the "donut-hole," nursing homes, and other types of medical expenditures.

Chapter Summary

Old age is a period of declining incomes and increasing medical costs for everyone; however, these economic constraints are even worse for the older cancer patient. Almost every older cancer patient is covered by Medicare and nearly 9% are covered by Medicaid. Medicare covers most hospitalization, outpatient, and physician services, but is less generous with prescription drugs and nursing home expenses. Changes in Medicare coverage for prescription drugs enacted in 2004 led to a 39% reduction in out-of-pocket expenditures by older cancer patients in 2006.

There is published evidence that many oncology healthcare professionals hold negative attitudes towards elderly people. Older cancer patients are more likely than younger cancer patients to believe that their physicians do not listen to them or show them the proper amount of respect. The economic and psychological costs of cancer care for the elderly are not restricted to the patients. Many informal caregivers suffer from depression and physical illnesses that are associated with their burdens.

 See expertconsult.com for a complete list of references and web resources for this chapter

SUGGESTED READINGS

1. Chang S, Long SR, Kutikova L, et al: Estimating the cost of cancer: results on the basis of claims data analyses for cancer patients diagnosed with seven types of cancer during 1999 to 2000, *J Clin Oncol* 22:3524–3530, 2004.
2. Chao LW, Pagán JA, Soldo BJ: End-of-life medical treatment choices: do survival chances and out-of-pocket costs matter? *Med Decis Making* 28:511–523, 2008.
3. Esbensen BA, Østerlind K, Hallberg IR: Quality of life of elderly persons with cancer: a 3-month follow-up, *Cancer Nurs* 29(3):214–224, 2006.
4. Given BA, Given CW, Stommel M: Family and out-of-pocket costs for women with breast cancer, *Cancer Pract* 2(3): 187–193, 1994.
5. Grunfeld E, Coyle D, Whelan T, et al: Family caregiver burden: results of a longitudinal study of breast cancer patients and their principal caregivers, *CMAJ* 170(12):1795–1801, 2004.
6. Haley WE, LaMonde LA, Han B, et al: Family caregiving in hospice: effects on psychological and health functioning among spousal caregivers of hospice patients with lung cancer or dementia, *Hosp J* 15(4):1–18, 2001.
7. Haley WE: Family caregivers of elderly patients with cancer: understanding and minimizing the burden of care, *J Support Oncol* 1(4 Suppl 2):25–29, 2003.
8. Haley WE: The costs of family caregiving: implications for geriatric oncology, *Crit Rev Oncol Hematol* 48(2):151–158, 2003.
9. Hayman JA, Langa KM, Kabeto MU, et al: Estimating the cost of informal caregiving for elderly patients with cancer, *J Clin Oncol* 19(13):3219–3225, 2001.
10. Kearney N, Miller M, Paul J, Smith K: Oncology healthcare professionals' attitudes toward elderly people, *Ann Oncol* 11(5):599–601, 2000.
11. Langa KM, Fendrick AM, Chernew ME, et al: Out-of-pocket health-care expenditures among older Americans with cancer, *Value Health* 7(2):186–194, 2004.
12. Ragan SL, Wittenberg E, Hall HT: The communication of palliative care for the elderly cancer patient, *Health Commun* 15(2):219–226, 2003.
13. Stommel M, Given CW, Given BA: The cost of cancer home care to families, *Cancer* 71(5):1867–1874, 1993.

14. Truong PT, Bernstein V, Lesperance M, et al: Radiotherapy omission after breast-conserving surgery is associated with reduced breast cancer-specific survival in elderly women with breast cancer, *Am J Surg* 191(6):749–755, 2006.

15. Valdimarsdóttir U, Helgason AR, Fürst CJ, et al: The unrecognised cost of cancer patients' unrelieved symptoms: a nationwide follow-up of their surviving partners, *Br J Cancer* 86(10):1540–1545, 2002.

16. Yabroff KR, Lawrence WF, Clauser S, et al: Burden of illness in cancer survivors: findings from a population-based national sample, *J Natl Cancer Inst* 96(17):1322–1330, 2004.

17. Yabroff KR, Davis WW, Lamont EB, et al: Patient time costs associated with cancer care, *J Natl Cancer Inst* 99(1):14–23, 2007.

18. Yabroff KR, Lamont EB, Mariotto A, et al: Cost of care for elderly cancer patients in the United States, *J Natl Cancer Inst* 100(9):630–641, 2008.

Page numbers followed by *b*, *t*, and *f* indicate boxes, tables and figures, respectively.

Turner 1775-1851

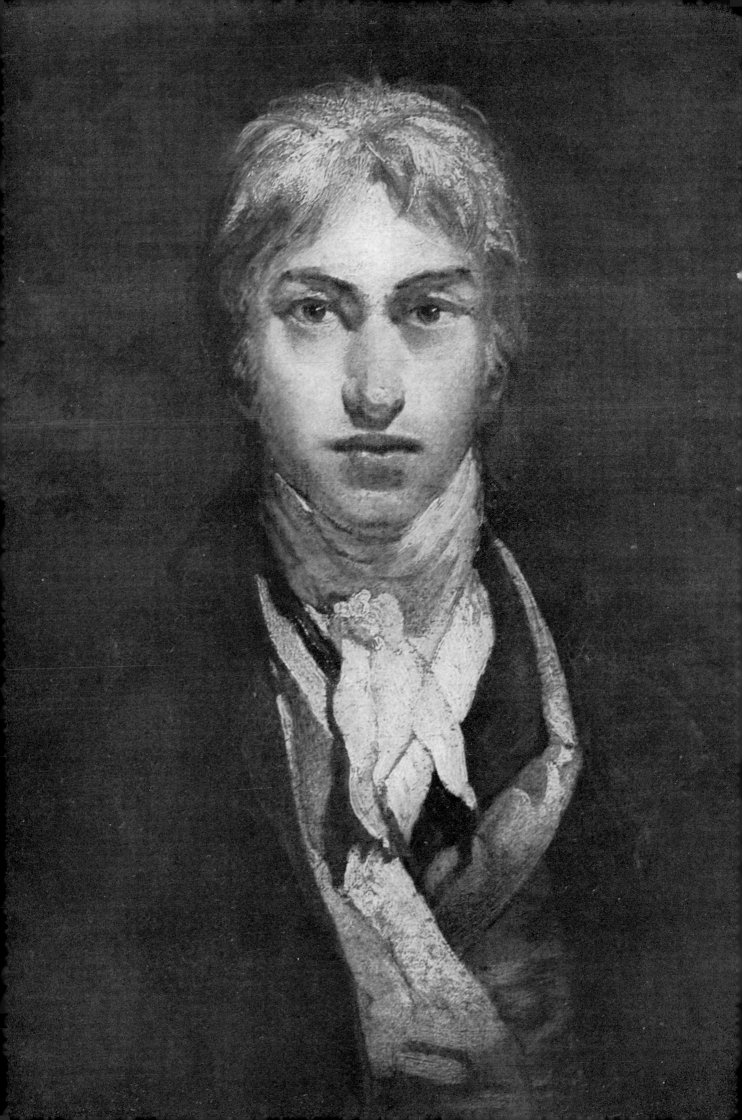

TURNER

1775-1851

Cover/Jacket
The Old Chain Pier, Brighton, c.1828 (details)
(catalogue No.328)

Frontispiece
Self-Portrait, c.1798 (detail)
(catalogue No.B1)

Exclusively distributed in France and Italy by Idea Books
24 rue du 4 Septembre, 75002 Paris and Via Cappuccio 21, 20123 Milan

ISBN 0 900874 84 8 paper 0 900874 85 6 cloth
Published by order of the Trustees 1974
for the exhibition of 16 November 1974 – 2 March 1975
organised jointly by the Tate Gallery and the Royal Academy of Arts
Copyright © 1974 The Tate Gallery

Designed and published by the Tate Gallery Publications Department,
Millbank, London SW1P 4RG
Blocks by Augustan Engravers Ltd, London
Colour separation by Gilchrist Ltd, Leeds
Printed in Great Britain by Balding & Mansell Ltd, Wisbech, Cambs.

Contents

Turner Exhibition

Committee

Sir Thomas Monnington *Chairman*
    President, Royal Academy

Sir Norman Reid
    Director, Tate Gallery

Martin Butlin
    Keeper of the British Collection, Tate Gallery

Michael Compton
    Keeper of Exhibitions and Education, Tate Gallery

Roger de Grey, R.A.
    Chairman, Exhibitions Committee, Royal Academy

John Gage
    Lecturer, Department of Fine Arts and Music,
    University of East Anglia

Sidney C. Hutchison, M.V.O.
    Secretary, Royal Academy

Philip James, C.B.E. (deceased)
    Librarian and Exhibitions Secretary, Royal
    Academy, until April 1974

Andrew Wilton
    Assistant Keeper, Department of Prints and
    Drawings, British Museum

Working Party

Sidney C. Hutchison, M.V.O. *Chairman*
    Secretary, Royal Academy

Iain Bain
    Publications Manager, Tate Gallery

Corinne Bellow, M.B.E.
    Head of Information Services, Tate Gallery

Martin Butlin
    Keeper of the British Collection, Tate Gallery

Hans Fletcher
    Assistant Secretary, Royal Academy

John Gage
    Lecturer, Department of Fine Arts and Music,
    University of East Anglia

Philip James, C.B.E. (deceased)
    Librarian and Exhibitions Secretary, Royal
    Academy, until April 1974

Kenneth J. Tanner
    Registrar, Royal Academy

Nicholas Usherwood *Exhibition Secretary*
    Assistant Secretary, Royal Academy

Robin Wade *Exhibition Designer*
    Robin Wade Design Associates

Andrew Wilton
    Assistant Keeper, Department of Prints and
    Drawings, British Museum

Foreword

Turner has good claim to be the most perceptive and creative artist that Britain has ever produced. His range of mood and the extent of his development from his early, traditional beginnings to his late masterpieces are perhaps wider than those of any other artist. It is our hope that something of the richness of his achievement will be visible in this exhibition. As the custodians of the majority of the oil paintings in the Turner Bequest, the Tate Gallery, where five rooms are normally devoted to his work, comes nearest to the Turner Gallery envisaged in the artist's will. The Royal Academy is the institution on which he rested his ambition and which saw his triumphs. It is therefore fitting that we should have organised this exhibition together and that it should take place in the Academy's galleries.

It is also appropriate that the team responsible for the selection and cataloguing of the exhibition should comprise the curators most closely concerned with the oil paintings and with the drawings and watercolours in the Turner Bequest, Martin Butlin and Andrew Wilton respectively, together with the leading young scholar of Turner in this country, John Gage. Although they have worked together, their individual opinions have been retained; no complete agreement can ever be reached on so complex an artist and it was thought best that their differences should not be masked but rather left to provoke discussion. The team has been complimented by the designers, Robin Wade Design Associates, who have coped, among other problems, with that of fitting an exhibition divided into twenty sections into a suite of only fourteen galleries. The catalogue has been designed by Pauline Key of the Tate Gallery Publications Department.

The degree of collaboration does not end with the people named above. The entries on the oil paintings exhibited by Turner during his lifetime would have been impossible without the readily forthcoming assistance of Evelyn Joll, who is preparing a complete *catalogue raisonnée* of Turner's oil paintings with Martin Butlin, to be published jointly by the Tate Gallery and the Paul Mellon Centre for the Study of British Art. Indeed, Mr Joll has gone further and the entries for Nos. 74, 79, 132, 142, 506, 515, 517, 568 and 620 are substantially his work; many others are based on entries supplied by him for earlier exhibitions, including that devoted to Turner at Agnew's in 1967. The entries on Turner's exhibited oil paintings also embody a considerable amount of new material in the shape of extracts from contemporary newspaper and magazine criticism, painstakingly researched by Frances Butlin in connection with the *catalogue raisonnée* mentioned above. We are grateful to Christopher White, Director of Studies at the Mellon Centre, for encouraging us to use material destined for this catalogue. Our debt to other Turner scholars is great, both to their published works and for information received more informally; in particular to Luke Herrmann who helped us with both information and suggestions following a recent visit to the United States.

Our debt is equally great to Sir Geoffrey Agnew and, in this field as well, Evelyn Joll for their help in securing loans of both oils and watercolours and for making available to us the resources of the archives of Thos. Agnew &

Sons, Ltd, whose first purchase of a work by Turner can be traced back to the year of the artist's death. We are similarly indebted to Hugh Leggatt and Paul Thomson for putting us in touch with private owners. We must also thank Mrs Patricia Barnden of the Mellon Centre for her generous assistance over photographs of works in private possession. Other photographs have kindly been supplied by the owners.

It is indeed to the owners that we owe our greatest debt of all. Their names appear at the end of this catalogue but we would like to thank especially Her Majesty The Queen for the loan of the original manuscript of Farington's Diary, all those private owners who have deprived themselves of their treasured possessions for such a long period, and those museums in the United States and elsewhere who have agreed to their pictures travelling overseas.

W. T. Monnington
President of the Royal Academy

Norman Reid
Director of the Tate Gallery

J. M. W. Turner: Art and Content

Turner is that relatively rare thing among British artists, a thorough-going professional whose motivation was above all visual. Not that his art did not have content, content that can to a certain extent be explained by reference to literary sources. Significant content, in fact, he regarded as essential to the highest forms of art and to make them worthy of the public's attention. But his relative carelessness over titles, his cavalier attitude to what might be called the proper documentation, suggests that it was the visual effect and the hint of underlying literary sources that were important to him, not an intellectual content of the kind that underlies the work of such an artist as Poussin. This is not to gainsay the importance of current research into Turner's literary sources; only to warn against an over-dependence on intellectual sources when dealing with a largely self-educated barber's son. In so far as Turner was an intellectual, he was an intellectual *manqué*, an amateur intellectual.

Amateur was just what Turner was not as an artist. He trained the hard, the thorough way, not just in the Royal Academy Schools but as a topographical draughtsman for the engraver and as a copyist of other men's works. This last task, the copying of drawings by J. R. Cozens and other artists for Dr Monro over a period of three years, was all-important to him in getting to know the alternative tradition: the imaginative use of landscape instead of the 'tame delineation' of an object beautiful, interesting or picturesque in itself. In an age before the creation of public collections, or the multiplicity of illustrated art books, he was also lucky that the times and his patrons gave him an opportunity for seeing a wide range of paintings by the Old Masters. The wars of the French Revolution led to the sending of many masterpieces to London, to be shown in the sale rooms. There they were bought by such early patrons of Turner as William Beckford and could be seen again when he was invited to produce topographical views of the patron's estate, views that soon became the most accomplished and the grandest of their kind.

The Academy was also important for its traditions, as well as its training. Founded seven years before Turner's birth it embodied, in general terms at least, the academic ideals of the seventeenth-century classicists, in themselves based on an idealisation of the achievements of the High Renaissance, in particular Raphael. By a happy chance two of the greatest artists in seventeenth-century Rome, the French-born Poussin and Claude, were landscape painters, but painters of idealised landscapes peopled with the embodiments of moral qualities. In Poussin in particular the very forms of the landscape became the means by which the virtues of Christian and Stoic morality could be expressed. In the Academic hierarchy of genres landscape could never rise to the topmost rank, occupied as that was by figure-paintings of moral subjects, but it could approach it by shedding the topographical or decorative associations of 'mere' landscape and replacing them by significant content. As a young artist of no social status Turner's ambitions naturally turned to the Academy, and he accepted wholeheartedly its assessment of what was most important in art, fortunate in that its traditions included an inculcation in just the sort of art to which he was most suited, the historical landscape.

Turner's most revolutionary accomplishments, as well as his seeming vagaries of taste, are based on his ambition to make his landscapes worthy of the grand tradition of the Old Masters. Right up to the last he continued to exhibit landscapes with morally important subjects, from mythology, the history of Rome and Carthage, and to a lesser extent the Bible. At one period, round about 1830, he even produced a whole series of Biblical and other pictures in which the figures predominated. But his ambition to produce historical landscapes led inevitably to a widening of what was historical, what was significant. His earlier exhibits can be fairly easily divided into categories according to subject, though already, in the first decade of the nineteenth century, he began to blur the distinctions with large pictures of classical weight which nevertheless dealt with contemporary subjects: the death of Nelson and shipwrecks and stormy sea-crossings, historical subjects to us but a very present reality in his own day. In this he was following the precedent set by two earlier leading Academicians, Benjamin West (actually the President of the Royal Academy at this time) and John Singleton Copley, who had painted the deaths of General Wolfe, Major Peirson and Lord Chatham in a style based on the seventeenth-century classicists in Rome.

Turner was to go further. By the end of his life he was to exhibit pictures of steamers in snowstorms, railway trains crossing viaducts and cataclysmic happenings in the Alps that carried the same weight as his more traditionally significant subjects. These new subjects were, and are, as significant as the old, embodying forces that act on man as much or more than the deeds of other men. In fact the tradition of mythology had always recognised this, gods, nymphs, dryads and so on being personifications of natural forces. Jove's thunderbolts represented thunder and lightning, but at the same time thunder and lightning represented an anger that had a moral force. By the 1840s 'Snow Storm – Steam-Boat off a Harbour's Mouth' had the universal significance of the Biblical Deluge, but Turner was also able to reinterpret the Deluge and its aftermath ('Moses writing the Book of Genesis') in the light of his own pessimistic philosophy. Paintings of Ancient Rome and Carthage pointed the moral of the decay of empires, very much in mind in a Britain that had been beleagured by the forces of Napoleon for twenty years, but at the same time pictures of contemporary Venice, the burning of the Houses of Parliament, or industrial activity on the Tyne proclaimed the same message.

All this Ruskin saw, as does the modern art historian; but Turner's moral philosophy was a matter of passion and visual expression, not of strict archaeology and attention to sources. If he called a Biblical Plague the Fifth when it was in fact the Seventh this was because he couldn't be bothered, because the expression of the destructive force of a deity (or could it be nature?) was what was important. The fumes of history filled his brain, not its dry facts. All was grist to his mill: the contemporary poetry of Byron, Shakespeare (transported from Verona to Venice though might be the setting of the magical 'Juliet and Her Nurse', unfortunately not available for this exhibition), Beale's book on whaling, classical and Biblical history, Cowes Week, his travels, the paintings of other artists – the 'sources' are endless. Had he been better educated his pictures might have been more scholarly, more literary – but they would have been less exciting.

Allied to this ambition to succeed in the Academic market-place was an immense skill and an immense visual appetite and visual memory, without which he would not have been the great artist that he was, perhaps the greatest that this country has ever produced. A true professional, he never stopped observing, recording. Over two hundred and fifty sketchbooks at the British Museum bear witness to this. Not for him the busy private life; his social life was confined to professional functions at the Royal Academy and basic, safety-valve affairs with his housekeepers. On his many tours abroad he did not take the waters, try his luck at the gaming tables, visit the opera or take the air for recreation; he sketched all day and worked up his watercolours back at his lodgings in the evenings. His visit to the Low Countries in 1817 is an example. He left London on 10 August, primarily intending to gather material for his next piece of contemporary history for the Academy, the 'Field of Waterloo' exhibited in 1818, only three years after the event. He reached Cologne on 18 August and went up the Rhine to Mainz, filling two sketchbooks with tiny thumb-nail sketches delineating its banks. He was back in Cologne by 29 August. Returning by sea via Rotterdam and probably Hull, he sketched Raby Castle and other places in County Durham and reached his patron Walter Fawkes at Farnley Hall on 15 November, by which date, or very soon after, he had completed fifty-one finished watercolours of Rhine views. Such concentration on his art was not exceptional. Even a mishap while crossing the Alps led to a watercolour.

His ambitions did lead him to literary expression, draft verses in some of his sketchbooks and the almost certainly non-existent epic poem *The Fallacies of Hope* from which he purported to quote in the catalogue entries for his Academy exhibits. But his overriding means of expression were visual, in the over 19,000 sketches and watercolours in the Turner Bequest, the hundreds of finished watercolours and well over five-hundred oil paintings. Drawings, watercolours and oils range from the scrappiest jottings to the fully-completed work for exhibition. Everything he touched, as with Leonardo or Picasso, bears the mark of genius. Fifty years ago, this was enough; formal values were all, content did not matter. Now the balance is swinging back towards a concern with content, with the artist's intentions. In particular, there is the question of the status of the oil paintings he never exhibited in his lifetime.

Turner certainly made a distinction between works for exhibition, 'finished paintings', and the others. The distinction is made in his will. Only because its terms were overturned by his relations, wresting the money that he left, £140,000 or so, from the poor artists to whom he had willed it, was the British nation so fortunate as to get all the works by him in his studio, whether finished or not (or so it would seem from most readings of his very unclear intentions in this respect; at one point he did talk of showing in sequence four selections of finished pictures, one of unfinished oils and one of unfinished drawings and watercolours – see Finberg 1961, p.444 n.1). The same distinction was made by his executors and the authorities of the National Gallery when they received the Bequest. Only 118 of the 285 oils were even given inventory numbers straight away, and of these only thirteen, so far as one can tell, had never been exhibited in his lifetime; even these were pretty conservative in style. These works can easily be picked out at the Tate and National Galleries: their numbers run from 458 to 562. It was not until the twentieth century that any further oils were numbered: 1857 to 1890 in 1901, 1980–2068 (including 'Norham Castle') in 1905, 2302–2707 in 1908 and 1910, 2857–3557 at intervals between 1911 and 1920, 4445–4665 in 1929 and 1932 and 5473–5546 in 1944. The last batch, as Lord Clark has described, were discovered in the cellars of the National Gallery, rolled up, and thought to be old tarpaulins. Even now the Conservation Department of the Tate Gallery, despite a special effort to concentrate on the magnificent holding of Turner's works, is still faced with a number of works remaining to be freed from over a hundred years of dirt and neglect, and exciting discoveries continue to be made, for instance Nos. 320, 484, 536, 537, 569 and 570 in this exhibition.

Turner's own attitude towards the survival of his works was fairly ambivalent. He would buy back works at the sales following the deaths of such important patrons as Sir John Leicester, and would refuse to sell certain key works such as 'The Fighting Temeraire' despite the importunities of would-be buyers. Yet the conditions in his own gallery were appalling. He willed the creation of a Turner Gallery, but never seems to have been quite clear as to what it was to contain.

Turner's natural mode of expression was visual; the pressure to create was obviously enormous. To this extent he was driven, obsessed by his art; he could not stop creating. Yet it is probable that the unexhibited pictures, the 'unfinished' pictures, represent working material or work in progress. Some are definitely sketches, drawings or oils used to try out ideas realised in separate, finished works. This traditional use of material is, not surprisingly, most common in the first part of his career, though there are composition sketches in oils apparently from as late as his second visit to Italy in 1828.

Turner's well-documented activities on Varnishing Days show another way of working. The Varnishing Days, which occurred at both the Royal Academy and the British Institution, were privilege days before the opening of the exhibitions to the public, designed for the artists, or in the case of the Academy full Members or Associates only, to make minor last-minute adjustments to allow for any special conditions resulting from the placing of their pictures, such as lighting, the vividness of a neighbouring picture and so on. Turner however exploited these days to the full, partly indeed to cope with the competition of over-bright or over-colourful neighbours – the anecdotes are plentiful – but partly to work up into finished pictures what were, very clearly, only the slightest of lay-ins. As an eye-witness, E. V. Rippingille, observed of one case, 'the picture when sent in was a mere daub of several colours, and "without form and void", like chaos before the creation'.

Today we would not accept that what was sent in was chaos. From all accounts these mere daubs were among what are now the most admired of all Turner's works, the delicate, watercolour-like dreams of pure colour such as 'Norham Castle'. This is perhaps an extreme case; the oils in the Turner Bequest range the full gamut from such delicate lay-ins to much more heavily painted yet still not 'finished' works such as 'Yacht Approaching the Coast'. Towards the end of Turner's life, in the 1840s, there is in fact very little difference in degree of finish between some of the works he did exhibit, such as 'Snow Storm – Steam-Boat off a Harbour's Mouth', and those he did not. Yet one sometimes feels a twinge of regret for the earlier state of the picture beneath the final exhibited work, the putative Norham Castles beneath the Carthage pictures exhibited in 1850, or the glow of glorious colour made ridiculous by the ill-drawn and impossibly tall figure of Napoleon regarding the rock-limpet in 'War', the companion to 'Peace – Burial at Sea' in the exhibition of 1842.

The unfinished pictures in fact embody, if sometimes in latent form, the content of the exhibited works. The stormy seas are none the less terrifying as expressions of the power of nature than those to which a few more specific details, of steam-boats or life-saving rockets, have been added. Rather more mystifying are 'Norham Castle' and other similar expressions of light and colour that seem to embody an optimistic, grateful acceptance of nature's bounty. In the exhibited works of the later years this is usually blighted, though sometimes there is little more than a clue in a passage from the *Fallacies of Hope* to make this clear. 'The Sun of Venice', which delighted Ruskin when he found its echo in an actual experience at Venice, is in fact about the delusion of hope, as is the 'positive' demonstration of Goethe's theory of colour, 'Light and Colour – the Morning after the Deluge'.

Turner's practise of working up existing paintings makes it difficult to date his late works; even the year of exhibition may only apply to the last touches.

In some cases, such as 'The Hero of a Hundred Fights' exhibited in 1847, the discrepancy between what was added and what lies beneath is so great that one is forewarned. 'Regulus' is known to have been painted and put on exhibition in Rome in 1828, but was not exhibited in London until 1837 and may have been considerably altered, particularly as 'Orvieto', similarly painted and exhibited in Rome, is known to have been worked on during the Varnishing Days in 1830. There may be other instances, and for the unexhibited picture the case is even more difficult. In the catalogue tentative dates are given, and some unfinished works are tentatively associated with exhibited works to establish slightly firmer points of reference, but not too much weight should be given to these suggestions.

Turner's general development is however fairly clear. He remarkably quickly reached proficiency in the tradition of the topographical watercolour, and soon, with Girtin, transformed the accepted techniques to produce a far less pre-determined process in the late 1790s. As Farington reported in 1799, Turner 'told me he has no systematic process for making drawings . . . By working and occasionally rubbing out, he at last expresses in some degree the idea in his mind'. This development is treated more fully in the essay on 'Turner's Drawings and Watercolours' elsewhere in this catalogue.

Turner's first oil paintings are, not surprisingly, rather tentative and reflect a number of different interests and influences. Significantly, the most important influence soon became that of Richard Wilson, Turner's chief predecessor among British artists as a painter of serious, moral landscapes, including historical landscapes. In Turner's paintings, however, Wilson's formal style was enriched by a subtlety of atmospheric effects that seem to reflect the influence of the landscapes of P. J. de Loutherbourg. In many ways, in their atmosphere and effects of light, and even in their composition, these early paintings embody qualities that were to distinguish Turner's work throughout his life.

Turner's accomplishment within existing traditions soon brought him success: election in 1799 as Associate of the Royal Academy at the earliest possible age and full membership only three years later. He immediately turned to the production of the archetypal Academy picture, the large machine on a moral subject, the historical landscape in the style of Poussin and Claude. At the same time he demonstrated that he could match the Dutch with seapieces in the manner of the Van der Veldes, sometimes on a similar large scale, and also with rather less ambitious landscapes that reflect the more domestic virtues of Cuyp, Ruisdael and Hobbema. At this time his style still varied considerably according to the kind of subject he was painting. His works attracted buyers, including such leading collectors as Lord Egremont, Sir John Leicester and William Beckford.

The creation of the big exhibiting bodies, particularly the Royal Academy, had revolutionised the relationship between artist and patron in Britain. Though commissions and work for engraving were still common the main market was now the annual exhibition; pictures were painted to attract potential purchasers, not on demand. Turner's ambitions and prodigious output were such that he soon found that the Academy did not give him enough scope: in addition internal politics made the outlook there a bit uncertain. He therefore opened in 1804 his own gallery adjacent to his studio in Harley Street, holding annual exhibitions, for some years with formal opening and closing dates and a catalogue, though later the arrangements became more casual. Here he tended to exhibit slightly less formal pictures, including unfinished works of topical subjects such as 'The Battle of Trafalgar' and works with the title 'Sketch . . .'.

Repeated tours of the country in connection with topographical engravings and to paint the homes of his patrons kept Turner in touch with nature, and two groups of oil sketches done on the Thames show him making a particularly determined effort to master its more intimate qualities by close observation. This, coupled with his interest in Dutch painting, led to a rapid development in the style of his less formal landscapes, first seen in 'Sun rising through Vapour', exhibited at the Royal Academy in 1807 and now in the National Gallery, and even more apparent in a whole group of Thames landscapes exhibited in his own gallery the following year.

From this time on his technique was capable of anything, though of course his style continued to develop. In addition, although these works seem very traditional today, he was already regarded as an advanced artist, particularly by conservative critics like Sir George Beaumont. The hostility of the critics throughout Turner's career has however been exaggerated, perhaps in part by Ruskin, who rushed so readily to Turner's defence that he tended to discount any encouragement Turner may have had from other quarters. Recent research, covering as many contemporary reviews as possible, has shown that criticism was usually balanced by praise, even within the same review and even late in Turner's career, when the regrets at Turner's departure from nature and his 'extravagances' were often accompanied by a deep if reluctant admiration of his sheer genius. Moreover, even the hostile criticisms show a considerable understanding of Turner's unique qualities, and pick out, admittedly for adverse comment, just those features that one now admires. There is often more truth in the observations, if not the judgments, of the contemporary critics than in the somewhat perverse enthusiasms of Ruskin.

In 1802 the Peace of Amiens had enabled Turner like many other artists to go abroad for the first time, and in particular to study in the Louvre, which was then bursting with extra treasures looted by Napoleon from the conquered countries of Europe. Here Turner increased his knowledge and admiration of the Old Masters, above all Titian and Claude. For the next fifteen years he was confined to Britain, for although peace was finally established in 1815 he did not get abroad again until 1817; apparently pressure of work for the engravers kept him too busy. Even when it came, this first trip after the war was, perhaps surprisingly, not to Italy but to the Low Countries and the Rhine. Again possibly he did not have time to go further, but perhaps his interest in Dutch art, an art so dependant on the particular qualities of the local sky and atmosphere, also drew him there. He also wanted to visit the site of the Battle of Waterloo; throughout his career he was always quick to make special trips in search of topical material.

The real turning-point in Turner's career was, however, his first visit to Italy in 1819. As Lawrence, among others, had realised, 'Turner should come to Rome. His genius would here be supplied with materials and entirely congenial to it . . . . The country and scenes, . . . Turner is always associated with them'; the only person who could do Tivoli justice was Turner who 'approaches, in the highest beauties of his noble works, nearer to the firm lines of composition, to the effects and exquisite combinations of colours, in the country through which I have passed, and that is now before me, than even Claude himself.' In the event, the revelation of Italian light and colour seems to have temporarily thrown Turner off course. The watercolours he produced first in Venice and then in and around Rome and Naples are among his masterpieces, but when it came to using this material for pictures for exhibition he seems to have encountered great difficulties. This was partly, perhaps, because, having established a new scale for his Academy pieces in 'Richmond Hill', exhibited just before he left for Italy, he felt he had to keep it up. In 'Rome from the Vatican' he succeeded, but it remains an isolated *tour de force* before which one is very conscious of the degree of effort that has gone into it. An equally large Venetian subject was abandoned. Turner exhibited only two further Italian subjects before he went back to Italy in 1828; in 1821 and 1824 he failed to exhibit any oils at all.

Meanwhile, one feels almost as light relief, he had moved in a very different direction. The foreground detail of 'Richmond Hill' had revealed a playful side of Turner's art, seen already in watercolours but not in oils, and this element was singled out in a number of small pictures beginning with 'What you will!', exhibited in 1822. This, and other examples, pay tribute to a very different kind of art than that hitherto challenged by Turner, the exquisite but delicate sensibility of the French eighteenth century as embodied in Watteau and, among Turner's contemporaries in England, Thomas Stothard. Hitherto Turner's challenges to other artists had been mainly the product of his ambition to show that he was the equal of the Old Masters, or in the case of David Wilkie, a slightly waspish attempt to show that he too could follow the current craze. His tributes in the 1820s and 1830s were more friendly, with the fellow-feeling of self-assurance. As well as fairly predictable allusions to Ruisdael, Van Goyen and, in 1833 when he started exhibiting oil paintings of Venetian subjects, Canaletto, there is a much more remarkable move towards Rembrandt, heralded by the title 'Rembrandt's Daughter' at the Academy in 1827 but leading to a more fundamental development in Turner's style in such figure subjects as 'Pilate washing his Hands'. Not only was the attitude to figures new – they now dominate the picture rather than merely acting as accessories – but this was accompanied by a much richer use of paint. Turner had always used paint like a virtuoso but now he seems to have begun to relish its actual texture, applying it more thickly and often working it with his fingers or the wrong end of the brush. This is also found in some of the sketches he did at Cowes in 1827 and in at least one Italian landscape of c.1828–30, and can be seen as early as 1822 in the picture of 'George IV at a Banquet in Edinburgh'. Turner's technique, despite the strictures of Ruskin and others, was usually very competent, apart from the occasional use of megilp, a medium that discolours, or the mixing of final glazes with varnish. His use of watercolour on some of his later oils, provided that they are sympathetically cleaned, has survived intact. But in certain pictures of this period, particularly the 'Interior at Petworth', possibly painted in 1837 in response to the death of his patron Lord Egremont, his technique has resulted in very bad cracking. This may have resulted from a combination of his interest in thick, worked up paint with the prodigious impatience that drove him to create.

Turner's tributes to both Watteau and Rembrandt were in part tied up with a renewal of his connections with Lord Egremont. Lord Egremont had been one of Turner's leading patrons in the first decade of the century, but now there was not only a new flow of works for him but Turner became a member of the lively and unconventional social life at Petworth. Recent evidence has shown that this happened as early as 1828, when at least some of the long landscapes of views at Petworth and nearby were installed in the Grinling Gibbons room. 'Watteau Painting' was exhibited in 1831 as a pair to a painting influenced by the Petworth Van Dycks and the Rembrandtesque 'Jessica', shown in 1830, was purchased by Egremont instead of an Italian landscape painted specially for him. These exhibited figure paintings were the public manifestation of a much greater activity in this field, comprising the wonderfully observed small studies in bodycolour of guests at Petworth and oil paintings of similar subjects such as 'Music at Petworth' and 'The Letter'. This activity seems to have continued well into the 1830s, culminating in the 'Interior at Petworth'.

Meanwhile, in 1828–9, Turner had paid a second visit to Italy, marked by a much greater activity in oils and, so far as one can judge, many fewer drawings and watercolours. Turner even exhibited three or more works in Rome. These mystified both the general public and professional artists, but Turner was obviously now able to reconcile the Italy he had always known from art with the reality of it as it actually was. He produced a succession of Italian landscapes, some historical, some more straightforward like 'Orvieto', for the next ten years, or considerably longer if one includes the special case of Venice.

Turner had stayed about a month in Venice in 1819, making lots of drawings but only very few watercolours. In 1820 and 1821 he completed three finished watercolours of Venetian subjects, apparently as inhibited by Venice as by Rome when it came to using his material for finished works. Suddenly, in 1833, in part as a challenge to Clarkson Stanfield, he exhibited two Venetian oils, the first of a succession that, with a break in the later 1830s, continued until 1846. Only after he had returned to Venice as a subject did he return to the city itself, later in the same year, 1833, as has recently been discovered. A further visit followed in 1840, again just after he had begun to exhibit Venetian subjects again after a break of two years. These pictures, aglow with light and colour and apparently regarded (though, as 'The Sun of Venice' shows, unjustifiably) as positive celebrations of the beauty of the city, remained popular even when Turner's more ambitious works were heavily criticised and largely unsold.

Turner's range of subjects continued to expand in the 1830s and 1840s. A wider variety of landscape and marine subjects, often depicting storms, avalanches and other manifestations of the destructive power of nature, was accompanied by historical and literary subjects, now often in pairs to point the moral, Ancient and Modern Italy, Ancient and Modern Rome, Peace and War, the Evening of the Deluge and the Morning after the Deluge, culminating in the four pictures of Aeneas at Carthage shown in 1850, the last time Turner was to exhibit. The Apocalyptic 'Angel standing in the Sun', four paintings of Whalers and, surprisingly, a fairy subject of the kind newly fashionable in the 1840s, 'Queen Mab's Cave', show his variety.

Turner also experimented with a new format, square, or sometimes circular or with the corners cut across, instead of the horizontal or upright rectangle. This was partly connected with his increased use of a vortex-like composition. His very first exhibited oil, 'Fishermen at Sea', had shown this in embryo, and 'Hannibal crossing the Alps' had exploited it to the full to demonstrate the power of the storm raging among the mountains, but its use now became much more frequent as Turner began to dissolve the distinction between solid forms and the forces of nature as made manifest in waves, vapour, spray or whirling clouds. The square concentrated the vortex, though this very concentration produced a problem of its own in making the unfilled corners much more obvious; hence Turner's frequent recourse to a circular or octagonal shape.

In the 1840s Turner's compositions became less disciplined, less clearly organised in different zones of light or colours, the treatment more overall and fragmentary. In the greatest of the pictures the effect is still as overwhelming, if not more so, but in others the decline noted by Ruskin is perhaps apparent. The frenzy is perhaps a bit too uncontrolled, the tonal relationships not quite so assured. The Apocalyptic 'Angel standing in the Sun', exhibited in 1846, is almost too apposite a symbol of the end of Turner's mastery. 'The sun is god' he is recorded as having said on his death-bed, but there is a hint in the verses in the Academy catalogue that the Angel is the Angel of Darkness. In 1847 and 1848 Turner sent in old, sometimes refurbished pictures for exhibition. Only in 1850, in a final gesture of his faith in the importance of the historical subject, did he summon up energy to produce four new works, on the destiny that drove Aeneas on to Italy, to the eventual destruction of

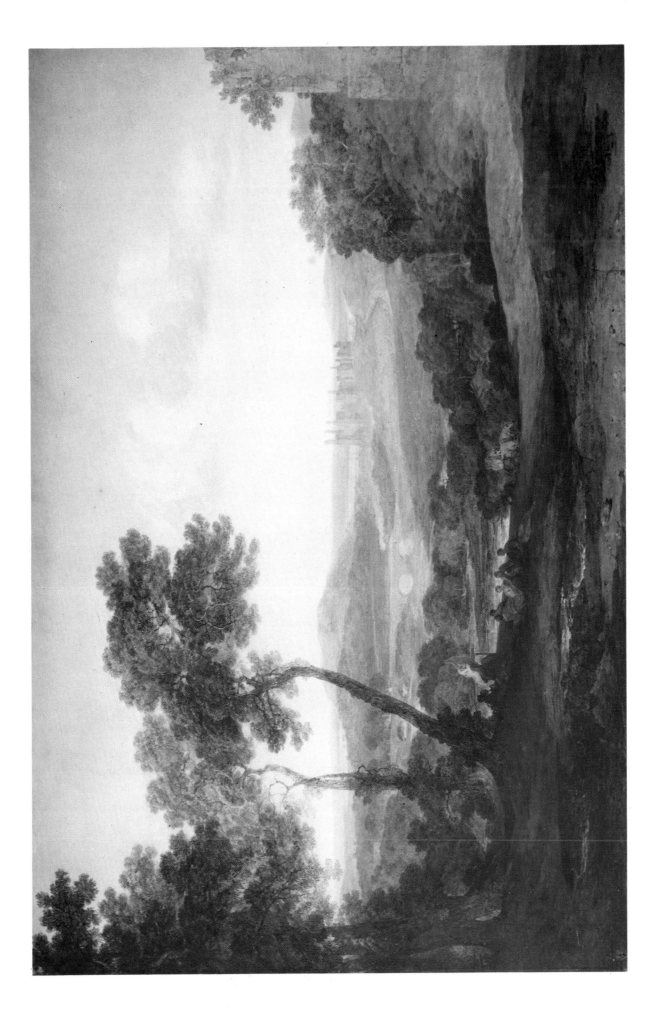

43 **Caernarvon Castle, North Wales** 1800 (entry on p.43)

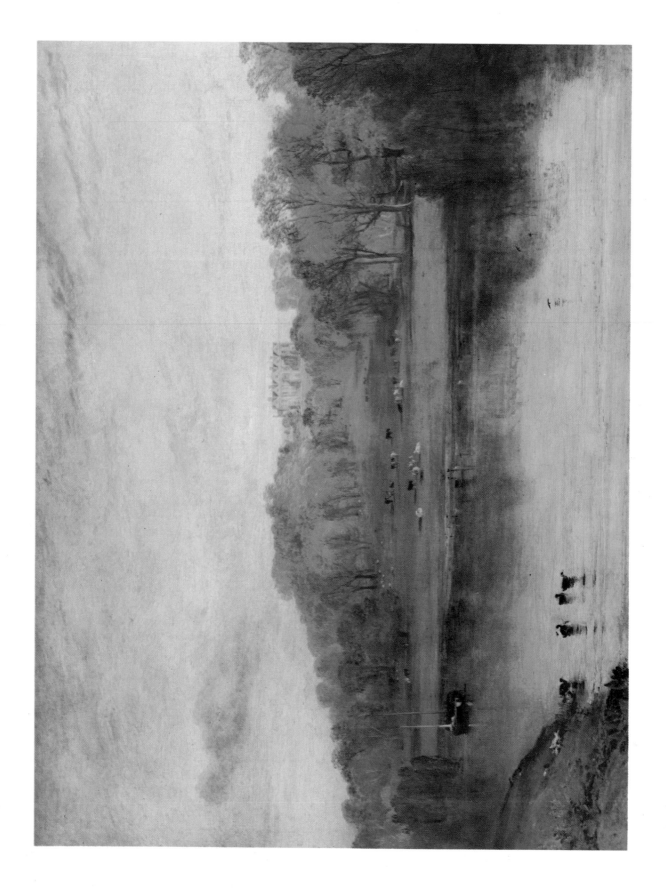

158 **Somer-Hill** 1811 (entry on p.75)

Carthage and the eventual decay of Rome. Both Rome and Carthage had been seen as prototypes of the British Empire, at its apparent height in the mid nineteenth century, but already doomed in Turner's pessimistic vision.

Perhaps however Turner's pessimism was, in the last resort, to a certain extent a literary affectation, belied in at least some of his pictures by the visual result. The unfinished paintings like 'Norham Castle' are life-enhancing and optimistic in their forms and colours. 'The Sun of Venice' is not a doom-laden picture until one reads the text; nor is 'Agrippina landing with the Ashes of Germanicus', until one works out its allusion to the seeds of decay in 'Ancient Rome'. Even the destructive fury of Turner's storms tempts one to recall that, in the words of a contemporary, 'Energy is Eternal Delight'.

Turner's Drawings and Watercolours

The act of drawing was for Turner an automatic response, a kind of nervous tic which never left him. Unstinting, uncompromising dedication to one particular activity is a characteristic of genius, and Turner's genius manifested itself unmistakably in this way. There is something wild, frenetic, in the sequences of pencil scribbles that we find in some of his sketchbooks: although many are, of course, admirably functional records of ideas, of places visited, large numbers of them are barely intelligible as drawings; dashed off with great speed, sometimes in awkward circumstances where there was nowhere to rest the book, or in a jolting carriage, they record nothing but Turner's passion for making drawings. Frequently these hasty scraps are sketches of subjects that he had drawn many times before, adding little or nothing to his previous knowledge; yet for him it was almost impossible to go anywhere, however familiar, without transcribing what he saw into line. It is as though drawing was an embodiment of the act of thinking.

But there was certainly nothing random or casual in Turner's attitude to the sketches he had made. They were generally done in stoutly bound notebooks or sketchbooks, and each book was carefully numbered, with a note of its contents, and added to a reference library of sketches which included, by the end of his active life, over 260 volumes. No other artist of Turner's stature has left such complete documentation of his development from the days of his studenthood until his final years of creation. The sketchbooks are amplified by numerous other drawings, made on separate sheets of paper but left with them to the Nation by the terms of Turner's Will. In all there are some nineteen thousand leaves of drawings in the Turner Bequest, which is now housed in the British Museum. This includes many of his finest watercolour studies, but hardly any of the highly finished watercolours which represent as important an aspect of his public output as do his paintings in oil.

It was as a watercolour painter that Turner began his career: indeed, the application of colour might be said to have preceded the drawing of outline: the earliest reports of his activity as a boy tell of him colouring prints which were exhibited for sale in his father's shop. This was a standard occupation for the young professional during his training (see No.B13). We also have examples of drawings copied complete from prints. But when he became a pupil of the architectural topographer Thomas Malton (1748–1804) in about 1789 he was automatically submitted to strict discipline in the matter of draughtsmanship. In the field he now entered accuracy and structural conviction were cardinal virtues, and the subject-matter with which he was concerned provided him with a stringent training of the eye. He began with simple buildings, country houses of uncomplicated design which gave him the opportunity to apply and master the laws of elementary perspective. His studies for these in the first sketchbooks are rather hesitant in the use of the pencil but show Turner's willingness to tackle each problem fully: at the same time he evolved a formula for representing the trees which surround such houses, a very adequate parallel to the hosts of similar formulae employed by all the topographical draughtsmen of the day. There are occasional figure drawings in these early

[21]

pages, too: a group of a man, a dog and a horse in pencil and watercolour seems to have been done simply for the interest Turner found in the subject, not for any specific undertaking; though the figures have the air of being all ready for service in the foreground of a topographical landscape.

The few sketchbooks which survive from these early years clearly do not represent the sum of Turner's youthful output. He had evidently not yet established the habit of preserving everything that he did for future reference; but at this stage his style was developing rapidly from that of a beginner to that of a professional exponent of the topographical watercolour and he must have drawn as prolifically then as at any other time. In 1790 he was admitted into the Royal Academy Schools; in that year his first watercolour was shown in the Academy's Exhibition, and in 1792 he produced a view of the 'Pantheon, Oxford Street, after the Fire' (No.7), which, taking a subject of topical interest that any reporter-artist of the moment would have drawn, sets out to be a full-scale topographical drawing in the style of one of the foremost practitioners of the genre, Edward Dayes. In its layout, in its use of large-scale figures, this drawing imitates Dayes' popular London views and succeeds so well that Turner had no need to produce another like it. It is perhaps the first instance of his deliberately imitating another master, to absorb the lessons he could teach and prove that Turner was capable of doing as well himself – a characteristic pattern for him.

Although the façade of the Pantheon that appears in the large watercolour bears only slight traces of the ruin which has overtaken it, Turner was particularly interested in the contorted remains of the fabric inside, and made studies of them which betray his early interest in the 'Picturesque' aspects of architecture. He had quickly graduated from the delineation of neat eighteenth-century houses to the drawing of 'Antiquities' – the ruins of Malmesbury Abbey in particular receiving a good deal of his careful attention when he visited them in 1791. It was this aspect of topography which was to dominate the first ten years of his career, and his sketchbooks of the period 1792–1800 are first and foremost collections of architectural outlines serving as notes of the appearance of buildings, either individually or in groups, which would provide material for topographical watercolours. The names of noblemen and gentlemen for whom watercolours were to be worked up from the drawings in the sketchbooks are often jotted in lists on the covers, or on the drawings themselves. There was a steady demand for views of famous buildings of general antiquarian interest, but often Turner's patrons commissioned drawings of their own property or of ruins associated with their families. So Edward Lascelles commissioned views of Harewood House, Dr York, Bishop of Ely, wanted a drawing showing the interior of his Cathedral, Lord Essex a series of views of Cassiobury Park, and William Beckford landscapes taken at Fonthill, with his new Abbey rising in the background.

One of the most interesting features of these drawings is their size. Although many are of modest dimensions several of them are as large as good-sized oil paintings, and they are pitched in deep tones which resemble those of oil far more than those of conventional eighteenth-century watercolour. The rivalry of watercolour with oil, which was to prompt endless large and brilliantly coloured drawings in the early nineteenth century, and which brought about the founding of the Water-Colour Society in 1804, was still in its early stages in the mid 1790s. There are few precedents for the enormous watercolours that Turner produced at that time; indeed we have to refer to continental masters like Ducros and Volpato for works of comparable power. The sense of scale which lends such impact to, say, the interior of Ely Cathedral (No.13) was something which he might have learnt from Thomas Malton, whose aquatints of London buildings display a highly dramatic use of steep perspective in order to achieve grandeur. The low viewpoint and plunging perspective of many architectural views by both Turner and Girtin seem to derive from Malton's example. But Malton did not work on Turner's gargantuan sheets of paper; nor, for that matter, did Girtin, whose largest watercolours are roughly of the size of Turner's views at Harewood (Nos.27 and 28) – Girtin made a similar view of the house at about the same time as Turner's. Girtin's name is always brought forward when the rise to prominence of watercolour at this period is discussed; but none of Girtin's achievements in the medium reaches Turner's level of sheer size and weight, though he may have progressed further at this time in the exploration of atmospheric effect. There are no other English watercolourists of the late eighteenth century from whom Turner can have learnt this particular and very striking quality; unless he had seen any of John Robert Cozens' largest drawings, which are in any case never architectural.

The influence of Cozens on Turner is however of great importance for another reason. It is well known how Turner and Girtin were taken up by Dr Thomas Monro, Surgeon to the King and amateur artist, who formed an 'academy' of his own in the Adelphi and set promising youngsters to draw, two to a candle, from his favourite masters. Cozens was one of the artists whose work Turner copied. Farington says that Girtin drew the outlines and Turner coloured them; it seems unlikely that either artist, or Dr Monro, would have allowed this arrangement to persist unchanged for long. At this moment in their careers, about 1794–6, Girtin and Turner became very alike in their drawing styles, adopting the half-cautious, half-florid system of lines punctuated with dots that Farington himself used, and seems to have got from Canaletto. The particular lesson that Cozens could teach both Girtin and Turner was the method of building up tones in watercolour by means of layers of carefully placed small brush-strokes, so that the whole structure of the design could be expressed in terms of mass rather than by outline. This process was cognate, in Cozens' own drawings, with an exceptional subtlety of response to atmosphere, and there can be little doubt that the close study of Cozens' landscapes enabled Turner to move faster in the direction of expressing his own sensitivity to atmosphere, even if, for the moment, he applied their lessons to the more prosaic business of drawing buildings. What is curious is that while Turner made probably hundreds of drawings after Cozens, colouring them either in blue and grey or green and yellow washes, he never, as far as can be judged, set out to imitate Cozens' style precisely. The other artists whose works Dr Monro offered as examples, especially Dayes and Hearne, became models whose manner Turner completely absorbed into his own style. Hearne in particular taught him a characteristic formula for the foliage of trees, which, like his cloudy skies, are always arranged in lateral or diagonal strips or streaks. The mannerism became the basis of Turner's technique when dealing with those parts of the drawing which surround and embellish the buildings themselves. It can be seen in his handling of foreground details at least up to 1800, gradually loosening towards greater and greater generalisation.

Turner's instinct for generalisation was very strong. He readily adopted the formulae of the eighteenth-century draughtsmen, and we do not find in his sketchbooks the careful drawings of individual plants which characterise Gainsborough's or Constable's formative exercises. That he observed and understood the details of natural life is clear from his output; Ruskin devoted much of *Modern Painters* to making the point; but this seems to have been something for which Turner was able almost entirely to trust his memory. Specific studies of weeds and grasses appear occasionally, for instance in the 'Thames' and 'Walmer Ferry' sketchbooks (Nos.262 and 259); it is significant that they can so easily be singled out, whereas studies of figures in costume, or performing particular actions, are commonplace. Hardly ever does he stop to sketch a tree; the studies of pines in the 'Devon Rivers' sketchbook No.2 (T.B.CXXXIII ff.35–37) are a rare exception.

By 1800 he had worked through the conventions of drawing to which he was brought up and remoulded them to suit himself. No sooner had he reached this point than he began to explore the use of the pencil in a totally new direction: his visit to Scotland in 1801 gave rise to a series of drawings which he referred to as his 'Scottish Pencils'. He made them on largish sheets of cartridge paper which he first washed over with a coat of grey colour. The drawing was executed in pencil; not, as always before, in outline, but in broad masses of tone, light, shade and texture, indicated with vigorous but finely controlled hatchings. Sometimes the lights were then scraped out, or a little chalk or bodycolour applied. In the apt use of simple pencil formulae to express wooded hillsides and distant rocky horizons, these drawings show Turner brilliantly taking over the drawing methods of J. R. Cozens, extending and broadening Cozens' technique but still heavily indebted to it. Turner did not make such elaborate drawings at the expense of his library of topographical information: he filled several small books with rapid outline sketches of views of Edinburgh, Stirling, and the Highlands. But he does seem to be thinking of the pencil drawing in a new capacity: as an area of experiment preparatory to making watercolours or paintings.

The appearance of his first oil painting at the Royal Academy in 1796 was paralleled by important changes in Turner's attitude to his sketchbooks. Those that he had used on his travels in the mid 1790s are full of fine pencil drawings, onto which he frequently pours light and air in the form of shimmering watercolour washes: these bring the outlines to life, giving them mass, colour and movement. Some of the studies of waterfalls and weed-grown ruins, half-finished so that we glimpse them, as it were, caught by a sudden shaft of light, are as exhilarating as any of his later feats of virtuosity. They show that in this respect too Turner had already gone further than anyone else along the road of conventional watercolour. Once he began to use oil paint, however, he recognised that a comparable process of building up tonality from dark to light was possible on paper. Several of the sketchbooks of this period have their pages washed with a grey or brown tone, and he worked on them with pencil or chalk, scratching-out and bodycolour, using several different media, if necessary, on one sheet, to obtain his effect. That effect is, of course, no longer merely one of carefully transcribed fact, but one of subjective mood superimposed on observed data. By the last years of the decade, Turner was applying these lessons to experiments on a much larger scale. The large preparatory study for 'Norham Castle' (No.639) gives evidence of the assiduity with which he built up a design with layer after layer of finely graded wash, blue, green, pink, yellow, one on top of another, rubbing through some or all of them as he went along in order to produce differentiated lights. This method was described by a contemporary:

> The lights are made out by drawing a pencil [i.e. a brush] with water in it over the parts intended to be light (a general ground of dark colour having been laid where required) and raising the colour so damped by the pencil by means of *blotting paper*; after which with crumbs of bread the parts are cleared. Such colour as may afterwards be necessary may be passed over the different parts. A white chalk pencil (Gibraltar rock pencil) to sketch the forms that are to be light. A rich draggy appearance may be obtained by passing a camel hair pencil [brush] *nearly dry* over them, which only *flirts* the damp on the part so touched and by blotting paper the lights are shown partially.

The 'Norham' experiment was repeated in various reworkings of the same idea, using different combinations of washes. His finished watercolours were subjected to similar attention: the large 'Caernarvon Castle' (No.43) shown at the Academy in 1800 was evidently mounted on a grey-coloured board when Turner had completed it, and then revised with a view to achieving a more integrated tonal scheme over the whole design: to do this, Turner has thrown broad, almost casual washes of blue, green and brown across the whole of the foreground.

This 'Caernarvon Castle' is significant in another respect: it is not topography in the sense that the views of cathedrals and castles and country houses of the 1790s had been, or even like the series of views of Fonthill at different times of the day, but a full-scale historical landscape, using a real view it is true, but using it as the starting-point for a landscape poem in the Classical tradition. The heroic verses that Turner inserted in the R.A. catalogue refer to the figures in the foreground, which strike a romantic, not a topographical note, as Claude's figures do. The whole design invokes the spirit of Claude in rather the way that the 'Opening of the Vintage' was to do in 1803. With the possible exception of 'Aeneas and the Sibyl' (No.46) which has not been precisely dated, this is Turner's first essay in classical landscape; there may be no coincidence that it is of a Welsh view, since the outstanding precedent for Claudian presentations of British scenery was the Welshman Richard Wilson, whose style 'Aeneas and the Sibyl' consciously copies. And in the delicate and subtle handling of detail in the background of this picture, Turner seems also to bring to its first fruition his intense study of Cozens.

He was to produce only one other large classical landscape in watercolour: the 'Composition of Tivoli' executed for John Allnutt in 1817 (No.181). This is a more explicit imitation of Claude than the 'Caernarvon', done in full awareness of his recent achievements in oil on similar lines: 'Dido', 'Crossing the Brook' and others. Another large watercolour, shown at the Academy in 1815, was the 'Battle of Fort Rock' (Turner Bequest, LXXX–G) which again points the fact that through the first decade and a half of the century Turner was equally ready to produce Academy pictures in either medium. The 'Battle of Fort Rock' also uses figures as properties in a historical landscape; though the battle in question was as recent as 1794, it is presented with a drama which is evidently intended to evoke the 'sublime' and to complement the sublimity of the natural setting. But it was in fact developed out of a much earlier composition showing 'Mont Blanc from the Val d'Aosta' which was one of a series of large watercolours featuring Swiss views inspired by Turner's continental tour of 1802.

These views are conceived on a scale comparable to that of the 'Ely' and other architectural drawings of the 1790s, and they make no claims to be historical: the heroic incident of the 1815 'Fort Rock' is absent here; only a few Swiss peasants give scale to the mountains; and some, like the 'Source of the Arveiron' (No.65) have no human staffage at all. Yet these rugged watercolours cannot be described as topographical. The mood they create forms a more important element in our response than the information they give us about Swiss geography. In them, as in the 'Caernarvon Castle', great delicacy of detail and subtlety of handling are combined with extraordinary power and breadth. Although he did not often again make such colossal watercolours, Turner united these qualities in nearly all the drawings that he finished for public exhibition or sale. The whole series of these watercolours, large and small, was acquired from Turner by Walter Fawkes of Farnley Hall, and constituted Fawkes' first major collection of Turner's work. It was not, apparently, conceived as a series but executed at various times over about five years after his return from the Continent. The subjects were all noted down during the tour, mostly in black chalk or pencil on a prepared grey surface, rather like the 'Scottish Pencils'; but some of the larger studies are coloured with greys, browns, blue-greens and yellow-greens, the lights scraped out or added in white bodycolour.

One important difference between the large watercolours of these years and their predecessors of the 1790s is that, whereas previously Turner's preliminary drawings were usually pencil outlines whose function was to fix accurately the detail of his subject, now he would begin a composition over the barest sketch, in colour alone, blocking in the principal masses and tones, establishing the overall structure of the design in colour, not in line. Sometimes this would serve as underpainting for the finished watercolour; sometimes, however, as in the case of the large sketch for 'Scarborough' (No.113) of about 1810, or in that for 'Tivoli' (No.182), or the 'Norham' studies already mentioned, the 'colour-beginning' is a separate exercise, exploratory, as it were, rather than preparatory. Later, indeed, it became an activity on its own, and Turner would make series of rapid studies in colour alone, based on a drawing taken from one of his sketchbooks, or on a picture he had already painted, and not necessarily intended as preliminary to any other work. The sequence of studies of 'Oxford High Street' (Nos.443 to 447) based on a pencil sketch of 1830 illustrates his practice clearly; the whole group was evidently done at one sitting, and differences between individual studies are limited to subtle variations in the play of light and shade, or the occasional introduction of roughly sketched figures. The figures suggest that Turner was in this case feeling his way towards a finished design – for the *England and Wales* series, perhaps – but no 'final version' exists. Such repeated exercises are a kind of equivalent in colour of the traditional method of working towards a final idea by repeating forms with slight modifications – Raphael, for example, could superimpose several thoughts in one pen drawing; while Turner, using colour alone, had to begin afresh with each restatement.

While he frequently made watercolour studies for his finished works in watercolour, Turner did not generally prepare his oil paintings in the same way. During the first years of his success at the Academy, however, he devoted much space in his sketchbooks to the planning of his canvases: the 'Calais Pier', 'Studies for Pictures' and 'Hesperides' sketchbooks (Nos.89, 94 and 117), for instance, are filled with drawings either directly related to the paintings on which he was currently engaged, or exploring possible themes for new pictures. Many of these are sketches of complete compositions, ranging in size from a few centimetres across to a foot or more. There are also large studies from the nude which indicates Turner's anxiety to conform to the academic standards of figure draughtsmanship set by his contemporaries in the field of historical painting: these figures were often transferred direct to the canvas, a process which he was not to employ at any subsequent period. In contrast to these single, carefully studied figures, there are complex groups, sketched in pen or chalks, for subjects such as the 'Deluge' of about 1804, in which bodies are piled and twisted together as if Turner were emulating a Baroque altarpiece.

Emulation of the old masters is a constant theme of these sketchbooks. The 'Louvre' sketchbook (No.91) testifies to the assiduity with which he examined the paintings of Poussin, Ruisdael, Rembrandt, Titian and others while he was in Paris: although his observations are mainly in the form of manuscript notes, he also made small drawings, some very lovely, reproducing the composition of pictures which particularly impressed him. And modern masters, even those younger than himself, received his serious attention: the 'Harvest Home' sketchbook (T.B.LXXXVI) contains sketches of a rustic festival clearly inspired by the arrival in London of David Wilkie, whose country genre subjects Turner immediately set himself to imitate.

The majority of the studies relating to paintings are in black and white chalks or pen and brown ink with wash, on a tinted ground – the 'Calais Pier' book has large pages of blue paper; the 'Studies for Pictures' book, of white paper, was prepared throughout with grey grounds on which Turner used pen and ink and watercolour – an extension of the technique of the Swiss studies. Many of the drawings in this book are of views at Isleworth, near Turner's home, but they alternate with more elaborate designs in which the features of the Thames landscapes are transformed into Classical scenes, with notes of possible alternative titles.

At about the same date as the work in the 'Studies for Pictures' sketchbook, perhaps 1806, Turner made a series of watercolour drawings of scenes on the Thames which do not in any way hanker after being Classical subjects. Technically, they are very like the coloured drawings in that book, but the grey ground is dispensed with in favour of plain white Whatman paper; what emerges is the first group of Turner's mature watercolour studies made for his own recreation and reference, not finished watercolour 'paintings' for the market. The technical experiments of the previous ten years, from the time of his first oil painting, seem to be summed up and brought to a consummation in the freshness and richness of these studies. There is no sense here of the artist labouring with his medium to increase its expressive power: light and colour flow easily and limpidly from his brush and the result retains the spontaneity of a sketch but achieves the weight and subtlety of a highly wrought and carefully considered work of art.

Turner's output in watercolour divides itself naturally into these two categories: elaborately finished works, for exhibition or sale through an agent, which he produced at irregular intervals even when working on a series of related views; and spontaneous watercolour sketches, equally fine, but evidently done together in groups for his own private use. To this second category belong not only the famous Italian watercolours of 1819, the Petworth and *French Rivers* studies of about 1829, the late Venetian drawings and the batch of Swiss views that Turner submitted to Thomas Griffith in 1841, but also the 'colour-beginnings' to which reference has been made. These series are distinguished from each other not only by subject-matter and format, but by the fact that Turner's technique varies constantly from one to another presenting new characteristics in response to changes of purpose and mood, and to his developing experience. It is not always easy, however, to understand why a particular medium was chosen to express certain ideas. For his series of fifty-one views on the Rhine, made after his Continental tour of 1817, Turner chose rather small sheets of paper prepared with his distinctive grey wash, on which he worked with bodycolour, scratching out highlights, as he had done in his first-hand colour sketches of the Alps in 1802. The drawings are curiously intimate in quality. They resemble the 'private' studies which Turner kept by him rather than finished works for sale to a patron; nevertheless, Walter Fawkes bought them all, and it was not until 1820 that some of the subjects were taken up and elaborated, as we might have expected them to be, in watercolour on white paper.

At about the time Fawkes acquired the Rhine views, Turner made another series for him in bodycolour on prepared paper, this time of scenes at Fawkes' home and the countryside in its neighbourhood. Turner had already been asked to make drawings relating specifically to Farnley: his album of watercolour sketches of the family collection of 'Fairfaxiana' was compiled in 1815; and something of the same spirit pervades many of the Farnley views. We have the feeling that Fawkes specified particular subjects, and Turner's drawings seem to express the affection that both men felt for the place, and for each other. The simplicity with which Turner records house and grounds harks back, of course, to his early purely topographical work, and yet within an unpretentious format he succeeds in conveying his personal response quite clearly. The warmth of the medium of bodycolour seems to have been particularly suitable for the expression of his warmer personal feelings.

The puzzling coexistence of watercolour and bodycolour as equal and parallel media in Turner's output becomes more problematical in the context of the first Italian journey of 1819. The fresh, luminous studies of Venice, the brilliantly clear panoramas of Naples and the Roman Campagna, seem perfectly to express the impact that Italian light must have had on the artist when he met it for the first time. It is almost as though he were beginning all over again – indeed, some of the unfinished watercolours of Naples and Rome are strangely reminiscent of the half-completed drawings of Welsh waterfalls and buildings made during his apprenticeship in 1795. In their directness, their unaffected exultation in the revelation of daylight, they are the work of a young man – a man reborn, as it were, in the discovery of Italy. And yet Turner did not, as one might have expected, abandon the grey ground that had served him so well in the north. On the contrary, there is a fine sequence of colour studies, made in Rome, on prepared paper and in bodycolour. Again, this may perhaps be explained by the 'warmth' of the medium: just as the Mediterranean light was clearer and brighter, requiring the brilliance of a ground of white paper, so it was also warmer, and had also to be noted in terms of hot, dense bodycolour which alone could convey the heaviness of the atmosphere. But it was not only in coloured drawings that Turner used his grey ground: many of the pencil studies, especially those in the 'Tivoli' sketchbook (No.226) are worked out in terms of black and white on grey. The effect is very much reminiscent of the soft, atmospheric drawings of Rome made by Richard Wilson for Lord Dartmouth in the 1750s, and it may be that Turner, visiting the city of Wilson's inspiration for the first time, consciously imitated his use of grey paper and black chalk.

The intensity of bodycolour seems to have led Turner to use it on a deliberately reduced scale, as if he sought to achieve maximum concentration: in the long series of bodycolour drawings which he made towards the end of the 1820s he attained an unprecedented degree of brilliance and power on surfaces much more restricted than he had previously employed. The small sketches of Petworth interiors are a continuation of the intimate, domestic theme of the Farnley drawings of 1818, but are far richer in their colour, and far more dramatic in their realisation of effects of interior lighting. It is probable that they were done shortly after the visit to East Cowes Castle in 1827, when Turner had made indoor studies on similar small sheets of blue paper, but in pen only: at Petworth, he abandoned the pen altogether and expressed everything in colour alone. But impressive as the Petworth series is, it does not appear to have been the climax of the progression: at about the same time, Turner was engaged on his *Wanderings by the Seine* and *Loire*; and for these illustrations, continuing to use the small sheets of blue paper, he evolved an even more expressive and flexible technique. Some of the French views are as precisely and minutely finished as any of his large-scale watercolours; he uses a pen dipped in colour to draw in quantities of fine detail, and makes the bodycolour comprehend an extended gamut of tonal and textural variation: the crowded scenes in Rouen and Paris in blazing sunshine; are presented as we should expect work for the engraver, as this was, to be presented. On the other hand, some of the other drawings in the series are of the airiest elusiveness, rapidly noted effects of atmosphere, early morning mists or fading daylight, handled as though the medium were pure watercolour. Even now Turner had not concluded his exploration of this path: he contemplated yet another series, dealing with the rivers Meuse and Moselle, and it seems likely that he wanted to add more, featuring the south coast of France: bodycolour studies exist of all these places, although no publication ever made use of them. For these sets, he worked on grey, not blue paper, and his colour became noticeably richer, corresponding less and less obviously to normal conditions of light. The Meuse/Moselle drawings, and those of Marseille and its neighbourhood, are dominated by a scheme of heavy scarlets, mauves and purples, shot through with dark green and royal blue. Many of them are extremely slight, and the whole group is much less extensive than the Seine and Loire series; but it is not clear why Turner discontinued this extraordinary experiment.

As usual, there is a kind of correspondence between what he was doing in bodycolour and his current work in watercolour: the years of the Petworth and *French Rivers* drawings were also the years of his most intensive activity as a book-illustrator. Between 1826 and 1836 he produced vignette designs for sixteen publications, beginning with Rogers' *Poems* and *Italy* and concluding with the illustrations to Campbell's *Poems* and White's *Views in India*. The vignettes were all executed in watercolour alone, but they exhibit almost as great a brilliance in the use of colour as the bodycolour designs we have discussed. It is astonishing to see him begin a drawing for an illustration to be interpreted in black and white only, by applying broad washes of contrasting scarlet and yellow (Nos.297 and 298). Even when working expressly for the engraver, Turner thinks first of all in vivid colour. It has even been held against these vignettes that their colour is capriciously unnatural. But the fact remains that the engraved results are usually extremely successful, works of great subtlety and beauty including an immense range of effects within a tiny area; and it seems likely that Turner realised that it was by means of colour, exaggerated if necessary, that he could most effectively draw his engravers' attention to the wealth of detailed effect which he wanted them to achieve.

Not all his illustrations were on the miniature scale of the vignette, however. Throughout his active life he supplied designs for 'Picturesque' publications larger than the *French Rivers*. The commissions of Whitaker for his *History of the Parish of Whalley* and *History of Richmondshire* called forth views on the scale of many of the watercolours Turner had made for Fawkes; and William Bernard Cooke's *Picturesque Views of the Southern Coast of England*, a particularly lengthy sequence of varied subjects exploring the interrelationship of sea and land in complex, multiple-focus panoramas, seems to have appealed profoundly to Turner's instinct for working in series. The shorter series of *Rivers* and *Ports of England*, which occupied him as the *Southern Coast* was coming to an end, led straight into the most extensive and ambitious of all his works for the engraver: the *Picturesque Views in England and Wales* on which he lavished much of his creative energies during the decade which also produced the vignettes, the Petworth and the *Rivers of France* drawings.

In the *England and Wales* watercolours Turner's fecundity both as a designer and as a technician is at its most impressive. The variety of these subjects, and the inexhaustible resource with which they are realised in the minutest detail, reveal a study of natural and human phenomena that goes far beyond the observations and notes to be found in Turner's sketchbooks. As a document of life in England at the period the series is Shakespearian in comprehensiveness, and, more particularly, in its concern not for landscape in the abstract, but for the 'moral landscapes' of the country. Turner always saw nature as the necessary setting and background for human life, and rarely showed a real place without demonstrating, with great accuracy, the economics of the view in terms of the industry, agriculture, entertainments and costumes of the people. Ruskin's strictures on the 'Horse Fair, Louth' (No.422) could not have missed more completely the overriding theme of Turner's finished watercolours (and many of his oil paintings as well). The space devoted in the sketchbooks to details of occupations, clothing, boats, waggons, shops and signboards and all the paraphernalia of everyday life provide ample proof of Turner's abiding interest in humanity; and in every one of the *England and Wales* set he makes a point of introducing some telling indication of human activity relative to the locality he depicts.

It is a curious irony that this remarkable series was, of all Turner's published works, the outstanding failure. Its original sponsor, Charles Heath, became bankrupt on account of it. And yet Turner had lavished on it not only his famous inventive powers, but his unremitting vigilance over the engraving of the plates, which are some of the most satisfactory to have been made from his designs. But they were made on copper, which was beginning to suffer from the competition of the more durable and therefore cheaper steel engraving; in addition, the fashion which Turner had set for such views was in the process of expending itself in multitudinous imitations by inferior artists, and prints alone could not adequately advertise Turner's superiority. As for the original watercolours, they were not so easily accessible to the public. Turner did not make it his habit to show watercolours at the Royal Academy after he had established himself there as a painter in oils; it is true that he occasionally exhibited his larger works – the 'Edinburgh, from Caulton-hill', for example, in 1804, and 'Fort Rock' and 'Tivoli' in 1815 and 1817; and he must have shown a certain number at his own gallery in Harley Street. But the exhibitions at which his watercolours could be seen in any numbers were rare. Fawkes displayed his own collection at Grosvenor Place in 1819 and 1820, and it was lent again to Leeds in 1839. The engraver-publisher William Bernard Cooke mounted exhibitions of work done for him by various artists including Turner in 1822, 1823 and 1824; drawings from the *England and Wales* series were shown at the Egyptian Hall, Piccadilly, in 1829, and sixty-six of the subjects appeared in Messrs. Moon, Boys and Graves' Exhibition in 1833, along with twelve of the Scott illustrations most of which had been shown in the same gallery in the previous year. Apart from certain incidental appearances, Turner's watercolours were not otherwise seen by the public. But the exhibitions proved highly successful, and added much to the artist's reputation; as long as he continued to produce work of the kind shown there, he did not lack purchasers for his watercolours, at least among a restricted group of connoisseurs. They were certainly remarkable works. No-one, at that high moment of the English watercolour school, was doing anything that even remotely approached them for complexity: their infinitely subtle, refined and nervous detail applied with countless tiny strokes of brilliant colour was almost the reverse of the usual practice of the bold and confident young movement which had come to life after the death of Girtin. They anticipated, indeed, the later generation of watercolourists – J. F. Lewis and the Pre-Raphaelites: there were many sound reasons why Ruskin associated Turner with the Pre-Raphaelite Brotherhood. What distinguishes the finished watercolours of Turner, however, is the fact that, while being worked out in careful detail with a technique like that of a miniaturist, they are at the same time, miraculously, very broad, boldly designed and freely executed. The combination of these two apparently opposite processes is unique to Turner. In order to achieve their union, he adopted executive processes of the most violent order: Hawkesworth Fawkes's description of the creation of the 'First-Rate taking in Stores' (see No.194) offers only a suggestion of the extent to which paper and paint were for Turner wholly malleable elements in his hands. Such descriptions, while leaving us baffled, only enhance a sense of Turner's extraordinary creative mastery of his medium.

The technical virtuosity of the watercolours reached a climax in about 1840, when Turner produced a number of unrelated continental views – 'Oberwesel' (No.583), 'Lake Nemi', 'Tancarville' (both B.M.) and others. Here the natural drama of the *England and Wales* subjects is replaced by a brilliance more artificial, more self-consciously 'pictorial' in the sense that it refers explicitly to the diffused golden atmosphere of Claude. The compositions are deliberately classical, the colouring hot, predominantly red and yellow. The scraping-out which Turner had always employed as an indispensable adjunct to watercolour, and which he could use with amazing skill, becomes in these drawings an omnipresent component of their texture: it is made to suggest a dazzling glitter of light reflected from practically every object in the scene. It is obviously an expression of the same preoccupation with diffused light which pervades the contemporary Venetian watercolours, but approaches the problem from the opposite direction, imitating the scumbling of white paint over the surface of an oil painting rather than allowing the white paper to 'speak' through a delicately applied watercolour wash.

As in so many other cases, the late Venetian watercolours came into existence side by side with a series of bodycolour studies. Some of these, on brown paper, explore yet another aspect of brilliant light, which again complements the theme of 'Oberwesel' and its companions. They are concerned with rendering the effect of small points of intense brightness in predominantly sombre surroundings – lamps in a dark street or a theatre, flambeaux or fireworks against a night sky. These studies, which are perhaps the freest of all Turner's exercises in bodycolour, can also be seen as a further development of the indoor dramas of light and colour that occur in some of the Petworth sketches.

'Oberwesel' and 'Lake Nemi' were both engraved in 1842 for Finden's *Royal Gallery of British Art*. They were the last of Turner's watercolours to achieve public success of this kind. During the remaining years of his career his style underwent certain modifications which rendered it less palatable to his admirers – admirers who had happily borne with all his protean manifestations in the past. Although there are innumerable watercolour sketches, studies and 'colour-beginnings' executed between 1840 and 1846, and many probably done even later, only a small number of finished works in the medium came to be made. Ruskin's account of how Turner asked his agent, Thomas Griffith, to solicit buyers for two series of Swiss views (see p.161) makes it clear that even Turner's most assiduous patrons had difficulty in understanding him by 1842. That the great Swiss subjects are different from their precursors is evident, but it is hard to identify in precisely what way they represented a 'falling-off' in contemporary eyes. In fact, Sir Walter Armstrong (1902, p.137) was probably right in suggesting that Turner's intentions in the last decade of his working life are more fully and clearly conveyed in the watercolours than in the oil paintings.

The majority of the late finished works are as elaborately and dexterously wrought as ever, with the same moulding together of light, colour, detail and atmospheric breadth that distinguishes the *England and Wales* drawings; though it is true that the moulding process seems still to be going on, rather than to have been brought to a stable resolution. They call to mind Turner's advice to a pupil to put a finished watercolour 'into a jug of water'. The feature in which these watercolours strikingly diverge from previous ones is their more dynamic principal of composition. A few of the *England and Wales* series attain something of the same quality (the 'Longships Lighthouse', No.431, for example; or 'Llanberis Lake', Edinburgh, Vaughan Bequest);

but 'Oberwesel' returns to a more static compositional type. In the Swiss drawings Turner seems altogether to abandon traditional notions of composition: he presents the massive formations of mountains and sky with a kind of inchoate negligence which, more vividly than ever before, expresses the grandeur of sublime landscape. Sometimes he treats the land almost as if it were the sea, in a state of fluid motion incapable of being arrested even for an instant: there are parallels with his late oil studies of breaking waves.

Even the detail with which he still willingly crams his foregrounds is incorporated more organically into the rhythmic life of the whole design; crowds surge among swarming buildings or over undulating open spaces as an integral part of the earth they inhabit. Turner's final view of man is an accurate reflection of his own life's work: he springs from and identifies himself irresistibly with the overwhelming and dynamic unity of nature.

J. M. W. Turner 1775–1851

Explanations and Abbreviations

Titles of works exhibited by Turner at the Royal Academy, etc., are given as first printed in the appropriate catalogue, save for slight changes to the punctuation and capitalisation.

Measurements are given in inches, followed by centimetres in brackets; height precedes width.

Exhibitions during Turner's lifetime only are listed.

All Turners lent by the National Gallery, London, the Tate Gallery or the British Museum are from the Turner Bequest unless otherwise specified; the abbreviation 'T.B.' is used before the reference numbers of British Museum works.

The catalogue numbers of works in the 'Life and Times' section are preceded by the letter 'B', e.g. 'B23'. Certain works from the Tate Gallery, allocated numbers in the catalogue, have had to be excluded for reasons of space.

Engravings are identified as 'Rawlinson No.00' if listed in his *Engraved Work* of 1908 and 1913 or, if from the *Liber Studiorum*, as 'R.00', the numbers used in both Rawlinson's and Finberg's books on the series.

I. Beginnings 1789–97

Turner's earliest works show his remarkably rapid assimilation of the technique of the topographical watercolour, based partly on copying or colouring the engravings of others, partly on short periods of study with architectural and topographical draughtsmen such as Thomas Malton and Edward Dayes, and partly on his own studies on the spot; the first of his regular tours in search of material was that to South Wales of 1792. He first exhibited a watercolour at the Royal Academy in 1790 (No.2) and the period ends with the first oils he showed there in 1796 and 1797 (see Nos. 19–21). See also the entries on Turner's Boyhood and Apprenticeship in the 'Life and Times' section (Nos. B1–B27).

1   Radley Hall from the South-East 1789
Pencil and watercolour with some pen and brown ink, $11\frac{9}{16} \times 17\frac{1}{4}$ (29.4 × 43.8)
Inscr. bottom right: 'Wm Turner pinxit'
Trustees of the British Museum (T.B.III–D)
A companion view of Radley Hall from the north-west is T.B.III–C; both were enclosed by Turner in grey and yellow washline borders. Pencil drawings of the house occur in the 'Oxford' sketchbook of 1789 (T.B.II–2ᵛ, 3, and 14). This book records country houses and scenery in the neighbourhood of Turner's uncle, who lived at Sunningwell near Oxford, where Turner often stayed.

2   The Archbishop's Palace, Lambeth R.A.1790
Pencil and watercolour, $10\frac{3}{8} \times 14\frac{7}{8}$ (26.3 × 37.8)
Exh: R.A. 1790 (644)
Indianapolis Museum of Art (Gift in Memory of Dr and Mrs Hugo Pantzer by their Children)
The first drawing to be shown by Turner at the Royal Academy, and one of two versions of the subject. Finberg (1961, p.18) suggests that this was a repeat, with modifications, of a drawing made for Thomas Hardwick in 1789, and that the marked advance it shows on the earlier version indicates the effects of his study under Thomas Malton. It was drawn for Turner's Bristol friend, Mr Narraway.

3   The Avon, near Wallis's Wall 1791
Pencil and watercolour, $9\frac{5}{16} \times 11\frac{1}{2}$ (23.7 × 29.2)
Inscr. on verso: 'View on the River Avon Near Wallis's Wall Bristol'
Trustees of the British Museum (T.B.VII–B)
A number of similar views are in the 'Bristol and Malmesbury' sketchbook of 1791 (T.B.VI) and are in pencil only; but that on f.24 is very close in mood and treatment, especially in the palette. This drawing and the next are typical of the work that Turner produced during a tour in the summer of 1791, when he visited Bristol, Bath and Malmesbury.

4   A View of the Avon 1791
Pencil, pen and brown ink and watercolour, $9\frac{1}{8} \times 11\frac{5}{8}$ (23.2 × 29.5)
Inscr. on verso: 'View of on [sic] the River' and 'View on the River Avon near Bristol Wm Turner'
Trustees of the British Museum (T.B.VII–G)
A rough pencil sketch of a landscape is on the verso.

5   Ruins of the Pantheon, Oxford Street 1792
Pencil, pen and brown ink and watercolour, $9\frac{5}{8} \times 7\frac{7}{8}$ (24.5 × 18.8)
Trustees of the British Museum (T.B.IX–B)

6   Ruins of the Pantheon, Oxford Street 1792
Pencil, pen and brown ink, $8 \times 12\frac{5}{8}$ (20.2 × 32.1)
Trustees of the British Museum (T.B.IX–C)

7   The Oxford Street Pantheon after the Fire of 14 January 1792 1792
Watercolour over pencil, $15\frac{9}{16} \times 20\frac{1}{4}$ (39.5 × 51.5)
Inscr. bottom left: 'W Turner Del'
Trustees of the British Museum (T.B.IX–A)
A smaller drawing of 'The Pantheon, the morning

2

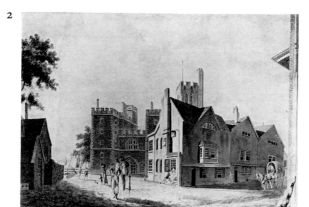

3

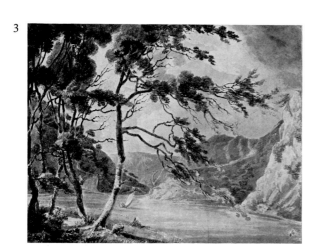

13

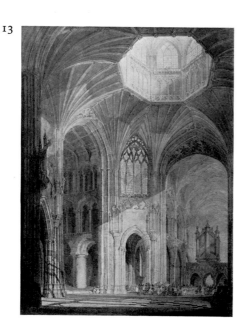

after the Fire' was exhibited at the Royal Academy 1792 (472) and bought by P. C. Hardwick, an architect who employed Turner. Two sketches of the ruins are in the Turner Bequest (Nos.5–6) and a third is in the collection of C. W. M. Turner, Esq. A pencil study of the whole façade of the burnt-out Pantheon, squared presumably for transfer to this sheet, is T.B.CXCV-156.

Gage (1969, p.23) suggests that the watercolour sketch of the interior, No.5, offers the earliest evidence of Turner's 'painterly' approach to colour; though at this date he had not begun to work in oils and was modelling himself on the leading topographical watercolourists of the time. The ambitious composition of No.7, and especially its many large-scale figures, suggests that Turner was consciously imitating the large London views of Edward Dayes, e.g. the 'Buckingham House, St. James Park' of 1790 (No.B14).

8   Oxford: St. Mary's Church and the Radcliffe Camera from Oriel Lane c.1793
Pencil and watercolour with some pen and brown ink, 10¾ × 8½ (27.3 × 21.7)
Inscr. bottom right: 'Turner ... [?]'
Trustees of the British Museum (T.B.XIV–C)
The same subject as the large unfinished view (No.9).

9   Oxford: St. Mary's Church and the Radcliffe Camera from Oriel Lane c.1793
Pencil and watercolour, 20⅞ × 15¼ (53 × 38.7)
Trustees of the British Museum (T.B.XXVII–X)
Unfinished, only a part of the grey under-painting and some blue and yellow washes applied. Apart from the figures the composition is the same as that of the smaller watercolour (No.8) which Finberg dates to c.1793. The front of Oriel College is on the right.

10   St. Anselm's Chapel with Part of Thomas-a-Becket's Crown, Canterbury Cathedral
R.A.1794
Pencil and watercolour, 20⅜ × 14¾ (51.7 × 37.4)
Inscr. bottom right: 'Turner 179.' (date cut)
Exh. R.A. 1794 (408)
Whitworth Art Gallery, Manchester (D.113.1892)
Turner seems to have visited Canterbury, perhaps for the first time, in the autumn of 1792; he exhibited a 'Gate of St. Augustine's Monastery, Canterbury' at the R.A. in 1793 (316). In the following August he made a tour of Kent, including Rochester, Canterbury, Dover, Maidstone and Tonbridge. Two more Canterbury views were shown in 1794: 'Christ Church Gate, Canterbury' (388) and a drawing with the present title. This drawing has been known as 'the East End of Canterbury Cathedral', but is identified by Finberg (1961, p.458, No.13) with the exhibited watercolour, which was presumably that in Dr Monro's sale, Christie's 26 June 1833 (122) as 'St. Anselm's chapel, upright, colours', bought back by Turner himself.

11   Llanthony Abbey 1794
Pencil and watercolour, 12⅞ × 16¹¹⁄₁₆ (32.7 × 42.4)
Inscr. bottom left: '1794' and 'W Turner' (name partly scratched out)
Trustees of the British Museum (T.B.XXVII–R)
Several smaller versions of the subject are known; one was engraved in aquatint by G. Hunt in 1823 (Rawlin-

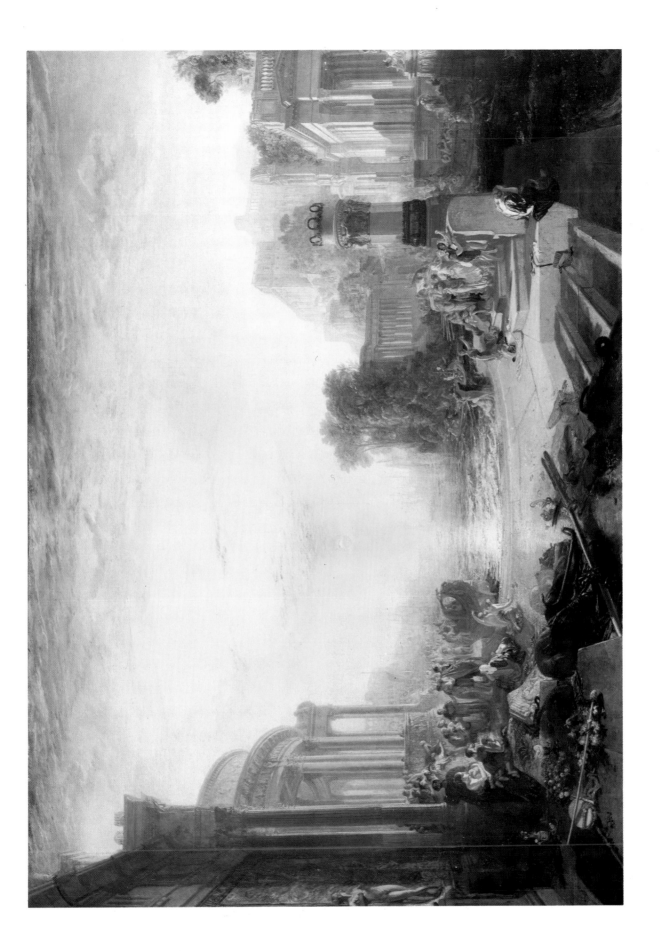

165 **The Decline of the Carthaginian Empire** 1817 (entry on p.77)

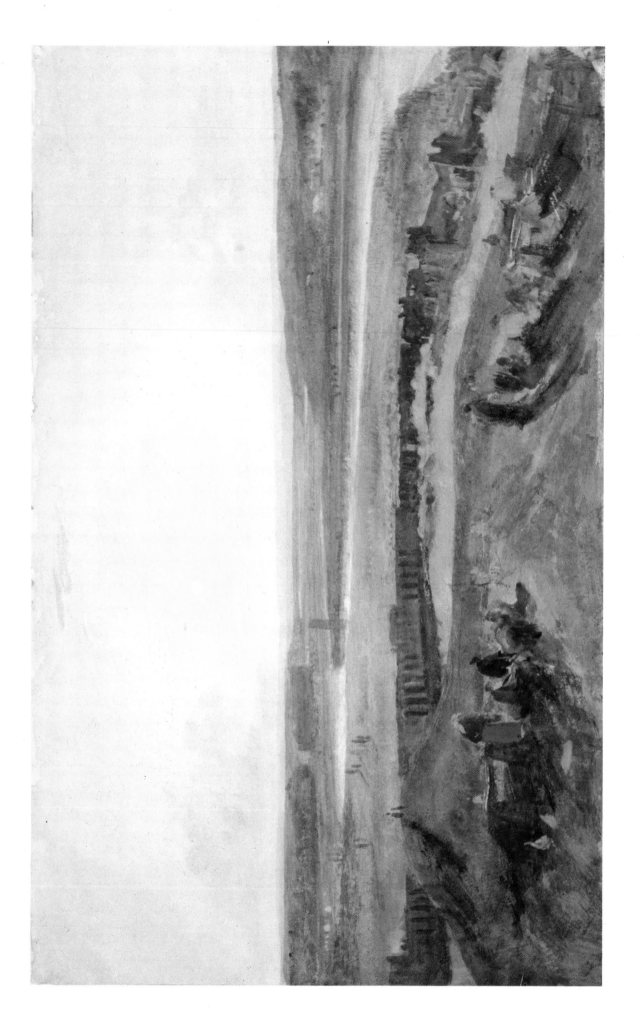

228 **A View over the Roman Campagna** 1819 (entry on p.91)

son No.827). The composition derives from a pencil drawing, probably of 1793 (T.B.XII–F). The version listed by Finberg (XXVII–Q) as 'unfinished' seems to be a crude copy of XXVII–R and is evidently not by Turner.

The design is among the earliest of Turner's attempts to translate topography into romantic landscape and with its bold composition, independent of horizontal and vertical stresses, and its misty atmosphere already approaches the 'Sublime', anticipating the north Welsh landscapes of the later part of the decade. It offers evidence that Turner had by this time seen and admired the watercolours of J. R. Cozens. Nevertheless the colour and drawing of this view are heavily influenced by the characteristic features of the style of Thomas Hearne. The composition was used again for an elaborate watercolour in the *England and Wales* series (No.430).

12 The Octagon, Ely Cathedral 1794
Pencil, $30\frac{3}{8} \times 23\frac{1}{8}$ (77.2 × 58.8)
Trustees of the British Museum (T.B.XXII–P)
Made during Turner's tour of the Midlands in 1794; a preparatory study for the watercolour exhibited at the Royal Academy in 1796 (711) (No.13).

13 Interior of Ely Cathedral: looking towards the North Transept and Chancel 1796
Watercolour, $24\frac{11}{16} \times 19\frac{1}{4}$ (62.7 × 49.1)
Exh: ?R.A. 1796 (711) as 'Trancept and Choir of Ely Minster'
Aberdeen Art Gallery
A full-scale pencil drawing made on the spot is T.B.XXII–P (No.12). In the catalogue of the Royal Academy exhibition of 1887 this watercolour, then owned by Mrs Winkworth, was identified with that shown at the R.A. 1797 (464) as 'Ely Cathedral, South Trancept', and the identification has remained. It seems unlikely, however, that Turner would have given such a title to a view which is evidently taken from the arch in the south-west pier of the crossing, looking across under the Octagon to the North Transept and Chancel. The sunlight falls in accordance with this orientation, i.e. from windows in the south wall of the Choir and South Transept. It is therefore reasonable to suppose that this drawing is the 'Trancept and Choir of Ely Minster' exhibited in 1796, or perhaps a version of it made, like the 'South Trancept' of 1797, for Dr Yorke, Bishop of Ely. Finberg records that the 'Trancept and Choir' was in the possession of R. Durning Holt, Liverpool. This seems certainly to have been at least the same composition as the present drawing, since he describes it (in a MS note, B.M.) as 'Transept and Choir from under the Crossing. Listening to Sermon'. C. F. Bell describes this same subject under both the 1796 and 1797 entries (p.32, No.31 and p.33, No.35), giving R. Chambers, R. Durning Holt as provenance for the first, and Dr Yorke, etc, for the second. It is improbable, however, that Turner would have shown two different versions of the same view in successive years and under different titles.

Farington, having just seen the 1796 drawing and other Turners among works submitted for the exhibition that year, said they 'are very ingenious, but it is a manner'd harmony which He obtains' (*Diary*, 2 April 1796).

14 Interior of a Cottage with a Woman seated before the Fire 1796
Watercolour over pencil, $7\frac{13}{16} \times 10\frac{11}{16}$ (19.8 × 27.1)
Inscr. bottom centre right: 'W Turner'
Exh: ?R.A. 1796 (686) as 'Internal of a cottage, a study at Ely'
Trustees of the British Museum (T.B.XXIX–X)
Finberg's conjecture (see 1961, p.459, No.27) that this was the 'study at Ely' exhibited in 1796 is supported by the unusual elaboration and neatness of finish of this watercolour of an otherwise informal subject.

15 The Interior of Salisbury Cathedral c.1797
Watercolour, $19\frac{1}{2} \times 26$ (49.6 × 66)
Inscr. bottom centre: 'TURNER RA' and bottom left: 'EPISCOP...SARUM'
Lady Agnew
This view, looking into the north Transept, is one of the views of Salisbury commissioned from Turner by Colt Hoare in about 1795 as illustrations for a history of Wiltshire which never appeared. A list of twenty Salisbury subjects, written out in Colt Hoare's own hand, is among Turner's papers, T.B.CCCLXVIII–A. This includes ten of the cathedral, though none of the titles clearly refers to the present view. A drawing of 'The Close Gate' was shown at the R.A. in 1796(369) and is now in the Fitzwilliam Museum, Cambridge; the 'Choir' and 'North Porch' appeared in 1797 (R.A. 450, 517); the 'Inside of the Chapter House' (now Whitworth Art Gallery, Manchester) and 'West Front' (now Harris Museum and Art Gallery, Preston) in 1799 (R.A. 327, 335). Another view of the Chapter House was shown in 1801 (R.A. 415) and is now in the Victoria and Albert Museum, which also owns a view of the Cloisters. A general view of the cathedral from the Bishop's Garden is at Birmingham City Art Gallery. Two pencil studies of the exterior of the cathedral occur in the 'Isle of Wight' sketchbook of 1795 (ff.16, 17; see No.18) which also has a short note of a commission:

Salisbury Porch – | Sr Richard Hoare
Front of Salisbury | Size of Ely.13

The 'Ely' referred to here may have been one of the large interiors (see No.13), or perhaps the view of the cathedral from the south which was in the family of Colt Hoare and on the market 1974, based on a sketch T.B.XX–Y.

16 Trancept of Ewenny Priory, Glamorganshire R.A.1797
Watercolour, $15\frac{1}{2} \times 22$ (39.1 × 56)
Exh: R.A. 1797 (427)
National Museum of Wales, Cardiff.
Turner's 'South Wales' sketchbook, used on his tour of 1795 (T.B.XXVI, No.17), contains an itinerary, written out by a friend, mentioning 'Ewenny or Wonny (as it is commonly called) . . . an ancient fortified Priory'; and the 'Smaller South Wales' sketchbook (T.B.XXV), used on the same tour, has in it (f.11ʳ) a summary pencil sketch of the subject of the watercolour, with a note in more detail of the effigy on the tomb of Moris de Londes which appears in the centre of the composition. The drawing was one of three important architectural interiors shown by Turner at the R.A. in 1797, and

although smaller than the others (compare Nos.13 and 15) achieves a more dramatic effect by its powerful and imaginative use of lighting. Whitley, in *Artists and their Friends in England*, 11, p.215, refers to a reviewer in the *St. James's Chronicle*, May 20–23, 1797, who wrote: 'In point of colour and effect this is one of the grandest drawings we have ever seen, and equal to the best pictures of Rambrandt.' Gage (1974, p.33) suggests that it was influenced by Piranesi, especially the 'Veduta dell'antico Tempio di Bacco' of 1767 (Hind 81). A replica by another hand is in the Walker Art Gallery, Liverpool.

17   'South Wales' Sketchbook 1795
    Bound in calf; four clasps
    The spine labelled 'SKETCHES' in gilt
    lettering
    94 leaves, the majority drawn on in pencil and
    watercolour, $10\frac{1}{4} \times 8$ (26.2 × 19.8)
    Watermarked: 1794
    Inscr. on spine: '49'; Finberg transcribes a label:
    'South Wales – Mon'
    Trustees of the British Museum (T.B.XXVI)

f.8ʳ Melincourt waterfall, near Abergarnedd
Pencil partially finished in watercolour

The inside front cover and first few leaves are occupied by an itinerary, not in Turner's hand, and a list of 'Order'd Drawings' including a set of five views of Hampton Court, Herefordshire, for Viscount Malden (later 5th Earl of Essex) and two of the same building for Sir Richard Colt Hoare. Most of the drawings are careful architectural studies, at Wells, Hereford, Monmouth, Gloucester and various Wye and Welsh castles, executed in pencil with watercolour partially added in some cases. There are also some studies of water, on the coast, at the edge of rivers, and waterfalls.

Turner used another sketchbook on this tour, the 'Smaller South Wales' book, T.B.XXV, in which the subject of 'Ewenny Priory' (No.16) was noted.

18   'Isle of Wight' Sketchbook 1795
    Bound in calf, four clasps
    55 leaves, nearly all drawn on in pencil and
    watercolour, $10\frac{1}{4} \times 8$ (26.2 × 19.8)
    Watermarked: 1794
    Inscr.: Finberg transcribes Turner's label on
    spine: '95, Isle of Wight'
    Trustees of the British Museum (T.B.XXIV)

f.51ʳ Extensive View from a Hill, with an Artist seated on the Ground sketching
Pencil and watercolour

Contains pencil outlines, some coloured, of Salisbury, Winchester, Southampton, Carisbrook, Newport, the Isle of Wight coast, etc. Finberg proposed (1961, p.29) that this tour took place in August or September 1795, after the South Wales tour (see No.17).

The watercolour study on f.51ʳ probably shows a scene in the Isle of Wight, near that of the preceding sheet (f.50ʳ).

19   Fishermen at Sea ('The Cholmeley Sea Piece') R.A.1796
    Oil on canvas, $36 \times 48\frac{1}{8}$ (91.5 × 122.5)
    Exh: R.A. 1796 (305)
    Tate Gallery (T.1585)

The identification of this picture with the work exhibited at the R.A. in 1796 is not fully documented but is strongly supported by the descriptions in two contemporary accounts of the exhibition and by that of the engraver E. Bell (who claimed to have got to know Turner as early as 1795). Reported by Thornbury (1862, 1, p.75 and 1877, p.44), Bell said that 'Turner's first oil picture of any size or consequence was a view of flustered and scurrying fishing-boats in a gale of wind off the Needles, which General Stewart bought for £10'. The Needles can be seen on the left of the painting, but unfortunately there is no evidence to prove that it passed from the General to the Fairfax-Cholmeley family, who owned it by the middle of the nineteenth century.

Turner toured the Isle of Wight in 1795, probably during August-September, but none of the sketches in the 'Isle of Wight' sketchbook (T.B.XXIV) are close to the oil painting. However, the painting is close to the larger watercolour apparently from the 'Cyfarthfa' sketchbook (T.B.XLI–37; the sketchbook is dated *c*.1798 by Finberg 1909, I, p.99, and 1799 by Wilkinson 1972, p.155, but is on paper watermarked 1794 and may have been used on Turner's tour in South Wales in June (?)1795). Turner later engraved the composition for the *Liber Studiorum*, R.85 (see p.61; repr. Finberg *Liber* 1924, p.340) but it was never published (the preliminary drawing is repr. Wilkinson 1974, p.118).

Unlike other early oil paintings such as Nos.33 and 45 this picture is very different in style from Turner's watercolours of the time. It is rather a highly accomplished example of the tradition of moonlight scenes established by Claude Joseph Vernet, P. J. de Loutherbourg and Joseph Wright of Derby. In particular it resembles the latter's 'Moonlight with a Lighthouse, Coast of Tuscany', exhibited at the Royal Academy in 1789, the year before Turner first showed there, and now at the Tate Gallery. This has the same contrast between the cold light of the moon and the warm light of the man-made lamp, in the lighthouse in the Wright, in the boat in the Turner. This rather intellectual, conceptual interest in light was to become a passionate obsession in Turner's later work. The reflections of light on the water are also close to those in Wright's picture, but Turner combines them with the illuminated break in the clouds above to create a lozenge-shaped surface pattern that anticipates the vortex-like compositions of so many of his later paintings. Thus, typically of Turner's whole achievement, this painting, while relying on earlier models, anticipates the revolutionary accomplishments of his most advanced work.

20   Moonlight, a Study at Millbank R.A.1797
    Oil on mahogany, $12\frac{3}{8} \times 15\frac{7}{8}$ (31.5 × 40.5)
    Exh: R.A. 1797 (136)
    Tate Gallery (459)

Another moonlight scene, less ambitious but more sensitive and personal than 'Fishermen at Sea'. Unlike the other oil exhibited in 1797 (see No.21) this picture does not seem to have attracted any critical attention.

William ANNIS (fl.*c.*1798–1812), J. C. EASLING
(fl.*c.*1807–1833) and TURNER

**21 Fishermen coming ashore at Sun Set
previous to a Gale ('The Mildmay Sea
Piece')** R.A.1797; published 1812
Etching and mezzotint, first published state,
$7\frac{1}{8} \times 10\frac{3}{8}$ (18 × 26.3); plate $8\frac{3}{8} \times 11\frac{1}{2}$ (21.2 × 29.1)
Inscr: 'M' [for Marine] above, and 'Picture in
the possession of Sir John Mildmay, Bar.'
'Published Feb.ʸ 11. 1812, by I. M. W. Turner,
Queen Ann Street West,' 'Drawn & Etched by
I. M. W. Turner,' and 'Engraved by W. Annis &
I. C. Easling' below; also bottom left: '3 Feet by
4 Feet'   *Royal Academy of Arts*
The plate, R.40, was issued in Part VIII of the *Liber*

Studiorum. The measurements engraved in the margin
refer to the painting exhibited at the Royal Academy in
1797 (344) and now untraced, of which this is the only
record. It was, therefore, in Turner's standard three-
foot by four-foot size, larger than 'Moonlight, a Study
at Millbank', the only other oil exhibited in 1797, and
may have been seen by Turner as a daylight pendant
to 'Fishermen at Sea' of the year before.

Contemporary reviews drew attention to the originality of Turner's view of Nature and singled out for
praise 'the sickly appearance of a setting Sun at Sea,
preparatory to a storm' (*Times*, 3 May) and the 'transparency and undulation' of the water (Anthony Pasquin
in the *Morning Post*, 5 May), and the painting probably
gave clearer evidence of Turner's advancing powers.

2. Exploration 1797–1801

This period saw Turner's most intensive exploration of
the British countryside and at the same time a great
widening of the technical resources of his art. To the
topographical tradition in which he was already a
master he added the lessons of the more generalised,
Italianate landscapes of J. R. Cozens, whose work he
copied at Dr Munro's (see Nos.B23–B25), and Richard
Wilson (see B37). The example of P. J. de Loutherbourg helped to develop his interest in effects of
weather and atmosphere and in sublime scenery.
Turner's drawings of the Scottish Highlands formed a
climax to this development which prepared him technically and aesthetically for his first visit to the Alps in
1802.

22 'Tweed and Lakes' Sketchbook 1797
Bound in calf with seven clasps
92 leaves (+one taken from cover) $14\frac{5}{8} \times 10\frac{1}{2}$
(37.1 × 26.6)
Watermarked 1796
Inscr. on cover: 'Yorkshire Tweed Lakes of
Cumberland – Westmoreland Lancashire York';
a fragment of parchment label from the spine
reads: 'Tweed and Lakes'; inside front cover
'Ambleside Mill – Mr Lambert Durham C Castle
Mr Hoppner'
Trustees of the British Museum (T.B.XXXV)

f.80ʳ Hubert's Tower, Fountains Abbey
Pencil partly finished in watercolour

The sketchbook contains architectural and landscape
studies in pencil, some finished or half-finished in
watercolour. Apart from making a series of views in the
Lake District, especially of Ullswater and Derwentwater to which he was often to turn for later subjects
(see No.428), Turner concentrated principally on major
ecclesiastical monuments: York, Ripon and Durham,
and the ruins of Kirkstall, Melrose, Bolton and Fountains. There are also some general views of Durham,

Lancaster, Richmond and other towns. This and the
'North of England' sketchbook (No.23) were to be
among the most permanently useful of all Turner's
early sketchbooks.

23 'The North of England' Sketchbook 1797
Bound in calf with four clasps
95 leaves, $10\frac{1}{2} \times 8\frac{1}{4}$ (23 × 27)
Inscr. on cover: 'Derbyshire Yorkshire Durham
Northumberland Tweedale Scot Lincolnshire
Northamptonshire'
Trustees of the British Museum (T.B.XXXIV)

f.45ʳ Dunstanborough Castle
Pencil

The sketchbook contains some of the most elaborate of
Turner's early architectural studies, some worked up
wholly or partially with colour. They include views of
Kirkstall, Egglestone, Warkworth, Bamborough and
Lindisfarne. On f.57 is a very slight sketch of Norham
Castle, used as the basis of the first of many treatments
of the spot (see p.639). There are also studies made at
Harewood (see Nos.27 and 28), and a drawing of Louth
used much later as an *England and Wales* subject
(No.422).

The drawing of Dunstanborough was the starting
point for a series of rough experiments in chalk, monochrome and coloured washes dating presumably from
shortly after the 1797 tour, and culminating in the
painting exhibited R.A. 1798 (322); this drawing was
also used as the basis for the *Liber Studiorum* plate
(R.14) and for the elaborate watercolour engraved for
the *England and Wales* series in 1829 (No. 423).

24 Dunstanborough Castle *c.*1797
Pencil, brush and black ink, watercolour and
bodycolour on buff paper, $7\frac{7}{8} \times 10\frac{7}{8}$ (20 × 27.7)
Trustees of the British Museum (T.B.XXXIII–S)
This and No.25 are connected with the painting ex-
hibited at the R.A. in 1798 (322) (National Gallery of

Victoria, Melbourne; repr. Rothenstein and Butlin 1964, pl.9); and with the later finished watercolour (No.423). All these designs appear to stem from the pencil drawing in the 'North of England' sketchbook (No.23).

25   Dunstanborough Castle *c.*1797
Pencil, grey wash and white bodycolour on buff paper, $10\frac{7}{16} \times 13\frac{5}{16}$ (26.5 × 33.8)
Trustees of the British Museum (T.B.XXXVI–S)

26   Derwentwater 1797
Watercolour, $19\frac{3}{8} \times 24\frac{13}{16}$ (49.3 × 63)
Trustees of the British Museum (T.B.XXXVI–H)
Looking south down the lake to Lodore Falls. The composition is an enlarged version of the partly coloured pencil drawing which appears on f.82 of the 'Tweed and Lakes' sketchbook (T.B.XXXV). On the back of this sketch is a note: 'Mr Farrington', and a finished watercolour of the subject was presented 'to Joseph Farrington, Esqr., with W. Turner's Respects'. Another drawing, T.B.XXXVI–I, shows the same view, though the waterfall is omitted. Turner later used the subject for one of the *England and Wales* series (B.M. 1958-7-12-442).

27   Harewood House from the South-East 1798
Watercolour, $18\frac{5}{8} \times 25\frac{3}{8}$ (47.4 × 64.5)
Inscr: 'W. Turner 98'
The Earl of Harewood
The 'North of England' sketchbook of 1797 (No.23) contains several pencil drawings made in the neighbourhood of Harewood, including one of the house in steep perspective (f.76); there is no study for the composition of this watercolour. Four views of the house were made presumably for Edward or Henry Lascelles after Turner's 1797 visit: from the north-east; from the south; from the south-east and from the south-west; also two of Harewood Castle (see No.28).

Girtin drew a similar view of the house from the south-east, probably at about the same date (the drawing is also at Harewood; Girtin and Loshak, *The Art of Thomas Girtin*, 1954, No.434, fig.75).

28   Harewood Castle from the North 1798
Watercolour, $18\frac{1}{2} \times 25\frac{1}{4}$ (47 × 64)
The Earl of Harewood
ff.67–9 and 71–4 of the 'North of England' sketchbook (No.23) have pencil studies of Harewood; this watercolour is clearly based on that on f.72. The inside front cover of the book is inscribed with a list of commissions including:
Mr Lacells Harwood Castle L
Mr Lacelles Harwood Castle L
Hon Mr Lacelles Kirkstall L
The two views of Harewood Castle, of which this is one, are at Harewood; that of Kirkstall, perhaps the best preserved of all Turner's topographical views of this period, is in the Fitzwilliam Museum, Cambridge. Finberg (1961, p.45) assumed that whereas Turner's 'Hon Mr Lacelles' refers to Edward Lascelles, his 'Mr Lacelles' is Edward's younger brother Henry, afterwards second Earl of Harewood. The letter 'L' stands for 'Large'.

29   The Cross at Stourton, Wiltshire *c.*1798
Pencil and watercolour, $15\frac{15}{16} \times 21\frac{3}{8}$ (40.5 × 54.4)
Inscr. on verso: 'Cross at Stourton Wilts'
Trustees of the British Museum (T.B.XLIV–e)
On his way to Wales in 1798 Turner probably visited Stourhead, whose owner, Sir Richard Colt Hoare, had commissioned him to make drawings of Malmesbury. Sketches for these, some inscribed with Hoare's name, appear in the 'Hereford Court' sketchbook (T.B. XXXVIII ff.1–9). This drawing of the medieval cross at Stourton, with Hoare's famous gardens with lake and temple behind, was presumably made at the same time. The garden itself became the subject of some of the elaborate technical experiments Turner began to make about 1798–9 (T.B.XLIV–f and g.).

**30   Buttermere Lake, with Part of
         Cromackwater, Cumberland, a Shower**
R.A.1798
Oil on canvas, $36\frac{1}{8} \times 48$ (91.5 × 122)
Exh: R.A. 1798 (527)
Tate Gallery (460).
Exhibited by Turner with a conflation of verses from 'Spring' from James Thomson's *Seasons*:
   Till in the western sky the downward sun
   Looks out effulgent – the rapid radiance
      instantaneous strikes
   Th'illumin'd mountains – in a yellow mist
   Bestriding earth – the grand ethereal bow
   Shoots up immense, and every hue unfolds.
This was the first year in which verses were allowed in the R.A. catalogue.

Based on a watercolour in the 'Tweed and Lakes' sketchbook (T.B.XXXV–84, repr. Wilkinson 1972, pp.48–9). Wilson's influence is still strong, as is that of P. J. de Loutherbourg in the Lake District subject and the interest in weather effects, but Turner's close dependence on a sketch made by him on the spot has introduced a personal element not to be found in his Wilsonian landscapes of about the same time, Nos.34, 35 and 36.

For John Hoppner, primarily a portraitist, but the painter of the dramatic 'A Gale of Wind' exhibited at the R.A. in 1794 (Tate Gallery), this picture and 'Morning amongst the Coniston Fells, Cumberland', also shown by Turner in 1798 (Tate Gallery 461), showed 'a timid man afraid to venture'.

31   Plompton Rocks *c.*1798
Oil on canvas, $48 \times 54\frac{1}{4}$ (122 × 137.5)
The Earl of Harewood
32   Plompton Rocks *c.*1798
Oil on canvas, $48 \times 54\frac{1}{4}$ (122 × 137.5)
The Earl of Harewood
Presumably painted for Edward Lascelles, Baron Harewood and later first Earl of Harewood (1740–1820) or his son Edward Lascelles, later Viscount Lascelles (1766–1814), in about 1798, the date of Turner's four finished watercolours of Harewood House (see No.27). Gage's unqualified dating to 1798 (1967, p.148), though likely, is not documented by any published account. They still normally hang each side of the fireplace in the library at Harewood House (see repr. in Gage, pl.32). There is a watercolour closely related to No.31 in the British Museum (T.B.CXCVII–L).

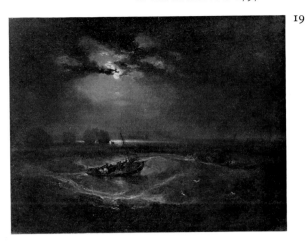

These direct uncompromising views of a fashionable picturesque feature on the Harewood estate, though owing something to Wilson, are much less sophisticated in composition and handling than Turner's other early oil paintings, presumably, as Gage suggests, because of their function and destination.

33   Shipping by a Breakwater *c.*1798
Oil on mahogany, $11\frac{7}{8} \times 7\frac{5}{8}$ (30×19.5)
Tate Gallery (469)

Not so far as is known directly related either to a water-colour sketch or drawing on the one hand, or to a larger oil painting on the other; this seems to be an independent composition in its own right. Formerly dated *c.*1802 (MacColl 1920, p.4) this painting seems very tentative by the side of the sea studies in the 'Calais Pier' sketchbook of that year (T.B.CXXI; see No.89) and is close to watercolours or gouaches in the 'Wilson' and 'Academical' sketchbooks (T.B.XXXVII and XLIII; examples repr. Wilkinson 1972, pp.57 and 82–3); these can both be dated *c.*1798.

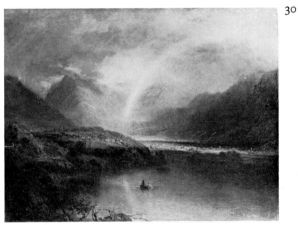

34   View of a Town *c.*1798
Oil on canvas, $9\frac{1}{2} \times 12\frac{3}{4}$ (24×32.5)
Tate Gallery (475)

A small but finished picture, close to Wilson in style and technique, particularly the large rock in the fore-ground, and perhaps derived, like the next example, from one of Turner's Welsh tours.

35   Mountain Scene with Castle *c.*1798
Oil on canvas, $17\frac{1}{4} \times 21\frac{1}{4}$ (44×54)
Tate Gallery (465)

Related to the sketches in the 'Dinevor Castle' sketch-book which seems to have been used, at least in part, in 1798 (T.B.XL–37^v and 38, repr. Wilkinson 1972, p.72, and 39^v and 40). Many years later, in a letter to Hawksworth Fawkes of 27 December 1847, Turner referred to how he felt when 'in the days of my youth . . . I was in search of Richard Wilson', apparent-ly on this tour of 1798 during which he seems to have done a drawing at Wilson's birthplace, Penegoes, near Machynlleth (T.B.XXXIX–1; see Finberg 1939, p.419 and Gage 1969, p.30), and this painting is again strong-ly Wilsonian in feeling.

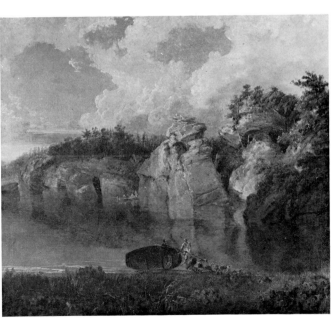

36   A Fishing Boat in a Choppy Sea *c.*1798
Watercolour and bodycolour on coarse grey
paper, $5\frac{1}{4} \times 8\frac{1}{4}$ (13.5×20.8)
Inscr. on verso. in an early nineteenth century
hand: 'Drawn by J. M. W. Turner|when giving
a lesson to Wm Blake (probably at the end of the
18th century)'
Private Collection

This drawing is one of a series of coastal or shore scenes executed on coarse paper in watercolour with white bodycolour. The majority are studies of fisher-men and their boats in breakers near the shore, and are in the Turner Bequest (XXXIII). XXXIII–K shows a boat (evidently the same one that appears here) with BRI . . . TON inscribed on its transom, so the series was presumably made during a visit to Brighton. The inscription on the back of this one is unlikely to be correct in its suggestion that Turner made the drawing during a lesson: he more probably showed the group to his pupil, who chose this drawing to keep. It remained in the family of William Blake of Newhouse until 1962. There are references to 'Wm Blake' in the 'North of England' sketchbook (No.23) f.67^v, and in the 'Hereford Court' sketchbook of 1798 (T.B.XXXVIII ff.47^v, 50a^v), and Turner was presumably teaching Blake then. It is not known how long the connection lasted. (See the drawing by Blake, No.B18.)

The style of this series of marines, with its sombre colour but spontaneous 'plein-air' treatment, is characteristic of the studies Turner made on tinted or prepared paper in conjunction with his first essays in oil painting; compare pages in the 'Wilson' sketchbook (T.B.XXVII) and in the slightly later 'Dunbar' sketchbook (No.54). The subjects have much in common with the two Dobree pictures, 'Fishermen on a Lee Shore' and the so-called 'Wave' (Kenwood, Iveagh Bequest and Southampton Art Gallery).

37 Builders working on the Construction of Fonthill 1799
Pencil, grey wash and watercolour,
sight $9\frac{11}{16} \times 16\frac{1}{8}$ (25 × 41)
C. W. M. Turner, Esq.

From the 'Smaller Fonthill' sketchbook, T.B.XLVIII, many leaves of which were distributed at an early date. See Nos.38 and 39.

38 View of Fonthill from a Stone Quarry 1799
Watercolour over pencil, $11\frac{3}{4} \times 17\frac{3}{8}$ (29.8 × 44.2)
Leeds City Art Gallery

It is not clear whether this watercolour ever belonged to Beckford; it does not form part of the series of large views of Fonthill shown at the R.A. in 1800. But for its slightly larger size, it resembles the watercolour studies made in the 'Fonthill' sketchbook (T.B.XLVII) when Turner was staying with Beckford in 1799.

39 Fonthill from the North-East 1799–1800
Pencil and watercolour, $40\frac{3}{8} \times 27\frac{1}{8}$ (102.5 × 69)
Exh: R.A. 1800 (?680) as 'North East View of the Gothic Abbey (sunset) now building at Fonthill, the seat of W. Beckford, Esq.'

Whitworth Art Gallery, Manchester (D.19.1904)

Commissioned from Turner by William Beckford as one of a series of five views of Fonthill at different times of the day, exhibited at the R.A. in 1800. They showed the Abbey in the light of morning (341), noon (663), afternoon (328), sunset (680) and evening (566). The title is that by which the present drawing is now known; but since the north-east view was specified as 'Sunset' and this drawing (though considerably faded) seems to represent a scene of full daylight, it may be that it should be identified with one of the other views, perhaps either 663 (noon) or 328 (afternoon). Turner stayed with Beckford in 1799, making numerous pencil and watercolour studies of the house, both in detail and seen at a distance, in the park and surrounding countryside; they are mostly in the 'Fonthill' sketchbook, T.B.XLVII, of which f.11 is closest to this view. The Abbey was still in course of construction while Turner was there (see No.37); many of the sketches indicate scaffolding round the tower which is shown here as completed, perhaps with the aid of architect's drawings. The architect was James Wyatt, whose own view of the 'building

now erecting at Fonthill' had been shown at the R.A. in 1799 (1016) as had Richard Westmacott's 'La Madonna della Gloria, a statue for Fonthill Abbey' (1006).

40 Oxford: Part of Balliol College Quadrangle
*c.*1802
Pencil and watercolour, $12\frac{3}{8} \times 17\frac{5}{8}$ (31.8 × 44.8)
Visitors of the Ashmolean Museum, Oxford

For the 'Oxford Almanack', though not used. The subject was re-drawn by Hugh O'Neill (1784–1824) and engraved by James Storer for the 1810 issue, on account of an objection by Dr Parsons, Master of Balliol, that Turner had shown the shadows in an impossible position. Turner's first design for the Almanack appeared in 1799, a 'South View of Christ Church'; he produced ten in all, receiving £73.10.0 in 1804 for the final seven of which 'Balliol College' was one. For a full account of Turner's relations with the Clarendon Press and of the Almanack series, see C. F. Bell 'The Oxford Almanacks', *Art Journal*, August 1904, and Luke Herrmann, *Ruskin and Turner*, 1968, pp.55–63. The present drawing is No.9 in Herrmann's catalogue.

A number of pencil studies of the architecture of Oxford, made at the time when Turner was working on the Almanack designs, are in the 'Smaller Fonthill' sketchbook (T.B.XLVIII, ff.2,7) and elsewhere (e.g. T.B. L–E, F, G, J).

41 Trees and Buildings seen over a Wall
?*c.*1800
Watercolour, $13\frac{1}{2} \times 16\frac{1}{8}$ (34.3 × 41)
Trustees of the British Museum (T.B.CXCVI–X)

Possibly derived from an Italian composition of J. R. Cozens. The palette and vigorous handling suggest that this drawing belongs to the same period as the experimental watercolours of *c.*1799–1800, T.B.LXX–N, O, Q etc.

42 Caernarvon Castle 1799
Watercolour over pencil, $22\frac{7}{16} \times 32\frac{1}{2}$ (57 × 82.5)
Inscr: 'Turner'
Exh: R.A. 1799 (340)
Private Collection

Shown at the R.A. with verses from David Mallet's 'Amyntor and Theodora', Canto I:

——Now rose,
Sweet Evening, solemn hour, the sun declin'd,
Hung golden o'er this nether firmament,
Whose broad cerulean mirror, calmly bright,
Gave back his beamy visage to the sky
With splendour undiminish'd.

The drawing was purchased by J. J. Angerstein. Farington (*Diary*, 27 May 1799) records that the price of 40 guineas 'was fixed by Mr. A. and was much greater than Turner would have asked'. A critic at the Academy was 'struck and delighted with . . . Caernarvon Castle, the sun setting in gorgeous splendour behind its shadowy towers . . . in water colours; to which he has given a depth and force of tone, which I had never before conceived attainable with such untoward implements' (quoted by Finberg, 1961, p.57).

43   Caernarvon Castle, North Wales

R.A. 1800   (repr. on p.17)

Watercolour, $26\frac{1}{16} \times 39\frac{1}{8}$ (66.3 × 99.4)

Exh: R.A. 1800 (351)

Trustees of the British Museum (T.B.LXX–M)

The verses appended to the entry for No.351 in the 1800
R.A. catalogue refer specifically to the Bard who figures
in the foreground of the view:

And now on Arvon's haughty tow'rs
The Bard the song of pity pours,
    For oft on Mona's distant hills he sighs,
Where jealous of the minstrel band,
The Tyrant drench'd with blood the land,
    And charm'd with horror, triumph'd in their cries.
The swains of Arvon round him throng,
And join the sorrows of his song.

The reference is to the extermination of the Bards by
Edward I, popularized by Gray in his poem 'The Bard'
and frequently used by painters as a theme for historical works (Thomas Jones, John Martin, etc). The same
subject may have suggested the armies which straggle
across the mountain valley in T.B.LXX–Q, a North
Welsh view on paper watermarked 1794. A study for a
similar historical subject, with a group of figures round
an old man, and distant armies, is LXX–N. Turner has
allowed himself the licence of incorporating an ana-
chronism – the tall-masted sailing ships moored round
the distant castle, which figure in many of his drawings
of Caernarvon.

The drawing was mounted on a grey washed mount
and appears to have been finished off afterwards. In
particular, it seems that Turner darkened the foreground and left and right repoussoirs with overlaid
glazes of blue, brown and ochre.

44   'Academical' Sketchbook *c.*1798

Bound in calf
51 leaves of blue paper almost all prepared with a
wash of reddish-brown, with white fly-leaves,
$8\frac{1}{2} \times 5\frac{1}{2}$ (21.5 × 13.8)
Inscr. on front cover: 'Academical'
Trustees of British Museum (T.B.XLIII)

f.39ᵛ   Caernarvon Castle at Sunset
Pen and black ink, watercolour and bodycolour
on blue paper prepared with a reddish-brown
wash

A series of Academy nude studies in pencil and watercolour begins from the front of the book, and from the
back, landscapes in chalk, watercolour and bodycolour.
The landscapes may all be Welsh subjects and have
much in common stylistically with a number of the
large experimental landscapes *c.*1798–1800. In addition
to f.39ᵛ, ff.41ᵛ, 42ʳ&ᵛ, 43ʳ&ᵛ and 44ᵛ also deal with
Caernarvon Castle. They display great freedom in the
manipulation of a variety of media, and demonstrate
Turner's rapidly increasing interest in the expressive
power of watercolour and bodycolour, probably suggested to him by his experience of painting in oils
(cf. No.45).

45   Caernarvon Castle ?1798

Oil on pine, $5\frac{13}{16} \times 9\frac{1}{16}$ (14.8 × 23)
Tate Gallery (1867)

This is related to a group of body-colours in the

'Academical' sketchbook (T.B.XLIII–39ᵛ, 41ᵛ, 42ᵛ, 43ᵛ
and 44ᵛ; all but the second repr. Gage 1967, pl.5 and
Wilkinson 1972, pp.82–3; see No.44) which were used
for the finished watercolour of 'Caernarvon Castle' exhibited at the R.A. in 1799 (No.42). Both body-colours
and oil seem therefore to have been painted on
Turner's tour of Wales in the late summer of 1798.

There is no difference here in style or purpose between the sketch in oil and those in body-colour; later
in his career Turner would differentiate between
different media. Turner, by covering the blue paper of
his sketchbook with a reddish-brown wash, has produced an effect very close to the use of a wood support
for the oil.

The finished watercolour was exhibited in 1799 with
some verses by the Scottish poet David Mallet (?1705-
1765). Turner's choice of these lines, similar in sentiment to *The Seasons* by Mallet's friend James Thomson, from which Turner had quoted the year before
(see No.30), again reflects his interest in the visual
effects of natural phenomena.

46   Aeneas and the Sibyl, Lake Avernus *c.*1798

Oil on canvas, $30\frac{1}{8} \times 38\frac{3}{4}$ (76.5 × 98.5)
Tate Gallery (463)

Based on a large pencil drawing in the British Museum
(T.B.LI–N) which is in its turn based on a drawing of
Lake Avernus made by Sir Richard Colt Hoare in 1786
(see No.B83). Turner did a considerable number of
watercolours for Colt Hoare between 1795 and 1800
and it is possible that this was a commission; in fact
John Gage has suggested (1974, pp.38–40) that Colt
Hoare put forward the subject partly to replace, as it
were, a Wilson in his collection which had turned out to
show not Lake Avernus but Lake Nemi with Diana and
Callisto.

Aeneas, in the sixth book of the *Aeneid*, is told by the
Cumaean Sibyl that he can only enter the Underworld,
where he seeks the shade of his father, with a golden
bough from a sacred tree as an offering to Proserpine.
A later version, practically the only case in which
Turner repeated one of his finished pictures in the
same scale and medium, was definitely painted for Colt
Hoare in 1814 (Mr and Mrs Paul Mellon collection)
and may have replaced the earlier painting in Hoare's
collection, though there is no evidence that this picture
ever left Turner's possession.

This picture again seems to have been painted *c.*1798
and is very Wilsonian in treatment, though in this case,
at Colt Hoare's suggestion so it seems, he was working
for the first time in the European tradition of the
historical landscape with a significant mythological or
historical subject, developed in Italy by Poussin and
Claude and brought to this country by Wilson. It is the
first of a long series of panoramic landscapes with
similar subjects (e.g. Nos.237 and 486). Lake Avernus
and the distant landscape reappear in 'The Golden
Bough', exhibited at the Royal Academy in 1834 and
now in the Tate Gallery (Vernon Collection, 371), the
story of which is connected.

47   Kilgarren Castle on the Twyvey, Hazy Sunrise, previous to a Sultry Day R.A.1799
Oil on canvas, 36 × 48 (92 × 122)
Exh: R.A. 1799 (305); Sir John Leicester's Gallery 1819 and subsequent years (27)
National Trust, from Wordsworth House

Turner exhibited a number of oil paintings of castles, mainly Welsh, from 1798 to 1800, including 'Harlech Castle, from Twgwyn Ferry, Summer's Evening Twilight' (Mr and Mrs Paul Mellon) in the same exhibition as this picture; see also No.48. There are a number of watercolours and drawings of both Kilgarren and Harlech in the 'Hereford Court' sketchbook including a watercolour of this composition (T.B.XXXVIII–88; see also 28–9, 100). There are other versions in oil, of greater or lesser authenticity, but this picture seems to be the one exhibited in 1799 and probably purchased by Sir John Leicester, apparently at Oxford, before 1804 from the painter William Delamotte.

The very titles of this landscape and that of the 'Harlech' reflect Turner's interest in the special light of a particular moment on a particular kind of summer's day. This interest, which accompanies and perhaps even eclipses the interest of the picturesque castle, was anticipated most fully by the works of P. J. de Loutherbourg, who used similar titles for such paintings as the Tate Gallery's picture of 'A Distant Hail-Storm coming on, and the March of Soldiers with their Baggage', exhibited the same year; an earlier example is 'Daybreak Dispelling a Mist', shown in 1783. The landscape is grander and rather more solidly constructed, and the fall of light more accentuated, than in the exhibits of the previous year (see No.30), and Turner's handling of paint is broader and less close to Wilson, whose own picture of the subject, from much the same view, is much less dramatic (see W. G. Constable, *Richard Wilson*, 1953, pl.30a). There is an extraordinary use of basic squares and triangles to indicate the little buildings on the right.

48   Dolbadern Castle, North Wales R.A.1800
Oil on canvas, 47 × 35½ (119.5 × 90)
Exh: R.A. 1800 (200); Diploma paintings, R.A. 1830 (Council Room 43)
Royal Academy of Arts

There are drawings of Dolbadern in the 'Hereford Court', 'North Wales' and 'Dolbadern' sketchbooks of 1798–9 (T.B.XXXVIII–47, XXXIX–33 and XLVI–21, 38ᵛ, 39) but the painting is based more directly on a remarkable series of six drawings in coloured pastels on blue paper in the 'Studies for Pictures' sketchbook (T.B.LXIX–103, 104, 108, 109, 112 and 113; four examples repr. in colour in Wilkinson 1972, pp.94–5). They are all variations of the main elements of the composition, silhouetting the castle tower against the glow of the sun setting under a glowering sky, an effect rather tamed in the final oil painting. In other respects, however, the painting shows a considerable advance in drama and concentration over the more Wilsonian landscapes of 1798 and 1799, and Turner's new aspirations are reflected in the Salvator Rosa-like figures in 'period' costumes and the verses in the Royal Academy catalogue:

How awful is the silence of the waste,
Where nature lifts her mountains to the sky.
Majestic solitude, behold the tower
Where hopeless OWEN, long imprison'd, pin'd,
And wrung his hands for liberty, in vain.

The verses appear for the first time to be by Turner himself, and Owen is presumably Owen or Owain Goch, the Welsh prince imprisoned in Dolbadern Castle from 1254 until 1277, though it could also be Owen Glendower (?1359–?1416) whose final end is however uncertain; he seems to have died in hiding rather than in prison.

Turner was elected an Associate of the Royal Academy in November 1799 at the lowest age allowed by the regulations, twenty-four, though in fact he had been proposed and nearly elected the previous year. In February 1802 he was elected a full Academician and chose this work for the obligatory 'Deposit' (now called Diploma) picture. However, he had second thoughts and subsequently offered another painting instead, but the first was chosen. Unfortunately it is not recorded what the second picture was, but it may have been something more ambitious.

49   The Vale of Earne 1801
Pencil and white bodycolour on white paper prepared with a grey wash, 13⅝ × 19⅛ (34.5 × 48.6)
Trustees of the British Museum (T.B.LVIII–44)

Finberg compares this view with that in the pencil sketch on ff.144ᵛ–5ʳ of the 'Scotch Lakes' sketchbook (T.B.LVI) which is inscribed 'Vale of Earne'; but apart from the conical hut in the foreground the two scenes have little in common.

50   View over a Valley 1801
Pencil, charcoal and white bodycolour on white paper prepared with a grey wash, 12 × 18⅞ (30.5 × 47.9)
Trustees of the British Museum (T.B.LVIII–6)

The view is tentatively identified by Finberg as 'near Arrochar'. It is typical of the elaborate 'Scottish Pencils' in the Turner Bequest which provided the first indication that Turner was beginning to explore the expressive possibilities of the monochrome drawing in the same way that he had already begun to experiment with watercolour and oil. The technique is, however, a development of that which Turner had learned from the pencil drawings of J. R. Cozens. There is a slight pencil sketch on the verso.

51   Loch Awe, with a Rainbow c.1801
Pencil and watercolour with some scraping out, sight, 8 × 11¼ (22.4 × 28.5)
Sir Edmund Bacon, Bart.

Probably made during or after Turner's visit to Scotland of 1801; the series of 'Scottish Pencils' in the Turner Bequest includes a number of views of Loch Awe (T.B.LVIII–13, 14, 15, 16), though the delicacy of handling and subtle evocation of atmosphere in this watercolour is unlike any of these. The watercolour of 'Kilchern Castle' shown at the R.A. in 1802 (377) seems to have included a view of Loch Awe with a rainbow, and this drawing may have been executed in connection with that work.

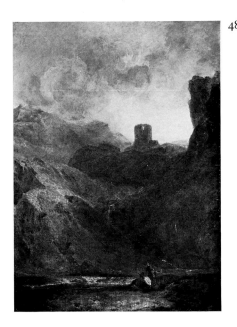

48

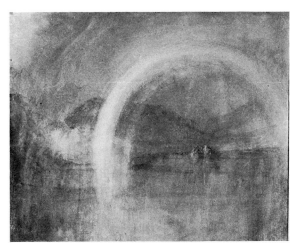

51

52 'Edinburgh' Sketchbook 1801
Bound in marbled cardboard with leather spine
78 leaves, the majority drawn on in pencil, some
with grey washes or watercolour, $7\frac{3}{4} \times 5$
(19.5 × 12.6)
Trustees of the British Museum (T.B.L V)

ff.5ᵛ–6ʳ View of Edinburgh from St. Anthony's Chapel
Pencil with blue and grey washes

This book contains sketches made in and around Edinburgh during Turner's visit to Scotland in July and
August 1801. Finberg (1961, p.74) points out the novel
freedom and rapidity of many of the drawings in the
Scottish sketchbooks, suggesting that they mark the
final disconnection from the topographical discipline of
Turner's youth. It seems likely that the atmosphere of
Scotland, especially of its mountains, contributed largely to his sense of emancipation; cf. some of his experiments with Welsh subjects of about this date.

Similar wash or watercolour views of Edinburgh to
that shown are on ff.1, 7ᵛ–8 (cont. on 9) and 10. The
remainder of the sketches are in pencil only.

53 'Scotch Figures' Sketchbook 1801
Bound in calf, one clasp
187 leaves, the majority blank; 16 at the front of
the book drawn on with figure studies in pencil
and watercolour, 5 at the back with studies of
boats and trees, $6\frac{1}{8} \times 3\frac{1}{2}$ (15.5 × 9)
Inscr. Finberg records a label on the spine
which reads: '50 Scotch f . . .'
Trustees of the British Museum (T.B.LIX)

f.5ʳ Study of Three Women, one stooping to fill a Jug at a Spring
Pencil and watercolour

Compare Turner's use of this book with that of the
'Swiss Figures' sketchbook (No.55). Although he made
so few detailed notes of Scottish costumes and occupa-

tions he was able to produce a large watercolour,
'Edinburgh, from Caulton-hill', for the R.A. in 1804
(373) which makes imaginative use of a number of fully-
realised figures engaged in appropriate pursuits (T.B.
LX-H). Three other watercolours of Scottish subjects
were shown at the R.A. in 1802: 'The fall of the Clyde,
Lanarkshire: Noon' (336; Walker Art Gallery, Liverpool, repr. Gage, 1969, pl.16); 'Kilchern Castle, with the
Cruchan Ben mountains, Scotland: Noon' (377; ex.
Beausire collection; see No.51); and 'Edinburgh New
Town, castle, &c. from the Water of Leith' (424; the
drawing of this title repr. Armstrong, 1902, fp.30 is not
by Turner).

54 'Dunbar' Sketchbook 1801
Bound in calf, one clasp
116 leaves of white paper, almost all prepared
with a wash of pink bodycolour, $4\frac{1}{2} \times 6\frac{1}{2}$ (11.5 ×
16.3)
Watermarked: 1794
Inscr. on label on spine: '90 Scotland'
Trustees of the British Museum (T.B.LIV)

ff.115ᵛ–116ʳ Study of Waves breaking on a Beach
Pencil, brown wash and white bodycolour with
scraping-out

The sketchbook was used by Turner en route for
Edinburgh in 1801, including sketches of Rievaulx, the
Bass Rock and Tantallon Castle; the drawings are
mostly in pencil with scraping out, with occasional use
of brown wash and white bodycolour.

The drawing shown is one of a series of studies of
waves on ff.109ʳ–16ᵛ. This drawing appears to be related to the painting known as 'The Wave' executed for
Samuel Dobree in 1802 and now in Southampton Art
Gallery. Similar studies of breakers, with a fishing-
boat, occur in the 'Calais Pier' sketchbook (No.89),
ff.84–7 etc. with the inscription 'Mr. Dobree's Lee
Shore'.

3. First Continental Tour 1802

The Peace of Amiens with France enabled Turner, like many other artists, to cross the Channel after years of war. Going first direct to the Alps, already known to him at second hand through the works of J. R. Cozens, he stopped on his way back at Paris, where the treasures of the Louvre were swelled by works of art looted from Napoleon's conquests (see No.91). As well as the large finished watercolours in this section the journey resulted in several oil paintings in which he treated places he had visited in the Grand Manner (see Nos.74–6).

55   'Swiss Figures' Sketchbook 1802
Bound in vellum
74 leaves, the first 18 only drawn on in pencil and watercolour, $7\frac{3}{4} \times 6\frac{1}{4}$ (19.5 × 16)
Inscr. on spine: '14'; and on label on spine: '69'
Trustees of the British Museum (T.B.LXXVIII)

f.1ʳ Two Nude Women lying on a Bed, with Swiss Costumes on the Floor beside them
Pencil and watercolour

Turner's use of this book – beginning with pencil and watercolour studies of figures in local costume, and leaving the majority of leaves unused – parallels that made of the 'Scotch Figures' sketchbook (No.53), though here there are one or two pencil studies of boats on a lake (?Thun), ff.9, 11.

56   Martigny 1802
Pencil, charcoal and white bodycolour on grey paper, $11\frac{3}{16} \times 8\frac{3}{8}$ (28.4 × 21.3)
Trustees of the British Museum (T.B.LXXIV–54)

57   Near the Gate of the Grande Chartreuse 1802
Pencil, charcoal and white bodycolour on grey paper, $11\frac{3}{16} \times 8\frac{5}{16}$ (28.4 × 21.2)
Trustees of the British Museum (T.B.LXXIV–36)

58   The Cascade of the Chartreuse 1802
Pencil and white bodycolour on grey paper, $11\frac{1}{8} \times 8\frac{3}{8}$ (28.2 × 21.3)
Trustees of the British Museum (T.B.LXXIV–31)

59   A Castle on a Wooded Promontory by a Lake 1802
Pencil and black chalk and white bodycolour on grey paper, $11\frac{3}{16} \times 8\frac{1}{2}$ (28.2 × 21.5)
Trustees of the British Museum (T.B.LXXIV–46)

Four drawings from the 'Grenoble' sketchbook, which was apparently dismembered by Turner himself; some of the leaves were mounted with his own titles, but these were cut off at a later date.

60   A Road among Swiss Mountains 1802
Pencil, watercolour and scraping-out on white paper prepared with a grey wash, $22\frac{3}{16} \times 28\frac{5}{8}$ (56.3 × 72.7)
Trustees of the British Museum (T.B.LXXIX–H)
Perhaps based on the pencil sketch on f.62ʳ of the

'Lake Thun' sketchbook (T.B.LXXVI). The series numbered LXXIX consists of nineteen large drawings of Swiss views, mainly in pencil heightened with white chalk. This example is unusually finished, but was evidently never intended to make one of the group of Swiss views sold to Walter Fawkes during the years following this tour (see Nos.65, 67, 68 and 69).

61   L'Aiguillette, Valley of Cluses 1802
Pencil and watercolour with scraping-out on white paper prepared with a grey wash, $18 \times 12\frac{7}{16}$ (45.8 × 31.6)
Whitworth Art Gallery, Manchester (D.59.1925)
From the 'St Gothard and Mont Blanc' sketchbook (T.B.LXXV); the sheet formerly belonged to Ruskin. A finished drawing of the subject, executed shortly after Turner's 1802 journey to Switzerland, is now in America.

62   The Pass of St. Gothard 1802
Pencil, watercolour and scraping-out on white paper prepared with a grey wash, $18\frac{1}{2} \times 12\frac{3}{8}$ (47 × 31.5)
Watermarked: 1801
Trustees of the British Museum (T.B.LXXV–33)
The basis for Fawkes' large watercolour No.67. A drawing of the scene looking back to the Devil's Bridge (from which Turner took this view) is LXXV–34.

63   The Lake of Thun 1802
Pencil and watercolour with scraping-out on white paper prepared with a grey wash, $12\frac{7}{16} \times 18\frac{5}{8}$ (31.6 × 47.3)
Whitworth Art Gallery, Manchester (D.58.1925)
A leaf from the 'St Gothard and Mont Blanc' sketchbook (T.B.LXXV). With No.61 formerly in Ruskin's collection.

64   The Mer de Glace, Chamonix 1802
Pencil, watercolour and bodycolour on white paper, prepared with a grey wash, $12\frac{3}{8} \times 18\frac{7}{16}$ (31.5 × 46.8)
Watermarked: 1801
Trustees of the British Museum (T.B.LXXV–22)
Used as the basis for one of the views bought by Walter Fawkes, 'Blair's Hut on the Montanvert and Mer de Glace' (Finberg, *Farnley*, 1912, No.12), now in the Courtauld Institute Galleries (Kitson, *Turner Watercolours from the Collection of Stephen Courtauld*, 1974, No.4).

65   Glacier and Source of the Arveiron c.1803
Watercolour, 27×40 (68.5 × 101.5)
Exh: R.A. 1803 (896); Grosvenor Place 1819 (39); Leeds 1839 (61)
Mr and Mrs Paul Mellon, Upperville, Virginia
The full title given to this drawing in the Royal Academy catalogue of 1803 is 'Glacier and source of the

Arveron, going up to the Mer de Glace'. Turner may have used studies in the 'St Gothard and Mont Blanc' sketchbook (T.B.LXXV), but no single one of them corresponds precisely to the whole composition. The closest is perhaps the study in black and white chalk on f.20^r which was used again as the basis for the *Liber Studiorum* plate (R.60). f.21^r of the same book is also apparently a view of the Source of the Arveiron. There is, however, a drawing in black chalk on grey prepared paper which gives the central motif of the design almost at its full scale (T.B.LXXIX–L). This was executed in series with the large and more finished 'Road among Mountains' (No.60) and with a group of similar chalk drawings under the same number in the Turner Bequest. The drawing was purchased by Walter Fawkes.

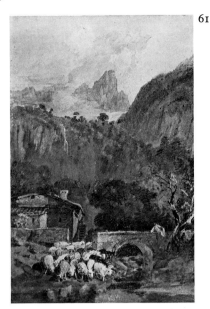

61

66 The Great St. Bernard Pass *c.*1803
  Pencil and watercolour, 26¼ × 39 (66.4 × 99)
  Trustees of the British Museum (T.B.LXXX–D)
The title is Finberg's; he suggests that the drawing may alternatively show the Jungfrau from the Lauterbrunnen road. The pencil sketch on which the drawing is based is in the 'Thun' sketchbook (T.B.LXXVI, f.66) though the view is somewhat extended laterally here. The pencil cross on the sketch may indicate that it had been chosen for treatment in this way. It may have been intended to be worked up uniformly with the other large Swiss views of this period, which were bought by Fawkes (see Nos.65, 67, 68 and 69), but no more finished version is known.

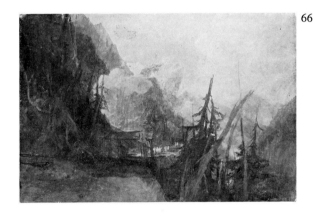

66

67 The Passage of Mount St. Gothard 1804
  Watercolour with scraping-out, 38⅞ × 27
  (98.5 × 68.5)
  Inscr. top left: 'I M W Turner R A 1804'
  Exh: ?Turner's Gallery 1804; R.A. 1815 (281);
  Grosvenor Place 1819 (4); Leeds 1839 (68)
  Abbott Hall Art Gallery, Kendal
Derived from the study in the 'St. Gothard and Mont Blanc' sketchbook (No.62). The watercolour was exhibited at least three times during Turner's life, always with the title 'The Passage of Mount St. Gothard, taken from the centre of the Teufels Broch (Devil's Bridge) Switzerland'; it was also probably one of the works to appear in Turner's first exhibition at his own gallery in 1804, from which it would have been purchased by Walter Fawkes, together with another large Swiss view, 'The Great Fall of the Reichenbach, in the valley of Hasle, Switzerland' (Cecil Higgins Art Gallery, Bedford; repr. Royal Academy, *British Art*, exhibition catalogue, 1934, No.763, pl.CLXXI).

68 The Lake of Thun *c.*1804
  Watercolour, 11 × 15½ (28 × 39)
  Private Collection
One of the Swiss drawings acquired by Walter Fawkes. Based on pencil studies in the 'Lake Thun' sketchbook (T.B.LXXVI ff.60, 61). A design for the *Liber Studiorum* follows the general composition of this watercolour: the sepia drawing is T.B.CXVI–R; the plate was published in 1808 (R.15).

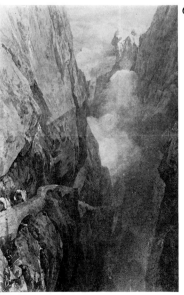

67

69 St. Martin and Sallenches, Savoy *c.*1805
Pencil and watercolour with scraping-out,
11 1/16 × 15 11/16 (28.1 × 39.9)
Inscr. bottom left: 'I M W Turner, R A'
Exh: Grosvenor Place 1819 (30)
Leger Galleries Ltd

The composition is closely based on the study in pencil and white bodycolour on f.12 of the 'St. Gothard and Mont Blanc' sketchbook (T.B.LXXV). The drawing was originally owned by Walter Fawkes.

4. Success at the Royal Academy 1801-12

Turner was elected as an Associate of the Royal Academy in 1799 and a full Academician in 1802 (for his Diploma picture see No.48). His success was marked by a series of imposing oil paintings, classical landscapes, dramatic historical subjects and turbulent sea-pieces that, despite some critical opposition, established him as the leading young painter of his day. At the same time he set out in his *Liber Studiorum* to establish an academic, theoretical framework for the various kinds of landscape (see p.61).

70 The Fifth Plague of Egypt R.A.1800
Oil on canvas, 49 × 72 (124.5 × 183)
Exh: R.A. 1800 (206)
Indianapolis Museum of Art

Apart, possibly, from the lost 'Battle of the Nile', exhibited the previous year and about which nothing is known, this is Turner's first real essay in the Grand Manner, an Old Testament scene of death and destruction painted in the manner of Poussin. In the Royal Academy catalogue Turner quoted the following lines from *Exodus* IX, 23:

> And Moses stretched forth his hands towards heaven,
>   and the Lord sent thunder and hail, and the fire ran
>   along the ground.

In fact the Plague shown is the seventh, which suggests that Turner was interested less in the text itself than in its possibilities for dramatic treatment and the chance of working in the manner of the artist who had done more than any other to raise landscape to the status enjoyed in the academic hierarchy by pictures of serious subjects. The picture was bought for 150 guineas by William Beckford, owner of the Altieri Claudes and builder of Fonthill Abbey, five watercolour views of which by Turner were exhibited at the Royal Academy the same year (see No.39).

There is a slight study among sketches of North Wales in the 'Dolbadern' sketchbook (T.B.XLVI-79), suggesting that, as in the case of 'Hannibal crossing the Alps' (No.88), Turner may have been partly inspired to paint a scene set in a distant place and time by a climatic experience in the British Isles. There is also a possible study for the standing man with arms raised in supplication on the right (could this be intended to be Moses?) in the 'Studies for Pictures' sketchbook (T.B.LXIX-22), and a nude study in the 'Calais Pier' sketchbook (see No.89).

The composition, somewhat condensed and altered,

was engraved for the *Liber Studiorum*, R.16, still as 'The Fifth Plague of Egypt', published 10 June 1808 (No.102). Meanwhile, in 1802, Turner had exhibited another Plague picture at the Royal Academy, this time correctly identified as 'The Tenth Plague of Egypt' (Tate Gallery 470).

71 Dutch Boats in a Gale: Fishermen endeavouring to put their Fish on Board ('The Bridgewater Sea Piece') R.A.1801
Oil on canvas, 64 × 87½ (162.5 × 221)
Exh: R.A. 1801 (157); *Old Masters*, British Institution 1837 (145)
His Grace The Duke of Sutherland

Commissioned by the Duke of Bridgewater for 250 guineas to hang as a companion to a sea piece of 'A Rising Gale' by Willem van der Velde the Younger (repr. illustrated souvenir, *Dutch Pictures 1450-1750*, R.A.1952-3, p.37). The van der Velde is, in fact, slightly smaller but Turner's composition is basically the same in reverse. There are, however, significant differences. In the van der Velde all the ships are placed diagonally to the surface of the painting, leading the eye into depth. In the Turner the distant ships are parallel to the surface and depth is suggested by the sweep of the clouds and the highly selective fall of light: the most distant ship and the far horizon are picked out in a sharp line of light and the ship in the middle distance is silhouetted against the lightest area of the sky. Turner's contrasts of light and shade are greater, but the general effect is more controlled, Neo-Classical as opposed to Baroque.

Despite Thornbury's story (1877, pp.291, 325) that Turner completely dead-coloured the large canvas the night he received the commission there are a number of sketches in the 'Calais Pier' sketchbook (T.B.LXXXI-106-9, 118-19, 126-7, 129; see No.89).

The painting was unanimously well received in the press, *The Porcupine* classing it 'as one of the greatest ornaments of the present Exhibition', though this praise was qualified here and in *The Monthly Mirror* by a desire for 'greater distinctness' in the foreground boats, a remarkably early foretaste of the perennial criticism of Turner's works. Farington's diary records the admiration of Sir George Beaumont, later to be one of Turner's fiercest critics, and Constable, and that Fuseli called it the best picture in the exhibition '- quite Rembrantesque'. The other oil exhibited by Turner in 1801, the lost 'Army of the Medes destroyed in the desert by a whirlwind', was less well reviewed.

In 1837 Lord Francis Egerton lent a number of pictures to the summer Old Masters exhibition at the British Institution, including van der Velde's 'A Rising Gale' and the painting by Turner, who thereby acquired Old Master status. This afforded *Blackwood's Magazine*, July–December 1837, the opportunity of comparing the two works: 'They are both fine pictures, but painted upon very different principles. The one is careful painting, smooth in execution, very transparent... The other is with a bold and dashing pencil, with little care for anything but effect. The texture of all parts is the same, the surface is plastered; accordingly the sky, even at a considerable distance, looks rocky, and the water certainly not liquid ... Still the picture is very forcible'. The *Literary Gazette* for 3 June came down solidly on the side of Turner: 'we put it to the most cynical and inveterate *laudator temporis acti*, whether there is a single point in which the old Dutch painter has the advantage over the modern English one? Our artists ought to feel much obliged to Lord Francis Egerton ... for the opportunity thus afforded of most unequivocally shewing that, at least in one department of the fine arts, there is in this country living merit, as high as that which is attached to the greatest name, in that department, of former days'.

72 Ships bearing up for Anchorage ('The Egremont Sea Piece') R.A.1802

Oil on canvas, 47 × 71 (119.5 × 180.5)
Exh: R.A. 1802 (227)
H.M. Treasury and the National Trust, from Petworth House (33)

The earliest and probably the first Turner to be purchased by his great patron the 3rd Earl of Egremont. There are a number of sketches in the 'Calais Pier' sketchbook (T.B.LXXXI–64–7, 72–3, 88–9).

Here, still more than in the Bridgewater Sea Piece, Turner applied the Poussinesque principles of composition first seen in 'The Fifth Plague' to the tradition of marine painting in England, which, based on the work of the van der Veldes in the later seventeenth century, had continued more or less unaltered until the end of the eighteenth. Once again, however, Turner uses the selective fall of light to clarify his design, particularly in the complex of overlapping ships in the centre. When Turner repeated the composition for the *Liber Studiorum* plate, R.10, published on 20 February 1808 (No.103), he condensed and simplified the composition and called it 'Ships in a Breeze'.

73 Jason R.A.1802

Oil on canvas, 35¼ × 47⅛ (89.5 × 119.5)
Exh: R.A. 1802 (519); British Institution 1808 (South Room 394); Plymouth 1815
Tate Gallery (471)

The title was given in the 1808 British Institution catalogue as 'Jason, from Ovid's Metamorphosis': Jason is shown slaying the dragon that guarded the Golden Fleece. Gage suggests (1969, pp.137–9) that the subject of this picture was chosen following P. J. de Loutherbourg's rare precedent because of its alchemical associations, but Turner's omission of the Fleece suggests that once again his choice was motivated by a desire to paint an essay in the manner of an admired Old Master, in this case Salvator Rosa. However, unlike the Rosa-like figures in 'Dolbadern Castle', the figure here plays a leading role for the first time in Turner's work. For a possible sketch see No.92.

The subject was engraved for the *Liber Studiorum*, R.6 (No.100). This plate was published in Part I on 11 June 1807 and was labelled 'H' for Historical.

74 Chateaux de St. Michael, Bonneville, Savoy R.A.1803

Oil on canvas, 36 × 48 (91.5 × 122)
Exh: R.A. 1803 (237); ?Turner's gallery 1804
Messrs Thos. Agnew & Sons Ltd

Turner exhibited two paintings of Bonneville at the R.A. in 1803, following his visit to Savoy in 1802. The other was entitled 'Bonneville. Savoy, with Mont Blanc' and was last shown at Agnew's 1967 Turner exhibition (4, repr.). A third picture, very close to the second, was exhibited at the R.A. in 1812 as 'A View of the Castle of St. Michael, near Bonneville, Savoy' and is now in the Johnson Collection, Philadelphia Museum.

Evelyn Joll, in the pamphlet accompanying the exhibition of this picture at Agnew's in July 1974, has discussed the related drawings and watercolours. There is a slight pencil sketch of the hills in the background (T.B.LXXIII–46ᵛ; repr. *loc. cit.*, pl.1), and a watercolour sketch (T.B.LXXX–H; repr. *loc. cit.*, pl.2, and, in colour, Wilkinson 1974, p.55), and two finished watercolours, both probably later than the oil, the first in the Courtauld Institute Galleries (repr. *loc. cit.*, pl.4), the other, dated 1817, formerly in the collection of Miss Julia Swinburne.

According to Farington, Lawrence observed to him on 4 May 1803, 'that in Turner's pictures there are his usual faults, but greater beauties'. This picture 'He thought remarkably fine'. It, rather than its companion, was almost certainly the work bought in 1804 by Samuel Dobree (1759–1827), perhaps from Turner's gallery. On 30 June 1804 Turner wrote to Dobree, 'and may I ask once more "am I to put out the cloud in the Picture of Bonneville?" If you can drop me a line decide[d]ly yes or no this Evening or tomorrow morning it shall be as you wish'. Evidently Turner's letter did not reach Dobree in time for him to reply as a second letter from Turner states that he has not yet heard from Dobree. Therefore the cloud was presumably left 'in' and it is certainly much more prominent in this picture than in the other picture of Bonneville (see Hilda F. Finberg 'Turner to Mr. Dobree', *Burlington Magazine*, XCV, 1953, pp.98–9). It subsequently belonged to William Young Ottley (d.1836) and the Earl of Camperdown; its most recent private owner was Sir Stephen Courtauld.

Here a very Poussinesque treatment is applied to a straightforward landscape without historical or mythological pretentions. Progression into depth is measured out by both solid forms and bands of light placed parallel to the surface of the picture, and the colours have a sharpness and clarity attuned to this classical composition. Evelyn Joll has demonstrated a particularly close relationship in general principles to Poussin's 'Landscape with a Roman Road' at Dulwich (repr. *loc. cit.*, pl.3). This passed through the London salerooms in 1802.

70

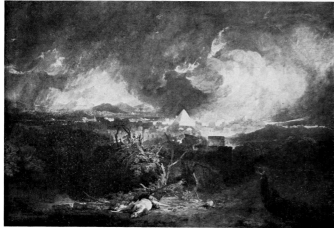

72

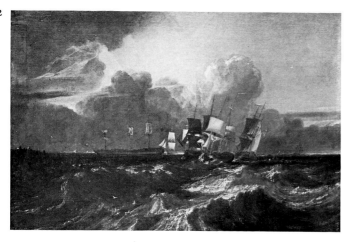

75

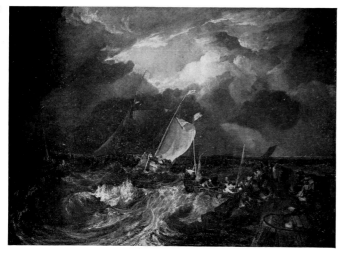

**75   Calais Pier, with French Poissards
preparing for Sea: an English Packet
arriving** R.A.1803
Oil on canvas, 68 × 95⅜ (172.5 × 242)
Exh: R.A. 1803 (146)
Trustees of the National Gallery, London (472)

In this picture Turner elevated a genre scene, coupled
with his own experiences on visiting France in 1802, to
an unprecedented scale, claiming for it equal rank with
the Biblical Plagues and great marines of this and the
previous two years. The personal experiences are en-
shrined in the 'Calais Pier' sketchbook which includes
several drawings with such inscriptions as 'Our Landing at Calais. Nearly swampt' and 'Our Situation at
Calais Bar' (T.B.LXXXI–58ᵛ and 59, 70, 71, 74ᵛ and 75,
76ᵛ and 77, 78ᵛ and 79). Despite its title, however, the
sketchbook only seems to contain one sketch directly
related to this picture, for the light-sailed boat in the
middle distance (LXXXI–151; cf. also 146–50).

The title in the 1803 exhibition catalogue is typically
slap-dash, Turner having made up the pseudo-French
word 'Poissards' from 'poissarde', which can mean a
fish-wife. Farington, whose sycophancy and reverence
for the accepted opinions of the old guard seems to have
led him to take considerable delight in recording negative opinions on Turner's work, records examples of
qualified praise from Benjamin West, Fuseli and Sir
George Beaumont. As usual it was the lack of finish in
the foreground that was criticised, even by so careless a
technician as Fuseli, who 'commended' the picture,
holding that it 'shewed great power of mind', but that
perhaps the foreground was 'too little attended to, – too
undefined'. John Britton in the *British Press* was readier
with praise, but criticised the opacity of the clouds,
certainly not a criticism that one could make of
Turner's later works.

Farington also recorded that 'Lord Gower asked the
price of the "Calais Harbour", & Turner signified that
it must be more than that for which He sold a picture
to the Duke of Bridgewater (*250 guineas*)' (see No.71).
The painting remained in Turner's possession and was
engraved much later, in 1827, by Thomas Lupton as a
companion to the print of 'The Shipwreck' but was left
unfinished as Turner insisted, on account of the change
in scale, on enlarging and adding to the boats.

**76   The Festival upon the Opening of the
Vintage at Macon** R.A.1803
Oil on canvas, 57½ × 93½ (146 × 237.5)
Exh: R.A. 1803 (110); ?Turner's Gallery 1804;
Old Masters, British Institution 1849 (43); Royal
Scottish Academy 1851 (158)
Sheffield City Art Galleries

Like 'Bonneville' and 'Calais Pier' this was based on
Turner's visit to France in 1802 but, typically of this
moment in his career, the composition is blown up into
an essay in the manner of Claude, the first of a long
series of panoramic landscapes that continue through
most of his life (e.g. Nos.237 and 486). The composition was developed in the 'Calais Pier' sketchbook (T.B.
LXXXI–54, 116–17, the last two pages, a single composition, repr. Wilkinson 1974, p.60).

William Seguier told Burnet (John Burnet, *Turner
and his Works*, 1852, pp.78–9) that Turner had begun
the picture 'with size colour on an unprimed canvas'

and that 'when first painted it appeared of the most vivid greens and yellows'. This vividness obviously shocked Sir George Beaumont who complained to Farington that 'the subject is borrowed from Claude but the colouring forgotten'.

On the other hand the critic of the *British Press* for 3 May 1803 praised the picture in a review that gives a good insight into how high Turner's reputation stood in some quarters. 'The productions of Mr. Turner's pencil are of that extraordinary kind, that they must inevitably call forth considerable praise or blame. . . . The effulgence of great genius is not to be looked at by mechanical eyes, nor are her sparks to be analized by simple processes. Mr. Turner has evidently derived improvement from his continental tour, and with wonderful labour and facility has produced four paintings and two drawings since his return in last October. A view of the French galleries has stimulated his native energy, and the scenery of Switzerland and Savoy has furnished sublime features for his powers and pencil [see No.65]. For truth of conception, and richness of execution, Mr Turner ranks with a Reynolds and a Wilson. . . .' This picture was described as 'without comparison; the first landscape of the kind that has been executed since the time of Claude Lorrain, on whose works, indeed, Mr. Turner has evidently and usefully fixed his eye; and we are bold to say, that he has even surpassed that master in the richness and forms of some parts of his pictures. The scene is singularly fine, and the figures, which are many, are drawn and grouped in a style far superior to any of this Artist's former productions. But perhaps the blues are rather too powerful in the distance. . .'.

The picture was the subject of another of the many incidents revealing Turner's tough attitude over prices. Sir John Leicester, a leading patron of the time, offered 250 guineas during the R.A. exhibition but for some reason the deal fell through. The following year he offered 300 guineas, but Turner now demanded 400, which Leicester refused; the price was, however, paid by Lord Yarborough. These transactions, recorded by Farington in May 1804, suggest that the picture was then on view in Turner's own gallery, newly opened at his own house at the corner of Harley Street and Queen Ann Street.

When Lord Yarborough's son lent the picture to the British Institution in 1849 the *Spectator* for 16 June saw it as having been a foretaste of things to come: 'yet even here the painter is beginning to aim at impossibility, and the centre of the sky ferments with an unsuccessful effort to dash at the brightness of the sun.'

77 **Holy Family** R.A.1803
Oil on canvas, 40¼ × 55¾ (102 × 141.5)
Exh: R.A. 1803 (156)
Tate Gallery (473)

78 **Venus and Adonis** c.1803
Oil on canvas, 59 × 47 (150 × 119.5)
Exh: R.A. 1849 (206)
Christopher Gibbs Ltd

Whereas 'Jason' shows Turner setting out to paint a picture in the manner of Salvator Rosa, these two paintings show him at his most Titianesque. The 'Holy Family' may have been inspired in general terms by Titian's 'Holy Family and a Shepherd', sold with the

W. Y. Ottley collection in London in January 1801 and now in the National Gallery (see Cecil Gould, *National Gallery Catalogues: The Sixteenth Century Venetian School*, 1959, pp.97–8), while 'Venus and Adonis' owes a still closer debt to Titian's now destroyed 'St. Peter Martyr' altarpiece. This painting from SS. Giovanni e Paolo in Venice (where Turner was later, in 1819, to copy a detail of the foreground foliage and the Martyr's leg) had been looted by Napoleon and was seen by Turner in the Louvre during his visit in 1802; his notes on the picture cover three pages of the 'Studies in the Louvre' sketchbook (T.B.LXXII–28ᵛ, 28 and 27ᵛ). Well-known in England already through engravings, Turner eulogised it in his 1811 lecture as Professor of Perspective at the R.A.: 'the highest honour that landscape has as yet, she received from the hand of Titian; . . . the triumph of Landscape may be safely said to exist in his divine picture of St. Peter Martyr' (see Jerold Ziff '"Backgrounds, Introduction of Architecture and Landscape": A Lecture by J. M. W. Turner', in *Journal of the Warburg and Courtauld Institutes*, XXVI, 1963, p.135).

Turner's work on the two pictures was indeed connected. A drawing in the 'Calais Pier' sketchbook shows the Holy Family in the setting, complete with flying putti above, of the Titian 'Peter Martyr' (T.B.LXXXI–63, repr. with both the Turners under discussion and Martino Rota's engraving after the Titian, by Gage 1969, pls.61–4; see also LXXXI–62). However, Turner decided on an oblong format, close even in size to the Ottley Titian, apparently following another drawing in the 'Calais Pier' sketchbook (T.B.LXXXI–60; there are further related drawings on LXXXI–44 and 47). The 'St. Peter Martyr' setting he then used for 'Venus and Adonis', dateable for stylistic reasons to c.1803–5.

The serpent that slides away on the right of the 'Holy Family' is presumably a traditional allusion to the Redeemer striking the serpent's head, though Gage also finds a connection with the confrontation of 'Apollo and the Python' (Tate Gallery 488, exhibited by Turner at the Academy in 1811 (81) but almost certainly painted c.1803–5, there also being sketches for this composition in the 'Calais Pier' sketchbook) and the nature symbolism of Jacob Boehme (*op. cit.*, pp.139–40).

The 'Holy Family' was not well received in the press. *The True Briton* for 6 May, attacking the figures, concluded that 'unless the artist can produce something better, we advise him to take an eternal farewell of History', and the *British Press*, for 9 May, while noting 'a bold and daring effort', agreed with 'a man of great taste, that Mr. Turner has . . . spoilt a fine landscape by very bad figures'.

'Venus and Adonis' was not exhibited by Turner until in 1849 he borrowed it back from its then owner, his friend and patron H. A. J. Munro of Novar, together with the 'Wreck Buoy' (now in the Walker Art Gallery, Liverpool) for his contribution to that year's exhibition. Unlike 'The Wreck Buoy' which was completely repainted, 'Venus and Adonis' was left in its early state. It had earlier belonged to John Green, 'the well-known amateur of Blackheath', before being bought in 1830 by Munro at Christie's for 83 guineas, the price apparently having been bid up by a 'ruddy-cheeked butcher's boy' acting for Turner.

When 'Venus and Adonis' was exhibited in 1849 the *Art Union* for June 1849 described it as 'A work that will bear comparison with the best of its class that ever emanated from the Venetian school'. 'Who would say that this picture was executed by the same hand, as, for instance, the other in the exhibition [the completely re-painted 'Wreck Buoy'] or even those all-beautiful Venetian subjects'. The *Athenaeum*, 12 May, spoke of the 'mythological theme, which, having been painted by Titian and sung by Shakespeare, has lost none of its beauty on Mr. Turner's canvas. It is full of fancy and of feeling'. The *Spectator* for 12 May, on the other hand, called it 'a strange work by Mr. Turner who does not wish us to forget that he can't paint the human form.'

79 Boats carrying out Anchors and Cables to Dutch Men of War in 1665 R.A.1804
Oil on canvas, 40 × 51½ (101.5 × 130.5)
Exh: R.A. 1804 (183)
Corcoran Gallery of Art, Washington, D.C.

According to Farington Turner painted most of this picture in one of the Keeper's rooms at the R.A., probably because his own studio was still occupied by builders. During the exhibition Farington reported that Turner was concerned about his seapiece being hung under the white drapery of Copley's portrait of 'Mrs Derby as St. Cecilia'. However, Turner sold the picture to Samuel Dobree and actually arranged for it to be delivered to Dobree on 2 July 1804. This is recorded in a letter from Turner to Dobree published by Hilda Finberg ('"Turner to Mr. Dobree": Two unrecorded letters' in *Burlington Magazine* XCV, 1953, pp.98–9) although the price seems not to have been agreed upon before the picture was sent. Hilda Finberg suggests that criticisms of the picture during the exhibition may have encouraged Dobree to try to get a reduction. The date of delivery means that Turner must have removed the picture before the end of the exhibition, which may have been one cause of his disagreement with the Council that year (see No.81; the exhibition opened on 30 April and ran for approximately three months.)

On the whole, the picture was not favourably received at the Academy although the *Star* and the *Monthly Mirror* both had something to say in its favour. The *St. James's Chronicle* (12–15 May) called it 'a fine sea-scape' but added 'but the sailors in the boats are all bald, and like Chinese'. *The Sun* (10 May) also had some harsh things to say: 'Why the scene before us should be placed so far back as in 1665, it is difficult to conceive, except by referring to that affectation which almost invariably appears in the work of the Artist. There is nothing in the subject to excite an interest. The figures are very indifferently formed, and the *Sea* seems to have been painted with *birch-broom* and *whitening*.'

Farington records that Opie said the water in Turner's seapiece looked like a 'Turnpike Road' over the sea. Northcote said he should have supposed Turner had never seen the sea.

It seems likely that Turner made a mistake in the date in his title and that the scene he portrayed refers to the end of 'The Four Days' Battle' of 1–4 June 1666. On this occasion the British fleet came upon the Dutch fleet at anchor seven leagues from Ostend. Admiral de Ruyter's Journal records, 'We saw the English fleet, about 70 sail in strength bearing down upon us. Owing to the heavy seas we could not weigh our anchors. At noon we all had to cut our cables, some losing a cable and a half, and some two whole ones. . . .'

80 Windsor Castle from the Thames *c*.1804–5
Oil on canvas, 35 × 47 (89 × 119.5)
Inscr. bottom right: 'J M W Turner RA Isleworth'
H.M. Treasury and the National Trust, from Petworth House (4)

In style and treatment this landscape is close both to the Bonneville pictures exhibited in 1803 (see No.74) and to 'The Goddess of Discord choosing the Apple of Contention in the Garden of the Hesperides' shown at the British Institution in 1806 (Tate Gallery 477), particularly the former. It is based on a watercolour sketch in the 'Studies for Pictures: Isleworth' sketchbook (T.B.XC–29ᵛ, repr. Reynolds 1969, pl.50, and, in colour, Wilkinson 1974, p.108; see No.94), which has Turner's name and Isleworth address inside the front cover: 'J. M. W. Turner, Sion Ferry House, Isleworth'. Turner used this address in a letter to Colt Hoare of 23 November 1805 and other notes inside the front cover of the sketchbook are dated 1804, so Turner may have had a *pied-à-terre* on the Thames in what was then outside London as early as 1804. Very little is known of what works Turner exhibited in his own gallery in the first two years it was open, 1804 and 1805, and it is quite likely that this could have been included.

This is the first of a large number of pictures showing places in and around Windsor (see Nos.139 and 156) but is distinguished from later examples by the way in which the vagaries of the site are submitted to the strict discipline of a classical landscape composition.

81 The Deluge *c*.1804–5
Oil on canvas, 56¼ × 92¾ (143 × 235)
Exh: ?Turner's Gallery 1805; R.A. 1813 (213)
Tate Gallery (493)

A note in the *British Press* for 8 May 1804 stated that 'Mr. Turner is engaged upon a very large picture of the Deluge, which he intends for the exhibition next year'. By 'the exhibition' is probably meant that at the Royal Academy, but, apparently owing to some dispute in the Academy Council, Turner told Farington on 21 February 1805 that he would 'not exhibit at the Royal Academy but at his own House'. It is likely therefore that 'The Deluge', like 'The Shipwreck', was on view in Turner's own gallery from early May to the beginning of July 1805.

When exhibited again at the Academy in 1813, the same year as 'Frosty Morning' (No.161), it must have looked rather strange, but the *Morning Chronicle* praised it as 'a good composition, and treated with that severity of manner which was demanded by the awfulness of the subject'. The catalogue contained the following lines from Milton's *Paradise Lost*:

Meanwhile the south wind rose, and with black wings
Wide hovering, all the clouds together drove
From under heaven————
————the thicken'd sky
Like a dark cieling [*sic*] stood, down rush'd the rain

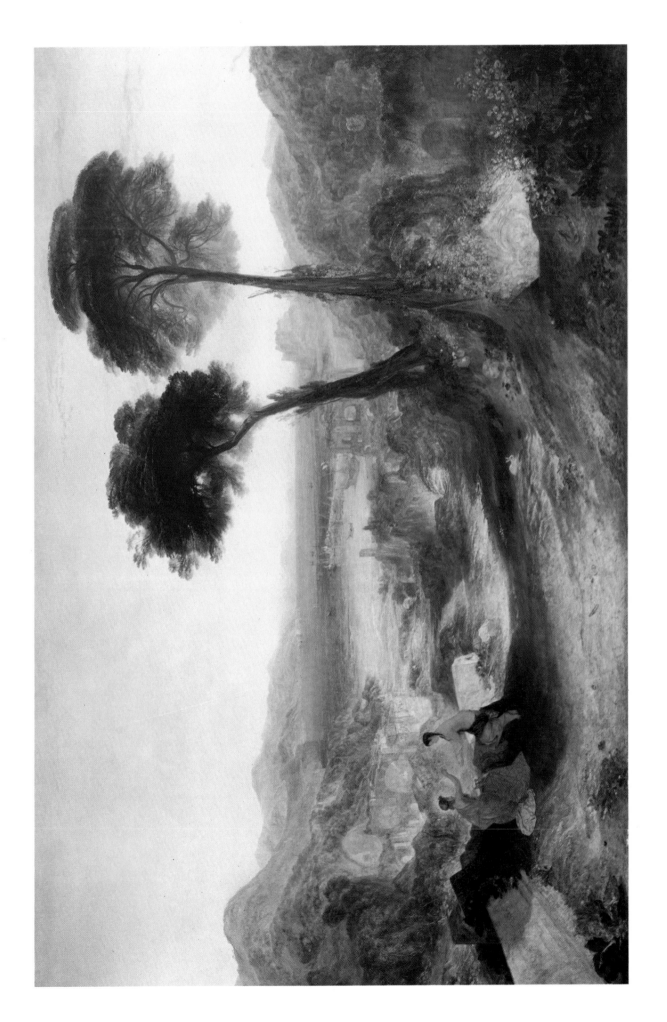

237 **The Bay of Baiæ, with Apollo and the Sibyl** 1823 (entry on p.92)

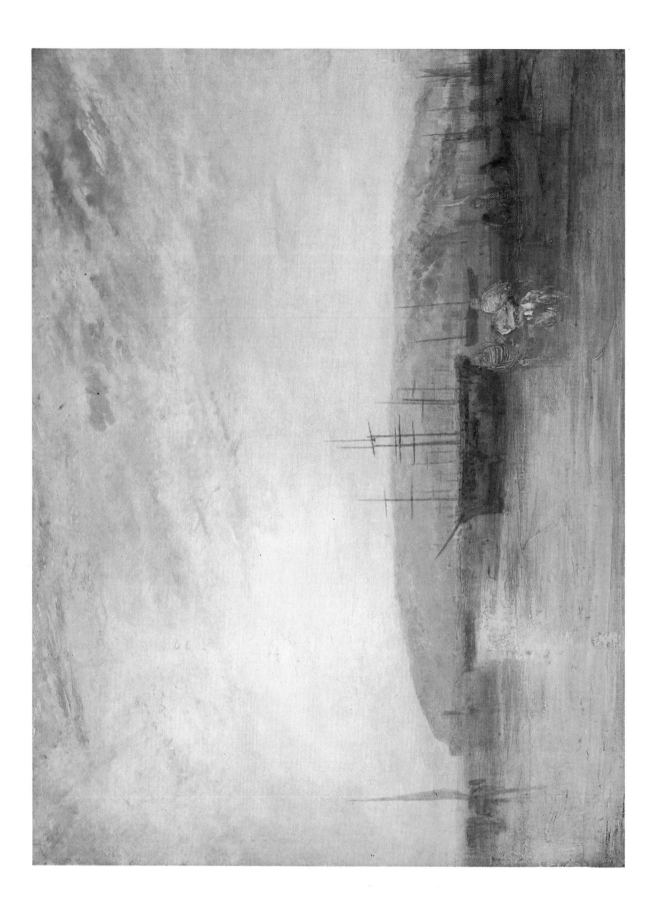

317 **Shipping off East Cowes Headland** 1827 (entry on p. 103)

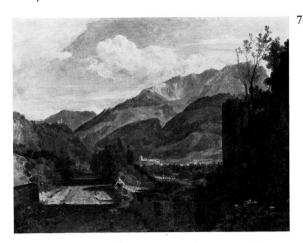

74

Impetuous, and continual, till the earth
No more was seen.

As in the case of his Plague pictures Turner may have
been spurred on by the example of Poussin, whose own
picture of the subject he had studied closely in the
Louvre in 1802 (for his notes see the 'Studies in the
Louvre' sketchbook, T.B.LXXII–41ᵛ, 42). But Turner's
main inspiration, particularly in the vivid colouring of
the figures on the right, came from Titian and Veronese.

The drawing inscribed 'Study for the Deluge' in the
'Calais Pier' sketchbook shows an alternative composition, and that inscribed as for the 'Whirlwind' is also
related (T.B.LXXXI–120, 121, 163). The group of a
negro supporting a girl on the right is close to a figure
study in the 'Studies for Pictures' sketchbook of c.1800–
2 (T.B.LXIX–66). The composition was subsequently
engraved by J. P. Quilley in 1828, perhaps significantly
only two years after John Martin exhibited the first of
his two large pictures of the subject, and again with
considerable alterations for the *Liber Studiorum* (R.88)
but never published.

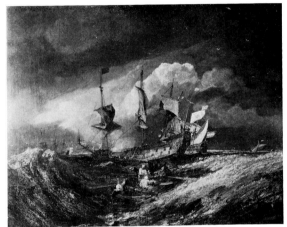

79

82   The Shipwreck Turner's gallery 1805
Oil on canvas, 67⅛×95⅛ (170.5×241.5)
Exh: Turner's gallery 1805
Tate Gallery (476)

This picture was bought at the opening of the exhibition in Turner's gallery by Sir John Leicester for
300 guineas, but the following year it was exchanged
for 'Fall of the Rhine at Schaffhausen' (R.A. 1806;
now at Boston), Turner receiving an additional 50
guineas. There are again drawings for the composition in the 'Calais Pier' sketchbook (T.B.LXXXI–2,
6, 132–3, 136–7 (repr. Wilkinson 1974, p.61), 140–1)
and slighter sketches, probably from actual wrecks,
in the 'Shipwreck No.1' sketchbook (T.B.LXXXVII–11,
16, repr. Kitson 1964, p.41 and Reynolds 1969, pl.41
respectively, as well as other sketches related in more
general terms; see No.93 and the examples repr. Wilkinson 1974, pp.66–7). This was the first of Turner's oil
paintings to be engraved, by Charles Turner in 1806
(No.B101).

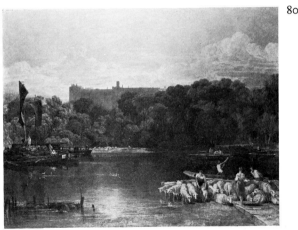

80

The composition, as compared with the 'Bridgewater Sea Piece' and 'Calais Pier', shows the rapid
advance of Turner's powers. The drama of the action
is at one with the composition, Turner's favourite
lozenge-shape transformed out of all recognition from
its first appearance in the 'Cholmeley Sea Piece'. The
jagged shape of the sail replaces the more artificial rent
in the clouds of 'Calais Pier' to add to the agony of the
scene.

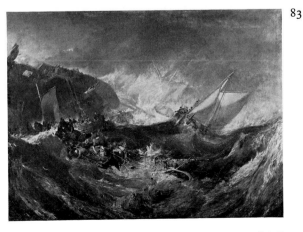

83

83   The Wreck of a Transport Ship *c.*1805–10
Oil on canvas, 68×95 (173×241)
Exh: *Old Masters*, British Institution, 1849 (38);
Royal Scottish Academy, 1851 (306)
Fundaçao Calouste Gulbenkian, Lisbon

Exhibited in 1851 as 'The Wreck of the Minotaur,
Seventy-four, on the Haack Sands, 22nd December
1810' with the note that it was 'Painted in 1811–12 for
the father of the Earl of Yarborough', the lender; in
1849 it was catalogued with the title given above, followed by 'purchased by the Father of the Earl of
Yarborough'. In May 1810 the Hon. Charles Pelham,
later 1st Earl of Yarborough, paid Turner approxi-

mately £300 for an unspecified picture. If this was this work it cannot show the wreck of the *Minotaur* which took place later in the year. However, although the price is less than the 400 guineas paid in 1804 by Pelham's father for 'The Festival upon the Opening of the Vintage at Macon', a picture of the same size (see No.76), there is no other candidate for the Pelham picture.

Turner used at least two of the studies in the 'Shipwreck No.1' sketchbook for this picture (T.B.LXXXVII–8, 23, the second repr. Wilkinson 1974, p.66). The sketchbook contains a list of subscribers to the 'Shipwreck' engraving of 1806 (see No.B101) which also suggests that this new painting grew out of the old rather than being inspired by the actual incident of December 1810.

The composition of the picture represents a further advance beyond that of 'The Shipwreck' in the way the whole picture conveys the tumult of the catastrophe. The elements of the composition are arranged in much the same lozenge-like shape, but they flow into each other and are given energy by a much looser handling of the paint, foreshadowing the all-engulfing vortex of 'Hannibal crossing the Alps' (see No.88).

When the picture was exhibited in 1849 the *Spectator* for 16 June saw it as already showing signs of decline by the side of 'Macon' (No.76): 'By the next generation ... Turner had grown more audacious, and had correspondingly lost power: the forms are looser, *all* are fermenting and dissolving – a partial foretaste of that dissolution which now decomposes all Turner's works even before they reach the canvas.' On the other hand, the *Athenaeum* for the same date was full of praise: 'For the credit of England and of Mr. Turner let it be said that the picture of most excellence and interest in this assemblage [of Old Masters] is from his hand ... We have no recollection of any production in its class – whether of the Dutch, the Italian, or the French school – which surpasses – or even equals – this artist's *Shipwreck*.' It showed 'a grasp of mind and a command of hand that have exhibited in a high moral sense the excitement and action of the tempest in its wrath.'

84 The Battle of Trafalgar, as seen from the Mizen Starboard Shrouds of the Victory
Turner's Gallery 1806
Oil on canvas, 67¼ × 94 (171 × 239)
Exh: Turner's gallery 1806; British Institution 1808 (South Room 359)
Tate Gallery (480)

The Battle of Trafalgar took place on 31 October 1805 and the *Victory*, bearing Nelson's body, anchored off Sheerness on 22 December. Turner made a special trip to sketch the *Victory* as she entered the Medway and subsequently made a large number of detailed studies on board the ship in the 'Nelson' sketchbook (T.B.LXXXIX; see Nos. 95–7 and Wilkinson 1974, pp. 68–9). Another result of all this activity was the smaller oil painting of 'The "Victory" beating up the Channel on its return from Trafalgar', probably shown in Turner's gallery the same year, subsequently in the Fawkes collection at Farnley Hall and now in the Mellon collection; here, however, he used his memories of the Needles (see No.19) for the background. Such journalist-like expeditions to sketch matters

of topical interest were common in Turner's career: he went specially to Portsmouth in 1807 before painting 'Two of the Danish Ships which were seized at Copenhagen entering Portsmouth Harbour', exhibited unfinished at his gallery in 1808 (Tate Gallery 481), to the Low Countries in 1817 for 'The Field of Waterloo' exhibited at the R.A. in 1818 (Tate Gallery 500), to Edinburgh in 1822 to cover George IV's state visit (see No.308), and again down the Thames Estuary in 1838 before painting 'The Fighting Temeraire' (National Gallery, London, 524).

Perhaps because he had been so keen to show the picture as soon as possible after the event Turner seems to have felt the need to work on it further before exhibiting it again in 1808. According to the writer, probably John Landseer, of a long review in *The Review of Publications of Art* for 1808, 'The picture appears more powerful both in respect of chiaro-scuro and colour than when we formerly saw it in Mr. Turner's gallery, and has evidently been since revised and very much improved by the author'. Describing the picture as 'a *British epic picture*' the writer called it 'the *first* picture of the kind that has ever, to our knowledge, been exhibited'. 'Mr Turner ... has detailed the death of *his* hero, while he has suggested the whole of a great naval victory, which we believe has never before been successfully accomplished, if it has been before attempted, in a *single* picture.' In fact there were precedents for the joint portrayal of a heroic death and a continuing battle in Benjamin West's 'Death of Wolfe' of 1771 and John Singleton Copley's 'Death of Major Peirson' of 1783 (Tate Gallery).

In this painting Turner broke away completely from the seventeenth- and eighteenth-century conventions of painting battles at sea. The only precedent for this close-up concentration on the details of the battle seems to have been John Singleton Copley's 'Siege of Gibraltar' of 1783 (Guildhall Art Gallery; a reduced-size replica in the Tate Gallery). The treatment however owes more to P. J. de Loutherbourg, in such works as his 'Battle of the Nile' of 1800 (Tate Gallery). The disappearance of Turner's own 'Battle of the Nile', exhibited in 1799, is all the more maddening in that it might have shown how early Turner displayed his own personality in this genre.

85 A Subject from the Runic Superstitions (?); Reworking of 'Rizpah watching the Bodies of her Sons' *c.*1808
Oil on canvas, 36¼ × 48 (91.5 × 122)
Exh: ? Turner's gallery 1808 (see below)
Tate Gallery (464)

This picture seems originally to have shown 'Rizpah watching the Bodies of her Sons' (2 *Samuel* XXI, 9–10) and was engraved as this subject for the *Liber Studiorum*, R.46 and published 23 April 1812 (No.86). In the engraving Rizpah is shown protecting the bodies of her two sons by Saul from predatory birds and beasts 'in the days of the harvest, in the first days, in the beginning of the barley harvest'.

Subsequent to the preparation of the *Liber Studiorum* engraving, which could have been at least begun any time after the scheme was first mooted in 1806, Turner seems to have overpainted the oil painting, replacing the bodies of Rizpah's sons by enormous insects dragging off the bodies of other creatures, adding another female figure behind that of Rizpah, and introducing several spectral figures and a mysteriously glowing light. The subject now seems to be a scene of incantation, possibly suggested by the encounter of Saul and the Witch of Endor during which the ghost of Samuel foretells the death of Saul and his sons (1 *Samuel* XXVII, 8–20). However, though one of the apparitions could well be Samuel, 'covered with a mantle', and the others are a soldier about to slay with a sword a child held by another, the putative Saul is a woman with bare breasts.

What was almost certainly this picture was shown at Turner's gallery in 1808 when it was described in *The Review of Publications of Art*. The reviewer, probably John Landseer, was obviously baffled by the subject which had presumably already been altered by Turner:

> Of an unfinished picture which hangs at the upper end of the room, the subject of which is taken from the Runic superstitions, and where the artist has conjured up mysterious spectres and chimeras dire, we forbear to speak at present.

The suggested title was not necessarily Turner's.

Robert DUNKARTON (1744–?) and TURNER

86   Rispah 1812
Etching and mezzotint, third published state, $7\frac{1}{8} \times 10\frac{3}{8}$ (18.1 × 26.3); plate $8\frac{1}{4} \times 11\frac{1}{2}$ (21 × 29.2)
Inscr: 'H' (for Historical) above, and with title and '2nd Book of Samuel. Chap.21.', 'Published April 23. 1812, by I. M. W. Turner, Queen Ann Street West', 'Drawn & Etched by I. M. W. Turner Esqr. R.A.', and 'Engraved by R. Dunkarton' below
Royal Academy of Arts

The drawing is with the Turner Bequest (Vaughan Bequest), CXVII–U. The print, R.46, was published in Part IX of the *Liber Studiorum* with the title spelt as above.

Although not published until 1812 this shows the original subject that seems to underlie the oil painting 'Subject from the Runic Superstitions' (No.85).

87   The Fall of an Avalanche in the Grisons
Turner's gallery 1810
Oil on canvas, $35\frac{1}{2} \times 67\frac{1}{4}$ (90 × 120)
Exh: Turner's gallery 1810 (14)
Tate Gallery (489)

Exhibited with the following lines, which anticipate those attributed by Turner to his *Fallacies of Hope*, first quoted in connection with 'Hannibal crossing the Alps':

> The downward sun a parting sadness gleams,
> Portenteous lurid thro' the gathering storm;
> Thick drifting snow, on snow,
> Till the vast weight bursts thro' the rocky barrier;
> Down at once, its pine clad forests,
> And towering glaciers fall, the work of ages
> Crashing through all! extinction follows,
> And the toil, the hope of man – o'erwhelms.

As Jack Lindsay has pointed out (1966, p.107) these verses and the reference to the Grisons recall a passage from 'Winter', one of Thomson's *Seasons*, and Turner was probably also inspired by two paintings of avalanches by de Loutherbourg in the collections of his

patrons, one, of *c*.1800, in the collection of Lord Egremont (still at Petworth; repr. illustrated souvenir *The First Hundred Years of the Royal Academy*, Royal Academy 1951–2, p.53), the other, dated 1803, exhibited at the Royal Academy in 1804 and sold to Sir John Leicester in 1805 (now Tate Gallery; see *The Tate Gallery Report 1965–66*, pp.19–20, repr.). However, as Ruskin noted in his *Notes on the Turner Gallery at Marlborough House* 1856, 'No one ever before had conceived a stone in flight'; de Loutherbourg's pictures and the verses of Thomson deal only with the power of falling snow. The crucial forms in the picture coincide with the main lines of the composition and the picture is given extra force by the extreme boldness of Turner's use of the palette knife. A contemporary review of Turner's gallery in *The Sun* for 12 June 1810 noted that the picture 'is not in his usual style, but is not less excellent'.

88   Snow Storm: Hannibal and his Army crossing the Alps R.A.1812
Oil on canvas, 57 × 93 (145 × 236.5)
Exh: R.A. 1812 (258)
Tate Gallery (490)

Turner's verses in the 1812 catalogue are described for the first time as coming from his 'MS. P[oem?] Fallacies of Hope', the source of most of his later quotations though almost certainly never a complete entity; Turner was content, as so often in his choice of subjects, to evoke the sonorous appeal of some epic event rather than bother himself with slavish accuracy of documentation.

> Craft, treachery, and fraud – Salassian force,
> Hung on the fainting rear! then Plunder seiz'd
> The victor and the captive, – Saguntum's spoil,
> Alike became their prey; still the chief advanc'd,
> Look'd on the sun with hope; – low, broad, and wan;
> While the fierce archer of the downward year
> Stains Italy's blanch'd barrier with storms.
> In vain each pass, ensanguin'd deep with dead,
> Or rocky fragments, wide destruction roll'd.
> Still on Campania's fertile plains – he thought,
> But the loud breeze sob'd, 'Capua's joys beware!'

Hannibal's crossing of the Alps in 218 B.C. was a common source of Romantic and proto-Romantic inspiration. Mrs Radcliffe's *The Mysteries of Udolpho*, 1794, describes the scene shown by Turner, who was also inspired by the lost oil painting by J. R. Cozens, which passed through the salerooms in 1802. This painting, however, showed the later, more hopeful moment when Hannibal showed his troops the fertile plains of Italy. Here Turner not only shows the hazards of the crossing but hinted at the enervating effect of Italian luxury: 'Capua's joys beware!'

The history of Carthage was to become a preoccupation of Turner's (see Nos.165 and 528). In this case John Gage has suggested that Turner saw a parallel between the struggle of Rome and Carthage and that between England and Napoleonic France (see exhibition catalogue, *La Peinture Romantique Anglaise et les Préraphaelites*, Petit Palais, Paris, 1972 No.262). On his visit to Paris in 1802 Turner had visited David's studio and seen his picture of *Napoleon on the St. Bernard Pass* in which Napoleon was shown as the modern Hannibal.

However, another source of inspiration for this

picture was a storm seen at his patron Walter Fawkes' house, Farnley Hall in Yorkshire, in 1810. According to Fawkes' son Turner even foresaw the use he would make of his sketch: '"There," said he, "Hawkey; in two years you will see this again, and call it Hannibal crossing the Alps."' There is a sketch for the foreground figures in the 'Calais Pier' sketchbook (T.B.LXXXI–38, 39) which suggests that Turner was thinking of the subject at least eight or so years earlier.

Farington, who was on the Hanging Committee of the Royal Academy in 1812, records Turner's concern over the hanging of this picture. It was first placed over a door in the Great Room and 'was thought was seen to great advantage'. But Turner objected and said that 'if this picture were not placed under the line He wd. rather have it back'. This was tried but 'it appeared to the greatest disadvantage' and was put back where it had been before. Turner persisted in his objection to its being hung high up and it was finally hung 'at the head of the *new room*'. After a second visit to make sure how it looked by daylight Turner finally 'approved of the situation of His large picture provided other members shd. have pictures near it'.

Turner's insistence that the picture should be hung low reveals his understanding of the novel effect of his vortex-like composition, which draws the spectator into its swirling depths. Here for the first time Turner's composition is based on an overriding circular force instead of the opposition of rectilinear, diagonal forces as in 'The Fall of an Avalanche'.

The picture was well received by the critics. For the *Examiner*, 7 June 1812, 'This is a performance that classes Mr. Turner in the highest rank of landscape painters, for it possesses a considerable portion of that main excellence of the sister Arts, Invention. . . . This picture delights the imagination by the impressive agency of a few uncommon and sublime subjects in material nature, and of terror in its display of the effects of moral evil.' The main body of the army is 'represented agreeably to that principle of the sublime which arises from obscurity' but 'An aspect of terrible splendour is displayed in the shining of the sun . . . A terrible magnificence is also seen in the widely circular sweep of snow whirling high in the air . . . In fine, the moral and physical elements are here in powerful unison blended by a most masterly hand, awakening emotions of awe and grandeur'. The critic of the *Repository of Arts, Literature, Commerce* for 12 June was 'almost led to describe it as the effect of magic, which this Prospero of the graphic arts can call into action, and give to airy nothing a substantial form . . . All that is terrible and grand is personified in the mysterious effect of the picture; and we cannot but admire the genius displayed in this extraordinary work'. According to the *St. James Chronicle* for 23–26 May the 'sun is painted with peculiar felicity, and the warm tinting from the great source of light struggling through the blackness of the storm, gives a fine relief to the subject, which is still further improved by the introduction of a corner of cloudless sky on the left'.

89 **'Calais Pier' Sketchbook** *c.*1800–5
Bound in marbled boards with leather spine and corners with two clasps
84 leaves of blue paper, all drawn on in pen and

brown ink and wash and black and white chalks, $17\frac{1}{8} \times 10\frac{3}{4}$ (43.6 × 26.7)
Trustees of the British Museum (T.B.LXXXI)

ff.106–7 **Study for the 'Bridgewater Sea Piece'**
Pen and brown ink and wash with some white chalk on blue paper
Inscr: 'Last Study of the Dutch Boats D of B'

The sketchbook is the only one of its size to be devoted entirely to the working out of the compositions of large-scale subject pictures and marines. The use of chalk and brown wash on blue paper indicates Turner's concern with the broadest problems of massing and pictorial organisation, though many of the designs are highly atmospheric as well. A number of large studies of nude figures in various positions probably relate specifically to historical pictures, rather than being routine Academic exercises as in the 'Academical' Sketchbook, T.B.XLIII (No.44). For example, the supine male nude on f.25 (the Inventory numbering is by pages, up to 170) relates to the 'Fifth Plague of Egypt' of 1800 (No.70). The pictures on which Turner was working principally in this book are:

'Shipwreck' (No.82), 'Jason' (No.73), 'Sun rising through Vapour', exh. R.A. 1807 (National Gallery, London, 479), 'The Parting of Venus and Adonis' (No.78), 'The Opening of the Vintage, Macon' (No. 76), 'Calais Pier' (No.75), 'The Egremont Sea Piece' (No.72), 'Fishermen on a lee Shore' exh. ?R.A. 1802 (Iveagh Bequest, Kenwood), 'The Deluge' (No.81), 'The Bridgewater Sea Piece' (No.71), 'The Holy Family – Rest on the Flight' (No.77).

The exhibited sketch is one of a series of preparatory drawings for 'Dutch Boats in a Gale: fishermen endeavouring to put their fish on board' commissioned by the Duke of Bridgewater, 1801, as a companion piece to a painting by Van de Velde (see No.71).

90 **'On a Lee Shore' Sketchbook No. 2** *c.*1801
No covers
8 leaves of white paper, prepared on both sides with a wash of grey, $4\frac{5}{8} \times 7\frac{1}{8}$ (11.6 × 18)
Watermarked: 1799
Inscr. on label on back: '103'
Trustees of the British Museum (T.B.LXVIII)

f.4ʳ **Fishermen hauling a Boat onto the Beach out of heavy Breakers**
Pen and brown ink and wash and scraping-out on white paper prepared with grey wash

One of two sketchbooks containing notes of fishing boats in surf, connected with the two paintings executed for Mr Dobree in 1802. Related sketches occur in the 'Dunbar' sketchbook (No.54).

91 **'Studies in the Louvre' Sketchbook** 1802
Bound in calf; one clasp
88 leaves of white paper prepared with a wash of grey, with two fly-leaves at each end, $5\frac{1}{16} \times 4\frac{3}{8}$ (12.9 × 11.2)
Watermarked: 1799
Inscr. Finberg records Turner's label on spine: '18 Studies in the Louvre'.
Trustees of the British Museum (T.B.LXXII)

f.31ᵛ **MS notes**
Pen
f.32ʳ **Copy of Titian's 'Entombment'**
Watercolour and scraping-out on white paper
prepared with a wash of grey

Contains MS notes on, and sketches from, paintings
seen by Turner in the Louvre on his way home from
Switzerland in September–October 1802. The works on
which he particularly concentrated were:
J. van Ruysdael; 'Landscape [?Coup de Soleil]', 'Sea
Port [?Une Tempête sur le bord des Digues de la
Hollande]'.
Titian; 'Alphonso di Ferrara and Laura de' Pianti
[Titian and his Mistress]', 'Christ crowned with
Thorns', 'The Entombment', 'Death of St Peter
Martyr'.
Poussin; 'Diogenes throwing away his Dish', 'Orpheus
and Eurydice', 'The Israelites gathering Manna in the
Wilderness', 'The Deluge'.
Caravaggio; 'St Jerome'.
Domenichino; 'Mars and Venus', 'Hercules and
Achelous'.
Guérin; 'Le Retour de Marcus Sextus'.
Rembrandt; 'The Good Samaritan', 'Susanna', 'The
Angel departing from Tobit'.
Rubens; 'Landscape with Rainbow'.
For a detailed account of the contents of this Sketch-
book, see Finberg 1961, pp.85–91.
The notes on f.31ᵛ refer to Titian's 'Entombment',
sketched opposite:
'This picture may be rank [ed] among the first of
Titian's pictures as to colour and pathos – of Effect
for by casting a brilliant light on the Holy Mother
and Martha the figures of Josephe and the Body
has the a [sic] Effect Sepulural [sic], the Expression
of Joseph is fine as to the care he is undertaking
but with out grandeur. The figure which is swathed
in striped drapery conveys the idea of silent distress,
the one in vermilion attention while the agony of
Mary and the solicitude of Martha to [?] prevent
her grief and View of the dead Body with her own
anguish by seeing are admirably described and on
the first view they appear'
here the page ends. Turner continues overleaf:
'but collateral figures yet the whole is dependent
upon them, they are the Breadth of and the
expression of the Picture . . .'

92 **'Rhine, Strassburg and Oxford' Sketchbook**
c.1802
Bound in striped boards
49 leaves, mostly drawn on one side only in
pencil, 6¹⁄₁₆ × 9½ (15.4 × 23.5)
Trustees of the British Museum (T.B.LXXVII)

ff.43ᵛ, 44ʳ **Two studies for Pictures**
Pencil

The book was used by Turner during his journey back
from Switzerland in 1802 and, at random unused
openings, at Oxford.
The study on f.43ᵛ is for 'Apollo and Python' (Tate
Gallery 488; see under Nos.77–8); that on f.44ʳ possibly
for 'Jason' (No.73) or, like that on f.45ʳ, for the 'Garden
of the Hesperides' (R.A. 1806; Tate Gallery 477).

93 **'Shipwreck' Sketchbook No. 1** *c*.1805
Marbled paper covers
30 leaves, the majority drawn on in pencil, pen
and brown ink and brown and grey wash,
4½ × 7¼ (11.6 × 18.5)
Watermarked: 1801
Inscr. on label on spine: '97 Shipwreck'; and on
front cover: 'Subscribers List'
Trustees of the British Museum (T.B.LXXXVII)

f.16 **A Shipwreck**
Pen and brown ink and blue-grey wash
f.17 **A sailing Boat in a Rough Sea**
Pencil, pen and brown ink

One of two books (the other is T.B.LXXXVIII) containing mainly pen and ink studies of a sinking ship, connected with the painting of 'The Shipwreck' shown at
Turner's gallery in 1805 (No.82).

94 **'Studies for Pictures: Isleworth' Sketchbo**
c.1804–6
Bound in calf, four clasps
80 leaves of white paper prepared with a wash of
grey, with two fly-leaves of white paper at each
end. The majority of sheets are drawn on in
pencil, pen and brown ink or watercolour, with a
little bodycolour, 10 × 5¾ (14.7 × 25.6)
Watermarked: 1794, 1799
Inscr. on label on spine: '37 Studies for Pictures
Isleworth'; and inside front cover: 'J. M. W.
Turner Sion Ferry House Isleworth'
Trustees of the British Museum (T.B.XC)

f.49ᵛ **Classical Composition**
Pen and ink and watercolour and bodycolour
with some scraping-out on white paper prepared
with a wash of grey
Inscr. top left: 'Jason: arrival at Colchis Ulysses
at Crusa'
f.50ʳ **Slight Sketch of Trees**
Pen and ink
Inscr: 'Females dancing and crowning the [?]
ropes with flowers or the foreground Figures
rejoicing the left – the Priests standing [?]
attending to receive the Fleece – Jason &
Argonauts on Board bearing the Fleece. Ulysses
with Orytus [?] . . . offering her to her Father'

The sketchbook contains a series of views on the
Thames, near Twickenham, Windsor and Weybridge.
A memorandum inside the front cover notes dates in
the summer of 1804; the sketchbook may have been in
use from that period. There is considerable homogen-
eity of style among the sketches, both in pen and in
watercolour; they have stylistic affinities with the
group of Thames watercolours of *c*.1806 (T.B.XCV;
Nos.114, 115). Some of the views identified by Finberg as Windsor, e.g. ff. 18, 19, 35 seem in fact to show
Richmond or Hampton Court.

95 **'Nelson' Sketchbook** *c*.1805
Marbled paper covers
32 leaves, almost all drawn on in pencil, 4½ × 7
(11.7 × 18.3)
Watermarked: 1804
Inscr. on label on spine: '105 Victory'

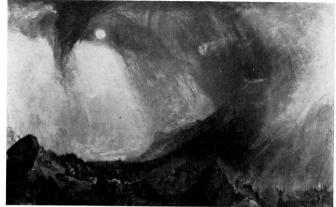

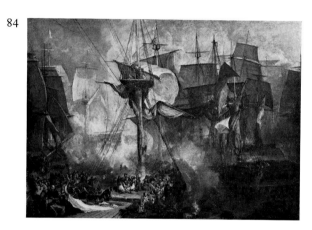

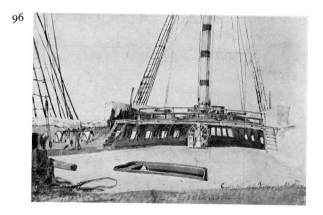

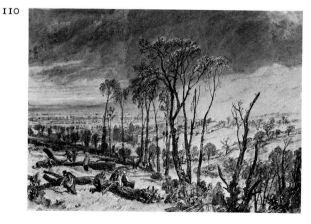

Trustees of the British Museum (T.B.LXXXIX)

f.28ᵛ The Bows of the 'Victory'
Pencil
f.29ʳ The Hull of the 'Victory'
Pencil

Turner seems to have visited the *Victory* almost as soon as she arrived off Sheerness with the body of Nelson, in December 1805. He made use of this small sketchbook and also of some larger, loose sheets of paper on which he made studies and notes of the ship from on board (Nos. 96, 97). The sketchbook contains several pencil studies of the flagship and other vessels, with notes of the uniforms of officers and men. This material was used for the picture of 'The Battle of Trafalgar' shown at Turner's gallery in 1806 (No.84).

96   Study of the Quarter-Deck of the 'Victory'
1805
Pencil, pen and brown ink and grey and brown wash with a little watercolour, $14\frac{15}{16} \times 21\frac{3}{4}$ (37.9 × 55.2)
Inscr. with various notes in pencil and pen, including: 'Quarter deck of the Victory.
J M W Turner'; 'Guns 12 lbers used in the ports mark i x'; 'Splinter hitting mark'd'; '9 Inch Mesh'; 'x Rail Shot away during the action'
Trustees of the British Museum (T.B.CXXI–S)
For the painting exhibited in 1806; see No.95. This drawing is said to have belonged to Dr Thomas Munro; it was also in the possession of Samuel Rogers, and, later, of Henry Vaughan, who bequeathed it to the British Museum where it is now placed with the Turner Bequest.

97   The 'Victory' from the Quarter-Deck 1805
Pencil, $18\frac{3}{8} \times 29\frac{11}{16}$ (46.7 × 75.4)
Trustees of the British Museum (T.B.CXX–c)
For the painting of the 'Battle of Trafalgar' exhibited in 1806 (No.84). See also the 'Nelson' sketchbook, No.95.

98   'Lowther' Sketchbook 1809–10
Bound in red morocco, one clasp
83 leaves, of which many have been wholly or partly cut or torn away, $3\frac{1}{4} \times 4\frac{1}{2}$ (8.3 × 11.5)
Watermarked: 1808
Trustees of the British Museum (T.B.CXIII)

f.40ᵛ Academy Study of a Female Nude
Pencil and watercolour

This book contains some pencil studies apparently of Lowther Castle, which Turner visited in the Autumn of 1809; f.26 has the word 'Lowther' written beside some sketches of Gothick details. There are also miscellaneous MS notes and some sketches connected with life on a canal. A series of Academy studies from a female model occurs spasmodically throughout the book.

A pencil study of the model in the same pose as in f.40ᵛ is on f.46ᵛ.

THE 'LIBER STUDIORUM'

The majority of Turner's grand series of compositions – the *Rivers* and *Ports of England*, for instance, or the *England and Wales* views – betray very little overall logic or comprehensive plan; they emerged casually, as it were, from the material by which Turner found himself inspired. The *Liber Studiorum* is very different. It was conceived from the first as a kind of visual treatise on landscape art, and is the central document of Turner the theorist of painting.

Its origins betray the academic purpose he had in mind: it imitates in its title and its medium (etched outline and mezzotint) the famous set of prints by Richard Earlom after the drawings in Claude's *Liber Veritatis*, published by Boydell in the 1770s (No.B28). Even Turner's careful drawings for the plates, for the most part in sepia or grey monochrome, evoke Claude's landscape studies. This historical allusion at once suggests that Turner was offering his own work in direct competition with that of Claude. But it had a more general purpose. Claude's *Liber Veritatis* was simply a convenient record made by the artist of all his own compositions, a kind of register of subjects. Turner, it is true, used many of his paintings as subjects for the *Liber Studiorum* plates; but he did not do so in order to record them – at least, not primarily for that purpose; they contribute to an overall plan, which was to illustrate with suitably designed examples the various 'branches' into which landscape painting could be divided. This scheme also demonstrated with great clarity the range and variety of Turner's powers, and was therefore an effective advertisement which would reach a far wider public than his paintings ever might.

The plates were issued in fourteen parts between 1807 and 1819, each part bearing the title: 'Liber Studiorum; Illustrative of Landscape Compositions, viz. Historical, Mountainous, Pastoral, Marine, and Architectural'; with the price, 1 guinea for prints, 2 guineas for proofs. Each part seems to have been intended to contain an example of each of the five branches of landscape, but in practice the pattern was somewhat erratic; Turner frequently uses 'E.P.' (probably standing for 'Epic' or 'Elegant Pastoral') as an additional category, at the expense of one of the others. It is, with 'Pastoral', the category which occurs most consistently; and, indeed, is the heading under which Turner's characteristic landscapes seem most naturally to place themselves. The branch in which he is least successful is the 'Pastoral', consisting mainly of rustic genre subjects which do not afford scope for dramatic invention, but of which Turner nevertheless was at pains to demonstrate his mastery (see No.B30).

All the parts contained five plates, and No.X, published 23 May 1812, included as an extra plate the frontispiece (No.99) to the whole series which thus comprised seventy-one plates in all. Twenty further designs were not published, though they were wholly or partly engraved, and a number of sketches in brown wash in the Turner Bequest are evidently related to Turner's plans for the work. The transfer of the outlines of the designs on to the plates was generally undertaken by Turner himself, who etched the majority, occasionally using soft-ground, before handing the plate over to the engraver. It seems that at one stage he had envisaged that the *Liber* would be executed in aquatint, and approached F. C. Lewis, who was engaged in making aquatint facsimiles of Claude's wash drawings; but the two men quarrelled and Turner decided to employ his namesake, Charles Turner, the engraver of his 'Shipwreck' in 1805 (No.B101), and to carry out his project in mezzotint.

Charles Turner was responsible for finishing all the plates in the first four parts: thereafter W. Say, R. Dunkarton, G. Clint, T. Lupton and others shared the work with him and with Turner himself, who contributed at least one plate to each of the parts from No.VI onwards. Among the later, unpublished plates are some by him in pure mezzotint, exploring a much richer tone than that commonly found in the earlier plates and anticipating the dramatic effects of the *Little Liber* (see p.95).

99 Frontispiece to the 'Liber Studiorum'
*c.*1811
Etched outline, brush and brown ink with scraping-out, 7⅜ × 10¼ (18.7 × 26.0)
Inscr. bottom right: 'H.V.' (initials of Henry Vaughan)
Trustees of the British Museum (T.B.CXVII–V)

One of numerous preparatory proofs of the etched outline for the plate, published in 1812 with part X of the *Liber* (R.I). Finberg (*Liber Studiorum*, 1924) describes the central design as drawn with pen and sepia: it is, in fact, etched in outline with brown wash added. The impression belonged to Henry Vaughan, who bequeathed it to the British Museum. For the published states mezzotint was added to Turner's etching by J. C. Easling.

Charles TURNER (1774–1857) and J. M. W. TURNER

100 Jason 1807
Etching and mezzotint, proof touched in pencil by the artist, 7¼ × 10¼ (18.3 × 25.8); plate 8¼ × 11½ (20.8 × 29.2)
Inscr. by the artist with MS notes of lettering to be engraved below the plate, and, top left, by C. Turner: 'No.2'
Royal Academy of Arts

The drawing is in the Turner Bequest, CXCI–E; and is derived from Turner's painting exhibited at the R.A. in 1802 (No.73). The plate, R.6, was issued in the first part of the *Liber Studiorum* which appeared on 11 June 1807; it was categorised as 'Historical'.

101 The Fifth Plague of Egypt *c.*1807
Pen and grey, brown and pink washes, 7 1/16 × 9 15/16 (18 × 25.3)
Trustees of the British Museum (T.B.CXVI–S)

Engraved in mezzotint by C. Turner (etched outline by J. M. W. Turner) for the *Liber Studiorum* part III, 1808 (R.16, No.102).

The subject is that of Turner's painting 'The Fifth Plague of Egypt', exhibited R.A. 1800 (206) and bought by William Beckford (No.70). It was categorised in the *Liber* as 'Historical' landscape.

A sketch for the subject is in the 'Dolbadern' sketchbook, T.B.XLVI f.79.

Charles TURNER (1774–1857) and J. M. W.
TURNER

102 The Fifth Plague of Egypt 1808
Etching and mezzotint, first published state,
$7\frac{1}{8} \times 10\frac{1}{4}$ (18×25.9); plate $8\frac{1}{4} \times 11\frac{1}{2}$ (20.8×29.1)
Inscr. above: 'H' [for Historical]; and below:
'The 5th Plague of Egypt the Picture late in the
Possession of W. Beckford Esqr.'; 'London
Published June 10. 1808 by C. Turner No.50.
Warren Street, Fitzroy Square'; 'Drawn &
Etched by J. M. W. Turner Esqr. R.A.P.';
'Engraved by C. Turner'; and bottom left in
scratched letters: 'Proof'
Royal Academy of Arts

The painting is No.70, and Turner's monochrome
drawing for the plate, R.16, is No.101.

Charles TURNER (1774–1857) and J. M. W.
TURNER

103 Ships in a Breeze 1808
Etching and mezzotint, proof, $7\frac{1}{8} \times 10$
(18.2×25.8); plate $8\frac{1}{8} \times 11\frac{3}{8}$ (20.7×29)
Inscr. in scratched letters: 'In the possession of
the Earl of Egremont' and signed bottom right by
C. Turner
Royal Academy of Arts

The plate, R.10. bearing the symbol 'M' for Marine,
was issued in Part II of the *Liber Studiorum* (R.10).
Turner's drawing of the subject is T.B.CXVI–M; it was
closely based on the 'Egremont Sea Piece', exhibited as
'Ships bearing up for Anchorage' in 1802 (No.72).

104 Holy Island Cathedral 1807
Pen and brown ink and wash, $7\frac{3}{16} \times 10\frac{5}{16}$
(18.3×26.2)
Trustees of the British Museum (T.B.CXVI–N)

Engraved in mezzotint by C. Turner (etched outline by
J. M. W. Turner) for part III of the *Liber Studiorum*,
1808 (R.11).

Transcribed almost without modification from the
pencil drawing of Lindisfarne Church in the 'North of
England' sketchbook (T.B.XXXIV f.54^r). Categorised as
'Architecture' in the *Liber* series.

105 London from Greenwich 1810
Etching, proof, $7 \times 10\frac{1}{2}$ (17.8×26.5); plate
$8\frac{1}{4} \times 11\frac{3}{8}$ (20.8×28.9)
Inscr. in scratched latters: 'In the Possession of
Walter Fawkes Esqr. Farnley'
Royal Academy of Arts

The inscription refers to the painting exhibited in
Turner's Gallery in 1809 (No.152); Turner's mono-
chrome drawing for the plate is in the Turner Bequest,
CXVII–13; another version of it is in the Whitworth
Art Gallery, Manchester.

The plate, R.26, was mezzotinted by Charles Turner
and published 1 January 1811 in Part V of the *Liber
Studiorum* (see No.106).

Charles TURNER (1774–1857) and J. M. W.
TURNER

106 London from Greenwich 1810
Etching and mezzotint, proof, $7 \times 10\frac{1}{2}$
Royal Academy of Arts

See the proof of Turner's etched outline, No.105. The
plate, R.26, was published with the symbol 'A' for
Architecture in Part V of the *Liber Studiorum*.

107 Calm 1812
Soft-ground etching, unique proof, $7 \times 10\frac{5}{8}$
(17.8×26.9), cut inside plate mark
Royal Academy of Arts

The plate was published 28 April 1812, in part IX of the
Liber Studiorum, R.44, with the symbol 'M' for Marine.
It was begun and completed by Turner himself. It is
one of a small number of the plates which have a
foundation of soft-ground rather than the normal
etched outline. No drawing is known, although two
paintings entitled 'Fishing-boats in a Calm' were
shown at Turner's gallery in 1809; these are now
untraced.

There is a faint off-print of 'Dunstanborough
Castle' (R.14) on the verso.

George CLINT (1770–1854) and TURNER

108 Peat Bog, Scotland 1812
Etching and mezzotint, 3rd published state,
$7\frac{1}{4} \times 10\frac{1}{4}$ (17.9×26); plate $8\frac{1}{4} \times 11\frac{1}{2}$ (20.8×29)
Inscr. above: 'M' (for 'Mountain'); and below
with title and: 'Published April 23, 1812, by
I. M. W. Turner, Queen Ann Street West',
'Drawn & Etched by I. M. W. Turner Esqr.
R.A.'; 'Engraved by G. Clint'
Royal Academy of Arts

The drawing is in the Turner Bequest, CXVII–T. The
plate, R.45, appeared in Part IX of the *Liber Studiorum*.

109 Mill near the Grande Chartreuse c.1815
Pen and brownish-black ink and red-brown
wash, $9\frac{1}{16} \times 13\frac{7}{16}$ (23×34.1)
Trustees of the British Museum (T.B.CXVIII–B)

Engraved in mezzotint over an etched outline by H.
Dawe for part XI of the *Liber Studiorum*, 1816 (R.54).

Categorised by Turner as 'Mountain' landscape. Although he made many drawings near the Chartreuse in
1802 ('Grenoble' sketchbook, T.B.LXXIV, ff.24–37)
none corresponds at all closely with the subject of this
design.

110 Crowhurst c.1816
Pen and brown ink and grey and brown washes
with scraping-out, $7\frac{13}{16} \times 10\frac{13}{16}$ (19.8×27.5)
Trustees of the British Museum (T.B.CXVIII–R)

Engraved in mezzotint by H. Dawe (etched outline by
J. M. W. Turner) for the *Liber Studiorum*, but unpublished (R.76).

A subject presumably inspired by Turner's visit to
Crowhurst for the *Views of Sussex* series, 1816. Although the plate bears no letters, a note in the 'Aesacus
and Hesperie' sketchbook of 1819 (T.B.CLXIX, inside
cover) indicates that a *Liber* subject of 'Snow', which is
almost certainly the 'Crowhurst', was undertaken by
Dawe. Rawlinson records the possibility that Turner
did some work on the mezzotint as well as providing
the etched outline.

III Isleworth *c.*1818
 Pen and brown ink and grey and brown washes
 over traces of pencil, $8\frac{1}{4} \times 11\frac{3}{8}$ (21 × 29)
 Trustees of the British Museum (T.B.CXVIII–I)

Engraved in mezzotint by H. Dawe (etched outline by
J. M. W. Turner) for part XIII of the *Liber Studiorum*,
1819 (R.63).

The plate is known as the 'Alcove, Isleworth', and
has been called 'Pope's Villa', 'Garrick's Temple' and
'Hampton Church'; all three titles are incorrect.
Turner categorised the subject as 'Epic Pastoral'. The
'Alcove', a shooting lodge in the form of an Ionic
temple, built by Robert Mylne for the second Duke of
Northumberland, occurs frequently in Turner's
sketchbooks as the focal point of his imaginary landscape compositions, for instance in the 'Studies for
Pictures, Isleworth' sketchbook (T.B.XC, ff.3, 4, 5, 6,
etc). It recurs in another *Liber* plate, 'Isis' (R.68).

112 Shipping Scene with Fishermen *c.*1815–20
 Pen and brown wash $8\frac{1}{2} \times 11\frac{1}{2}$ (21.7 × 29.1)
 Private collection

One of the drawings in sepia wash which Turner made
in connection with the *Liber Studiorum*, but not actually
used as the basis of an engraved design. The subject has
affinities with 'Shipping at the Entrance of the Medway', a drawing similar in size and handling to this in
the Turner Bequest, CXVIII–b* (presented by W. G.
Rawlinson, 1913), also unused by Turner; it was later
engraved by Sir Frank Short (R.98).

5. England 1805–15

At the same time as Turner was rivalling the Old
Masters in the large pictures he sent in to the Royal
Academy, there occurred a great deepening of his
understanding of nature in all its subtleties. A new
generation of patrons, such as Walter Fawkes and John
Fuller, who among other things commissioned Turner
to paint their houses, led him to a more intimate connection with the countryside. This was revealed particularly in his studies of the Thames in both oils and
watercolours, and led to a series of domestic landscapes,
mainly exhibited at his own gallery adjacent to his
home in Queen Ann Street (see Nos.B71–B75). The
most crucial example of his new understanding of
atmosphere, albeit partly inspired by the Dutch
masters, was 'Sun rising through Vapour; Fishermen
cleaning and selling Fish', exhibited at the Royal Academy in 1807; this can be seen at the National Gallery.

113 Scarborough *c.*1810
 Watercolour, 27 × 40 (68.7 × 101.6)
 Exh: ?R.A. 1811 (392) as 'Scarborough Town
 and Castle: Morning: Boys catching Crabs';
 Leeds 1839(17)
 Mrs William Crabtree

Acquired by Walter Fawkes, who probably bought the
drawing from the Academy exhibition in 1811. When
it was exhibited at Agnew's in 1967 (No.43) Joll
reiterated Finberg's suggestion (*Farnley*, 1912, No.76
pl.IV) that a smaller version, without the boats, and
dated 1809, now in the Wallace collection, was that
shown in 1811; but it seems altogether more probable
that this very large and elaborate watercolour was
intended by Turner for the walls of the Academy. A
large 'colour-beginning' the size of the finished watercolour, with the main view lightly indicated and more
detailed treatment of the posts and pool to the left, is
T.B.CXXVI–C; a smaller one is CXCVI–B. Turner used
a similar view of the town, though from a nearer viewpoint, for a drawing in the *Ports of England* series
(T.B.CCVIII–I)

**114 Scene on the Thames with Barges and a
 Punt** *c.*1806
 Watercolour, $10\frac{1}{16} \times 14\frac{1}{2}$ (25.6 × 36.8)
 Trustees of the British Museum (T.B.XCV–49)

From a roll sketchbook watermarked 1797 and labelled
by Turner: 'Thames from Reading to Walton'. The
small building on the far bank of the river, to the right
of the composition, may be the 'Alcove' at Isleworth;
see No.111.

The series of forty-eight drawings in this book, many
of them in watercolour, has been associated with the oil
sketches of the Thames in the Turner Bequest (see
Nos.135–141 and 143–146), usually dated to about 1807.
Finberg gives 1806–7 as the date of the sketchbook,
which has close stylistic affinities with the 'Studies for
Pictures: Isleworth's ketchbook (No.94) in use from
1804.

115 Kew Bridge *c.*1806
 Pencil and watercolour, $10\frac{1}{16} \times 14\frac{3}{8}$ (25.6 × 36.5)
 Trustees of the British Museum (T.B.XCV–42)

From the 'Thames from Reading to Walton' sketchbook; see also No.114.

116 'Boats, Ice' Sketchbook *c.*1807
 Inscr.: 'Green'; 'Blue'; 'Greenish Blue'
 Bound in calf, one clasp
 88 leaves, ff.42–58, 60–84 blank, almost all of the
 remainder drawn on in pencil, $4\frac{1}{4} \times 7\frac{1}{16}$
 (10.6 × 17.9)
 Inscr.: Finberg records Turner's label on spine:
 '51, Boats, Ice'
 Watermarked: 1805
 Trustees of the British Museum (T.B.CI)

f.4ʳ **Sky Study**
 Pencil

The title of the sketchbook refers to a series of studies of
boats in ice; ff.10, 12, 14 show small boats apparently
on the frozen Thames; ff.15, 16, 17, 18 are presumably
imaginary scenes of pack-ice with sailing vessels caught

in it. A famous frost on the Thames was that of January 1814, and it is possible that the sketchbook dates from that time; but there is no strong evidence to contradict Finberg's dating of *c*.1806–8.

117 **'Hesperides' Sketchbook No.1** *c*.1805–7
Bound in marbled boards, leather spine and corners; two clasps
40 leaves of white paper prepared with a wash of grey (except the first leaf) and two fly-leaves at each end; nearly all drawn on in pencil, pen and brown ink, black and white chalk and watercolour, $10\frac{3}{8} \times 6\frac{3}{4}$ (26.2 × 17.2)
Watermarked: 1799
Inscr. on label on spine: '71 H [esperides Bk' added by another hand]
Trustees of the British Museum (T.B.XCIII)

f.23ᵛ **A Group of Figures seated by Lamplight among [?] Carts**
Pen and brown ink and wash

The sketchbook is named after the painting shown at the British Institution in 1805 (55): 'The Goddess of Discord choosing the apple of contention in the Garden of the Hesperides' (Tate Gallery, 477), for which some of the sketches appear to be studies; in particular a pen drawing on f.3ᵛ is for the dragon in that picture, and is inscribed 'the Garden of the Hesperides'. There are also drawings for other subjects, and a series of studies on the Thames similar to those in the 'Isleworth' sketchbook (No.94).

The page shown is one of a series of rustic figure subjects on ff.22–5 which seem to reflect the success of Wilkie's 'Village Politicians' shown at the R.A. in 1806 (145). Similar designs occur in the 'Harvest Home' sketchbook (T.B.LXXXVI, ff.2,3,4). See also No.133.

Inscribed on the first front fly-leaf is: 'Varnish| Razor|Blue Black|Bt Sienna|Fishing Rod. Flies|Pallet Knife|Shoes'.

118 **'Tabley' Sketchbook No.1** *c*.1808
Bound in marbled boards, leather spine
28 leaves, 27 used (ff.21, 22 mounted)
$9 \times 11\frac{3}{4}$ (22.7 × 29.6)
Watermarked: 1801
Trustees of the British Museum (T.B.CIII)

f.18ʳ **View of Tabley House**
Oil and gum arabic

Mostly careful pencil drawings in Lancashire, especially around Whalley where Turner made studies for his illustrations to Whitaker's *History of Whalley* during his stay with Sir John Leicester at Tabley in the summer of 1808. f.8 has the study which formed the basis of 'Whalley Bridge and Abbey, Lancashire', shown at the R.A. 1811 (244) and now in the Lloyd collection.

The leaf shown has been extracted from the book and folded twice. It is a worked up version of the pencil drawing on f.15ᵛ–16ʳ. The view on f.22 (now mounted separately) is in watercolour over pencil with some pen and ink and also has a coat of gum arabic over its surface.

119 **'Tabley's Sketchbook No.3** 1808–18
Bound in calf, one clasp
92 leaves, the majority drawn on in pencil, $4\frac{1}{4} \times 7\frac{1}{4}$ (10.7 × 18.3)
Trustees of the British Museum (T.B.CV)

f.17ʳ **The Lake at Tabley**
Pen and brown ink

This sketchbook contains several drawings made at or near Tabley, including sketches of a picture gallery, probably that at Tabley, with notes and diagrams relating to Turner's own remodelled gallery in Harley Street, eventually opened in 1820.

A series of pencil sketches of London, centring on Waterloo Bridge and Somerset House (ff.72–8), are close in spirit and composition to the series in the so-called 'Scotland and Venice' sketchbook of 1818 (T.B. CLXX; No.203) which also contains material relating to Turner's visit to Scotland in that year. Waterloo Bridge was opened in 1817. A further group of views on the Thames, showing the old Custom House and the church of St Magnus at London Bridge, CV ff.39–41, are also closely paralleled in CLXX (esp. f.41ʳ which is the same general view as CLXX f.10ʳ). Since the Tabley drawings in this sketchbook include studies for the paintings shown at the R.A. in 1809 (Nos.150 and 151) it must be proposed that the book was in use over a period of ten years.

Shown is a preparatory sketch for the painting 'Tabley, the Seat of Sir J. F. Leicester, Bart: Windy Day'. Pencil studies for the companion view of Tabley, 'Calm Morning', are on ff.5ᵛ–6ʳ and 8ʳ.

120 **The Garreteer's Petition** *c*.1808
Pen and brown ink and wash with a little watercolour, $7\frac{1}{4} \times 11\frac{7}{8}$ (18.4 × 30.2)
Inscr. on recto: 'Translation & Vide [?] Art of Poetry', 'Hints on an Epic Poem', 'Reviews Torn upon Floor', 'Paraphrase of Job', 'coll of odds & ends'; and on verso: 'The Garreteer petion [sic] to the [caret: his] Muse'; with three fragments of verse, including: 'The hard urged Garretteer whose [?stout] brains|shake hands with penury and [gap] pain|Inverted looks for inspiration to the ground|Sinking from thought to thought a vast profound'
Trustees of the British Museum (T.B.CXXI–A)
A study for the picture shown at the Royal Academy in 1809, No.134; see also No.121.

121 **The Amateur Artist** *c*.1808
Pen and brown ink and wash with some watercolour and scraping-out, $7\frac{1}{4} \times 11\frac{7}{8}$ (18.5 × 30.2)
Inscr. on recto:
'Pictures either ⎰Judgment of Paris
⎱Forbidden Fruit
Old Masters scattered over ye floor
Stolen hints from celebrated Pictures Phials,
Crucibles retorts label'd Bottles . . . Varnish quiz (?)'; and on the verso with a draft of eleven lines of verse beginning: 'Please[d] with his Work he views it o'er and o'er And finds fresh beauties never seen before . . .'
Trustees of the British Museum (T.B.CXXXI–B)

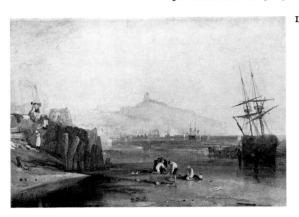

113

It has been suggested that this subject is related to the painting of 'An Artist's Colourman's Workshop' in the Tate Gallery (5503); but in style and conception it is obviously a companion piece to the 'Garreteer's Petition', No.120, and must therefore have subject-matter complementary to that. These drawings appear to have been motivated at least in part by the genre pictures of David Wilkie (see No.117), but they are primarily satires in the manner of Hogarth: the 'Garret-eer' can be compared with Hogarth's print of the 'Distressed Poet' of 1736 (Ronald Paulson, *Hogarth's Graphic Works*, 1965, No. 145, pl.156). Turner's line 'Sinking from thought to thought a vast profound' appears on Hogarth's plate, with its original context, altered from Book I of Pope's *Dunciad*. Turner's use of symbolic pictures in the 'Amateur Artist' is also a device characteristic of Hogarth. It may even be that the medium of pen and brown wash was suggested by Hogarth's drawings.

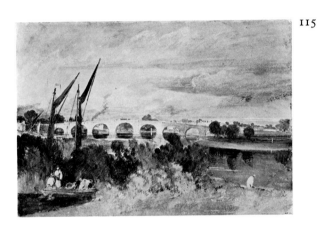

115

122 Petworth from the Lake 1809
Pencil, 9 × 14¾ (22.8 × 37.5)
Trustees of the British Museum (T.B.CIX–4)
Used for the painting 'Petworth, Sussex, the seat of the Earl of Egremont: Dewy Morning', shown at the R.A. 1810 (115) and still at Petworth (repr. Rothenstein and Butlin 1964, pl.46).

123 Malham Cove, Yorkshire *c*.1810
Watercolour, 11 × 15⁹⁄₁₆ (27.9 × 39.6)
Inscr. bottom right: 'I M W Turner RA'
Trustees of the British Museum (1910-2-12-277)
The pencil study on which this composition is based is in the 'Tabley' sketchbook No.1, T.B.CIII f.10. This book was in use during a visit to Tabley in the summer of 1808 (see Finberg 1961, p.151). The early history of this drawing is not clear, and it may have been executed a little later than the date suggested, perhaps in connection with Whitaker's *Richmondshire* (see No.180) or a similar project.

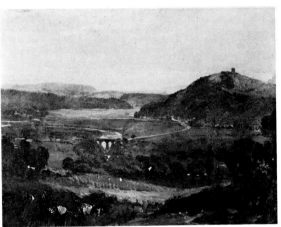

126

124 View over Falmouth Harbour *c*.1813
Oil on paper prepared with a buff ground,
6⅜ × 10¼ (16.3 × 25.7)
Trustees of the British Museum (T.B.CXXX–C)
125 A Devon Hillside, with a Quarry *c*.1813
Oil on paper prepared with a buff ground,
5⅝ × 10¼ (14.3 × 25.7)
Trustees of the British Museum (T.B.CXXX–D)
126 A Valley in Devonshire *c*.1813
Oil on paper, 9⅝ × 12¹⁄₁₆ (24.5 × 30.6)
Trustees of the British Museum (T.B.CXXX–E)
Although the series of oil studies made in Devonshire in 1812 or 1813 have the appearance of open-air sketches, Turner apparently executed some of them indoors, for an acquaintance, Cyrus Redding, records a picnic on Mount Edgecumbe at which Turner 'showed the Ladies some of his sketches in oil, which he had brought with him, perhaps to verify them'. On the other hand, Sir Charles Eastlake gives circumstantial evidence of work in this medium out of doors. He records a visit to Plymouth in '1813 or perhaps 1814': 'Turner made his sketches in pencil and by stealth. His companions, observing his peculiarity, were careful not to intrude on him. After he returned to Plymouth, in the neighbour-

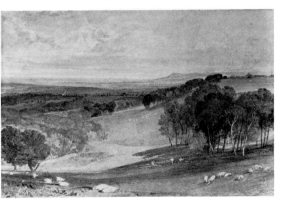

127

hood of which he remained some weeks, Mr Johns fitted up a small portable painting-box, containing some prepared paper for oil sketches, as well as the other necessary materials. When Turner halted at a scene and seemed inclined to sketch it, Johns produced the inviting box, and the great artist, finding everything ready to his hand, immediately began to work. As he sometimes wanted assistance in the use of the box, the presence of Johns was indispensable, and after a few days he made his oil sketches freely in our presence. Johns accompanied him always; I was only with them occasionally. Turner seemed pleased when the rapidity with which these sketches were done was talked of; for, departing from his habitual reserve in the instance of his pencil sketches, he made no difficulty of showing them. On one occasion, when, on his return after a sketching ramble, . . . the day's work was shown, he himself remarked that one of the sketches (and perhaps the best) was done in less than half an hour.' (Quoted in Thornbury, 1862, I, pp.219–20.)

127　The Vale of Pevensey c.1816
　　Watercolour, $15\frac{1}{2} \times 22\frac{1}{4}$ (39.4 × 56.5)
　　Lady Agnew
A pencil drawing of the subject is in the 'Views of Sussex' sketchbook (T.B.CXXXVIII f.19ʳ); that book, and the 'Vale of Heathfield' Sketchbook (No.130), were in use c.1815-16 when Turner was collecting material for the series of Sussex views commissioned by John Fuller of Rosehill Park, of which 'The Vale of Pevensey' is one. Four of the designs were aquatinted by J. C. Stadler c.1818 (see No.B102); this subject appeared as 'Rosehill' (Rawlinson No.822).

William Bernard COOKE (1778–1855) after
TURNER

128　Pevensey Bay from Crowhurst Park 1816
　　Engraving, proof corrected by Turner, $17\frac{1}{2} \times 11\frac{1}{16}$ (19 × 28.2); trimmed inside plate-mark
　　Inscr: 'Drawn by J. M. W. Turner Esq. R.A.'
　　'Engraved by W. B. Cooke, 1816' and 'Crowhurst Sussex'; in MS 'Second' and 'touched by Turner – W. B. Cooke'
　　Trustees of the British Museum (1861-5-18-82)
　　(Rawlinson No.132)
One of eight plates engraved by W. B. Cooke after designs by Turner for *Views in Sussex* (later called *Views in Hastings and its Vicinity*) commissioned by John Fuller in 1810, which appeared between 1816 and 1820. Turner himself etched an emblematical vignette for the cover of Part I (Rawlinson 128). No.127 is one of Turner's drawings for the series. See also the aquatint by J. C. Stadler (No.B102) and No.130.

William Bernard COOKE (1778–1855) after
TURNER

129　The Vale of Ashburnham 1816
　　Engraving, proof touched by Turner, $7\frac{3}{8} \times 11\frac{1}{16}$ (18.7 × 28.1); trimmed inside plate-mark
　　Inscr. bottom left: 'Drawn by J. M. W. Turner Esq. R.A. 1815'; and bottom right: 'Engraved by W. B. Cooke 1816'; 'Ashburnham Park'; also, in Cooke's hand: 'Touched by Turner with his observations W B Cooke'; and in Turner's hand: 'Hop-poles in bundles' (with sketch) and '3

windows each side the Entrance'
　　Trustees of the British Museum (1861-5-18-85)
　　(Rawlinson No.131)
From the drawing now in the B.M. (1910-2-12-272).

130　'Vale of Heathfield' sketchbook ?1809–16
　　Bound in green boards with green leather spine and corners
　　Contains two fly-leaves and 72 leaves, the majority drawn on in pencil, occasionally with watercolour, $7\frac{1}{4} \times 9\frac{1}{4}$ (18.2 × 23)
　　Inscr. on label on spine: '113'; inside front cover and front fly-leaf with notes on the geography, history, etc, of Dorset and Devon.
　　Trustees of the British Museum (T.B.CXXXVII)

　　ff.68ʳ–69ᵛ　**The Vale of Ashburnham**
　　Pencil

ff.3ᵛ–4ʳ have a pencil drawing of Somer Hill which Turner used for his painting of the house, seat of Major Woodgate, which appeared at the R.A. in 1811 (No.158). Finberg suggests (1909, I, p.392) that the sketchbook was in use from this time until about 1816, when Turner was working on the series of views in Sussex commissioned by John Fuller. But although the 'Hastings' sketchbook, connected with that commission, is watermarked 1815, a commission for 'three or four views' had come from Fuller as early as 1810 (see Farington, *Diary*, 21 April 1810). The views of Heathfield and Ashburnham (ff.41ᵛ–42ʳ and 68ʳ–69ʳ) were used for two of the Fuller watercolours, the latter signed and dated 1816. The MS notes were presumably written into the sketchbook prior to the tour of Dorset, Devon and Cornwall in July, August and September of 1811. Some of the views (e.g. those on ff.64ᵛ and 63ᵛ) suggest the Lake District, where Turner was in 1809 (see Finberg 1961, p.159).

In support of Finberg's view that the sketchbook went on being used until about 1816 it should be noticed that the studies of sea and sky in watercolour on ff.38ʳ and 39ʳ are of a freedom normally associated with the late 1810s, or even later (cf. the 'Skies' sketchbook, T.B.CLVIII, No.177), though Finberg identified some of them as the Eddystone lighthouse which, as Wilkinson notes (1974, p.132), Turner must have visited in either 1811 or 1813. Furthermore, the style of many of the pencil drawings is close to that of the 'Yorkshire' sketchbooks of 1815–18 (T.B.CXLIV–CXLIX). It is evident too that Turner was in the habit of retaining sketchbooks for several years, especially at this period; compare the 'Tabley No.3' sketchbook, T.B.CV, apparently used in 1808 and in 1818 (No.119).

The drawing exhibited was used for the watercolour of the Vale of Ashburnham (see No.129), one of a series of thirteen executed for Fuller and sold by Sir Alexander Acland Hood at Christie's, 4 April 1908 (85–98).

131　Walton Bridges c.1806
　　Oil on canvas, $36\frac{1}{2} \times 48\frac{3}{4}$ (92.5 × 123.5)
　　Exh. ? Turner's gallery 1806
　　C. L. Loyd, Esq.

132 Walton Bridges *c.*1806
Oil on canvas 36¼ × 48⅛ (92 × 122.5)
Exh: ? Turner's gallery 1806
National Gallery of Victoria, Melbourne

The first of these two views of Walton Bridges was bought by Sir John Leicester for £280. Turner's receipt is dated 18 January 1807, which suggests that the picture could well have been seen by Leicester in Turner's gallery the previous year. The Melbourne picture, which was bought by the Earl of Essex, seems to be a pendant to the other and was probably painted at the same time. There are drawings for both pictures in the 'Hesperides (2)' sketchbook (T.B.XCIV–4, 6 and 7 for No.131, 5ᵛ for No.132) and for the Loyd one also in the 'Thames from Reading to Walton' sketchbook (T.B.XCV–22 (repr. Wilkinson 1974, p.75), 23).

The double bridge at Walton seems to have been a well-known attraction in the eighteenth and nineteenth centuries. The old, wooden bridges were painted by Canaletto (e.g. the picture at Dulwich) and Turner did several later sketches (see No.138). The bridges are also the basis of one of the *Liber Studiorum* plates, 'The Bridge in the Middle Distance', R.13, published 10 June 1808 and marked 'EP' for Epic (?) Pastoral (see p.61). This in its turn was the basis for the later oil, often thought to be an Italian subject, in the collection of Henry Morgan, New York. A much later watercolour, engraved in 1830 by J. C. Varrall for *Picturesque Views in England and Wales*, follows very closely the composition of No.132.

133 A Country Blacksmith disputing upon the Price of Iron, and the Price charged to the Butcher for shoeing his Poney R.A.1807
Oil on pine, 21⅝ × 30⅝ (55 × 78)
Inscr. bottom left: 'J.M.W. Turner RA'
Exh: R.A. 1807 (135); Sir John Leicester's gallery 1819 and subsequent years (19)
Tate Gallery (478)

Turner here stepped outside his usual range of subjects to paint a genre interior in the manner of Teniers. In this he was almost certainly inspired by the success of the young David Wilkie, ten years his junior, with his first exhibit at the Royal Academy the year before, 'Village Politicians', also in the Teniers manner. In 1807 Wilkie exhibited 'The Blind Fiddler' (Tate Gallery; repr. illustrated souvenir *David Wilkie*, R.A. 1958, pl.5), another interior, and visitors to the exhibition drew the obvious comparisons, some favouring Turner, others Wilkie.

On 8 May Farington recorded that Sir George Beaumont 'sd. Sir John Leicester had told him that He had asked Turner the price of His picture of a Forge. Turner answered that He understood Wilkie was to have 100 guineas for *His Blind Fiddler* & He should not rate His picture at a less price'. Turner, as his receipt of 9 January 1808 shows, got his price. The painting returned to Turner's possession in 1827 when he bought it back for 140 guineas at the sale following the death of Sir John Leicester, later 1st Lord de Tabley. Apart from 'London from Greenwich', which also left Turner's possession, this is the only picture in the Turner Bequest to bear a signature; presumably Turner only signed his paintings when he sold them.

There are a number of drawings of figures engaged in various indoor activities in the 'Hesperides (1)' sketchbook of *c.*1805–7, one being used for this picture (T.B.XCIII–22ᵛ). A rebate round the edge of the picture shows that it was finished in its frame.

134 The Garreteer's Petition R.A.1809
Oil on mahogany, 20⅞ × 30¾ (53 × 78)
Exh: R.A. 1809 (175); Turner's gallery 1810 (17)
Tate Gallery (482)

This work was painted on a panel already covered with what is apparently ordinary household paint, an example among several of Turner using the first material to come to hand (see also Nos.333 and 334). When exhibited again in 1810 it was entitled 'Poet's Garrett', and in 1809 it was exhibited with the following verses:

Aid me, ye Powers! O bid my thoughts to roll
In quick succession, animate my soul;
Descend my Muse, and every thought refine,
And finish well my long, my *long-sought* line.

These verses, with the possible exception of those for 'Dolbadern Castle' and 'Caernarvon Castle' shown at the Royal Academy in 1800, are the first of his own to be published by Turner in an exhibition catalogue. There are drafts on the back of the study for the picture (see No.120). For a companion sketch of an artist's studio see No.121.

Pasquin, writing in *The Morning Herald* for 4 May 1809, attacked Turner for imitating Wilkie and attempting a genre to which he was not suited, concluding with 'the insulted Garrateer thus indignantly admonishing the Royal Academician . . .'

Avaunt! presumptuous, proud R.A.
What wouldst thou here, so pert, so gay?
May thine own Gods forsake thee:
You've spoil'd the tadpole of a thought,
Which Genius from Apollo caught,
For wich [sic] the Devil take thee!

135 Guildford from the Banks of the Wey
Oil on mahogany veneer, 10 × 7¾ (25 × 20)
Tate Gallery (2310)

136 Godalming from the South
Oil on mahogany veneer, 8 × 13¾ (20 × 35)
Tate Gallery (2304)

137 Sunset on the River
Oil on mahogany veneer, 6¹⁄₁₆ × 7⁵⁄₁₆ (15.5 × 18.5)
Tate Gallery (2311)

138 The Thames near Walton Bridges
Oil on mahogany veneer, 14⅝ × 29 (37 × 73.5)
Tate Gallery (2680)

139 Windsor Castle, from Salt Hill
Oil on mahogany veneer, 10⅞ × 29 (27.5 × 73.5)
Tate Gallery (2312)

140 Eton from the River
Oil on mahogany veneer, 14½ × 26⅛ (37 × 66.5)
Tate Gallery (2313)

141 Tree Tops and Sky, Guildford Castle (?), Evening
Oil on mahogany veneer, 10⅞ × 29 (27.5 × 73.5)
Tate Gallery (2309)

A selection from the eighteen sketches on mahogany veneer of various sizes in the Turner Bequest (Tate Gallery 2302–13, 2676–81). The subjects are all on the Thames or its tributary the Wey; several of the Guildford and Godalming views were identified in 1970 by Mr Christopher Pinsent, including No.141, formerly thought to show Windsor Castle. The same area, with the exception of Walton Bridges, is covered by drawings in the 'Windsor, Eton' and the 'Wey, Guildford' sketchbooks, though none of the viewpoints are identical (T.B.XCVII and XCVIII).

The small oil sketches, like these sketchbooks, were dated c.1807 by Finberg (1961, p.137) but, being less closely connected with Turner's exhibited paintings, are more difficult to date precisely. John Gage divides them into three groups. The first, which includes Nos.135–7, he associates with the Wey and Guildford sketchbook but dates c.1809–10; the second, including No.138, he dates c.1811–12; and the third, including Nos.139–41, later still, c.1813 or later, as more accomplished even than the small Devonshire oil sketches of 1813 (see Nos.124–6). The Devonshire sketches, however, are not strictly comparable in either technique or general approach, and again it may be that, as is argued in the case of the large Thames sketches on canvas, the whole group represents a single campaign playing a crucial part in the rapid development of Turner's approach to nature in 1807 and 1808 (see Nos.143–6).

These sketches were probably done out-of-doors, perhaps from a small boat as the younger Trimmer described, though he talks of Turner using 'a large canvas' (see Nos.143–6). In them Turner approaches nearest to what Constable termed 'a natural painter', but, unlike Constable, Turner always seems to have been interested in making a complete pictorial composition even when he came closest to recording a direct experience of nature.

142 Rosehill Park, Sussex c.1810–15

Oil on canvas, 35 × 47 (89 × 119.5)
Inscr: 'J.M.W. Turner R.A.'
Lt Col Sir George Meyrick, Bart.

Probably painted for the owner of Rosehill, Mr John Fuller, M.P. for Sussex, whose son Augustus Elliott Fuller married Clara Meyrick, heiress of Bodorgan; their son assumed the surname of Meyrick in addition to that of Fuller. On the other hand, family tradition has it that the picture was only acquired from Turner later, when he brought it to Bodorgan and sold it to the son, Owen Fuller Meyrick, for as much as 1,000 guineas. Turner is said to have asked for half a guinea for his cab fare as well, which would date the visit to about 1849 when the railway to Anglesey was opened.

A visit by Turner to Rosehill is documented in Farington's *Diary* for 21 April 1810. Farington records that Fuller had engaged Turner 'to make drawings of three or four views. He is to have 100 guineas for the use of his drawings, which are to be returned to him.' A small but accurate pencil study for the picture occurs on pages 20ᵛ and 21 (composition continued on p.22) of the 'Hastings' sketchbook (T.B.CXI, listed by Finberg merely as 'View on the Sussex Downs'). Unfortunately this cannot be precisely dated, but another pencil drawing of Rosehill occurs in the later 'Hastings' sketchbook (T.B.CXXXIX–33aᵛ and 34), watermarked 1815, which suggests a further visit or visits, and other Turner watercolours that belonged to Fuller are dated 1816. The terms of the commission must therefore have been altered or extended later, for Fuller finally owned thirteen Turner watercolours. See also under No.130.

This picture must therefore have been painted between 1810 and 1816 and on stylistic grounds it would seem closer to the two views of Lowther Castle (exhibited 1810) than to the Raby Castle of 1818 (Walters Art Gallery, Baltimore). Indeed, the absence of human figures, a rarity in Turner's work which does however occur around 1810, points to a dating about then. It was in that year that Fuller bought his other oil by Turner, the 'Fishmarket on the Sands, Hastings' (William Rockhill Nelson Gallery, Kansas City) and there are several references to payments from Fuller in Turner's sketchbooks at this time. It seems possible that an outstanding amount of £200, which it appears that Fuller owed Turner at the end of 1810, refers to the oil of Rosehill.

Rosehill Park (now renamed Brightling Park) is in East Sussex about four miles from Battle. It was bought in 1697 by John Fuller's ancestor and later passed by inheritance to Sir Alexander Acland Hood, Bart, on whose death in 1908 the Turner watercolours and the picture of Hastings were dispersed at Christie's (4 April).

143 Hampton Court from the Thames c.1807–8

Oil on canvas, 33¾ × 47¼ (86 × 120)
Tate Gallery (2693)

144 Washing Sheep c.1807–8

Oil on canvas, 33¼ × 45⅞ (84.5 × 116.5)
Tate Gallery (2699)

145 Cleeve Mill (?) c.1807–8

Oil on canvas, 33¾ × 45¾ (85.5 × 116)
Tate Gallery (2704)

146 Willows beside a Stream c.1807–8

Oil on canvas, 33⅞ × 45¾ (86 × 116.5)
Tate Gallery (2706)

These are a selection from the group of seventeen large oil sketches of subjects on or near the Thames in the Turner Bequest (Tate Gallery 2691–700, 2702–7, 5519); see also No.154. All, though carried to a different degree of finish, are similar in technique, lightly painted over a dry chalky ground, and all are roughly similar in size save for the sketch for 'Harvest Dinner, Kingston Bank', which only measures 24 × 36 in (Tate Gallery 2696). This last was used for the painting exhibited at Turner's gallery in 1809 and again in 1810 (Tate Gallery 491). Others are more loosely related to finished oil paintings exhibited in 1808, 1809 and 1810. A number of them are also related to drawings in the 'Thames from Reading to Walton' sketchbook, datable c.1807 (T.B.XCV; cf. for example, pp.31 and 37 with No.144, and p.35 with No.146; there is a different view of Cleeve Mill, apparently the subject of No.145, on p.18, repr. Wilkinson 1974, p.78), while the composition of one example, 'Trees beside a River, with a Bridge in the Middle Distance' (Tate Gallery 2692), is very close to that in the rather earlier 'Studies for Pictures: Isleworth' sketchbook, sandwiched between lists of classical and Biblical subjects (T.B.XC–55ᵛ and 56; see Nos.80 and 94 for the dating of this sketchbook).

There is reason to suppose that, contrary to Turner's usual practice, some of these sketches were at least begun out-of-doors. Thornbury (1862, I, p.169) prints some reminiscences of the son of Turner's 'oldest friend the Rev. Mr Trimmer', who had been out fishing with Turner when a child. 'He had a boat at Richmond

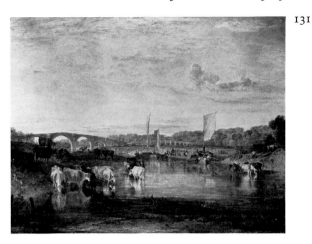
131

... From his boat he painted on a large canvas direct from Nature. Till you have seen these sketches, you know nothing of Turner's powers. There are about two score of these large subjects, rolled up, and now national property . . . There is a red sunset (simply the sky) among the rolls'. The last, probably the sadly darkened 'Sunset' (Tate Gallery 1876), is different in character from the works under discussion and is probably later, but the folded battered condition of many of the Thames sketches such as No.144 supports the identification with the works mentioned by Trimmer. Though Turner did not complete his own cottage at Twickenham, across the river from Richmond, until 1813, he already had a second home at Isleworth, not that much further from Richmond, in 1804 or 5 (see No.80), and at Upper Mall, Hammersmith probably from late 1806 until 1811.

John Gage has suggested (1969, pp.37–8) that this group of sketches was executed over a number of years, from about 1807 to as late as 'Crossing the Brook' (No.164), but it seems equally possible that despite the differences between them they were all done at more or less the same time, Turner only trying this rather unusual size and technique for this sort of sketch as a limited experiment. Despite their differences they all seem to show the fresh approach to simple, everyday subjects that is reflected in the great change in his exhibited pictures in 1807 and 1808, after which such an elaborate recourse to nature would no longer have been necessary. The range is indeed wide. 'Cleeve Mill' is treated just like a topographical watercolour, the centre being finished in detail while much of the primed canvas is left untouched. The direct, almost clumsy trees of 'Washing Sheep' are in strong contrast to the feathery 'Willows beside a Stream' with its flurry of action in the left foreground, perhaps dogs attacking a stag, reminiscent of one of Rubens' paintings of Boar Hunts.

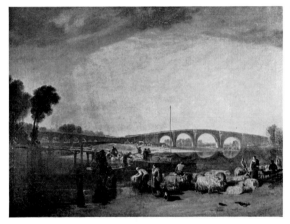
132

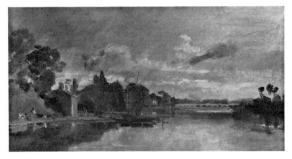
138

147 Windsor Forest: Reaping c.1807–8
  Oil on oak, $35\frac{7}{16} \times 48$ (90 × 122)
  Tate Gallery (4663)

Very similar to the large Thames sketches (Nos.143–6) but painted on wood instead of canvas; this presumably must have been painted indoors. In the related pen and wash drawing in the British Museum (T.B.CXX–D) the building in the background could well be Windsor Castle, but that in the oil has been identified as the Cranbourne Tower in Windsor Great Park.

148 View of Pope's Villa at Twickenham,
  during its Dilapidation Turner's gallery 1808
  Oil on canvas, 36 × 48 (91.5 × 122)
  Exh: Turner's gallery 1808; Sir John Leicester's
  gallery 1819 and subsequent years (17)
  *Trustees of the Walter Morrison Picture Settle-
  ment, from Sudeley Castle*

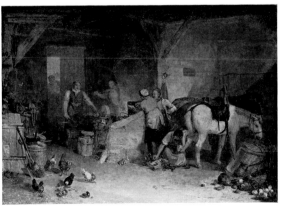
133

One of four views of the Thames above London exhibited at Turner's own gallery in 1808. Together with 'The Forest of Bere', three Thames Estuary scenes, and a 'View of Margate' now at Petworth House these must have given the public a fascinating insight into Turner's developing style in which, as opposed to paintings of earlier in the decade, classical formulae and a rather dry palette gave way to a much greater naturalism and feeling for atmosphere. Luckily, for no catalogue of the exhibition survives, it provoked an eighteen-and-a-half page review, almost certainly by John Landseer, in *The Review of Publications of Art* for 1808. 'The show of landscape is rich and various, and appears to flow from a mind clear and copious as that noble river on whose banks the artist revels, and whose various beauties he has so frequently been delighted to display.' In comparison with other artists Turner depends 'on the manifestation of mind. . . . The science which regulates his various art', however, 'appears to flow with spontaneous freedom and in an ample stream'. The reviewer noted the novelty of Turner's approach to colour. 'The brightness of his lights is less effected by the contrast of darkness than that of any other painter whatever, and even in his darkest and broadest breadths of shade, there is – either produced from some few darker touches, or by some occult magic of his peculiar art – a sufficiency of natural clearness. . . . In the pictures of the present season he has been peculiarly successful in seeming to mingle light itself with his colours. Perhaps no landscape-painter has ever before so successfully caught the living lustre of Nature herself . . .'.

Over three pages were devoted to 'Pope's Villa' itself. 'The artist has here painted not merely a portrait of this very interesting reach of the Thames, but all that a poet would think and feel on beholding the favourite retreat of so great a poet as Pope, sinking under the hand of modern improvement.' The artist 'has represented with unprecedented success, the poetic hour of pensive feeling on a tranquil autumnal evening', and the figures add to the prevailing sentiment of the picture, pensive tranquillity. The reviewer even detected a hint at what was to become perhaps Turner's most important subject, the comparison of 'the permanency of Nature herself with the fluctuations of fashion and the vicissitudes of taste; . . . not even the taste, and the genius, and the reputation of Pope, could retard the operations of Time, the irksomeness of satiety, and the consequent desire of change!'

The reviewer concluded, 'In adding this picture to his collection, Sir John Leicester has added much to his former reputation as a tasteful collector of modern art.' The purchase was also noted by *The Examiner* for 8 May, and Turner's receipt for 200 guineas survives. The picture was engraved in 1810 for inclusion in John Britton's *Fine Arts of the English School*, 1811-12 (repr. Gage 1969, pl.43), and at the sale of Sir John Leicester's paintings in 1827 it was bought by James Morrison for 210 guineas.

Pope's Villa had been demolished in 1807 and there is a draft of an 'Invocation of Thames to the Seasons – upon the Demolition of Pope's House' in the 'Greenwich' sketchbook (T.B.CII-11ᵛ onwards). There is also a more finished poem on the subject in the Poetry Notebook in the possession of C. M. W. Turner (see Jack Lindsay *The Sunset Ship*, 1966, p.117). The same Notebook also contains a poem on 'Thomson's Æolian Harp', the subject of the large oil painting exhibited in Turner's gallery the following year, 1809, with further verses also referring to Pope's Villa; this picture was also bought, probably in the 1820s, by James Morrison.

149 The Forest of Bere Turner's gallery 1808
Oil on canvas, 35 × 47 (89 × 119.5)
Inscr. '. . . Turner R.A. . . .'
Exh: Turner's gallery 1808
H.M. Treasury and the National Trust, from Petworth House (39)

The identification with the Petworth picture, which has also been called, among other things, 'Evening: the Drinking Pool', is made certain by the description in *The Review of Publications of Art*, probably by John Landseer. *The Examiner* for 8 May 1808 confirms that 'At Mr Turner's private Gallery the Forest of Bere has been bought by the Earl of Egremont'. The picture shows men barking chestnut branches for caulking and tanning, an important activity on Lord Egremont's estate.

The picture, like many at Petworth, has alas, suffered from injudicious cleaning in the past, so it is particularly interesting to note that the *Review of Publications* described this picture as 'rich, golden-toned' and said that it glowed 'with a warmer sun than any other picture in the room: yet it is not the tropical heat that Mr. Turner has here painted but the milder radiance of a warm English summer's evening'. It concluded by claiming that 'The pride of Cuyp . . . would be humbled, we conceive, by a too near approach to this picture of Turner'. It is interesting to find a contemporary review appreciating the new feeling for light that was already apparent in 'Sun rising through Vapour' of the previous year (National Gallery, London, 479).

The painting, despite its debt to Gainsborough and Dutch landscape painters, also shows a return to Turner's interest in atmosphere and light that had characterised such works of the later 1790s as 'Buttermere Lake'. One is probably justified in seeing this 'return to nature' as the result of a new campaign of painting in oils out-of-doors, resulting in the two groups of Thames sketches, large and small. Turner would have passed through the Forest of Bere, a few miles north of Havant, on his way to Portsmouth in October 1807 to see the arrival of the Danish ships captured at the Battle of Copenhagen (the subject of the large painting first exhibited, unfinished, at Turner's gallery also in 1808; Tate Gallery 481). There is a drawing related to the white horse in the 'River' sketchbook, probably also done in 1807 (T.B.XCVI-45ᵛ).

150 Tabley, the Seat of Sir J. F. Leicester, Bart: Windy Day R.A.1809
Oil on canvas, 36 × 47½ (91.5 × 120.5)
Inscr. bottom right: 'J M W Turner RA'
Exh: R.A. 1809 (105); Sir John Leicester's Gallery 1819 (68)
Lt Col J. L. B. Leicester-Warren, T.D.

151 Tabley, Cheshire, the Seat of Sir J. F. Leicester, Bart: Calm Morning R.A.1809
Oil on canvas, 36 × 46 (91.5 × 117)
Inscr. bottom right: 'J M W Turner RA'
Exh: R.A. 1809 (146); Sir John Leicester's Gallery 1819 (43)
H.M. Treasury and the National Trust, from Petworth House (8)

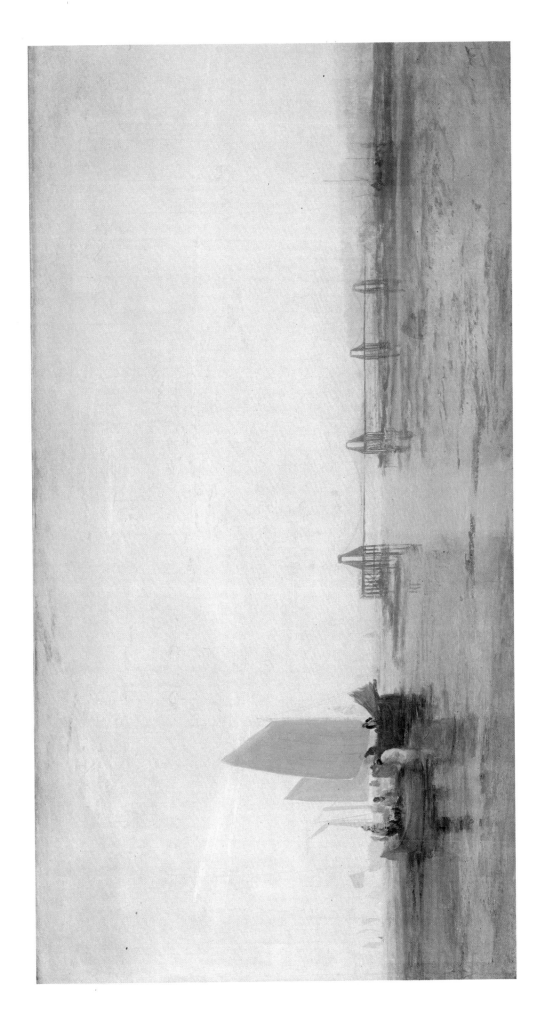

328 **The Old Chain Pier, Brighton** c.1828 (entry on p.105)

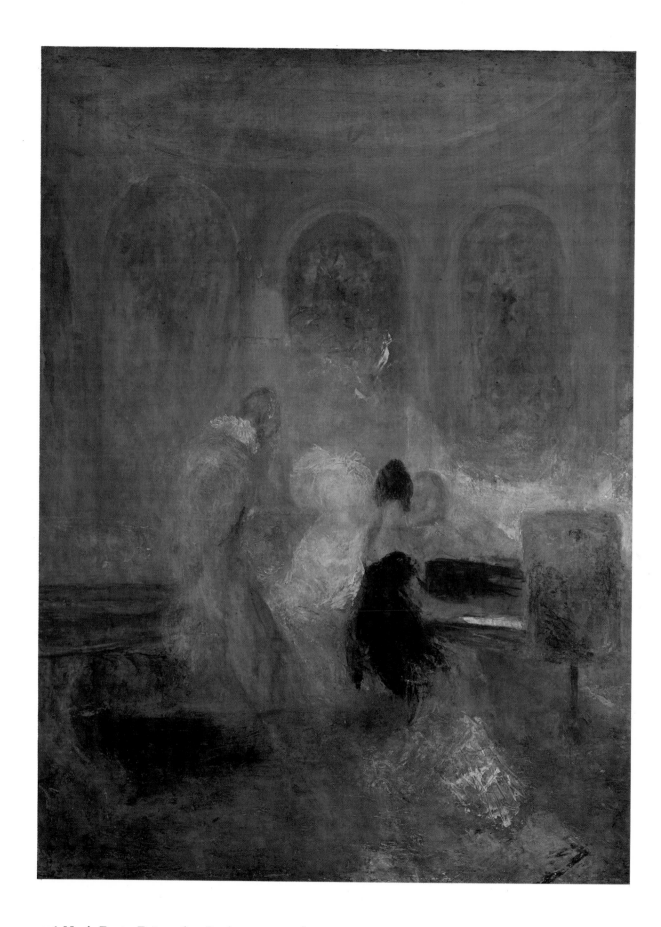

336 **Music Party, Petworth** *c.*1835 (entry on p.110)

These two views of his seat, Tabley House, near Knutsford, Cheshire, were commissioned by Sir John Leicester. Turner went there in the summer of 1808. According to Farington, writing on 11 February 1809, 'Calcott [the painter Sir Augustus Wall Callcott, R.A., 1779–1844] told me Turner while He was at Sir John Leicester's last Summer painted two pictures for Sir John, views of Tabley, of His 250 *guineas* size, yet Thomson [Henry Thomson, R.A., 1773–1843] who was there said, That His time was occupied in *fishing* rather than painting'. There are a number of drawings of the house in the 'Tabley' sketchbooks Nos.1 and 3 (T.B.CIII–15ᵛ and 16 (close to No.151 though lacking the water-tower; repr. Wilkinson 1974, p.92) and T.B.CV–7, 8 and 17, the last (repr. Wilkinson 1974, p.95) being a sketch of the composition of No.150) but it is not clear whether Turner actually painted the finished oils there. The 'Tabley' sketchbook No.1 also includes a finished oil sketch of the house from the same general viewpoint (though without the water-tower) that has been cut out and folded as if for dispatch through the post (T.B.CIII–18, repr. E. T. Cook, *Hidden Treasures at the National Gallery, A Selection of Studies and Drawings by J. M. W. Turner, R.A.*, 1905, p.34; see No.118).

Turner would have felt the challenge of Wilson's view of Tabley, painted for Sir John's father, just as in 1814 James Ward responded to the challenge of Turner's paintings, and was only paid £150 for his picture (see exhibition catalogue *Landscape in Britain*, Tate Gallery 1973–4, Nos.40 and 219, the Wilson and Ward pictures repr.). At the de Tabley sale in 1827 only No.151 was sold, being bought by Lord Egremont for 165 guineas.

The pictures were well received by the critics, again in terms that reveal some understanding of Turner's new feeling for light. Anthony Pasquin in *The Morning Herald*, 4 May 1809, having ended his attack on 'The Garreteer's Petition' in verse (see No.134), was able to

. . . satisfactorily exclaim

Joseph, William, Mallord, is himself again!

He goes on, speaking of No.151, 'the Artist has evidently taken Cuyp for his study and it is but just to aver, that he has preserved the aerial perspective better than any other Artist within our remembrance, at least in this country. There is such *repose* in the whole composition . . .'. The success of these pictures led to further commissions, from Lord Egremont for 'Cockermouth Castle', exhibited at Turner's gallery in 1810, and 'Petworth, Sussex, the Seat of the Earl of Egremont: Dewy Morning', R.A. 1810, both now at Petworth, and from Lord Lonsdale for two views of 'Lowther Castle, Westmorland', also shown at the R.A. in 1810 and still at Lowther; see also No.158.

One or other of these pictures was also exhibited at the Liverpool Academy in 1811 (9), as 'View of Tabley, the seat of Sir John Leicester, Bart'.

152 London Turner's gallery 1809
Canvas, 35½ × 47¼ (90 × 120)
Inscr. bottom right: 'J M W Turner RA PP [?]
1809'
Exh: Turner's gallery 1809 (16)
Tate Gallery (483)

Exhibited in Turner's gallery in 1809 with the following

verses:
Where burthen'd Thames reflects the crowded sail,
Commercial care and busy toil prevail,
Whose murky veil, aspiring to the skies,
Obscures thy beauty, and thy form denies,
Save where thy spires pierce the doubtful air,
As gleams of hope amidst a world of care.

There is a preliminary drawing for the whole composition in the British Museum (T.B.CXX–N, repr. Finberg 1910, pl.30), and also some related studies of deer in the 'Thames from Reading to Walton' sketchbook (T.B.XCV–43, 44). The composition was engraved for the *Liber Studiorum*, R.26, and published 1 January 1811, as 'in the possession of Walter Fawkes, Esq, of Farnley', who however returned it to the artist at some unknown date in exchange for another work (Thornbury 1862, I, p.293).

The signature is inscribed in brown; the date, to the left and slightly higher, more carefully in black, perhaps on the picture's return to Turner; it is painted on a distinctly thinner area of paint. The letters 'PP', of which traces seem to remain at the end of the signature, would stand for Professor of Perspective at the Royal Academy, a post to which Turner was elected in December 1807 (see p.181). Unevenly discoloured retouchings in the sky were removed in 1973; in particular the heavy plume of smoke rising just to the right of the right-hand dome of Greenwich Hospital was found not to be original.

Turner has taken one of the classic views of English art, painted innumerable times from the seventeenth century onwards, and transformed it with his sense of atmosphere. At the same time this wide panoramic view, full of incident, is held together in a carefully controlled composition based on a criss-cross of diagonals and the sweeping curve of the Thames. Even the rising plumes of smoke, seen by Ruskin as particularly characteristic of Turner's pictures, play their part.

153 Guardship at the Great Nore, Sheerness, &c.
Turner's gallery 1809
Oil on canvas, 36 × 49 (91.5 × 124.5)
Inscr. bottom right: 'J M W Turner RA [?]'
Exh: Turner's gallery 1809 (11); ?Turner's gallery 1810 (7); Society of British Artists 1834 (33)
Major General E. H. Goulburn, D.S.O.

Turner exhibited no fewer than three sea-pieces set in the Thames Estuary at his gallery in 1808 and three more the following year and the year after that (to say nothing of the large 'Spithead: Boat crew recovering an anchor' first exhibited in 1808 as showing Portsmouth but re-named for the Academy exhibition in 1809 to conceal the original subject of the captured Danish ships, the Danes having now become allies). The 1808 exhibits, the titles of which are known from the *Review of Publications of Art*, were 'Purfleet and the Essex Shore, as seen from Long Reach', which was bought by Lord Essex, 'The Confluence of the Thames and Medway', now at Petworth (665), and 'Sheerness as seen from the Nore', the rather larger picture, 41½ × 59 in, probably bought by Samuel Dobree and now in the Loyd collection (see Leslie Parris *The Loyd Collection* 1967, p.42, No.60, repr.). The 1809 works, known from Turner's printed catalogue, the first to survive,

152

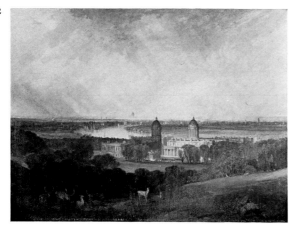

153

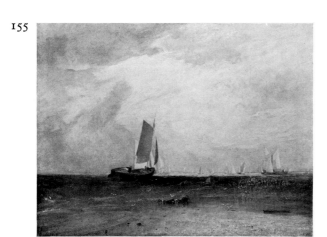

155

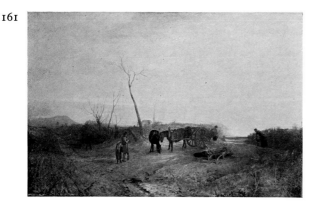

161

were Nos.153, 155, and 'Shoeburyness Fishermen hailing a Whitstable Hoy', bought by Walter Fawkes and now in the National Gallery of Canada. The 1810 works, 'Blythe Sands' (No.155), 'Sheerness, from the Great Nore' and 'Shoeburyness, Essex', may all have been those shown the year before, but there is a further example, in the larger 42¾ × 56½ in format, in the National Gallery of Art, Washington (what seems to have been the large 'Spithead' also reappeared this year). A letter from Turner to Sir John Leicester of 2 December 1810, headed by a slight pen and ink sketch that shows he is referring to No.153, gives it yet another title, 'Old Sandwich, G. Ship at the Nore'.

Though the compositions of this group are a development of the grand sea-pieces of 1801 and 1802 by way of 'The "Victory" beating up the Channel on its Return from Trafalgar', probably shown at Turner's gallery in 1806, and the large so-called 'Spithead', the immediate inspiration of this unmatched concentration on an only slightly varied theme seems to have been Turner's activity making sketches on the Thames. Just as the group of large oil sketches includes two estuary scenes (No.154 and Tate Gallery 2698) as well as views on the river above London, so too does the 'Hesperides' sketchbook include drawings and watercolours of both estuary and river subjects (for the estuary subjects see T.B.XCIII–16 (a sketch for the Washington picture), 17–18ᵛ, 41). There are further Thames Estuary drawings in the 'River and Margate' sketchbook (T.B.XCIX; see especially 25, 31, 56ᵛ–59ᵛ, the last inscribed 'Guardship at the Nore' but not specifically related to No.153). The finished pictures show an endless variety of skies and weather conditions, and also endless permutations and combinations of ships, large and small; Turner perhaps used his models as well as observation on the spot (see No.B77).

154 Shipping at the Mouth of the Thames
c.1807–8
Oil on canvas, 33¾ × 46 (86 × 117)
Tate Gallery (2702)

One of the group of large oil sketches of Thames subjects from the Turner Bequest (see Nos.143–6). However, even though some of the sketches may have been painted on the spot, it is difficult to imagine Turner managing a canvas of this size in the middle of the Thames Estuary. As in most of the finished oils discussed under No.153 the distant town appears to be Sheerness, but none of the details of this sketch are repeated in the finished works. It is presumably therefore an essay on the same theme done before Turner turned to painting it for exhibition, which supports the traditional dating of c.1807 or 1808 at the latest.

155 Fishing upon the Blythe-Sand, Tide
setting in Turner's gallery 1809
Oil on canvas, 35 × 47 (89 × 119.5)
Exh: Turner's gallery 1809 (7); Turner's gallery 1810 (4); R.A. 1815 (6); Plymouth 1815
Tate Gallery (496)

The title given above is that of the 1809 exhibition catalogue. In 1810 it was called simply 'Blythe Sand', but at the R.A. in 1815 'Bligh Sand, near Sheerness: Fishing Boats trawling'. The picture is the distillation of the elements of the other Thames Estuary pictures (see Nos.153 and 154). Neither the different types of shipping nor the town on the distant shore are of interest any more, only the everyday activity of fishing, paralleling that of ploughing up turnips in 'Slough', and the mood of sea and sky under particular weather conditions.

As in the case of the more conventional Thames Estuary pictures there is a related oil sketch among the large Thames sketches, even less specific and with no precise details in common (Tate Gallery 2698). There is also a wash drawing at the British Museum, closer in the placing of the nearest sailing boat but again not exactly the same (T.B.CXX–Q).

The picture is one of the four mentioned, presumably as available for sale, in a letter to Sir John Leicester of 12 December 1810, accompanied by slight pen sketches of the subjects. According to Thornbury Turner had 'the proud pleasure of refusing to sell "this picture" to his old enemy Sir John [*sic* for George] Beaumont' (1862, I, p.297).

156 Ploughing up Turnips, near Slough
Turner's gallery 1809
Oil on canvas, 40⅛ × 51¼ (102 × 130)
Exh: Turner's gallery 1809 (9)
Tate Gallery (486)

Often known as 'Windsor', even in the schedule of the Turner Bequest; Turner's somewhat perverse title suggests that for him the agricultural activity in the foreground was more interesting than the royal castle that looms through the haze behind. The contrast with the earlier 'Windsor Castle from the Thames' at Petworth (No.80) could not be more marked and stresses the revolution in Turner's approach to landscape in the few years that had elapsed.

Turner made innumerable studies at and around Windsor. In the 'Windsor and Eton' sketchbook there is a small sketch from the same viewpoint and related but not exactly corresponding drawings of cows and figures (T.B.XCVII–2; 22, 87, 89 etc; 27, 81ᵛ, 82ᵛ, etc; examples repr. Wilkinson 1974, p.82).

157 Dorchester Mead, Oxfordshire
*c.*1810
Oil on canvas, 40 × 51¼ (101.5 × 130)
Exh: ?Turner's gallery 1810 (12)
Tate Gallery (485)

Catalogued in the George Hibbert sale at Christie's on 13 June 1829 (24), where it was bought back by Turner for £120.15.0, as 'Abingdon, taken from the River – Cattle cooling themselves, Group of Lighters in half-distance, figures loading a Timber Waggon on right Bank, Sultry Sun in Mist', and listed in the schedule of the Turner Bequest as 'Abingdon', this picture nevertheless seems to be the otherwise lost 'Dorchester Mead' exhibited by Turner at his own gallery in 1810. The title is somewhat misleading in that Dorchester Mead is some two miles from Abingdon church, the spire of which is seen in the distance, but not much more perverse than the title of the picture to which it may well have been intended as the companion, 'Slough', exhibited the year before (No.156). There is a pencil sketch in the 'Hesperides (2)' sketchbook (T.B.XCIV–4ᵛ, repr. Wilkinson 1974, p.74).

158 Somer-Hill, near Tunbridge, The Seat of W. F. Woodgate, Esq. R.A.1811 (repr. on p.18)
Oil on canvas, 36 × 48 (91.5 × 122)
Exh: R.A. 1811 (177)
Trustees of the National Gallery of Scotland

In April 1810 John Fuller asked Turner to make three or four watercolours in and around his seat, Rosehill Park, Sussex (see No.142), and it was probably on this same trip that Turner drew the view of Somer Hill in the 'Vale of Heathfield' sketchbook (T.B.CXXXVII–3ᵛ and 4; see No.130). The painting does not seem to have been a commission; its early history is unknown until 1851, when it was sold from the collection of J. Alexander.

This painting is probably the most exquisite example of Turner's transformation of the tradition of the topographical house-portrait. The house itself is pushed into the extreme background, but every device of lighting and composition makes it the focal point of the picture. A pentimento shows that Turner continued to modify his composition up to the last moment: the bank in the left foreground has been raised to prevent the tunnel-like effect of the avenue of trees beyond the lake from dragging the eye into depth too abruptly.

159 View of the High-Street, Oxford
Turner's gallery 1810
Oil on canvas, 27 × 39¼ (68.5 × 99.5)
Inscr. bottom right: 'J M W Turner R A'
Exh: Turner's gallery 1810 (3); R.A. 1812 (161)
C. L. Loyd, Esq.

160 View of Oxford, from the Abingdon Road
R.A.1812
Oil on canvas, 26 × 38½ (66 × 97.5)
Exh: R.A. 1812 (169)
Private collection

The 'View of the High-Street' was commissioned by the Oxford dealer and frame-maker James Wyatt in November 1809 as the basis for an engraving. Late in December Turner went to Oxford to make a drawing, perhaps that now in the British Museum though this was probably done considerably earlier and lacks the buildings in the immediate foreground, having been taken from slightly further west (T.B.CXX–F). The picture was finished in March 1810, sent to Oxford before 6 April but returned in time for the opening of Turner's gallery on 7 May. Some alterations were made to the figures and the spire of St. Mary's was raised at Wyatt's request. It was subsequently engraved by John Pye and S. Middiman, with figures by C. Heath, and published by Wyatt on 14 March 1812. A smaller print by W. E. Albutt was published in Paris in 1828.

The later companion picture of 'Oxford from the Abingdon Road', also commissioned by Wyatt, was painted between Christmas 1811 and April 1812, in time to be shown with the other at the Academy in 1812. It was engraved by Pye and Heath and published by Wyatt on 13 February 1818. There is a large annotated pencil drawing of the composition in the British Museum (T.B.CXCV(a)–A), said by Finberg to be watermarked 1814 (1909, I, p.597); if so, it was presumably done for the engraving.

As in the case of 'Hannibal crossing the Alps' Turner had trouble over the hanging of these two pictures at the Academy in 1812. On 13 April he wrote to

Wyatt that 'Your Pictures are hung at the Academy, but not to my satisfaction'. He suggested that he should withdraw them and show them at his own gallery or the British Institution the following year, but left the final decision to Wyatt who presumably preferred them to remain in order to help the sale of the engravings'. The *St. James' Chronicle* for 23–26 May, after reviewing 'Hannibal', mentioned that 'Mr. Turner has three other fine views', these two and the later version of the second Bonneville picture (see No.74).

For later watercolours of Oxford High Street see Nos.443–7.

161 Frosty Morning R.A.1813
Oil on canvas, 44¾ × 68¾ (113.5 × 174.5)
Exh: R.A. 1813 (15); Turner's gallery 1835
Tate Gallery (492)

Exhibited with the following line from Thomson's *Seasons*:

The rigid hoar frost melts before his beam.

According to the younger Trimmer the picture immortalised Turner's 'old crop-eared bay horse, or rather a cross between a horse and a pony'. 'The "Frost Piece" was one of his favourites . . . He said he was travelling by coach in Yorkshire, and sketched it *en route*' (Thornbury 1862, I, p.170).

The picture was praised in *The Morning Chronicle* for 3 May 1813 and, more significantly, by Constable's great patron Archdeacon Fisher who singled it out as the only picture to be preferred to Constable's in the exhibition: 'But then you need not repine at this decision of mine; you are a great man like Bounaparte & are only beat by a frost' (R. B. Beckett (ed.), *John Constable's Correspondence*, VI, 1968, p.21). In May 1818 Turner offered the picture to Dawson Turner for 350 guineas, but it was never sold.

Just as 'Blythe Sands' represents the ultimate fining down of the early Thames Estuary sea-pieces to their basic elements, so too does 'Frosty Morning' in relation to the earlier naturalistic landscapes. Here, on a grander scale than usual, Turner concentrates on the simplest elements of countrymen at work on a cold early morning; any feature of picturesque or topographical interest has been omitted.

6. Synthesis 1814–19

The middle of the second decade of the century saw a synthesis of Turner's previous discoveries and strivings in a series of masterpieces. 'Crossing the Brook', an English scene painted with all the sensitivity of Turner's studies on the Thames but composed in the manner of Claude, typifies this. In the large watercolour of 'Tivoli' (No.181) Turner demonstrated his command of Italianate landscape and prepared himself, as it were, for his first visit to Italy in 1819.

162 Apullia in Search of Apullus – Vide Ovid
B.I.1814
Oil on canvas, 57½ × 93⅞ (146 × 239)
Inscr. bottom left: 'Appulia in Search of Appullus learns from the Swain the Cause of his Metamorphosis', and 'Appulus' on the tree.
Exh: British Institution 1814 (South Room 168); Turner's gallery 1835
Tate Gallery (495)

The reference in the title 'Vide Ovid' refers to his *Metamorphoses*, Book XIV of which contains the story of the transformation of the Apulian shepherd. In Garth's translation this became the transformation of 'Appulus', and Turner seems to have invented a mythical wife 'Apullia', to whom the swain points out the name 'Appulus' carved on the tree.

The painting was submitted for the British Institution's annual competition for a work 'proper in Point of Subject and Manner to be a Companion' to a landscape by Claude or Poussin, and is almost a copy of Lord Egremont's Claude of 'Jacob with Laban and his Daughters' (repr. exhibition catalogue *Pictures and*

Works of Art from Petworth House, Wildenstein's, 1954, No.6); Thornbury even suggests that it was painted as a pendant for Lord Egremont (1862, I, p.296). Turner has varied the architectural forms and some of the figures, but all the main elements of the composition are the same. Turner failed to win the premium because, as has been recently discovered, the picture did not arrive on time.

William Hazlitt, writing in the *Morning Chronicle* for 5 February 1814, found Turner's dependence on Claude an advantage. 'All the taste and all the imagination being borrowed, his powers of eye, hand, and memory, are equal to any thing'. He attacked the figures as even worse than Claude's and found 'the utter want of a capacity to draw a distinct outline with the force, the depth, the fulness, and precision of this artist's eye for colour . . . truly astonishing'.

There are composition sketches in the 'Woodcock Shooting' and 'Chemistry and Apuleia' sketchbooks and a drawing for the group of figures in the latter (T.B.CXXIX–41 and CXXXV–66ᵛ–68ᵛ; and CXXXV–65ᵛ and 66). The composition was engraved for the *Liber Studiorum*, R.72, but never published.

163 The Eruption of the Souffrier Mountains, in the Island of St. Vincent, at Midnight, on the 30th April, 1812, from a Sketch taken at the Time by Hugh P. Keane, Esq. R.A.1815
Oil on canvas, 31¼ × 41¼ (79.5 × 105)
Exh: R.A. 1815 (258)
University of Liverpool

Exhibited in 1815 with the following lines, presumably from the *Fallacies of Hope*, but not attributed to them:

Then in stupendous horror grew
The red volcano to the view,
And shook in thunders of its own,
While the blaz'd hill in lightnings shone,
   Scattering their arrows round.
As down its sides of liquid flame
The devastating cataract came,
With melting rocks, and crackling woods,
And mingled roar of boiling floods,
   And roll'd along the ground!

As well as using a drawing made by an amateur on the spot Turner probably read the long account in the *Gentleman's Magazine* for October 1812. The explosion was a particularly violent one and could be heard over a hundred miles away, the Barbados Islands being covered with dust. See also No.B116. Volcanoes had been painted fairly frequently in the eighteenth century, among others by Wright of Derby, and would have had a special appeal to Turner although he did not see one until he went to Italy in 1819 (but see No.184).

The suitability of the subject for Turner was recognised by the *Repository of the Arts* for June 1815. 'It appears that there is no record existing of a volcanic irruption on so mighty a scale as this of St. Vincent. Those who were on the ocean supposed the whole island was destroyed, and this opinion lasted for several days. To represent the grand phenomena of nature in painting, requires the powers of a mind like that of Mr. Turner, whose daring flights have often surprised the connoisseur. This wonderful effort of his pencil is said, by those who witnessed the effects of the eruption of the Souffrier mountains, to convey a faithful resemblance of the awful scene.'

The picture was engraved by Charles Turner but apparently never published, an inscription on a tinted copy in the British Museum suggesting that it was done privately for 'a gentleman who took it – copper-plate, impressions and all, abroad with him.' The early history of the painting is not known.

164   Crossing the Brook R.A.1815

   Oil on canvas, 76 × 65 (193 × 165)
   Exh: R.A. 1815 (94); Turner's gallery 1835
   Tate Gallery (497)

This highly Italianate, Claudian landscape is in fact a product of Turner's visit to Devon in 1813 (see Nos. 124–6), as was recognised in a review known from a press-cutting in the Victoria and Albert Museum, annotated 5 May 1815 but without the name of the publication: 'Notwithstanding the buildings are Italian, the scene is found in Devonshire.' Further evidence comes from two people who were with Turner for part of this tour. Cyrus Redding 'traced three distinct snatches of scenery on the river Tamar' when he saw the picture later in Turner's gallery and mentions how 'Turner was struck with admiration at the bridge above the Wear, which he declared altogether Italian'. According to Charles Eastlake, 'The bridge . . . is Calstock Bridge; some mining works are indicated in the middle distance. The extreme distance extends to the mouth of the Tamar, the harbour of Hamoaze, the hills of Mount Edgcumbe, and those on the opposite side of Plymouth Sound. The whole scene is extremely faithful' (Thorn-

bury 1862, I, pp.210–11, 219). There are drawings of the countryside represented but not actually copied in the picture in the 'Plymouth, Hamoaze' sketchbook (T.B.CXXXI), and a small composition sketch in the 'Woodcock Shooting' sketchbook (T.B.CXXIX–52), but the composition is really a development of one of Turner's paintings of classical subjects in an Italian setting, the 'Mercury and Hersé' exhibited at the Royal Academy in 1811 (sold at Christie's 16 June 1961 (65), where repr., bought by Agnew's). Here however the foreground is occupied merely by an unpretentious genre scene.

The painting was well received in the press but Sir George Beaumont was not mollified by its traditional appearance, Farington reporting him as saying on 5 June 1815 that 'it appeared to Him *weak* and like the work of an Old man, one who no longer saw or felt colour properly; it was all of *peagreen* insipidity'. Referring bitterly to 'the Portrait Painters who are particularly loud in their praise' he could only repeat 'that I never knew a Portrait Painter excepting Sir Joshua Reynolds who had a right feeling and judgment of Landscape Painting'. Perhaps because of the criticism from this influential connoisseur Turner failed to sell the picture, though Dawson Turner asked about it in 1818 when the price was 550 guineas.

165   The Decline of the Carthaginian Empire – Rome being determined on the Overthrow of her Hated Rival, demanded from her such Terms as might force her into War, or ruin her by Compliance: the Enervated Carthaginians, in their Anxiety for Peace, consented to give up their Arms and their Children R.A.1817   (repr. on p.35)

   Oil on canvas, 67 × 94 (170 × 239)
   Exh: R.A. 1817 (195); Turner's gallery 1835
   Tate Gallery (499)

In 1815 Turner had exhibited 'Dido building Carthage; or the Rise of the Carthaginian Empire' (National Gallery, London, 498). This picture of two years later shows the end of the story, Turner's verses for the catalogue stressing the significance of the setting sun:

****** At Hope's delusive smile,
The chieftain's safety and the mother's pride,
Were to th'insidious conqu'ror's grasp resign'd;
While o'er the western wave th'esanguin'd sun,
In gathering haze a stormy signal spread,
And set portentous.

John Gage (1974, pp.41–4) has pointed out that such comparisons of the rise and fall of empires, and their application to the contemporary situation, were a commonplace in the late eighteenth and early nineteenth centuries, as in Oliver Goldsmith's *Roman History* and Edward Gibbon's *Decline and Fall of the Roman Empire* (both writers had been Professor of Ancient History at the Royal Academy). The then well-known guide to Italy, J. C. Eustace's *Classical Tour through Italy* of 1813, even draws the parallel between Carthage and England. Claude's paintings had been interpreted in a similar way, the two pictures at Longford Castle having been engraved in 1772 as 'The Landing of Aeneas in Italy: The Allegorical Morning of the Roman Empire' and 'Roman Edifices in Ruins: the Allegorical Evening of the Empire'. Turner's two large Claudian harbour scenes seem therefore to have been deliberate essays in this tradition.

Contemporary reviews do not, however, seem to have noted any connection between the two pictures though, with rare exceptions, they were high in praise of both. The *Repository of Arts* for June 1817 even praised Turner's verses: 'The awful description of the setting sun, so exquisitely described by the poet in the three last lines of the extract above, has been chiefly attended to by Mr. Turner; and never has so bold an attempt been crowned with greater success. . . . The colouring of every part of the picture is full of extreme richness. . . . It is impossible to pass over the execution of the architectural parts of this picture: they are drawn with purity and correctness; the Grecian orders are carefully preserved, and the arrangement of the buildings in perspective is formed with so much adherence to geometrical rule, that the eye is carried through the immense range of magnificent edifices with such rapidity, that we entirely forget the artist, and merely dwell on the historic vision. Mr. Turner has here embodied the whole spirit of Virgil's poetical description of the event, its awful grandeur, and solemnity of effect.' The *Annals of the Fine Arts* wrote 'Mr. Turner has only one, but that one is a lion, . . . excelling in the higher qualities of art, mind and poetical conception, even Claude himself'.

In an earlier issue of the *Annals* the critic John Bailey had already said that 'I wish the Directors of the British Institution would purchase it. When shall we see a National Gallery, where the works of the old masters and the select pictures of the British school, may be placed by the side of each other in fair competition, then would the higher branches of painting be properly encouraged?'. Could this have been the inspiration to Turner to bequeath two of his paintings to hang next to two Claudes in the National Gallery? In his first will, drawn up in 1829 five years after the National Gallery first opened at 100 Pall Mall, Turner left the two Carthage pictures to be 'placed by the side of Claude's "Sea Port" and "Mill" that is to hang on the same line same height from the ground'; later, in 1831, 'The Decline of Carthage' was replaced by the earlier painting 'Sun Rising through Vapour' (R.A. 1807; National Gallery 473).

There are composition sketches in the 'Yorkshire No.1' sketchbook (T.B.CXLIV–101ᵛ (repr. Reynolds 1969, pl.68) and 102ᵛ) and perhaps also in the 'Hastings to Margate' sketchbook (T.B.CXL–73ᵛ), and studies for the architectural setting in the 'Hints River' sketchbook (T.B.CXLI–32ᵛ and 33).

166 Entrance of the Meuse: Orange-Merchant on the Bar, going to Pieces; Brill Church bearing S.E. by S., Masensluys E. by S. R.A.1819

Oil on canvas, 69 × 97 (175 × 246.5)
Exh: R.A. 1819 (136)
Tate Gallery (501)

More or less the subject of 'The Wreck of a Transport Ship' (No.83) reinterpreted following Turner's first experience of Dutch light on his journey to and from the Rhine in 1817, this is one of a series of large coast or harbour scenes in Northern Europe painted in a style and tonality that owes much to Cuyp. The first is the

'Dort' exhibited the previous year (Mellon collection), and it was followed by 'Harbour of Dieppe (changement de domicile)', R.A. 1825, and 'Cologne, the Arrival of a Packet Boat. Evening', R.A. 1826 (both in the Frick Collection, New York). This example is particularly notable for its high key and almost obsessive variety of cloud formations. The title embodies a typical pun, the 'Orange Merchant' not only hailing from the country once ruled by the House of Orange but having spilled its cargo of oranges. 'Masensluys' is Maassluis, the other side of the Maas from Brill.

The picture was singled out for praise in the *Repository of Arts* for June 1819 in a review beginning 'To speak of the extraordinary powers of this artist would indeed be a work of superogation', though the *Annals of the Fine Arts* for the year found it 'Too scattered and frittered in its parts to be reckoned among Turner's happiest productions. Compared with himself, this picture suffers, – compared with others, it maintains Turner's rank uninjured'. It was the first Turner to be seen be the young Samuel Palmer and made an indelible impression upon him. See also No.188.

167 England: Richmond Hill, on the Prince Regent's Birthday R.A.1819

Oil on canvas, 70⅞ × 131¾ (180 × 335)
Exh: R.A. 1819 (206); Turner's gallery 1835
Tate Gallery (502)

Exhibited with the following lines, attributed to Thomson:

Which way, Amanda, shall we bend our course?
The choice perplexes. Wherefore should we chuse?
All is the same with thee. Say, shall we wind
Along the streams? or walk the smiling mead?
Or court the forest-glades? or wander wild
Among the waving harvests? or ascend,
While radiant Summer opens all its pride,
Thy Hill, delightful Shene?

The large size of this picture is all the more surprising in view of its domestic, pastoral subject. Like the later 'What you will!' (No.307), this may reflect in part the effect of French eighteenth-century painting: Jerold Ziff has pointed out that several of the figures are based on a sketch in the 'Hints River' sketchbook after Watteau's 'L'Ile Enchantée' (T.B.CXLI–26ᵛ and 27; see Ziff's review of Gage 1969 in *Art Bulletin*, LIII, 1971, p.126). The same sketchbook also contains drawings of the general view from Richmond Hill, a gift to the Claudian artist and next in popularity in the eighteenth and nineteenth centuries to that from Greenwich Park (10ᵛ–13). For other versions of this view see Nos.174, 256, 257, 434 and T.B.CCLXIII–348 (repr. in colour in Wilkinson 1974, p.30).

The Turner Bequest also contains an unfinished oil of the same view in Turner's normal large format, 58 × 93¾ in (Tate Gallery 5546). There are only a few figures in the foreground and the painting was presumably abandoned when Turner turned to the unprecedented scale of the finished picture, perhaps inspired by the idea of doing homage to the Prince Regent, a possible and highly desirable patron.

This is the first of Turner's Royal Academy exhibits in connection with which there is some hint at his activities on the three 'varnishing days', granted to Academicians to give final touches to their pictures

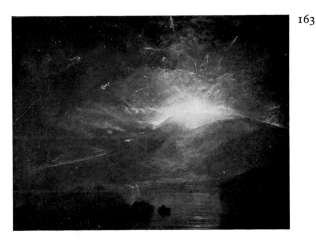

163

before the exhibition opened to the public. On 2 May 1819 Farington recorded criticism of the effect of 'the flaming colour of Turner's pictures' on their neighbours, immediately following this with a reference to 'the pernicious effects arising from Painters working upon their pictures in the Exhibition by which they often render them unfit for a private room' (unpublished; see Gage 1969, p.167). The *Repository of the Arts* for June 1819, though liking the picture less than 'Entrance of the Meuse', praised 'the fore-ground beautifully worked up, and the azure blue of the distances modified in all the gradations of aerial perspective'. The *Annals of the Fine Arts*, on the other hand, recommended Turner 'to pummice it down, give it a coat of priming, and paint such another picture as his building of Carthage' (R.A. 1815; National Gallery 498).

William Bernard COOKE (1778–1855) after TURNER

168 Plymouth Dock seen from Mount Edgecumbe 1816

Engraving, proof, $6\frac{5}{16} \times 9\frac{5}{8}$ (16×24.3) cut inside plate-mark

Inscr. on left: 'Drawn by J. M. W. Turner R.A.'; on right: 'Engraved by W. B. Cooke 1816' and 'Plymouth Dock from Mount Edgecumbe'; below, with MS notes in W. B. Cooke's hand: 'Touched by Turner with his remarks, sent by Post from Mr Fawkes's seat in Yorkshire – W. B. Cooke'; and in Turner's hand on left: 'too strong in tone all above the pencil line make lighter'; 'X Houses [sketch], Lines of Fortifications'; 'Line of Horizon'; 'the distance and the sky more blended by the [sketch] hill'; on right: 'Sheep too White', and below, 'I will talk to you about Hastings when I return which will not now be long – can you make the Fiddle more distinct' [sketch]

Trustees of the British Museum (1861-5-18-99)

This proof of 'Plymouth Dock' (Rawlinson No.99) was folded and addressed on the back to 'Mr W B Cooke, 12 York Place Penton-ville London', postmarked 'Otley 14 Sep 1816'; as Cooke notes, Turner made his corrections while staying at Farnley. The plate was No.60 in Vol.II of Cooke's *Picturesque Views of the Southern Coast of England*; the drawing was on the market in London in 1973. The *Southern Coast* series consisted of eighty plates by several different engravers, principally William Bernard Cooke and his brother George. Forty of them were after watercolours by Turner, the remainder from designs by William Westall, Samuel Owen, Peter de Wint, William Havell, William Collins and others. They were issued in sixteen parts spasmodically between 1814 and 1826, but the completed series was bound into two volumes arranged topographically from Kent to Somerset. The series was the first of the extended sequences of designs for engraving which occupied much of Turner's maturity, culminating in the *Picturesque Views of England and Wales* (Nos. 417–34).

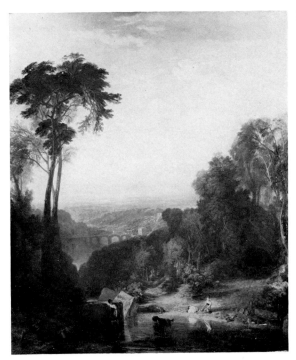

164

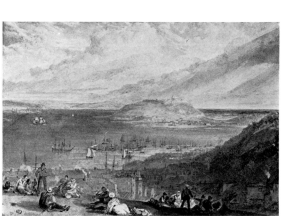

169

169 **Falmouth** *c.*1815
Watercolour with some bodycolour, sight $6 \times 9\frac{1}{16}$ (15.2 × 23)
Trustees of the Lady Lever Art Gallery, Port Sunlight (WHL 4507)
Engraved by W. B. Cooke for the *Southern Coast*, 1816 (Rawlinson 98). See No. 168.

170 **'Hastings' Sketchbook** 1816
Bound in boards, leather spine and corners
41 leaves, many blank including ff.7–15, the remainder drawn on in pencil, 5 × 8 (12.8 × 20.5)
Watermarked: 1815
Trustees of the British Museum (T.B.CXXXIX)

ff.19^{v}–20^{r} **Hythe**
Pencil

The book contains drawings relating to Cooke's *Southern Coast* and to the commission for views of Sussex by 'John' Fuller of Rosehill. ff.1 and 2 and 35^{v} to 41 have sketches made near Farnley. ff.3–6 have studies for a classical composition with many figures.

'Hythe' was used as the basis for the design for Cooke's *Southern Coast* (No.171). See No.168.

171 **Hythe, Kent** 1824
Watercolour, sight $5\frac{1}{2} \times 8\frac{15}{16}$ (14 × 22.7)
Guildhall Library and Art Gallery (1259)
Engraved by G. Cooke for *Picturesque Views of the Southern Coast*, 1824 (Rawlinson No.118). Based on the pencil sketch in the 'Hastings' sketchbook (T.B.CXXXIX–19^{v}, 20^{v}). The watercolour was evidently made several years after the sketch, since, according to Thornbury, Cooke paid Turner 10 guineas for it in 1824 (1862 Vol.II, p.424).

George COOKE (1781–1834) after TURNER
172 **Hythe, Kent** 1824
Engraving, first published state, $5\frac{15}{16} \times 9\frac{3}{16}$ (15.1 × 23.3); plate $9\frac{1}{2} \times 12\frac{1}{4}$ (24.2 × 31.3)
Inscr: 'Drawn by J. M. W. Turner, R.A.' on left, 'Engraved by George Cooke. 1824' on right, and 'Hythe, Kent' below
Trustees of the British Museum (1849-4-21-310)
The plate (Rawlinson No.118) appeared as No.5 of Vol.I in Cooke's *Picturesque Views of the Southern Coast of England.* The watercolour is No.171 and a pencil study No.170. Turner corrected the proofs of this plate from Farnley where he was staying in November 1824 (see also 'Plymouth Dock', No.168). One is annotated: 'You ask me for my opinion; first, I shall say in general, very good: secondly, the figures at Barracks, excellent, but I think you have cut up the bank called Shorncliff too much with the graver, by lines which are equal in strength and width and length that gives a coarseness to the quality, and do not look like my touches or your work . . . The marsh is all swamp; I want flickering lights upon it up to the sea, and although I have darkened the sea in part, yet you must not consider it to want strength but that the whole marsh and sea down to the Barracks lies dark and not clear; get it into one tone, flat by dots or some means, and let the sea and water only appear different by their present lines'. On a subsequent proof, Turner wrote: 'I fear you mistook my meaning, let the water be distinguishable only by its lines, therefore strengthen all the horizontal lines of the Sea which you have to do for I would prefer overtones to the lines [sketch] in the marsh. I do not want more work but filling in to make it flat, and a flickering light somewhat like the *Brixham* plate [Rawlinson No.111] where marked [sketch] too dark. I shall not want to see another proof but save me my No four and etching.'

173 **Plymouth** *c.*1824
Watercolour, $6\frac{1}{4} \times 9\frac{5}{8}$ (16 × 24.5)
Fundaçao Calouste Gulbenkian, Lisbon
Engraved in mezzotint by T. Lupton for the *Ports of England* (Rawlinson No.788), but the plate was not published until 1856 when it appeared in Gambart's *Harbours of England* (see No.243). Numerous pencil sketches of Plymouth occur in the 'Plymouth, Hamoaze' sketchbook (T.B.CXXXI).

174 **The Thames from Richmond Hill** ?*c.*1815
Pencil and watercolour, $7\frac{3}{8} \times 10\frac{7}{16}$ (18.8 × 27.1)
Trustees of the British Museum (T.B.CXCVII–B)
An unfinished watercolour study of the same view, dating from about 1795, is in the Turner Bequest, XXVII–K. Compare also the later compositions related to the 1825 and *England and Wales* designs (Nos.256–7 and 434). As Turner lived in the neighbourhood of Richmond he made many drawings of the famous view; numerous studies in the sketchbooks may or may not relate directly to particular watercolours. It is possible that the pencil study on f.76^{r} of the 'Hastings to Margate' sketchbook of *c.*1815 (T.B.CXL) was used for this watercolour.

175 **Sheet of Studies** ?*c.*1817
Watercolour, $17\frac{1}{2} \times 21\frac{7}{8}$ (44.5 × 55.5)
Trustees of the British Museum (T.B.CCLXIII–369)
Three separate landscape compositions on a large sheet which appears to have been folded down the centre, along the border common to all the designs. The largest is apparently a view of Hardraw Force. The finished watercolour of 'Hardraw Fall', made for *The History of Richmondshire* in about 1817, is now at the Fitzwilliam Museum (PD227–1961).

The motif of the outlined mansion or castle on the skyline recurs in a rough watercolour study, T.B. CCLXIII–380.

176 **Two Studies on One Sheet: a Cloudy Sky over the Sea; and a Stormy Landscape** ?*c.*1817
Watercolour, $19 \times 11\frac{7}{8}$ (48.2 × 30.2)
Trustees of the British Museum (T.B.CCCLXV–27a and b)
Compare these two studies (on one sheet of paper) with those in the 'Skies' sketchbook (No.177) and such 'colour-beginnings' as the 'Landscape with a low Hill and a Group of Trees' (No.178) and the sheet of studies connected with *The History of Richmondshire* (No.175).

177 **'Skies' Sketchbook** *c.*1818
Bound in white parchment
69 leaves, $5 \times 9\frac{3}{4}$ (12.4 × 24.6)
Watermarked: 1814
Trustees of the British Museum (T.B.CLVIII)

f.54ʳ Sunset with a Crescent Moon
Watercolour

The book contains a series of sky studies in watercolour, and some pencil sketches: f.69ᵛ, an interior which may be at Farnley; ff.67ᵛ–68ʳ, a view of London from Lambeth (not from Greenwich as suggested by Finberg, 1909 I, p.453); studies at Eton on 4 June and at Windsor. Turner was at Eton for the Fourth of June 1818: see Finberg 1961, pp.252–3.

178 Landscape with a Low Hill and a Group of Trees ?*c.*1817
Pencil and watercolour, approx. $11\frac{3}{16} \times 19\frac{1}{4}$ (30 × 48.5)
Trustees of the British Museum (T.B.CCLXIII–76)
Called by Finberg 'River Scene with Trees', this drawing appears to show an English view, possibly in Sussex. It is not clear that the central band of green is intended to represent water. The technique, using watercolour very unctuously and fluidly, is similar to that in some of the studies of skies dating from *c.*1817–20 in the 'Skies' sketchbook (No.177) and in certain 'colour-beginnings' probably associated with them.

179 Lancaster Sands *c.*1818
Watercolour, $11 \times 14\frac{7}{16}$ (28 × 36.6)
Exh: Grosvenor Place, 1818 (21); Leeds 1839 (77)
City Museums and Art Gallery, Birmingham
(*By courtesy of Mrs Keith*)
A drawing made in connection with the series of north country views executed *c.*1818 for Whitaker's *Richmondshire*, though not one of the engraved subjects. It was acquired by Walter Fawkes.

Turner made studies around Lancaster in the 'Yorkshire' sketchbook No.5 (T.B.CXLVII ff.32ʳ etc.) A different view on Lancaster sands was made *c.*1826 for inclusion in the *Picturesque Views in England and Wales* (No.419).

180 Kirby Lonsdale Churchyard *c.*1818
Watercolour, $11\frac{1}{8} \times 16\frac{5}{16}$ (28.6 × 41.5)
Private Collection
Engraved by C. Heath for Whitaker's *History of Richmondshire*, 1822, Vol II, p.277 (Rawlinson No.186). Turner had contributed subjects to Whitaker's earlier publications, the histories of Whalley, Craven and Leeds; *Richmondshire*, intended as part of a large work on Yorkshire as a whole which never materialised, was begun in 1817 and Turner's twenty illustrations appeared between 1819 and 1823. The book was a great success. Turner made extensive tours of the north of England in connection with the project, and the six 'Yorkshire' sketchbooks, T.B.CXLIV, CXLV, CXLVI, CXLVII, CXVLIII, CXLIX, in use between about 1815 and 1818, contain many of the *Richmondshire* and related subjects. A pencil sketch showing a view of Kirby Lonsdale is on f.58ʳ of the 'Yorkshire' sketchbook No.2 (T.B.CLXV); it is continued on f.58ᵛ with a note 'the Continuation of K. L. Cyd View', but the subject does not correspond with 'Kirby Lonsdale Churchyard'.

181 Landscape: Composition of Tivoli 1817
Watercolour, 26 × 40 (67.6 × 102)
Inscr. bottom right: 'I M W Turner 1817'
Exh: R.A. 1818 (474); Old Water-Colour Society (Loan Exhibition) 1823 (88)
Simon Day Esq.
Engraved by R. Goodall for John Allnutt, 1827 (Rawlinson No.207). This large watercolour was executed before Turner's first visit to Italy; hence the rather periphrastic title which exemplifies Turner's care in specifying the topography of his subjects – a habit instilled into him by his early training. The large 'colour-beginning' in the Turner Bequest (No.182) appears to be a preparatory study for this work. An account of Allnutt's sale in *The Times* of 20 June 1863 states that the drawing was 'painted especially for Mr Allnutt'.

A companion 'The Rise of the River Stour at Stourhead' is supposed to have been executed in the same year, but was not exhibited until 1825 (R.A.465). It is now untraced.

182 Colour-Beginning: Tivoli *c.*1817
Pencil and watercolour $26\frac{1}{8} \times 39\frac{3}{8}$ (66.4 × 100.1)
Trustees of the British Museum (T.B.CXCVII–A)
Evidently a design related to Turner's large 'Landscape – A Composition of Tivoli' No.181, though here the Temple of the Sibyl on the right has not yet made its appearance. Traces of a pencilled tree at that point in the composition suggest that Turner was searching for some taller form to balance the group of dark trees opposite. The reversal of the distant view in the final design also serves to broaden and smooth out the rhythms of the composition. All these points seem to show that the drawing must have been executed immediately before Turner tackled the final watercolour. Dark greens and ochres are characteristic of a number of 'colour-beginnings' which, on the evidence of this one, may be dated to about the same period. Turner apparently was in the habit of planning his large-scale water colours with full-size studies like this from a comparatively early stage in his development: compare the 'Norham' colour-beginning (No.639). There is also a full-scale preparatory study in colour for the large 'Scarborough' of *c.*1810 (No.113).

183 Tivoli: the Temple of the Sibyl ?*c.*1817
Watercolour over pencil, $19\frac{7}{8} \times 15\frac{3}{8}$ (50.5 × 39)
Trustees of the British Museum (T.B.CXCVI–U)
The mood of this drawing is somewhat akin to that of the large 'Tivoli' of 1817 (No.181) with which it may be connected, but it is possible that it was done during, or after, the Italian tour of 1819.

184 Vesuvius in Eruption 1817
Watercolour, $11 \times 15\frac{1}{8}$ (28 × 38.5)
Inscr. on verso: 'Mount Vesuvius in Eruption J M W Turner R A 1817'
Exh: Cooke's Gallery 1822 (8); Music Hall, Leeds 1839 (80)
Mr and Mrs Paul Mellon, Upperville, Virginia
From Walter Fawkes's collection. Turner is known to have been engaged on a pair of views of Vesuvius 'In Repose' and 'In Eruption' for W. B. Cooke in about 1817 and it has been supposed that this drawing is one of them. It is said to have been engraved by Cooke for

189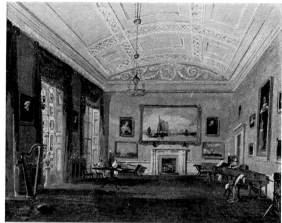

193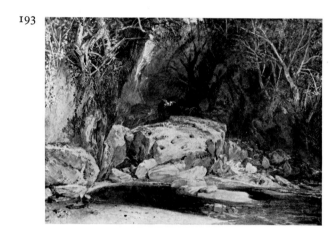

194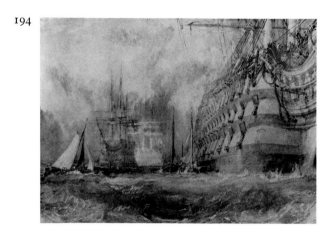

196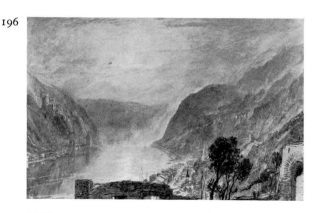

Delineations of Pompeii. But it seems more likely that Cooke's drawings were the two in the John Dillon sale, Christie 17 April 1869 (36 and 37), both bought by Ruskin. It is possible that one of them was the subject engraved by Thomas Jeavons in 1830 for *Friendship's Offering* (Rawlinson 339). A small watercolour $6\frac{7}{8} \times 11\frac{1}{8}$ in which is radically different in design from the present drawing, of Vesuvius with shipping in the foreground, is now in a private collection in London and is probably the companion; it corresponds exactly with the subject reproduced in Ruskin's *Lectures on Landscape*, 1897 fp.16. If this identification is correct, the Dillon/Ruskin pair were much smaller than the single Fawkes 'Vesuvius'.

Turner was working on several views of Italy from drawings by J. Hakewill published in 1818–20, and Hakewill may have supplied him with sketches on which these scenes were based, although no view of Vesuvius appears in Hakewill's *Picturesque Tour of Italy*. The format, with the bay sweeping in a curve to the left, suggests a reminiscence of J. R. Cozens. As a work showing Turner's interest in Italy before he went there, it may be placed with the large 'Composition of Tivoli' also of 1817 (No.181).

185 A Frontispiece: Fairfaxiana 1815
Pencil and watercolour with some pen, $7 \times 9\frac{1}{2}$
(17.8×24.2)
Inscr. bottom right: 'I M W Turner R A 1815'
Visitors of the Ashmolean Museum, Oxford
Intended as the frontispiece to the volume of drawings made by Turner of the collection of Fairfax relics at Farnley. Ruskin acquired the drawing 'in exchange for some *Liber* proofs from Mr Stokes of Gray's Inn'. Stokes (Turner's stockbroker, who was responsible for the catalogue of Turner's engraved works in the appendix to Thornbury's *Life*, 1862, 11, p.352 ff.) supplied Ruskin with a note reporting that Turner had told him 'Fairfaxiana are a set of drawings I made for Mr Fawkes of subjects relating to the Fairfax property which came into Mr Fawkes' family and I did this for the frontispiece. The helmet, drinking cup and sword were those of a knight of that family who was called Black Jack.' Ruskin regarded the drawing as 'faultless' in its use of 'pure watercolour' and recommended his students to copy it. The 'Fairfaxiana' album is still at Farnley; it is not clear why the frontispiece became separated from it. See Herrmann 1968, p.77.

186 Leeds 1816
Watercolour, $11\frac{3}{8} \times 16\frac{3}{4}$ (29×42.5)
Inscr. bottom left: 'J M W Turner R A 1816'
Mr and Mrs Paul Mellon, Upperville, Virginia
The view of the town is taken directly from a pencil drawing of the whole panorama in the 'Devonshire Rivers' sketchbook No.3, T.B.CXXXIV, ff.79ᵛ and 80ʳ (continued on f.38ʳ). On f.38ᵛ is a rough sketch of the view with some foreground incident; ff.45ʳ and 37ᵛ have smaller compositions for the whole design. It has been supposed that the drawing was made specifically for Whitaker's *Loidis and Elmete* for which Turner produced other designs, etched or engraved c.1816 (Rawlinson Nos.83–87) but the only known print of the subject, the lithograph by J. D. Harding (No.B105), does not in fact seem to have been used for that purpose.

187 Study of a Ship in a Violent Storm *c.*1817
Watercolour, $12\frac{3}{16} \times 18\frac{1}{8}$ (31×46)
Watermarked: 1816
Inscr. bottom left: 'Begun for Dear Fawkes of Farnley'
Trustees of the British Museum (T.B.CXCVI–N)

A preparatory study for the watercolour of about 1818 'Loss of a Man o'War', on the art market in London in 1974, which, as Turner's inscription indicates, was in Fawkes' collection, perhaps having been painted as a companion to 'A First-Rater taking in Stores', No.194. The MS comment was perhaps added after Fawkes' death in 1825.

188 'Farnley' sketchbook *c.*1818
Bound in buff boards, leather spine, one clasp
90 leaves, ff.18–40, 42–88 blank; the remainder drawn on in pencil, $4\frac{1}{2} \times 7\frac{1}{2}$ (18.7×11)
Watermarked: 1813
Inscr. on label on spine: '122'; and on back cover: 'Farnley'
Trustees of the British Museum (T.B.CLIII)

ff.15^v and 16^r **Interior of the Library, Farnley, with Details of the Ceiling and Two Women at a Table**
Pencil
Inscr. with colour notes

A few of the sketches in this book seem to be preparatory to the painting 'Entrance of the Meuse: Orange Merchant on the Bar' of 1819 (No.166); the rest are studies made at Farnley and in the surrounding countryside, and were used for a number of the finished drawings executed for Walter Fawkes in about 1818.

The drawing on ff.15^v and 16^r is continued to the right on f.17^r. Through the open door in the left-hand wall can be glimpsed the drawing room (see No.189).

189 The Drawing Room, Farnley Hall 1818
Bodycolour on grey paper, sight $12\frac{3}{8} \times 16\frac{1}{4}$ (31.5×41.2)
Nicholas Horton-Fawkes, Esq.

Compare the pencil drawing of the Library at Farnley on ff.15^v and 16^r of the 'Farnley' sketchbook (No. 188); where the drawing room (including the harp) can be glimpsed through the doorway on the left. The majority of Turner's Farnley views are now hung in the drawing room there. In this drawing the 'Dort' can be seen in the centre of the far wall; its colouring is distinctly more blue here than now appears in the painting itself, which was installed in 1818. Turner is known to have made this drawing during his stay at Farnley in November of that year; it seems probable that many, if not all, of the views at Farnley (see also Nos.190–192) were made at that time. Many of the Farnley subjects do not seem to be related to specific drawings in the Turner Bequest, but some of the sketchbooks contain material connected with them, especially the 'Farnley' and 'Large Farnley' sketchbooks, T.B.CLII and CXXVIII, the 'Woodcock Shooting' sketchbook, T.B.CXXIX, the 'Devon Rivers' sketchbook No.2, T.B.CXXXIII, and 'Devonshire Rivers No.3 and Wharfedale' sketchbook, T.B.CXXXIV. The sketches made at Farnley in these books may have been done over a period of several years, from about 1812 onwards. The Farnley interiors precede those drawn at Petworth probably by about ten years. They are larger and, generally, more elaborate; but the medium is the same (bodycolour) and Turner's approach to the depiction of rooms, and to interior lighting, is often similar in each series.

190 The Oak Staircase, Farnley Hall *c.*1818
Bodycolour on grey paper, sight $12\frac{1}{2} \times 16\frac{3}{16}$ (31.8×41.1)
Nicholas Horton-Fawkes, Esq.

See No.189.

191 The West Lodge, Farnley *c.*1818
Bodycolour on grey paper, $12\frac{15}{16} \times 17\frac{1}{2}$ (32.9×44.4)
Nicholas Horton-Fawkes, Esq.

The pencil drawing for this subject is in the 'Farnley' sketchbook (T.B.CLIII ff.14^v–15^r, see No.188).

192 The Wharfe from Farnley Hall *c.*1818
Bodycolour on grey paper, sight $11\frac{5}{8} \times 16\frac{1}{4}$ (29.6×41.3)
Nicholas Horton-Fawkes, Esq.

See No.189. The technique of this drawing is characteristic of many of the outdoor views of Farnley and its environs. It is very close to the style of the Rhine drawings done late in 1817, and may help to date the group.

193 A Rocky Pool with Heron and Kingfisher ?*c.*1818
Watercolour, $12 \times 15\frac{3}{4}$ (30.9×40)
Leeds City Art Gallery (5/57)

Finberg relates this watercolour with a study of rocks in the 'Scottish Pencils' series (T.B.LVIII–52); it has, therefore, been suggested (e.g. by Martin Hardie, *Mezzotints of Sir Frank Short*, 1939, p.29, No.65) that the subject is 'A Scottish Dell'. It is difficult to find more than a broad similarity between the two compositions, however, and the traditional title 'A Lonely Dell, Wharfedale' may perhaps retain a correct identification though it is unlikely to have been Turner's own.

The drawing seems to date from about 1818, when the *Richmondshire* series were executed; it has strong affinities with these, and with 'Weathercote Cave' (B.M. 1910-2-12-281) in particular; though if it represents a scene in Scotland it may date from somewhat earlier.

194 A First-Rate taking in Stores 1818
Pencil and watercolour, $11\frac{1}{4} \times 15\frac{5}{8}$ (28.6×39.7)
Inscr. bottom right: 'I M W Turner 1818'
Cecil Higgins Art Gallery, Bedford

This drawing was made at Farnley Hall during Turner's stay there in November 1818, and by family tradition was the only one that the artist executed in the presence of anybody at the house.

The circumstances of its genesis are recorded in an account by Edith Mary Fawkes, wife of a grandson of Walter Fawkes: 'One morning at breakfast Walter Fawkes said to him [Turner], "I want you to make me a drawing of the ordinary dimensions that will give some idea of the size of a man of war". The idea hit Turner's fancy, for with a chuckle he said to Walter Fawkes' eldest son, then a boy of about 15, "Come along Hawkey, and we will see what we can do for Papa", and the boy sat by his side the whole morning and witnessed the evolution of "The First Rate Taking in Stores". His description of the way Turner went to work was very extraordinary; he began by pouring wet paint on to the paper till it was saturated, he tore, he scratched, he scrabbled at it in a kind of frenzy and the whole thing was chaos – but gradually and as if by magic the lovely ship, with all its exquisite minutia, came into being and by luncheon time the drawing was taken down in triumph.' The subject seems to be an adaptation of a watercolour study of about 1798 (T.B.XXXIII–e) in which the hull of a large boat occupying the right-hand edge of the design similarly dwarfs smaller boats beside it.

195   Marxburg 1817
Watercolour and bodycolour on white paper prepared with a wash of grey, $7\frac{7}{8} \times 12\frac{5}{8}$ (20 × 32)
Indianapolis Museum of Art (Gift in memory of Dr and Mrs Hugo O. Pantzer by their Children)
A small pencil sketch inscribed 'Marxburg' occurs in the 'Waterloo and Rhine' sketchbook (T.B.CLX f.77ᵛ); other studies of Braubach and Marxburg are on ff.18–20 of the 'Rhine' sketchbook (T.B.CLXI); none corresponds exactly with the view shown in this drawing, which is one of fifty-one small Rhine subjects executed on a prepared grey surface from sketches made during Turner's tour of August-September 1817. Thornbury's account of how Turner immediately travelled to Farnley and 'before he had even taken off his great coat . . . produced these drawings, rolled up slovenly and anyhow, from his breastpocket' has been shown to be false (Finberg 1961, p.249). The drawings were probably made at Farnley while Turner was there in November, perhaps at the same time as the 'Wharfedale' series still mainly at Farnley (Nos.189–192), but they may have been begun beforehand, and Finberg suggests that they were possibly executed at Raby while Turner was working on studies for his painting of Raby Castle for Lord Strathmore (see No.202). A study in the same medium which appears to be a preliminary or unfinished drawing related to the series is in the Courtauld Institute Galleries. For other drawings from this series see Nos.196–199. The subject of 'Marxburg' was one of those re-used by Turner in slightly larger format, on white paper without a ground, for the Swinburne family, c.1820; that version is now in the British Museum (1958–7-12-422).

196   From Rheinfels, looking over St. Goar to Katz 1817
Watercolour and bodycolour with scraping-out on white paper prepared with a wash of grey, $7\frac{13}{16} \times 12\frac{5}{16}$ (19.5 × 31.3)
Private collection
One of the fifty-one Rhine views made in the autumn of 1817 and bought by Walter Fawkes (see No.195). The subject is based on two pencil studies in the 'Rhine' sketchbook (T.B.CLXI, No.201): one on ff.22ᵛ and 23ʳ is taken from beneath the castle of Rheinfels, at river level; the other, on f.42ʳ, shows the view from the castle itself, though from a viewpoint slightly further to the right than that of the watercolour.

197   Rüdesheim looking to Bingen Klopp 1817
Bodycolour and scraping-out on white paper prepared with a grey wash, $8\frac{3}{4} \times 13\frac{1}{2}$ (21.4 × 34.5)
National Museum of Wales, Cardiff
A small pencil sketch in the 'Waterloo and Rhine' sketchbook (T.B.CLX, f.66ʳ) is inscribed 'Rüdesheim' but is not of this view. It is probable, however, that the bottom drawing on ff.70ᵛ – 71ʳ is a panoramic sketch of the scene, which occurs again at the top of the next opening 71ᵛ – 72ʳ; another little composition sketch in the same place, inscribed 'Rüdesheim', shows the buildings to the right in greater detail. The subject was one of the fifty-one Rhine views acquired by Fawkes (see No.195), and was sold at the Ayscough Fawkes sale, Christie's, 27 June 1890 (4).

198   The Loreleiberg 1817
Watercolour and bodycolour with scraping-out on white paper prepared with a wash of grey, $7\frac{3}{4} \times 12\frac{1}{16}$ (19.7 × 30.7)
Whitworth Art Gallery, University of Manchester
One of the fifty-one Rhine drawings acquired by Fawkes in 1817 (see No.195). Three drawings entitled 'Lurleiberg' were sold at the Ayscough Fawkes sale, Christie's, 27 June 1890, lots 11, 12, 13. This view is based on a slight pencil sketch in the 'Waterloo and Rhine' sketchbook, T.B.CLX–1ʳ.

199   The Loreleiberg 1817
Watercolour and bodycolour on white paper prepared with a wash of grey, $7\frac{15}{16} \times 11\frac{7}{8}$ (20.2 × 30.2)
Leeds City Art Gallery (13.219/.53)
One of the fifty-one Rhine subjects acquired by Fawkes in 1817 (see No.195).

200   'Waterloo and Rhine' sketchbook 1817
Bound in calf with one clasp
93 leaves drawn on in pencil $6 \times 3\frac{3}{4}$ (15 × 93)
Watermarked: 1816
Inscr. on back cover: 'Rhine'
Trustees of the British Museum (T.B.CLX)

ff.70ᵛ–1ʳ   Johannisberg, Edrich, Elfelt, etc: six panoramas on the Rhine
Pencil
Inscr.with some place-names: 'Clows' etc.

This book was used during August 1817 at Bruges, Ghent, Brussels, Waterloo and along the Rhine. The series of tiny sketches noting the successive panoramas of the Rhine as Turner travelled up it provided much of the material from which the famous fifty Rhine views for Walter Fawkes were created (see No.195).
    The watercolour of 'Johannisberg' is now in the British Museum (1958-7-12-418).

201   'Rhine' sketchbook 1817
Bound in calf; one clasp
61 leaves, almost all drawn on in pencil, $8 \times 10\frac{1}{2}$ (26.3 × 20.1)
Watermarked: 1816
Inscr. on label on spine: '19 Rhine'; and on front cover: 'Rhine'
Trustees of the British Museum (T.B.CLXI)

ff.21ᵛ and 22ʳ **Rheinfels, with the Castle of Thurnberg in the Distance**
Pencil
Inscr. bottom left: 'Wood Timber Trees' (?)

The drawings in this book, showing scenes on the Rhine from Bingen down to Cologne, contrast strongly with the masses of tiny sketches in the little 'Waterloo and Rhine' book used on the same journey (No.200); they are much larger in scale, making full use of the large leaf size and frequently occupying a double page.

202 'Raby' Sketchbook 1817
Bound in mottled boards with leather corners and spine
32 leaves nearly all drawn on in pencil with some watercolour, 9⅛ × 13 (23.1 × 32.7)
Watermarked: 1816
Inscr. on spine: '115 Raby'
Trustees of the British Museum (T.B.CLVI)

ff.23ᵛ and 24ʳ **View of Raby Castle**
Pencil and watercolour

One of numerous studies of Raby and the surrounding countryside, including Bishop Auckland and Streatlam, made in 1817 preparatory to the painting of 'Raby Castle, the Seat of the Earl of Darlington' exhibited at the R.A. 1818 (198; now Walters Art Gallery, Baltimore). A more detailed view in pencil only on ff.21ᵛ and 22ᵛ (continued on f.11ʳ) was directly used as the basis for the painting, which is the last and grandest of Turner's topographical house-portraits in the eighteenth-century tradition (repr. Rothenstein and Butlin 1964, pl.58).

203 'Scotch Antiquities and London' Sketchbook 1818
Bound in pink grained boards with leather spine and corners
42 leaves, the majority blank; a drawing in pencil and watercolour on stiff card has been inserted at the back (f.42), 7 × 10⅛ (17.8 × 25.7)
Watermarked: 1815
Inscr. on label on spine: '109'
Trustees of the British Museum (T.B.CLXX)

f.7 **Waterloo Bridge**
Pencil and brown wash

This book was called by Finberg 'Scotland and Venice'. It contains two pencil studies related to the Borthwick Castle design for the *Provincial Antiquities of Scotland* (See No.204) on ff.1, 2 and a watercolour sketch of Crichton Castle for the same work; and, as C. F. Bell pointed out, the sketches which Finberg mistook for Venice on ff.10, 11 and 42 show the Custom House and Monument at London Bridge. They seem to relate to the watercolour drawing of London Bridge in the 'Hesperides' sketchbook of about 1805–7 (T.B. XCIII f.12), which Finberg described as a 'Study for a Picture' not executed and which Turner seems to have considered painting at various different times. See also the 'Tabley No.3' sketchbook (T.B.CV, No.119). There are also two very bold 'colour beginnings' on ff.12, 13.

f.7 is one of a series in this medium, ff.5–9, which relate to pencil sketches in the 'Tabley No.3' sketchbook (T.B.CV ff.72, 78). The low viewpoint (even more

exaggerated on the preceding leaf, f.6) reverts to topographical types used by Thomas Malton in his *Picturesque Tour through the Cities of London and Westminster*, 1792.

204 'Scotch Antiquities' Sketch Book 1818
Bound in buff boards
90 leaves, the majority drawn on in pencil, 4½ × 7⅛ (11.2 × 18.4)
Inscr. on cover: 'Scotch Work' and on label on spine: '89 Scotch Antiquities'
Trustees of the British Museum (T.B.CLXVII)

ff.39ᵛ, 40ʳ **View of Edinburgh from Calton Hill**
Pencil

The sketchbook was used by Turner on his journey to Scotland in October and November 1818 to gather material for the *Provincial Antiquities of Scotland* to be published in Edinburgh with text by Sir Walter Scott. It includes studies of Edinburgh, Roslin, Crichton, Borthwick, Tantallon and Dunbar. Most of the ten finished watercolours used as illustrations to the work are based on studies in this sketchbook (see No.206). In addition Turner designed two vignettes and other artists also contributed. Scott kept Turner's drawings, eight of which he hung together in an oak frame in his breakfast room at Abbotsford. They were later purchased by Thomas Brocklebank.

'Edinburgh from Calton Hill' was the basis of the watercolour engraved for Vol.1, p.83 by George Cooke, 1820 (Rawlinson No.193).

205 The Bass Rock 1821
Watercolour, 6¹¹⁄₁₆ × 9⅞ (17 × 25) (sight)
Trustees of the Lady Lever Art Gallery, Port Sunlight
Engraved by W. Miller for *The Provincial Antiquities of Scotland*, Vol.II, p.181, 1826 (Rawlinson No.200)

There are several studies of the subject in the 'Bass Rock and Edinburgh' sketchbook of 1818 (T.B.CLXV–5–8, 37ᵛ, 38ʳ) with a sequence of rapid sketches made as Turner sailed round the rock.

206 Hawthornden c.1821
Watercolour with some bodycolour, 6⅞ × 10⁷⁄₁₆ (17.5 × 26.5)
Inscr. bottom left: 'Turner'
Indianapolis Museum of Art (Gift in memory of Dr and Mrs Hugo O. Pantzer by their Children)
Engraved by W. R. Smith for *The Provincial Antiquities of Scotland*, 1822, as 'Roslin Castle' (Rawlinson No. 196).

Based on a pencil sketch of Roslin Castle in the 'Scotch Antiquities' sketchbook of 1818, T.B.CLXVII–66ʳ (see No.204). Other views of Hawthornden with the Castle occur in the same book. Turner had already visited the spot during his 1801 tour of Scotland; see the 'Edinburgh' sketchbook, LVI–62, etc. (No.52).

7. First visit to Italy 1819

Turner's first visit to Italy, like his first visit to the continent in 1802, was long delayed by war. When it came Turner was well prepared, both in the narrow sense, with guide books and lists of places to visit (see Nos.B84–B86), and mentally through his knowledge of the Old Masters and of contemporaries who had recorded the Italian scene such as James Hakewill (see No. B87). The visit led to a magnificent outpouring of watercolours and drawings, but when it came to oil paintings Turner seems to have been inhibited by the wealth of new experience, and only three of Italian subjects were exhibited before his second visit in 1828.

During the four months he spent in Italy between August 1819 and January 1820, Turner used no less than nineteen sketchbooks. The sheer quantity of the studies which they each contain bears witness to the immense importance that he attached to his journey. The majority of the books – fourteen of them – are fairly small and are crammed with pencil studies recording every aspect of the landscape, architecture, habits and costumes of Italy and the Italians, as well as details of works of art of all kinds encountered in museums and public buildings, especially the Vatican. Each book was carefully labelled both on its spine and on its cover, to provide easy reference, and it is clear that Turner's first object was to compile a library of notes for future use. He did not execute any finished watercolours while he was in Italy, though a few, mainly of Roman subjects, were made subsequently and purchased by Fawkes.

It was not possible, of course, to record everything about Italy in terms of the pencil alone and Turner made some fifty watercolour studies in which he catches with breathtaking conviction the luminous atmosphere of Naples, the Campagna, Venice and Lake Como. Although his watercolours of the years immediately preceding the Italian journey give evidence of his steadily developing power and subtlety in the medium, the progress reaches a climax in this series, which is all the more remarkable in that it represents his first reactions to a new climate and environment.

Although many of these colour studies are executed simply in watercolour on white paper, the medium in which one would expect Turner to respond to Mediterranean light, he also worked extensively, as he had done in Switzerland in 1802, on a prepared grey ground. The 'Tivoli' sketchbook, for instance, contains dramatically contrasted studies on both white and grey grounds (No.226); and the series of 'Rome: Colour Studies' (T.B.CLXXXIX) includes many pencil drawings on grey, together with elaborate exercises in watercolour and bodycolour, also on the prepared surface. In some cases this use of a tinted ground, combined with rather soft pencil work, evokes the Roman drawings of Richard Wilson, which Turner cannot have failed to recall as he saw Rome for the first time; though it was no doubt with subtler and more particular motives than the mere imitation of Wilson's grey paper and delicate atmospheric drawing that he adopted this manner (see B37).

It is not clear whether the coloured drawings were made out of doors or not; one contemporary in Naples reported Turner's comment that 'it would take up too much time to colour in the open air – he could make 15 or 16 pencil sketches to one coloured'. On the other hand there is an account of Turner sketching in Italy with the amateur artist R. J. Graves: 'At times . . . when they had fixed upon a point of view, to which they returned day after day, Turner would content himself with making one careful outline of the scene, and then, while Graves worked on, Turner would remain apparently doing nothing, till at some particular moment, perhaps on the third day, he would exclaim "there it is" and seizing his colours, work rapidly until he had noted down the peculiar effect he wished to fix in his memory.' (See Finberg, 1961, p.262 and Armstrong, 1902, p.96.)

The freshness and spontaneity of the pure watercolours seem to support this account; but the drawings which employ mixed watercolour and bodycolour, and often attempt complicated atmospheric effects, may well have been among those for which Turner had 'no time' while he was engaged in his unremitting task of record-taking.

207 **'Turin, Como, Lugano, Maggiore' Sketchbook** 1819
Bound in buff boards, leather spine; one clasp
93 leaves (f.23 missing) nearly all drawn on in pencil, $4\frac{1}{2} \times 7\frac{1}{2}$ (11.2 × 18.4)
Inscr. on front cover: 'Turin Como Lugarno [sic] Maggiore'
Trustees of the British Museum (T.B.CLXXIV)

ff.62ᵛ–63ʳ (?)**The Duomo, Como**
Pencil; with studies of architectural details
Inscr. with notes of architectural details and costumes, largely illegible.

This book shows Turner sketching as he progressed from the Southern Alps to Turin, where he made many architectural studies, and on to Lakes Como and Maggiore.

208 **'Milan to Venice' Sketchbook** 1819
Bound in buff boards, leather spine; one clasp
91 leaves, all drawn on in pencil, $4\frac{1}{2} \times 7\frac{1}{2}$ (11 × 18.4)
Watermarked: 1813
Inscr. on front cover: 'Milan to Venice' and '3'; on spine: '3'
Trustees of the British Museum (T.B.CLXXV)

ff.78ᵛ–79ʳ **Venice: the Rialto Bridge**
Pencil
Inscr. with a few notes

Cf. the large unfinished oil painting, Tate Gallery 5543.

209 'Como and Venice' Sketchbook 1819
Bound in marbled boards 45 leaves, some
now removed, 9 × 11½ (22.4 × 28.5)
Watermarked: '1816'
Inscr. on label on spine: '67 Como'
Trustees of the British Museum (T.B.CLXXXI)

f.10 Colour-beginning
Watercolour

The extreme delicacy and subtlety of this colour
scheme is characteristic of the light palette employed by
Turner in his first short series of Venetian watercolours
(see Nos.212–4) which were all made in this book.

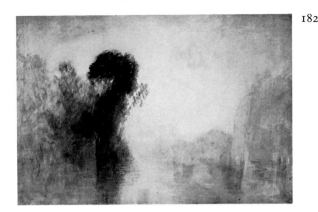

182

210 'Venice to Ancona' Sketchbook 1819
Bound in buff boards, leather spine, one clasp
90 leaves (one torn out) nearly all drawn on in
pencil, 4½ × 7½ (11 × 18.5)
Inscr. on label on spine: '9 Venice to Ancona';
and on front cover: 'Venice to Ancona'
Trustees of the British Museum (T.B.CLXXVI)

**ff.28ᵛ–29ʳ Studies of Venice from the
Lagoons**
Pencil
Inscr. with numerous notes, including: 'The
Lower part of the Canal from the Madona della
Salute'; 'very dark Reflect[ions] of the Boats'
and with memoranda of colour.

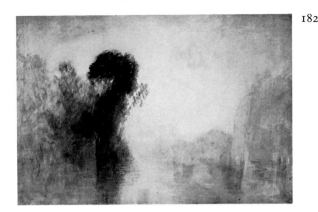

The view at the top of f.29ʳ is of S. Giorgio Maggiore
and the Zitelle from the Riva degli Schiavoni.

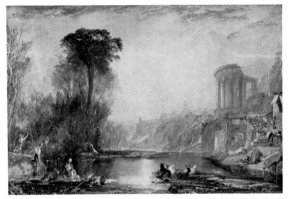

181

211 Lake Como 1819
Watercolour, 8⅞ × 11⁷⁄₁₆ (22.5 × 29.1)
Trustees of the British Museum (T.B.CLXXXI–1)
A similar watercolour of the Lake is T.B.CLXXXI–2,
also from the 'Como and Venice' sketchbook (No.209).

**212 Venice: S. Giorgio Maggiore from the
Dogana** 1819
Watercolour, 8¹³⁄₁₆ × 11⁵⁄₁₆ (22.4 × 28.7)
Trustees of the British Museum (T.B.CLXXXI–4)
Regarded by Finberg as the first watercolour Turner
made in Venice.

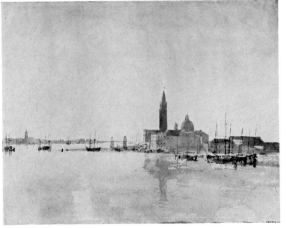

212

**213 Venice: looking East from the Giudecca;
Sunrise** 1819
Watercolour, 8¾ × 11⁵⁄₁₆ (22.2 × 28.7)
Trustees of the British Museum (T.B.CLXXXI–5)

**214 Venice: the Campanile of St. Mark's and the
Doge's Palace** 1819
Pencil and watercolour, 8⅞ × 11⁵⁄₁₆ (22.5 × 28.7)
Trustees of the British Museum (T.B.CLXXXI–7)
Finberg (*Venice*, 1930, p.23) considered that all the
watercolours made in Venice in 1819 were done from
memory, except this one which 'may have been painted
direct from nature. . . . As a study it was perhaps the
most useful drawing Turner made in Venice on this
occasion, as it fixed upon his mind for the remainder of
his life that vision of a city of gleaming marble rising
from the sea which we find in his later paintings.'

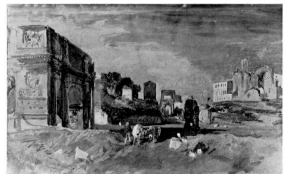

220

215 'Tivoli and Rome' Sketchbook 1819
Bound in buff boards, leather spine, one clasp
92 leaves almost all drawn on in pencil, $4\frac{1}{2} \times 7\frac{1}{2}$
(11.1×18.4)
Watermarked: 1813
Inscr. on label on spine: '6 Tivoli Raffele's Logi
Castello St. Ange'; and on back cover: 'Tivoli
Raffaelo's Logi Castello St. Ange'
Trustees of the British Museum (T.B.CLXXIX)

**f.13ᵛ View along One of the Loggie of
Raphael in the Vatican**
Pencil
Inscr: 'Red lined (?) Marble|White Base and
small plinth|Dark the Lower'
**f.14ʳ Studies of Details of the Decoration of
the Loggie**
Pencil
Inscr. with many notes on details of colour and
content

216 'Rome Colour Studies' Sketchbook 1819
Bound in buff boards, leather spine and corners
63 leaves of white paper prepared on one side
with grey wash; many sheets have been removed
and mounted separately, $14\frac{1}{2} \times 9$ (36.9×22.4)
Watermarked: 1816
Inscr. Finberg transcribes label on spine: '14
Rome C. Studies'; and on back cover: 'Rome'
Trustees of the British Museum (T.B.CLXXXIX)

**f.43ʳ Rome: The Forum with the Arch of
Titus**
Pencil and scraping-out on white paper prepared
with grey wash

217 'Small Roman Colour Studies' Sketchbook
1819
Bound in buff boards, with leather spine and
corners; one clasp
68 leaves of white paper prepared on one side
only with grey wash; nearly all drawn on, in
pencil with scraping-out, or watercolour and
bodycolour, $5\frac{1}{4} \times 10\frac{1}{8}$ (13.2×25.5)
Watermarked: 1814
Inscr. on back cover: 'Roma'; Finberg records a
label on the spine which read: '9. Roma:
C. Studies'
Trustees of the British Museum (T.B.CXC)

f.64 View of a Garden
Watercolour and bodycolour with wiping and
scraping-out on white paper prepared with grey
wash

All the drawings in this book are of Rome or the Campagna; the 'Moonrise' on f.65 and 'Sunset' on f.54
were both presumably observed in the neighbourhood
of Rome, although there is no evidence in either drawing to identify the location exactly.

218 'Naples, Rome Colour Studies' Sketchbook
1819
Bound in buff boards, leather spine and corners:
two clasps
70 leaves of white paper, many now removed and
mounted separately; some prepared with grey

wash on one side only, 16×10 (40.4×25)
Watermarked: 1814 and 1816
Inscr. on label on spine: '15. Naples: Rome C
Studies'
Trustees of the British Museum (T.B.CLXXXVII)

f.53ʳ Interior of a Large Church
Watercolour

Many of the drawings from this sketchbook are mounted
separately, see Nos.227–8, 233–5. f.53 is perhaps St.
Peter's. Compare the watercolour interiors of Eu Cathedral dating from 1845 (T.B.CCCLIX–7, 10; see No.631).

**219 Rome: View from the Janiculum with the
Palazzo Corsini in the left foreground** 1819
Pencil and scraping-out on white paper prepared
with grey wash, $9\frac{1}{8} \times 14\frac{1}{2}$ (23.1×36.8)
Trustees of the British Museum (T.B.CLXXIX–12)

**220 Rome: the Forum, with the Arches of
Constantine and Titus** 1819
Pencil, watercolour and bodycolour on white
paper prepared with grey wash, $9 \times 14\frac{7}{16}$
(22.8×36.7)
Trustees of the British Museum (T.B.CLXXXIX–40)

**221 Rome: the Arch of Titus, with the
Colosseum beyond** 1819
Pencil and scraping-out on white paper prepared
with grey wash, $9\frac{1}{8} \times 14\frac{9}{16}$ (23.1×37)
Trustees of the British Museum (T.B.CLXXXIX–44)

**222 Rome: the Baths of Caracalla from the
Aventine** 1819
Pencil, watercolour and bodycolour with some
pen and brown ink on white paper prepared
with grey wash, $9 \times 14\frac{1}{2}$ (22.8×36.8)
Trustees of the British Museum (T.B.CLXXIX–8)

**223 Rome: The Piazza of St. Peter from the
Vatican** 1819
Pencil, pen and brown ink and white bodycolour
on white paper, prepared with grey wash
(discoloured), $9\frac{3}{16} \times 14\frac{1}{16}$ (23.3×37)
Trustees of the British Museum (T.B.CLXXXIX–41)

**224 Rome: The Fountain in front of the Villa
Medici** 1819
Pencil and scraping-out on white paper prepared
with grey wash, $9\frac{1}{4} \times 14\frac{9}{16}$ (23.5×37)
Trustees of the British Museum (T.B.CLXXXIX–5)

225 Rome: the Church of SS. Giovanni e Paolo
1819
Watercolour and bodycolour on white paper
prepared with grey wash, $9\frac{1}{16} \times 14\frac{7}{16}$ (23×36.7)
Trustees of the British Museum (T.B.CLXXXIX–39)

226 'Tivoli' Sketchbook 1819
Bound in buff boards, leather spine and corners,
one clasp
82 leaves of white paper, prepared on one side
with grey wash, 10×8 (25.2×19.5)
Watermarked: 1814
Inscr. Finberg transcribes label on spine:

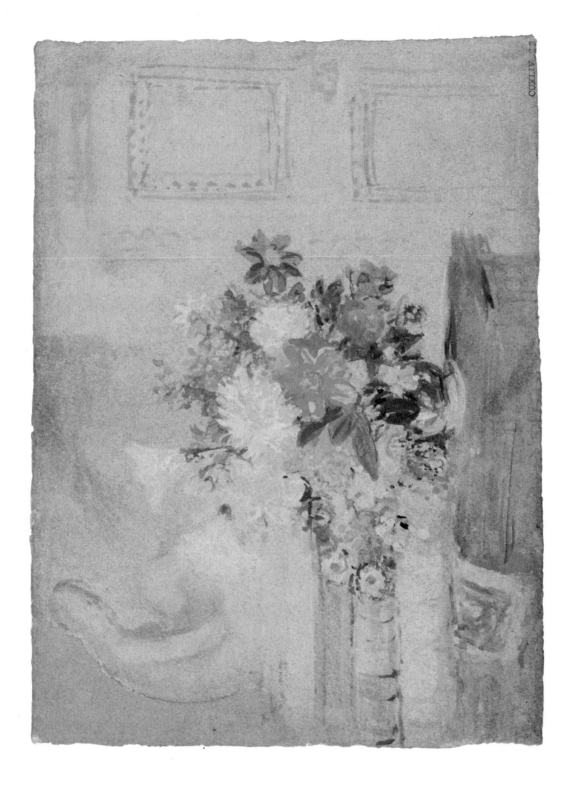

348 **Petworth: A Vase of Lilies, Dahlias and other Flowers** ? *c.*1828 (entry on p.112)

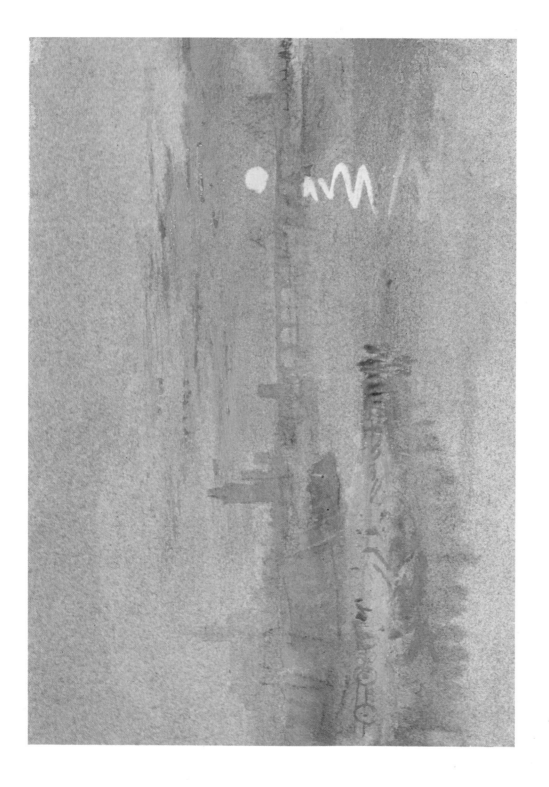

396 **Sunset: Rouen?** *c.*1829 (entry on p.116)

'13. Tivoli'
Trustees of the British Museum (T.B.CLXXXIII)

f.46ᵛ The Temple of the Sibyl seen from Below
Pencil

f.47ʳ The Temple of the Sibyl seen from Below
Pencil and scraping-out on white paper prepared with grey wash

The book is devoted solely to studies of the buildings at Tivoli, and the immediately surrounding countryside.

227 General View of Tivoli 1819
Pencil and watercolour, $10\frac{1}{16} \times 15\frac{7}{8}$ (25.6 × 40.4)
Trustees of the British Museum (T.B.CLXXXVII–28)
There is a similar view of Tivoli in the same series, CLXXXVII–32. A number of studies of the town occur in the 'Tivoli' and 'Tivoli and Rome' sketchbooks (Nos. 226 and 215), but the two watercolours do not apparently derive from any specific sketch, and may have been among those executed by Turner on the spot.

228 A View over the Roman Campagna with a low Sun 1819 (repr. on p.36)
Watercolour and bodycolour, $10 \times 15\frac{7}{8}$ (25.4 × 40.3)
Trustees of the British Museum (T.B.CLXXXVII–43)

229 Rome: the Claudian Aqueduct with the Temple of Minerva Medica 1819
Watercolour and bodycolour on white paper prepared with grey wash, $9\frac{1}{16} \times 14\frac{1}{2}$ (23 × 36.8)
Trustees of the British Museum (T.B.CLXXXIX–36)

230 'Albano, Nemi, Rome' Sketchbook 1819
Bound in boards with leather back, one clasp
89 leaves, all drawn on in pencil, one, f.48a, torn out, $4\frac{1}{2} \times 7\frac{1}{2}$ (11 × 18.4)
Watermarked: 1818
Inscr. on front cover: 'Albano Nemi Rome'
Trustees of the British Museum (T.B.CLXXXII)

ff.9ᵛ–10ʳ A wooded hillside with buildings near Albano; view of Lake Albano with sketch of the Pope's Villa
Pencil
Inscr. to left: 'Wood'

231 'Gandolfo to Naples' Sketchbook 1819
Bound in calf, with one clasp
92 leaves, all drawn on in pencil, $5 \times 7\frac{3}{4}$ (12.2 × 19.8)
Inscr. on back cover: 'Castello Gondolfo to Napoli Baeia Pozzoli Naples', and inside front cover: 'This Book contains – Gandolfo to Naples – Baie (?) and Puzzolio'.
Trustees of the British Museum (T.B.CLXXXIV)

ff.60ᵛ–61ʳ View of Naples with the Castel dell'Ovo Pencil

The book contains principally pencil studies of views and architecture in and around Naples, with a series of drawings of the Bay of Baiae (ff.82ᵛ–90) used in the evolution of the painting 'The Bay of Baiæ' (No.237).

232 'Naples, Paestum and Rome' Sketchbook
1819
Bound in buff boards, leather spine, with one clasp
92 leaves, almost all drawn on in pencil, $4\frac{1}{2} \times 7\frac{1}{2}$ (11.3 × 18.5)
Watermarked: 1813
Inscr. on label on spine [almost entirely removed; transcribed by Finberg]: '12 Vesuvius, Napoli. V. Tomb. 1 Rt to Salerno. Paestum, and Return from Naples to Rome'; and on front cover: 'Vesuvius. Napoli Virgils Tomb 1 Journey to Salerno. Paestum Return from Naples to Rome'
Trustees of the British Museum (T.B.CLXXXVI)

ff.30ᵛ–31ʳ Two studies of the Group of Temples at Paestum, with four composition sketches
Pencil
Inscr. with brief notes

The sketchbook is largely devoted to sketches at the places indicated by Turner's inscriptions, but there is a drawing of Windsor Castle on f.90ᵛ and the study of plants on f.89ᵛ, which is reminiscent of those in the 'Walmer Ferry' sketchbook (T.B.CXLII), may also have been made near the Thames.

233 Capri from Naples, with the Castel dell'Ovo 1819
Pencil and watercolour, $10\frac{1}{8} \times 15\frac{13}{16}$ (25.8 × 40.5)
Trustees of the British Museum (T.B.CLXXXVII–21)
A view taken from the same spot as CLXXXVII–2 (No.234). A further study in watercolour of the distant promontory and island is CLXXXVII–20, where the Castle in the foreground is omitted.

234 The Castel dell'Ovo, Naples, with Capri and Sorrento in the Distance; Early Morning
1819
Pencil and watercolour, $10\frac{1}{4} \times 15\frac{7}{8}$ (25.7 × 40.3)
Trustees of the British Museum (T.B.CLXXXVII–2)
A view taken, in more serene conditions, from the same spot as CLXXXVII–21 (No.233).

235 The Bay of Naples 1819
Pencil and watercolour, $9\frac{15}{16} \times 15\frac{13}{16}$ (25.3 × 40.2)
Trustees of the British Museum (T.B.CLXXXVII–13)
The subject is not, as Finberg states (1909, I, p.555), a view of the 'Castle of the Egg', though the Castel dell'Ovo is in fact just visible in the centre of the drawing.

236 Rome from the Vatican. Raffaelle, accompanied by La Fornarina, preparing his Pictures for the Decoration of the Loggia
R.A.1820
Oil on canvas, $69\frac{3}{4} \times 132$ (177 × 335.5)
Exh: R.A. 1820 (206)
Inscr. on plan bottom centre: 'Pianta del Vaticano'
Tate Gallery (503)
Turner's first visit to Italy in 1819, though resulting in a few exquisite watercolours of Venice (see Nos.212 and 213) and a much larger number of fine sketches and

watercolours in and around Rome and Naples (see Nos.219–35), seems to have had a detrimental effect on his painting of exhibitable oil paintings. This was the only work shown in 1820, in 1821 he showed nothing, in 1822 the small 'What you will!' (No.307), in 1823 the larger 'Bay of Baiæ' (No.237), in 1824 nothing, and in 1825 only one oil and one watercolour; only in 1826 did he again begin to show more than one oil. The large pictures of these years are, however, major statements, and none more so than 'Rome from the Vatican', perhaps intended, as Ron Parkinson has suggested, as a tribute to Raphael on the three-hundredth anniversary of his death.

Although Raphael's mistress, La Fornarina, is present this is far more than just an anecdotal painting. As his first exhibit after visiting Italy and one of such large dimensions, one would expect this picture to sum up his reactions to both the country and all that it had meant in the history of art. However, as John Gage has shown (1969, pp.92–5), the painting is more specifically biographical, with Turner identifying himself with the universal artist of the Italian Renaissance. When visiting the Louvre in 1802 Turner had ignored Raphael but by 1820 there was a growing appreciation of Raphael as a colourist as well as a draftsman; Turner himself noted in the 'Route to Rome' sketchbook that the frescoes in the Villa Farnesina were 'Exquisite colored' (T.B.CLXXI–14ᵛ). Raphael was also being increasingly appreciated as a painter of landscape, hence the inclusion of the surprisingly Claudian landscape in the foreground. John Gage suggests that Turner deliberately included inaccurate and anachronistic details to stress the autobiographical character of the picture. Raphael's great decorative schemes, painted in fresco direct on the wall, are represented by an easel painting on canvas of one of the Loggie subjects. Bernini's colonnades in front of St. Peter's, not built until the seventeenth century, are included to represent Turner's ambitions as an architect, fulfilled to some extent by his designs for his own gallery in Queen Ann Street, which he was re-building at this time, and his cottage near Twickenham. Sculpture is also included.

In the 'Tivoli and Rome' sketchbook of 1819 there are a number of sketches of the Loggie, including one general view as they appear in the finished picture as well as several detailed studies, two general composition sketches which were considerably modified, and a drawing of the distant snow-capped Apennines (T.B.CLXXIX–13ᵛ (No.215), 14–21ᵛ, 25ᵛ and 26 (repr. Wilkinson 1974, p.188), and 25 respectively). There is a finished drawing in pen and ink, finished in Chinese white, in the 'Rome: C[olour]' sketchbook (T.B. CLXXXIX–41). A fascinating recent discovery among the unfinished oils in the Turner Bequest is that another large picture, equal in size to this one and to 'Richmond Hill', shows the Grand Canal, Venice, with the bridge of the Rialto arching across the foreground somewhat like the arch in 'Forum Romanum' but filling much more of the picture (Tate Gallery 5543). This seems to be an unfinished project for a Venetian counterpart to the Rome picture.

Although Finberg quotes two unfavourable reviews (1939, p.264) the reception of the picture was not entirely negative. Two unidentified cuttings at the Victoria and Albert Museum speak of 'a grand view of

Rome' and of its 'possessing all the magical effects, the clear and natural atmosphere, and the glorious lights which give such a beauty and a charm to all his compositions' (Vol.V, p.1217, and Vol.IV, p.1178). The *Repository of Art* for June 1820 described it as 'a strange, but wonderful picture', criticising 'the crossing and re-crossing of reflected lights about the gallery', the figures and 'the perspective of the fore-ground', but praising the distance and the 'richness and splendour of the colouring'. The *Annals of the Fine Arts* said that 'Turner has not gone back, he only stands where he did', praised the 'grandeur of conception', but attacked the 'excessive yellowness, which puts everything out of tune that hangs by it'.

237 The Bay of Baiæ, with Apollo and the Sibyl

R.A.1823 (repr. on p.53)
Oil on canvas, 57¼ × 94 (145.5 × 239)
Inscr. on stone bottom left: 'Liquidæ Placuere Baiæ'
Exh: R.A. 1823 (77); Turner's gallery 1835
Tate Gallery (505)

The second of the large finished pictures resulting from Turner's first visit to Italy, exhibited two years after 'Rome from the Vatican' with the line: 'Waft me to sunny Baiæ's shore'. The Latin inscription on the picture comes from Horace's *Ode To Calliope* and alludes to the poet's delight in the waters of Baiae. Though the district had been painted by Wilson this is the first time it had been used for a subject picture. Apollo granted Deiphobe, the Cumeaen Sibyl, that she should live as many years as she held grains of sand in her hand, but she failed to ask for perpetual youth and wasted away until only her voice was left (Ovid, *Metamorphoses*, Book XIV). Baiae had been renowned for its luxury under the Romans and, as John Gage has pointed out (1974, pp.44–7), Turner probably followed his early patron Colt Hoare in drawing the lesson of its decline through profligacy and degeneracy. While the white rabbit alludes to Venus, to whom one of the local temples was dedicated, the snake is symbolic of the latent evil.

Turner visited Baiae from Naples in 1819 and there are many drawings in the 'Gandolfo to Naples' and 'Pompeii, Amalfi, Sorrento and Herculaneum' sketchbooks, including one in the former of the same view as the picture (T.B.CLXXXIV–82ᵛ and 83; see also CLXXXV). In this picture the Claudian panorama that had characterised so many of Turner's previous landscapes is composed in flowing curves rather than the more distinct zones and linear stresses of the earlier examples.

The adjective almost universally applied to this picture by the critics was 'gorgeous'. The writer in the *European Magazine* for May 1823 was 'much annoyed by a cold-blooded critic . . . who observed that it was not natural. Natural! No, not in his limited and purblind view of nature. But perfectly natural to the man who is capable of appreciating the value of a practical concentration of all that nature occasionally and partially discloses of the rich, the glowing and the splendid'. According to the *Repository of Arts* for June 1823 'Mr Turner's answer, and perhaps a sufficient one' to the 'somewhat monotonous effect produced by the unclouded richness of the landscape . . . may be, that he has painted the landscape as nature and the poets have given it'. *The Literary Gazette*, in its second notice of the picture on 17 May 1823, had a slightly different answer: 'The seductive influence of colours, and the necessity of painting up to the standard of an exhibition, where the spread of gold is more than that of canvas, will prevent, if it does not annihilate, the study of nature . . . Though we have no eye for criticism on this splendid piece, it is only when considered as a vision, or a sketch, or as a variety in a large collection, – in one word, it is not painting.'

238 Forum Romanum, for Mr Soane's Museum R.A.1826

Oil on canvas, 57⅝ × 93½ (145.5 × 237.5)
Exh: R.A. 1826 (132)
Tate Gallery (504)

Painted, to judge by the title in the Royal Academy catalogue, for Turner's fellow-Academician the architect Sir John Soane (1753–1837). Soane designed three adjacent houses in Lincoln's Inn Fields and moved from No.12 to the central one, No.13 in 1813, turning it also into a setting for his considerable collection of antiquities and works of art, particularly after the death of his wife in 1815. In 1833 he obtained a private Act of Parliament setting up the Museum under a body of trustees. The space is very constricted and it was probably because of this that he did not in fact take the picture. There is a letter from Soane to Turner of 9 July 1828 with a draft for 500 guineas and a request that 'you will have the goodness to take charge of the picture until I can find a suitable place for it or a purchaser'. The picture is not specified but the sum of money suggests a work of this size. The letter and draft, however, are still at the Soane Museum; presumably Turner did not hold his old friend to their bargain and just took the picture back. Soane later acquired one of Turner's standard three-by-four foot canvases, 'Admiral van Tromp's Barge at the Entrance of the Texel, 1645', exhibited at the Academy in 1831.

This, the third of Turner's great pictures resulting from his first visit to Italy in 1819, concentrates on the monuments of Ancient Rome and so would have had a particular interest for Soane. There is a composition sketch from a slightly different view in the 'Small Roman Colour Studies' sketchbook (T.B.CXC-1). In this painting Turner stresses the monumental quality of the Arch of Titus and the Basilica of Constantine on the right by the close viewpoint and consequent foreshortening, and even more by the massive arch which frames the picture at the top. The contrast between the *gravitas* of this picture and the lush curvilinear composition of 'Bay of Baiæ' was perhaps deliberate. However, though there are contrasts of light and shade, the whole painting glows with colour, as the critic of *The Literary Gazette* for 13 May 1826 noted, not altogether approvingly: 'The artist, we can readily perceive, has combated a very difficult quality of art, in giving solidity without strong and violent opposition of light and shade. . . . Mr. Turner . . . seems to have sworn fidelity to the Yellow Dwarf, if he has not identified himself with that important necromancer.'

Some letters have been inscribed down the left-hand edge near the bottom, scratched into the wet paint, some of it apparently added specially in small squares. They seem to read 'A[?]GM[?]SRMPA'.

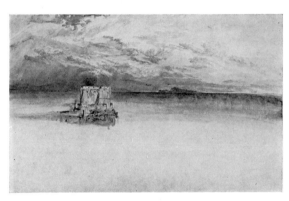

233

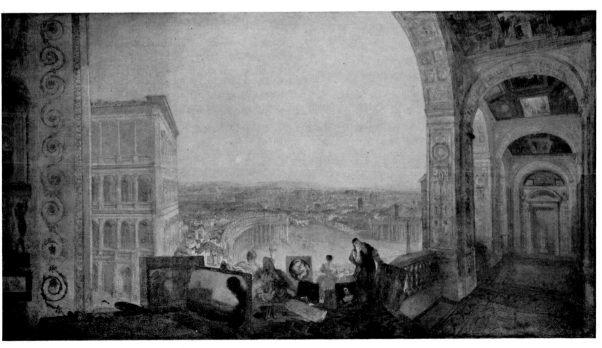

236

8. Work and Play 1820–36

During the years when Turner was struggling with his large pictures of Italian subjects he seems to have sought relaxation in small, more informal, almost playful pictures; the title 'What you will!' typifies his approach. A visit to the architect John Nash on the Isle of Wight led to a renewed interest in the sea in all its moods, but again with a new emphasis on its role in social life and recreation. Meanwhile Turner carried on his incredibly industrious activity for the engraver, embarking on a series of schemes for illustrating books of literature and travel that were to occupy him for a decade.

239   Kirkstall Abbey on the River Aire c.1824
Watercolour, $6\frac{5}{16} \times 8\frac{7}{8}$ (16 × 22.5)
Trustees of the British Museum (T.B.CCVIII–M)
Engraved in mezzotint by J. Bromley for *The Rivers of England* 1826 (Rawlinson 761). Studies of the Abbey from this angle, though from further down the river Aire, are in the 'Kirkstall' sketchbook of about 1808 (T.B.CVII–1 and 2). Turner had been at Kirkstall subsequently; see the 'Kirkstall Lock' group of drawings of about 1816 (T.B.CLV) and further studies of 1824 in the 'Brighton and Arundel' sketchbook (T.B.CCX) in which f.48 bears a sketch followed fairly closely by this watercolour. Kirkstall Lock itself, with the Abbey in the background, is the subject of another of the *Rivers of England* designs (T.B.CCVIII–L).

The *Rivers of England* or *River Scenery* series was planned in about 1822 as a sequel in mezzotint to the *Southern Coast* published by W. B. Cooke. It was inspired by the development of mezzotinting on steel, and by Thomas Lupton's print in that medium after Girtin's 'White House, Chelsea' (No.B43). Four subjects after Girtin were used and William Collins, R.A. contributed one design. Rawlinson lists seventeen plates after Turner (Nos.752–768).

240   More Park, near Watford, on the River Colne c.1823
Watercolour, $6\frac{3}{16} \times 8\frac{11}{16}$ (15.7 × 22.1)
Trustees of the British Museum (T.B.CCVIII–H)
Engraved in mezzotint by C. Turner for *The Rivers of England*, 1824 (Rawlinson 754). Based on a pencil sketch in the 'River' sketchbook T.B.XCVI 76ʳ (continued on 49ʳ) inscribed 'More Park' or 'For More Park'. Since the address Turner has written in the front of this book is 'West End Upper Mall Hammersmith', it has been dated to c.1807–11, when the artist lived there; it seems likely then that for this view he relied on a slight sketch which was some ten years old. The still life of foliage in the bottom right-hand corner may also have been derived from a study in the 'River' sketchbook, that on f.2ʳ; though such plant studies occur elsewhere, eg. in the 'Walmer Ferry' sketchbook (No.259).

Charles TURNER (1773–1857) after J. M. W. TURNER
241   Shields on the River Tyne 1823
Mezzotint, second published state, $6\frac{1}{16} \times 8\frac{1}{2}$ (15.3 × 21.7); plate $7\frac{9}{16} \times 10\frac{1}{16}$ (19.2 × 25.6)
Inscr: 'Drawn by J.M.W. Turner R.A.' and 'Engraved on Steel by Chas. Turner.'; with title and: 'Rivers of England Plate I', 'London Published June 2 1823, by W. B. Cooke 9, Soho Square'
Trustees of the British Museum (1850-1-14-128)
Rawlinson No.752. The drawing, signed and dated 1823, is in the Turner Bequest, No.CCVIII–V.

Small in size but large in scale, this design recreates the classic Claudian 'Sea-Port' composition as an industrial scene, and transforms the sun into the moon. A 'colour-beginning' in the Turner Bequest (T.B. CCLXIII–192) may be related to the subject and seems to connect it, in mood at least, with the *Little Liber* mezzotints (see No.252). Compare the painting 'Keelmen heaving in Coals by Night' of 1835 (No.513).

242   The Medway c.1824
Pencil and watercolour, $6\frac{1}{8} \times 8\frac{9}{16}$ (15.6 × 21.8)
Trustees of the British Museum (T.B.CCVIII–P)
Listed by Finberg among designs for the *Rivers and Ports of England* but not engraved for either series. A modified version of the design was mezzotinted by Turner for the *Little Liber* c.1825 (Rawlinson No.809a).

243   Portsmouth c.1824
Watercolour, $6\frac{5}{16} \times 9\frac{7}{16}$ (16 × 24)
Trustees of the British Museum (T.B.CCVIII–S)
Engraved in mezzotint by T. Lupton for *The Ports of England*, 1828 (Rawlinson No.784). For the print, see No.244. Ruskin, in his note on the mezzotint in the *Harbours of England*, 1856 (p.41), points out that this design uses the same view of Portsmouth from the sea as appears in the *Southern Coast* series (Rawlinson 120); only the shipping in the foreground is substantially different. Small but detailed pencil studies of Portsmouth from the sea appear in the 'London Bridge and Portsmouth' sketchbook (T.B.CCVI– 1ᵛ, 2ʳ&ᵛ, 3ᵛ, 5ᵛ, 9ʳ&ᵛ, etc.), and a colour study for that design is T.B.CCIII–A.

The *Ports of England* was a series of twelve plates conceived as a sequel to the *Rivers of England* (see No. 239), engraved, again, by Thomas Lupton and issued between 1826 and 1828; only six of the plates appeared, however, at that time (with a wrapper design etched, perhaps by Turner himself, from a drawing now in the Fitzwilliam Museum) – Rawlinson Nos.778–784. The remaining six were not published until Gambart reissued the whole set, with descriptive notes by Ruskin, in 1856 under the title *The Harbours of England*.

Thomas Goff LUPTON (1791–1873) after
TURNER

244   Portsmouth 1828
Mezzotint, $6\frac{5}{16} \times 9\frac{7}{16}$ (16 × 24); plate $7\frac{15}{16} \times 10\frac{1}{2}$
(20.1 × 26.7)
Inscr. on left: 'drawn by J.M.W. Turner, Esq.
R.A.'; on right: 'Engraved by Thos. Lupton';
and below: 'Portsmouth', 'Ports of England
Plate VI', 'London, Pubd. May 1, 1828, by Thos.
Lupton, 7 Leigh Street Burton Crescent;
Deposé à la Bibliothèque, et se vend à Paris, chez
Shroth, Rue de la Paix, No.18'
Trustees of the British Museum (1850-1-14-107)
Rawlinson No.784. From a drawing in the Turner
Bequest, CCVIII-S (No.243). Published as one of the
Ports of England series issued by Lupton between 1826
and 1828, and reprinted in Gambart's *The Harbours of
England . . . with Illustrative Text by J Ruskin*, 1856.

THE 'LITTLE LIBER'

Nothing is known of the circumstances under which
the series of mezzotints known as the *Little Liber* or
Sequels to the Liber Studiorum came to be engraved.
They are all by Turner himself and generally deal with
night scenes. Since some of the mezzotints were engraved on steel, which was not in use before 1820, a
date in the 1820s has been suggested. There is no
apparent connection with the *Liber Studiorum* itself
apart from the fact that mezzotint was employed in
both series; but here, in the hands of Turner himself,
the medium has an expressive power, a richness and
intensity lacking from even the finest of the *Liber*
plates. This intensity is much enhanced by the choice
of dramatically lit night and storm subjects; and it
may be noted that the later plates of the *Liber Studiorum* seem to show an increasing preoccupation with
extreme effects of light: 'Stonehenge' (R.81), 'The Lost
Sailor' (R.84), 'Moonlight on the Medway' (R.86) in
particular having affinities with the *Little Liber*. Few
impressions were taken, and prints and plates remained
in Turner's studio until his death; they were dispersed
at Christie's in 1873 and 1874. See Rawlinson, 1908, I,
pp.xliv–xlv.

245   Gloucester Cathedral *c.*1824
Watercolour and pencil, $9\frac{1}{16} \times 11\frac{3}{4}$ (23 × 29.8)
Trustees of the British Museum (T.B.CCLXIII–307)
The two drawings on the verso are possibly connected
with the *Ports of England* series (perhaps 'Catwater') of
about 1824.
   The scene on the recto is related to that of the drawing T.B.CCLXIII–246: both seem to be preliminary to
the *Little Liber* plate known as 'Gloucester Cathedral'
or 'Boston Stump' (No.246).

246   Gloucester Cathedral *c.*1825
Mezzotint, $5\frac{15}{16} \times 8\frac{7}{8}$ (15.1 × 21.3) (trimmed close
to engraved surface)
Trustees of the British Museum (1940-6-1-35)
One of the *Little Liber* series, Rawlinson No.809, trial
proof (a). The subject is also known as 'Boston Stump'
and 'The Hare', as Turner added a hare in the left

foreground (trial proof (b)). Two related drawings are
in the Turner Bequest, CCLXIII–246 and 307 (see No.
245).

**247   A Stormy Landscape with an Obelisk and
Classical Portico** ?*c.*1825
Watercolour, $8\frac{5}{8} \times 11\frac{3}{4}$ (21.9 × 29.8)
Trustees of the British Museum (T.B.CCLXIII–252)
Finberg suggests that this was a design for the *Little
Liber*; it has much in common with the 'Catania' and
'Paestum' plates (Nos.251 and 253).

248   The Evening Gun *c.*1825
Mezzotint, $5\frac{7}{8} \times 8\frac{1}{4}$ (15 × 21); plate $7\frac{1}{2} \times 9\frac{15}{16}$
(19 × 25.3)
Trustees of the British Museum (1912-10-14-3)
One of the *Little Liber* series, Rawlinson No.800, trial
proof (a). Rawlinson records a slight preparatory
sketch from the collection of J. E. Taylor.

249   Shields Lighthouse *c.*1825
Mezzotint, $5\frac{15}{16} \times 8\frac{3}{8}$ (15.1 × 21.2)
Trustees of the British Museum (1912-10-14-4)
One of the *Little Liber* series, Rawlinson No. 801, trial
proof (a). A later proof shows the moon much reduced
in size and the formation of the clouds considerably
modified. There is a watercolour of the subject in the
Turner Bequest, CCLXIII–308.

250   The Mew-Stone, Plymouth Sound *c.*1825
Mezzotint, $6\frac{3}{16} \times 8\frac{13}{16}$ (15.8 × 22.4); plate $7\frac{3}{8} \times 9\frac{15}{16}$
(18.6 × 25.2)
Trustees of the British Museum (1919-6-14-4)
One of the *Little Liber* series. The single known proof
described by Rawlinson, No.804. The design is a
modification of that used for the *Southern Coast*, en-
graved 1815, now National Gallery of Ireland, Vaughan
Bequest. A watercolour study in the Turner Bequest,
CXCVI-F, appears to be related specifically to this plate.

251   Catania, Sicily *c.*1825
Mezzotint, $6\frac{1}{16} \times 8\frac{7}{16}$ (15.4 × 21.4); plate $7\frac{5}{8} \times 10$
(19.3 × 25.3)
Trustees of the British Museum (1912-10-14-7)
One of the *Little Liber* series, Rawlinson No.805. An
early trial proof; later a boat and distant view of Mount
Etna were added on the left. Turner did not visit
Sicily and the subject may have been derived from a
sketch by another artist. Turner's drawing for the
plate, similar in size and technique to that for 'Paestum'
(No.252), is in the Museum of Fine Arts, Boston and
is called 'A Storm over St Peter's, Rome'.

252   Paestum in a Thunderstorm *c.*1825
Watercolour with pencil, $8\frac{3}{8} \times 12$ (21.3 × 30.5)
Trustees of the British Museum (T.B.CCCLXIV–224)
Related to Turner's mezzotint 'Paestum' for the *Little
Liber*. A number of pencil drawings of Paestum are in
the 'Naples, Paestum and Rome' sketchbook (No.232).
Turner used the motif of lightning playing round the
temples at Paestum for a vignette in Roger's *Italy*
(No.274).

253 Paestum *c*.1825
Mezzotint, $6\frac{1}{16} \times 8\frac{1}{2}$ (15.4 × 21.6); cut to edge of engraved area
Trustees of the British Museum (1940-6-1-30)
One of the *Little Liber* series Rawlinson No.799, trial proof (d). A watercolour drawing for the subject is T.B. CCCLXIV–224.

254 A Castle on a Headland *?c*.1824
Watercolour, $10\frac{1}{8} \times 10\frac{5}{8}$ (25.3 × 27)
Trustees of the British Museum (T.B.CCCLXIV–148)
Finberg dates this drawing, and CCCLXIV–149 which may perhaps show the same castle, to the 1830s; it is apparently a smaller variant of the subject of CCLXIII–54 which Finberg assigns to the 1820s. The two studies seem to have been executed at about the same time. The lower bands of blue, red and yellow in this one may in fact form a separate study of sunset sky and sea, intended to be read the other way up. The wiping-out technique in the castle itself suggests an early date, but Turner evidently continued to employ this device, which is characteristic of his experimental watercolours of about 1799, until late in his career. The drawing also has some stylistic affinities with work related to the *Little Liber*. The view is evidently Welsh, perhaps of Harlech, or as Finberg suggests, Criccieth.

255 Three Studies of a Hulk and Sailing Boats
?c.1822
Watercolour, $10\frac{1}{8} \times 9\frac{7}{8}$ (56.2 × 25)
Trustees of the British Museum (T.B.CCLXIII–384)
Perhaps connected with the *Ports of England* series (see No.243) for which Turner made several slight colour studies similar to the upper two on this sheet. The lowest study, with its washes of pink and green, is akin to some of the 'colour-beginnings' provisionally dated *c*.1817, but also has similarities with 'colour-beginnings' of *c*.1830, e.g. 'Tamworth Castle' (T.B. CCLX–184).

256 View from Richmond Terrace *?c*.1825
Watercolour, $14\frac{3}{8} \times 23$ (36.5 × 58.4)
Watermarked: 1824
Trustees of the British Museum (T.B.CCLXIII–385)
At the top of this sheet is a strip of colour belonging to another 'colour-beginning', perhaps of the same subject. This drawing and T.B.CCLXIII–348 may both have been executed as late variations of the large painting 'England: Richmond Hill on the Prince Regent's Birthday' of 1818 (No.167); but it seems more probable that they are to be associated with the large watercolour of 'Richmond Hill' of *c*.1825 (No.257) or even with the smaller view for the *England and Wales* series (No.434).

257 Richmond Hill *c*.1825
Watercolour and bodycolour, $11\frac{11}{16} \times 19\frac{1}{16}$
(29.7 × 48.4)
Trustees of the Lady Lever Art Gallery, Port Sunlight
Engraved by E. Goodall for *The Literary Souvenir*, Pl.III, 1826 (Rawlinson No.314). The largest and most splendid of Turner's watercolours relating to this subject, this drawing seems to have been executed in conjunction with a series of 'colour-beginnings' developing a theme which had appeared in some early watercolour

studies (see No.174) and which he developed very fully in one direction when he painted the large 'England: Richmond Hill on the Prince Regent's Birthday' in 1818 (No.167).

258 Virginia Water *c*.1829
Watercolour, $11\frac{7}{16} \times 17\frac{1}{2}$ (29 × 44.3)
Exh: Egyptian Hall, Piccadilly, 1829
Private collection
Engraved by R. Wallis for *The Keepsake* 1830 (Rawlinson 323). Turner made several sketches of Virginia Water, nearly all including the Chinese Pavilion, in the 'Kenilworth' sketchbook of *c*.1829–30 (T.B.CCXXXVIII; No.442). A sketch corresponding to the left half of this watercolour is on f.73^r.

One of a pair of views of Virginia Water made for George IV, who, it is said, refused to pay for them; the pendant is untraced. It also was engraved for *The Keepsake* (Rawlinson No.322).

259 'Walmer Ferry' Sketchbook *?c*.1820
Bound in leather with one clasp
96 leaves of white Whatman paper prepared with a dark grey-brown wash, and four fly-leaves,
$6\frac{1}{4} \times 4\frac{1}{2}$ (16 × 11)
Watermarked: 1794 and 1813
Trustees of the British Museum (T.B.CXLII)

ff.5^v–6^r Study of Plants
Pen and brown ink with scraping-out on white paper prepared with a wash of dark grey-brown
Inscr: 'Plantain Nettle Cats Tail' 'Daisy Lsmock Grass' 'Willow' and 'May'

Finberg's identification of Walmer Castle on f.1^v seems difficult to maintain; the bridge in the distance suggests Richmond or Kew. The remainder of the book is apparently devoted to views on the Thames both in London (ff.18–27) and higher up, e.g. Syon House, f.97^r. The book is difficult to date, in spite of its two watermarks; Finberg suggests *c*.1815–17, while admitting that some of the drawings may be later; it may well have been in use in the 1820s.

ff.5^v–6^r show one of several such studies in the book, of wild flowers and other plants, probably seen on the Thames. Compare the studies perhaps done near Windsor in the 'Naples, Paestum and Rome' sketchbook of 1819 (No.232).

260 The Ports of England Sketchbook *?*1818–23
Bound in boards, leather spine and corners; one clasp
31 leaves almost all drawn on in black chalk, pencil and watercolour, $7 \times 10\frac{1}{4}$ (17.8 × 26.1)
Watermarked: 1815
Inscr. Finberg transcribes Turner's label on spine: '108'
Trustees of the British Museum (T.B.CCII)

f.30^v Composition Study for a Classical Subject, with three studies showing (?) Greenwich Park with London in the distance beyond
Pencil

The free watercolour sketch on f.22 is close in spirit to those on ff.12 and 13 of the 'Scotch Antiquities and

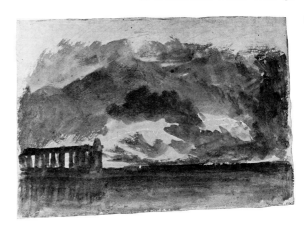

252

London' sketchbook (T.B.CLXX). The watercolour studies of skies, eg. on f.8ʳ are similar to those in the 'Skies' sketchbook (T.B.CLVIII) which also appears to have been in use in 1818 and those of ports are close in colour and treatment to the study of Crichton Castle in CLXX. Finberg dates the book c.1822–3, presumably on account of the presence in it of coloured designs which seem to relate to the *Ports of England* series undertaken for Cooke and published from 1823 onwards. If these drawings are indeed for that publication, the sketchbook may have continued in use until that time.

The small study at the bottom right of f.30 bears some resemblance to the architectural compositions on ff.1, 2 of the 'Mouth of the Thames' sketchbook (T.B. CCLXXVIII) and in T.B.CCCLXIV–243.

ff.25ᵛ–31ᵛ of this book are taken up with composition studies of classical scenes.

261 'Old London Bridge' Sketchbook *c.*1823
Bound in marbled boards, leather spine
44 leaves of pencil sketches with some sky
studies in grey wash, 4 × 6½ (9.8 × 16.1)
Watermarked: 1821
Inscr. Finberg records Turner's label on spine:
'91 London Bridge'
Trustees of the British Museum (T.B.CCV)

f.21ᵛ Studies of boats moored near St. Olave's, Southwark (Southwark Cathedral)
Pencil
f.22ʳ Study of a Sunset Sky
Grey wash

A note of Rubens's picture 'Le Chapeau de Paille', shown in London in March and April 1823, is on f.44ʳ. Other pencil sketches include studies of plants, shipping and views on the Thames near London Bridge. The sketchbook also contains a note of R.A. accounts 'from Xs 1818 to L day 1819'

262 'Thames' Sketchbook 1825
Bound in grey boards, with leather spine, one
clasp
91 leaves, ff.50–69 blank, the majority of the rest
drawn on in pencil or watercolour, 4½ × 7½
(11.3 × 18.8)
Watermarked: 1819
Trustees of the British Museum (T.B.CCXII)

f.9ᵛ Sketch of an Officer
Pencil
f.10ʳ Scene on a River
Watercolour

Sketches on the inside front and back cover and first two or three leaves at each end of the book may have been made on Turner's trip to Belgium and Cologne in August and September of 1825. Most of the remainder apparently show scenes on or near the Thames.

263 Looking down from Otley Chevin into the Valley of the Wharfe ?*c.*1828
Watercolour, 13 7/16 × 19 1/8 (34.2 × 48.5)
Trustees of the British Museum (T.B.CCLXIII–97)
The subject may be related to the pencil study, T.B. CLIV–J (on mount with No.B.137), presumably made

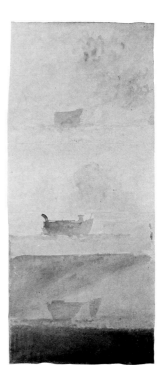

255

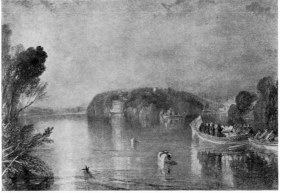

258

about 1817. The light tonality and palette of pure red, yellow and blue, however, suggest a later period for this 'colour-beginning', perhaps 1825–30.

264 Study of an Evening Sky over the Sea *c.*1825
Watercolour, $12\frac{1}{8} \times 19\frac{15}{16}$ (30.3 × 49)
Trustees of the British Museum (T.B.CCLXIII–79)
One of the 'colour-beginnings' dated by Finberg to between about 1820 and 1830. Compare with No.267.

265 Stormy Sky over a Jetty ?*c.*1825
Watercolour over traces of pencil, $6\frac{1}{4} \times 9\frac{1}{16}$ (15.8 × 23)
Sir Edmund Bacon, Bart.

266 Sunset over the Sea (crimson, yellow, blue, green) ?*c.*1825
Watercolour, $9\frac{3}{4} \times 13\frac{5}{8}$ (24.7 × 35)
Inscr. top left illegibly upside down
Trustees of the British Museum (T.B.CCLXIII–207)
Since the sheet has evidently been cut down on three sides (not the left) the inscription may refer to a drawing that has been removed. In any case, Turner has not worked to the edge of the paper, defining an area surrounded by margins to try out colours.

267 Rainclouds over the Sea (grey, pink, blue and green) ?*c.*1825
Watercolour, $7\frac{1}{2} \times 10\frac{3}{4}$ (19 × 27.3)
Trustees of the British Museum (T.B.CCLXIII–226)
The central band of pink and blue colour in this study is treated rather similarly to the peacock and mauve clouds in the 'Evening Sky over the Sea' (No.264).

268 Study of a Sunset (brown, orange, red and purple) ?*c.*1833
Watercolour, $12\frac{5}{16} \times 9\frac{7}{16}$ (31.3 × 24)
Trustees of the British Museum (T.B.CCCLXIV–146)
Nos.45, 107 and 113 of this group appear to have been executed at the same time as this study; No.113 includes an indication of land suggesting Venice as the location.

269 Study of Three Mackerel *c.*1825
Pencil and watercolour, $8\frac{7}{8} \times 11\frac{5}{16}$ (22.5 × 28.8)
Visitors of the Ashmolean Museum, Oxford
Compare No.271. In addition to this one, which he presented to the Ruskin School, Ruskin owned two other studies of mackerel by Turner, which he described in the catalogue of his own collection, shown in 1878 (Nos.106, 107), as 'Study on his kitchen dresser at Margate, splendid', and 'just a dash for three more. Cook impatient'. A note by Ruskin on one of the drawings says that he bought them from Mrs Booth, Turner's housekeeper at Margate. The J. E. Taylor sale, (Christie, 8 July 1912) included two drawings of mackerel, one with prawns; these are apparently identifiable with two drawings at Christie's 4 June 1974 (179, 180).

270 Study of a Teal with Outspread Wings ?*c.*1825
Pencil and watercolour, $12\frac{5}{8} \times 18\frac{1}{2}$ (31.5 × 47)
Trustees of the British Museum (T.B.CCLXIII–340)
Another study of a teal is T.B.CCLXIII–341. See also the *Farnley Book of Birds*, No.B127.

271 Study of Four Fish *c.*1825
Pencil and watercolour, $10\frac{13}{16} \times 18\frac{1}{2}$ (27.5 × 47)
Trustees of the British Museum (T.B.CCLXIII–339)
Another sheet, T.B.CCCXIII–338, contains slight pencil outlines of fish and a watercolour study of perch like that at the top of this group; it has the watermark 1822. A group of different fish is on T.B.CCLXIII–342; see also No.269 and B125.

The Book Illustrations

In about 1826 Turner's work as an illustrator opened out on two contrasting fronts: that of the large, elaborate designs for Charles Heath's *Picturesque Views in England and Wales* on the one hand: and on the other, that of the vignettes for Rogers' *Italy* (1830) and *Poems* (1834). The size of these vignettes is smaller than that of any drawings Turner had previously made for the engraver (the small plates which appeared in the *Keepsake*, the *Literary Souvenir* and other periodicals and annuals during the 1820s were all made from large drawings); and, for the first time, Turner's contribution embellishes the letterpress rather than existing separately, parallel to it. For the circumstances of Turner's employment by Rogers see Adele M. Holcomb, 'A Neglected Classical Phase of Turner's Art,' *Warburg Institute Journal*, Vol.XXXII, 1969, pp.405–410.

The fifty-eight Rogers vignettes were followed in the early 'thirties by a series of commissions for small-scale illustrations, including seventy-seven vignettes and small views for the *Life*, *Prose Works* and *Poetical Works* of Scott; twenty-six designs each for Moxon's *Byron* (1832–4) and Finden's *Landscape Illustrations of the Bible* (1836); and the twenty-one vignettes for Moxon's *Campbell* (1837). The final commission was apparently for Macrone's edition of Tom Moore's *The Epicurean*, which appeared with four designs by Turner in 1839.

The majority of the finished illustrations were dispersed during Turner's lifetime, or shortly after his death, but a large number, including nearly all the Rogers designs, are still in the Turner Bequest, which also contains a great many preparatory sketches (CCLXXX). For most of his designs Turner had recourse to material already existing in his sketchbooks; but the Scott illustrations were treated as a special case and prompted visits in 1831 and 1834. On the first of these journeys Turner filled several sketchbooks (see Nos. 449–453). Turner's work for Scott and Cadell is discussed in Adele M. Holcomb, 'Turner and Scott', *Warburg Institute Journal*, Vol.XXXIV, 1971, pp.386–397; and in Gerald E. Finley, 'J M W Turner and Sir Walter Scott: Iconography of a Tour', *Warburg Institute Journal*, Vol.XXXV, 1972 pp.385–390, and 'Turner's Illustrations to Napoleon', *Warburg Institute Journal*, Vol.XXXVI, 1973, pp.390–396.

272 Aosta ?1826
Pencil and watercolour, vignette approx. $5\frac{1}{2} \times 6\frac{7}{8}$ (14 × 17.5) on sheet $9\frac{3}{8} \times 11\frac{7}{8}$ (23.9 × 30.1)
Inscr. on cross in foreground: '1826'
Trustees of the British Museum (T.B.CCLXXX–145)

Engraved by H. le Keux for Rogers' *Italy*, 1830, p.25 (Rawlinson No.354) as headpiece for the section 'Marguerite de Tours'. In the engraving the date on the cross in the foreground is altered to '1814'. Although *Italy* was not published until 1830, some of the engravers' proofs of the vignettes are dated 1828 and 1829. Finberg says (1961, p.307) that Turner had finished at least most of his vignettes for Rogers' *Italy* by the end of 1828. It seems likely that Turner's share of the work was under way at least a year, perhaps more, before that and it is therefore possible that the date 1826 on the drawing is that of its execution.

273   Marengo *c.*1827
   Pencil and watercolour with some pen and brown ink, vignette approx. $4\frac{7}{8} \times 7\frac{7}{8}$ (12.5 × 20) on sheet $8\frac{5}{16} \times 11\frac{1}{2}$ (21.2 × 29.3)
   Inscr: 'Battle MARENGO 18...' and 'LODI'
   Trustees of the British Museum (T.B.CCLXXX–146)
Engraved by E. Goodall for Rogers' *Italy*, 1830, p.17 (Rawlinson No.353), as headpiece to 'The Descent'.

274   Paestum *c.*1827
   Watercolour with some pen and brown ink, vignette approx. $3\frac{5}{16} \times 6\frac{7}{8}$ (8.5 × 17.5) on sheet $9\frac{7}{16} \times 12$ (24 × 30.6)
   Trustees of the British Museum (T.B.CCLXXX–148)
Engraved by J. Pye for Rogers' *Italy*, 1830, p.207 (Rawlinson No.369), as headpiece to the section entitled 'Paestum'. A preliminary sketch of the subject is T.B.CCLXXX–92. Turner's drawing contains only one somewhat faint flash of lightning; the engraved vignette shows three against a black cloud. Compare this design with the *Little Liber* drawing and mezzotint (Nos.252 and 253).

275   Isola Bella, Lake Maggiore *c.*1827
   Pencil and watercolour with pen and brown ink, vignette approx. $5\frac{1}{8} \times 7\frac{7}{8}$ (13 × 20) on sheet $9\frac{5}{8} \times 12$ (24.4 × 30.5)
   Trustees of the British Museum (T.B.CCLXXX–150)
Engraved by R. Wallis for Rogers' *Italy*, 1830, p.233 (Rawlinson No.372 as 'A Farewell – Lake of Como II').

276   The Roman Forum *c.*1827
   Pencil and watercolour with pen and brown ink, vignette approx. $5\frac{1}{8} \times 5\frac{3}{4}$ (13 × 13.5) on sheet $9\frac{1}{4} \times 12$ (23.6 × 30.5)
   Inscr: 'Roma'
   Trustees of the British Museum (T.B.CCLXXX–158)
Engraved by E. Goodall for Rogers' *Italy*, 1830, p.137 (Rawlinson No.363); used as headpiece to 'Rome'.

277   The Villa Madama, Moonlight *c.*1827
   Watercolour, pen and black and brown ink, vignette approx. 5 × 5 (12.5 × 12.5) on sheet $9\frac{7}{16} \times 11\frac{5}{8}$ (24 × 29.6)
   Trustees of the British Museum (T.B.CCLXXX–159)
Engraved by H. le Keux for Rogers' *Italy* 1830, p.135 as tailpiece to the section 'An Interview' (Rawlinson 361).

278   Traitors' Gate, Tower of London *c.*1832
   Pencil and watercolour, vignette approx. $5 \times 5\frac{1}{4}$ (12.5 × 13.5) on sheet $7\frac{1}{4} \times 12$ (18.5 × 30.5)
   Trustees of the British Museum (T.B.CCLXXX–177)

Engraved by E. Goodall for Rogers' *Poems*, 1834, p.88 (Rawlinson No.383) as an illustration to 'Human Life':
   ...On he moves...
   On thro' that gate misnamed, thro' which before
   Went Sidney, Russell, Raleigh, Cranmer, More,
   On into twilight within walls of stone...
A preliminary sketch in pencil with some watercolour is T.B.CCLXXX–93.

279   Greenwich Hospital *c.*1832
   Pencil and watercolour, vignette approx. $4\frac{1}{8} \times 5\frac{7}{8}$ (10.5 × 15) on sheet $7\frac{9}{16} \times 9\frac{7}{8}$ (19.2 × 25.2)
   Trustees of the British Museum (T.B.CCLXXX–176)
Engraved by E. Goodall for Rogers' *Poems*, 1834, p.33 (Rawlinson No.377) as an illustration to the 'Pleasures of Memory' Part II:
   Go, with old Thames, view Chelsea's glorious pile...
   Go, view the splendid domes of Greenwich – Go...
   Hail noblest structures imaged in the wave!
   A nation's grateful tribute to the brave.
   Hail, blest retreat from war and shipwreck, Hail!
   That oft arrest the wondering stranger's sail...
A slight preliminary sketch of the subject in pencil and wash is T.B.CCLXXX–94.

280   Shipbuilding (an Old Oak dead) *c.*1832
   Pencil and watercolour, vignette approx. $4\frac{1}{8} \times 5\frac{1}{4}$ (10.5 × 13.5) on sheet $7\frac{1}{2} \times 9\frac{13}{16}$ (19 × 24.9)
   Trustees of the British Museum (T.B.CCLXXX–175)
Engraved by E. Goodall for Rogers' *Poems*, 1834, p.178 (Rawlinson No.392), and used as a tailpiece to lines 'To an Old Oak' for which Turner also designed a headpiece, T.B.CCLXXX–174 (Rawlinson No.391).

281   The Rialto Bridge, Venice – Moonlight *c.*1832
   Watercolour, vignette approx. $4\frac{3}{4} \times 5\frac{3}{4}$ (12 × 14.5) on sheet $9\frac{7}{16} \times 12$ (24 × 30.5)
   Trustees of the British Museum (T.B.CCLXXX–196)
Engraved by W. Miller for Rogers' *Poems*, 1834, p.95 (Rawlinson No.386). Rogers' lines seem to describe a daylight scene:
   Now the sun shifts to Venice – to a square
   Glittering with light, all nations masking there,
   With light reflected on the tremulous tide,
   Where gondolas in gay confusion glide...
A study in pencil and grey wash only is T.B.CCLXXX–108.

282   Datur Hora Quieti *c.*1832
   Watercolour, vignette approx. $3\frac{3}{4} \times 5\frac{1}{2}$ (9.6 × 13) on sheet $9\frac{1}{2} \times 12\frac{1}{16}$ (24.2 × 30.7)
   Trustees of the British Museum (T.B.CCLXXX–199)
Engraved by E. Goodall for Rogers' *Poems*, 1834, p.296 (Rawlinson No.405). The 'Cul de Lampe' or tailpiece of the book.

283   The Evil Spirit *c.*1832
   Pencil and watercolour, vignette approx. $4\frac{5}{8} \times 6\frac{1}{4}$ (11.8 × 16) on sheet $9\frac{9}{16} \times 12\frac{1}{2}$ (24.3 × 30.9)
   Trustees of the British Museum (T.B.CCLXXX–202)
Engraved by E. Goodall for Rogers' *Poems*, 1834, p.264 (Rawlinson No.403) as the tailpiece to Canto XII of the 'Voyage of Columbus'. Two pencil studies for the design are in the 'Berwick' sketchbook (T.B.CCLXV–29ᵛ, 30ʳ).

275

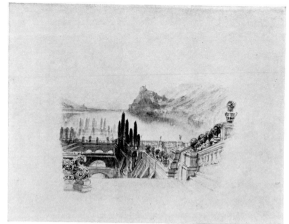

284

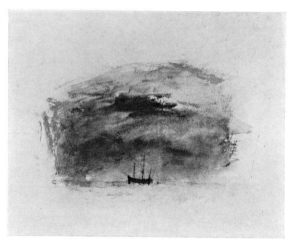

293

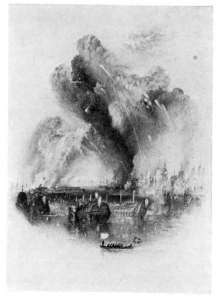

284 The Black Boat *c.*1832
Watercolour, vignette approx. 4¾ × 6½ (12 × 16)
on sheet 8⅝ × 10 15/16 (21.1 × 27.8)
Trustees of the British Museum (T.B.CCLXXX–209)
According to Finberg (1909, II, p.905) this sketch is a
design for Rogers' *Poems*, but it was not used.

285 The Castle of St Angelo *c.*1831
Watercolour, vignette approx. 6¾ × 8¼ (17 × 21)
on sheet 9¼ × 8⅞ (23.5 × 22.5)
Tate Gallery (5243)
Engraved by E. Finden for Murray's *Life and Works of
Byron*, Vol. VIII, 1832 (Rawlinson No.419).

286 The Tomb of Caius Sestus *c.*1831
Watercolour, vignette approx. 5¾ × 7⅝
(13.5 × 19.5) on sheet 9⅛ × 11 3/16 (23.2 × 28.5)
Tate Gallery (5242)
Engraved by E. Finden for Murray's *Life and Works of
Byron*, Vol. XIII, 1832 (Rawlinson No.423). For the
engraved vignette, see No.287.

Edward Francis FINDEN (1791–1857) after
TURNER
287 The Walls of Rome (Tomb of Caius Sestus)
1833
Engraving, proof, vignette, 2 9/16 × 3 9/16 (6.5 × 9);
plate 9⅛ × 6 15/16 (23.2 × 17.5)
Trustees of the British Museum (1868-8-22-4625)
Rawlinson No.423; a vignette for Vol. XIII of Murray's
Life and Works of Byron, published between 1832 and
1834. It is much reduced in size from No. 286.

288 The Drachenfels *c.*1832
Watercolour over pencil, 5 × 7 7/16 (12.7 × 20.2)
City Art Gallery, Manchester
Engraved by W. Finden for Murray's *Life and Works of
Byron*, Vol. XI, 1833 (Rawlinson No.412).

289 Edinburgh Castle *c.*1835
Watercolour, 3 7/16 × 5 9/16 (8.7 × 14.1)
Tate Gallery (4953)
Engraved by T. Higham for Fisher's *Illustrations to the
Waverley Novels* 1836; illustrating the 'March of the
Highlanders', from *Waverley* (Rawlinson No.560).

290 Dryburgh Abbey *c.*1833
Watercolour, 3 1/16 × 5⅞ (7.8 × 14.9)
Tate Gallery (5241)
Engraved by W. Miller for Cadell's *Scott's Poetical
Works*, 1834 (Rawlinson No.501), and used as the
frontispiece to Vol. V, illustrating 'Sir Tristram'. The
pencil drawing on which this watercolour is based is in
the 'Abbotsford' sketchbook (No.450 ff.8ʳ and 9ʳ).
The loop of the river is much less evident there; cf. the
composition of the 'Crook of Lune' (Courtauld Institute
Galleries; Kitson, *Turner Watercolours from the Collection of Stephen Courtauld*, 1974, No.6) and some of
Turner's studies in the Roman Campagna (No.471),
which show a similar interest in meandering rivers
seen from high viewpoints.

291 Rievaulx Abbey *c.*1835
Watercolour, 4 13/16 × 8⅛ (12.2 × 20.7)
Tate Gallery (5615)

Engraved by J. C. Bentley for the *Gallery of Modern British Artists c.*1835 (Rawlinson No.571).

292 Distant View of Rouen *c.*1835
Watercolour and bodycolour with some scraping-out over traces of pencil, $3\frac{1}{4}\times5\frac{3}{4}$ (8.3×14.6)
City Art Gallery, Manchester
Engraved by W. Richardson for *Scott's Prose Works*, 1836, *Tales of a Grandfather* (Rawlinson No.553). The drawing belonged to H. A. J. Munro of Novar. See 'Rouen from St Catherine's Hill' in the *French Rivers* series, No.415.

293 Battle of the Baltic *c.*1836
Watercolour with some pen over traces of pencil, vignette approx. $5\frac{7}{8}\times5\frac{1}{8}$ (15×13)
Mrs M. Fergusson
Engraved by E. Goodall for Moxon's *Campbell's Poetical Works*, 1837, p.81 (Rawlinson No.620).
This and No.294 are two of twenty-four designs made by Turner for Moxon's 1837 edition of Campbell's *Poems*. Rawlinson recounts the story of the commission as he heard it from the engraver's son: Turner was to receive £30 per drawing; 'Goodall was to engrave the plates, and . . . he and Moxon were to divide all the costs and risks and share the profits equally. A draft agreement to that effect was shown by Moxon to Goodall, and later on, the latter signed the document without reading it. Afterwards he discovered that it differed materially from the original proposal as he had understood it and that it would probably mean a very serious loss to him . . . Goodall . . . was advised to ask the painter to cancel the commission for the drawings. He did so, but at first met with a refusal; shortly afterwards, Turner called at Goodall's house late one night, and would come no further than the hall. On Goodall's going to him, he said: "You ask me too much – see what a sum I lose!" Goodall replied: "You could always get equally good pay for your time, Mr Turner." Turner said: "He did not see that he could be expected to forego such a sum." Then Goodall's little daughter happened to come into the hall, and going up to Turner asked him, "if he was the great Mr Turner?" Turner was pleased and said: "I am Mr Turner, don't know about *great* Mr Turner," and patted her head. Finally he agreed to give up the commission, and said: "This is the greatest act of generosity I have ever done in my life". In the end he made the drawings, charged the publisher £5 each for the loan of them, and retained them in his possession until his death.'

294 Camp Hill, Hastings *c.*1836
Watercolour, vignette approx. $5\frac{3}{4}\times4\frac{7}{8}$ (14.5×12.5)
Inscr: 'Over Hauberk and helm|As the sun's setting splendour was thrown|Thence they looked o'er a realm|And tomorrow beheld it their own'
Mrs M. Fergusson
Engraved by E. Goodall for Moxon's *Campbell's Poetical Works*, 1837, p.216 (Rawlinson No.629). See No.293.

295 A Shrine on a Cliff-Top – Study for a Vignette *c.*1835
Pencil, watercolour and brown chalk, $9\frac{3}{8}\times6\frac{1}{4}$ (23.8×15.9)
Trustees of the British Museum (T.B.CCLXXX–121)

296 ? A Ruined Temple – Study for a Vignette *c.*1835
Pencil and watercolour, $9\frac{3}{8}\times6\frac{3}{16}$ (23.8×15.8)
Trustees of the British Museum (T.B.CCLXXX–122)
Both this drawing and No.295 have been thought to be connected with Moxon's edition of *Campbell's Poetical Works*, 1837, though it is not apparently connected with any of the finished designs. The style and colour of both drawings is similar to some pages in the 'Colour Studies' sketchbook No.1 (No.455) which may have been for illustrations, but Turner usually worked out his vignette designs on separate sheets of paper or, as in this case, thin card.

297 A Sunset – Study for a Vignette *c.*1835
Pencil and watercolour, $8\frac{7}{8}\times7$ (22.6×17.7)
Trustees of the British Museum (T.B.CCLXXX–82)

298 A Scarlet Tower – Study for a Vignette *c.*1835
Pencil and watercolour, $9\times6\frac{15}{16}$ (22.8×17.6)
Trustees of the British Museum (T.B.CCLXXX–77)
This and No.297 are similar in technique, and in the type of card used, to the series of preparatory studies for *Campbell's Poetical Works* published by Moxon in 1837.
They also illustrate the important point that Turner conceived these designs for the engraver in brilliant colour from the outset.

299 Part of the Ghaut at Hurdwar *c.*1835
Watercolour, $5\frac{1}{2}\times8\frac{5}{16}$ (14×21.1)
Leeds City Art Gallery
One of seven small designs after drawings 'from nature' by George Francis White for *Views in India, Chiefly among the Himalaya Mountains*, published in 1838. Various engravers were employed; this subject (plate 4) was executed by T. Higham in 1836 (Rawlinson No.606).

300 'Holland' Sketchbook 1825
Bound in calf, one clasp
The spine stamped in gilt lettering:
'ITINERARY No. 1'
282 leaves, all drawn on in pencil, $6\times3\frac{1}{2}$ (14.9×8.8)
Trustees of the British Museum (T.B.CCXIV)

ff.65ᵛ–66ʳ **Studies of Shipping**
Pencil

Crammed with inumerable small pencil sketches of architecture, ships, costume, mostly in Holland, with a series of studies made at Dover and Folkestone, Walmer and Deal, ff.1–23, 243–282.

301 'Mortlake and Pulborough' Sketchbook 1825
Bound in buff boards, with leather spine, one clasp

91 leaves, ff.54–70 blank, the majority of the rest drawn on in pencil, with one or two sketches touched in watercolour, $4\frac{1}{2} \times 7\frac{1}{2}$ (11.2 × 18.7)
Watermarked: 1820
Trustees of the British Museum (T.B.CCXIII)

ff.10ᵛ–11ʳ **William Moffatt's House, Mortlake**
Pencil
Inscr. lower right: 'Tuscan 4 Trigliphs'
(note relating to the portico facing the river, visible from the side in this drawing)

The study is continued at the right on about an inch of f.12ʳ. A view of the river from the garden wall is on ff.12ᵛ and 13ʳ, with sketches of the portico of Moffatt's house. Further studies of the house and garden are on ff.13ᵛ–14ʳ and 15ᵛ–16ʳ. The latter was used as the basis of Turner's painting 'Mortlake Terrace, the seat of William Moffatt, Esq., Summer's Evening', shown at the R.A. 1827 (No.310). The drawing on ff.10ᵛ–11ʳ became the companion, 'Early (Summer's) Morning', shown at the R.A. 1826, now in the Frick Collection.

302 **'Windsor and Cowes' Sketchbook** 1827
Bound in grey boards with leather spine; one clasp
94 leaves, the majority drawn on in pencil, with watercolour studies on ff.8ʳ, 9ʳ, 10ᵛ, $4\frac{1}{2} \times 7\frac{1}{2}$ (9.2 × 11.2)
Watermarked: 1820
Inscr. on spine: 'Windsor'
Trustees of the British Museum (T.B.CCXXVI)

ff.47ᵛ–48ʳ **Sketches of Shipping off Cowes**
Pencil

The sketches in this book include scenes at Windsor and Eton as well as a long series of slight sketches of boats moored or sailing at Cowes, where, in July 1827, Turner visited John Nash who had commissioned him to paint pictures of the Regatta. These were shown at the R.A. in 1828 (see No.321).

303 **A Harbour seen beyond Trees beside a Road** 1827
Pencil, pen and brown ink and white chalk on blue paper, $5\frac{1}{2} \times 7\frac{1}{2}$ (14 × 19)
Trustees of the British Museum (T.B.CCXXVII(a)–57)

304 **East Cowes Castle: Figures in a Walled Garden with Fountains and Statues** 1827
Pen and brown ink and white chalk on blue paper, $5\frac{3}{8} \times 7\frac{1}{2}$ (13.7 × 19)
Trustees of the British Museum (T.B.CCXXVII(a)–47)

305 **East Cowes Castle: A Drawing Room with several figures** 1827
Pen and brown ink and white chalk on blue paper, $5\frac{9}{16} \times 7\frac{11}{16}$ (14.1 × 19.4)
Trustees of the British Museum (T.B.CCXXVII(a)–48)

306 **East Cowes Castle: Figures Seated in a Drawing Room** 1827
Pen and brown ink and white chalk on blue paper, $5\frac{1}{2} \times 7\frac{1}{2}$ (13.9 × 19)
Trustees of the British Museum (T.B.CCXXVII(a)–49)

Some of the series of drawings made while Turner was staying with John Nash at East Cowes Castle between July and October 1827; see Nos.302, 311–319 and 321.

The paper used for these sketches, and the pen and brown ink in which they are executed, occur again in the preparatory drawings for the *French Rivers* series, and it has been suggested that the date, 1827, which can with some certainty be attached to the East Cowes Castle drawings, may be that of all Turner's work in similar format and medium. Finberg listed a number of drawings which almost certainly show East Cowes subjects among the *French Rivers* material in the Turner Bequest, e.g. CCLX–5, 11, 12, 26, 29, 32 etc.

307 **What You Will!** R.A.1822
Oil on canvas, $19 \times 20\frac{1}{2}$ (48 × 52)
Exh: R.A. 1822 (114)
Sir Michael Sobell

This was Turner's only exhibit at the Royal Academy in 1822 and is in strong contrast to the large pictures resulting from his Italian visit in 1819 and shown in 1820, 1823 and 1826. Rather it develops the playful mood of the foreground figures in 'Richmond Hill', approaching closer to their source in Watteau. This was realised by the critics, who otherwise seem to have been baffled by Turner's change of tack. *The Literary Gazette* for 25 May 1822 described it as 'a garden-scene, and nothing else; a sketch, and no more. It is a pretty bit of colouring, something in the style of Watteau', and the *Repository of the Arts, Literature, Fashions* for 1 June called it 'a whimsical attempt at Watteau'. For *The Examiner* of 13 May 'Mr Turner has nothing of Art this season in the Exhibition. He has only a piece of coloured canvas, called . . . What you will!' All made great play with the title, Shakespeare's alternative title for *Twelfth Night*, and it is probably another of Turner's puns. For a later tribute to Watteau see No.334.

308 **George IV at a Banquet in Edinburgh** 1822
Oil on mahogany, $27 \times 36\frac{1}{8}$ (68.5 × 92)
Tate Gallery (2858)

In August 1822 George IV paid a state visit to Edinburgh, the first friendly visit by a monarch since the union of the two kingdoms. Wilkie, who had hopes of painting a scene from the visit for the King, was at the royal landing with William Collins, when 'to our surprise, who should start up upon the occasion to see the same occurence, but J. M. W. Turner, Esq., R.A. P.P.!!! who is now with us we cannot tell how'; so he wrote to his sister on 16 August. No finished paintings of the visit were subsequently exhibited, but Turner did paint this work and another of 'George IV at St. Giles's, Edinburgh' (Tate Gallery 2857), in which the figures, though somewhat caricature-like, are painted with a bravura and a sense of character that look forward to the sketches in body-colour done at Petworth a few years later (see Nos.341–362). There is what seems to be a rapid sketch of the scene in the 'King's Visit to Scotland' sketchbook (T.B.CC–22ᵛ). The visit also provided material for some of the plates for *Provincial Antiquities of Scotland*, published 1819–26, and some of Turner's later illustrations to Sir Walter Scott (see Nos.289–92). Turner travelled both ways by sea, making sketches for *The Rivers of England*, 1823–7, and *The Ports of England*, 1826–8 (see Nos.239–44).

309 View from the Terrace of a Villa at Niton, Isle of Wight, from Sketches by a Lady
R.A.1826
Oil on canvas, 18 × 24 (45.5 × 61)
Exh: R.A. 1826 (297)
William A. Coolidge

Painted for Lady Willoughby Gordon, formerly Julia Bennet, who had been a pupil of Turner in 1797 (see Hilda F. Finberg, 'With Mr Turner in 1797' in *Burlington Magazine*, XCIX, 1957, pp. 48–51). What seems to be a companion picture, though never exhibited, is the 'View in the Isle of Wight near Northcourt' (Musée de Québec), Northcourt having been inherited in 1818 by Lady Gordon and her elder sister, the wife of Sir John Swinburne, another of Turner's patrons. Turner had visited the Isle of Wight, including Niton, in 1795 but did not go there again, it seems, until 1827. This painting, after Lady Gordon's sketch, seems to have re-awakened his interest and led to his visit the following year, just as his first Venetian oil paintings, exhibited in 1833 (see No.529), led to his second visit to Venice. Like 'What you will!' it shows a delightfully light-hearted side to Turner's art, hitherto confined to his watercolours.

310 Mortlake Terrace, the Seat of William Moffatt, Esq. Summer's Evening R.A.1827
Oil on canvas, 36¼ × 48⅛ (92 × 122)
Exh: R.A. 1827 (300)
National Gallery of Art, Washington (Andrew Mellon Collection)

Painted as a companion to 'The Seat of William Moffatt, Esq., at Mortlake. Early (Summer's) Morning', exhibited at the Royal Academy the previous year, in which the house itself is seen from the west with the river on the left (Frick Collection, New York). There are sketches at Mr Moffatt's house, including the views seen in both paintings, in the 'Mortlake and Pulborough' sketchbook (T.B.CCXIII-10ᵛ to 14, 15ᵛ and 16ᵛ (that for this picture), 43ᵛ to 45; see No.301).

The dog on the parapet was an afterthought, perhaps not even Turner's. Tom Taylor adduced 'this dog as a proof of Turner's reckless readiness of resource when an effect in art was wanted. It suddenly struck the artist that a dark object here would throw back the distance and increase the aerial effect. Turner instantly cut a dog out of black paper and stuck him on the wall, where he still remains' (Thornbury 1862, I, p.305). But Frederick Goodall, R.A., whose father had engraved some of Turner's pictures, claimed that it was the work of Edwin Landseer, who would have been twenty-five years old at the time: 'He cut out a little dog in paper, painted it black, and on Varnishing Day, stuck it upon the terrace . . . All wondered what Turner would say and do when he came up from luncheon table at noon. He went up to the picture quite unconcernedly, never said a word, adjusted the little dog perfectly, and then varnished the paper and began painting it. And there it is to the present day' (William T. Whitley, *Art in England 1821–1837*, 1930, p.282).

In these two pictures Turner returned to the study of differing lights at differing times of day of the Tabley pictures of 1809 (Nos.150 and 151) but much of the press, particularly in 1827, was critical, especially of the painting's yellowness. According to *The Morning Post*

for 15 June 1827 'Turner's *View of Mortlake Terrace* is desperately afflicted with the disease of *yellow fever*', while *John Bull* for 27 May likened Turner to a cook afflicted with a mania for curry: 'That the Lord Mayor's barge, which is introduced only for the sake of the colour, should look yellow in its gingerbread decorations, is natural, and that the Aldermen's wives and daughters should look yellow, from sea-sickness, is also natural – but that the trees should look yellow, that the Moffatt family themselves, and all their friends and connexions, birds, dogs, grass-plots, and white stone copings of red brick walls, should be afflicted with the jaundice, is too much to be endured.' For *The Literary Magnet* however the picture was 'instinct with the brightness of Claude'.

311 Sketch for 'East Cowes Castle, the Regatta beating to Windward' No.1 1827
Oil on canvas, 11¾ × 19¼ (30 × 49)
Tate Gallery (1995)

312 Sketch for 'East Cowes Castle, the Regatta beating to Windward' No.2 1827
Oil on canvas, 17¾ × 23⅞ (45 × 60.5)
Tate Gallery (1994)

313 Sketch for 'East Cowes Castle, the Regatta beating to Windward' No.3 1827
Oil on canvas, 18¼ × 28½ (46.5 × 72)
Tate Gallery (1993)

314 Sketch for 'East Cowes Castle, the Regatta starting for their Moorings' No.1 1827
Oil on canvas, 18⅛ × 23⅞ (46 × 60.5)
Tate Gallery (1998)

315 Sketch for 'East Cowes Castle, the Regatta starting for their Moorings' No.2 1827
Oil on canvas, 17½ × 29 (44.5 × 73.5)
Tate Gallery (2000)

316 Sketch for 'East Cowes Castle, the Regatta starting for their Moorings' No.3 1827
Oil on canvas, 17¾ × 24 (45 × 61)
Tate Gallery (1997)

317 Shipping off East Cowes Headland 1827
Oil on canvas, 18⅛ × 23¾ (46 × 60) (repr. on p.54)
Tate Gallery (1999)

318 Between Decks 1827
Oil on canvas, 12 × 19⅛ (30.5 × 48.5)
Tate Gallery (1996)

319 Study of Sea and Sky, Isle of Wight 1827
Oil on canvas, 12 × 19⅛ (30.5 × 48.5)
Tate Gallery (2001)

Turner revisited the Isle of Wight in late July and August 1827, staying with the architect John Nash at East Cowes Castle. In an undated letter he asked his father to send one or if possible two pieces of unstretched canvas, either a piece measuring six by four feet or a 'whole length', and it was on a six by four-foot canvas, cut into two, that he painted these nine sketches. The two rolls of canvas were rediscovered at the National Gallery in 1905 and divided into separate pictures. One roll contained Nos.311, 313, 315, 318 and 319, the other Nos.312, 314, 316 and 317. No record was made of the placing of the sketches on the two rolls on canvas, but to a certain extent this can be reconstructed. On the first roll the two largest sketches, Nos.315 and 313, were one above the other, flanked on the left by Nos.318, 311 (both upside down) and 319. On the other Nos.317

and 314 were at the top, Nos.316 and 312 below; No.312 was definitely to the right of No.316, and No.317 seems to have been above No.316.

It has been suggested that at least some of these sketches were painted on the spot (Graham Reynolds in *Victoria and Albert Museum Yearbook*, 1, 1969, pp. 67–72), though the practical difficulties, especially when out at sea, would have been considerable. It is interesting that the three sketches for 'The Regatta beating to Windward' seem to have been painted alternately on each roll, No.311 on the first, No.312 on the second and No.313 again on the first; this could have been to allow an assistant time to adjust the roll for a new sketch. The 'Windsor and Cowes' sketchbook contains drawings of boats racing, boats stationary, views of the coast and figure studies, though none directly related to the oil sketches, which to a certain extent supports the suggestion that they were done on the spot. It also contains a list of the boats with their names, the names of their owners, and their colours, showing just how detailed was Turner's interest in the Regatta (T.B.CCXXVI-80ᵛ; see No.302).

The two groups of sketches of the Regatta were used for the pictures commissioned by John Nash and exhibited the following year (see No.321). The other three are of three different subjects. 'Between Decks' may be just a scene of visitors on board the naval guard ship that can be seen in the background of Nos.311–313 though it may reflect the practice, at least up to about 1805 if not later, of accommodating sailors' wives between the upper and lower decks when a ship was in port. The 'Study of Sea and Sky', in which the distant coast can just be seen on the horizon, may well be Turner's first oil painting to concentrate on these two elements; it hardly prepares one for the stormy sea-pieces to come (see Nos.490–506)! The smooth handling contrasts strongly with the vigorous sketches for 'The Regatta beating to Windward', but with 'Shipping off East Cowes Headland' one returns to a mood of exquisite calm.

320 Three Seascapes on One Canvas c.1827
Oil on canvas, 35¾ × 23¾ (91 × 60.5)
Tate Gallery (5491)

This canvas is not precisely datable but is fairly close to the 'Study of Sea and Sky' of 1827 (No.319) and serves to give some idea of how the two rolls of canvas used at Cowes must have looked before they were cut up. Here, however, Turner painted three sea-scapes, one of them to be seen with the canvas turned upside down so that two of the compositions share a single sky, and the smaller size of the canvas would have made it much more manageable.

321 East Cowes Castle, the Seat of J. Nash, Esq: the Regatta beating to Windward R.A.1828
Oil on canvas, 36¼ × 48 (92 × 122)
Exh: R.A. 1828 (113)
Indianapolis Museum of Art

This picture and its companion, 'East Cowes Castle, the Seat of J. Nash Esq; The Regatta starting for their Moorings', similarly exhibited in 1828 and now in the Victoria and Albert Museum (repr. in colour by Reynolds in *Victoria and Albert Museum Yearbook*, 1, 1969, p.69 pl.111a), were commissioned by the archi-

tect John Nash to commemorate the second year that the Royal Yacht Club held races at Cowes, and were based on the sketches painted while Turner stayed with Nash in 1827. At the sale after Nash's death in 1835 they were bought for 190 and 270 guineas respectively by the dealer Tiffin, in the second case almost certainly on behalf of John Sheepshanks whose collection passed to the Victoria and Albert Museum in 1857.

Most reviewers liked these pictures though there was a general criticism that the yachts were over-sailed, as for instance in the *Repository of Art* for June 1828: 'carrying such a spread of canvas in the channel in the like breeze would upset some of these yachts; but the canvas being Mr. Turner's they are safe; and perhaps the width of the sheet was necessary for pictorial effect'. Only the *Morning Herald* for 26 May was altogether critical, describing 'The Regatta beating to Windward' as 'as far from Nature in its way' as works showing Turner's more usual 'fiery and exaggerated colouring; ... the composition is a cold grey character throughout, particularly the part intended for the sea, which is more like marble dust than any living waters. The cutters of the regatta are quite out of drawing and just proportion.'

322 Boccaccio relating the Tale of the Birdcage
R.A.1828
Oil on canvas, 48 × 35⅝ (122 × 90.5)
Exh: R.A. 1828 (262)
Tate Gallery (507)

Once again Turner chose his title for general effect rather than to give a specific reference, there being no story about a birdcage in the *Decameron*. Turner was, in fact, inspired by Thomas Stothard's illustrations to an edition of the book published in 1825; the plate of 'Giornata Seconda' is particularly close with its Watteauesque figures sitting on the grass amidst trees (repr. A. C. Coxhead, *Thomas Stothard R.A.*, 1906, facing p.140). According to C. R. Leslie Turner painted the picture 'in avowed imitation' of Stothard and told him, while actually working on it during one of the Varnishing Days prior to the opening of the 1828 Royal Academy, that 'If I thought he liked my pictures half as well as I like his, I should be satisfied. He is the Giotto [sic: perhaps 'Watteau'] of England'. There is a further link with Watteau in that Turner here illustrates the text from Du Fresnoy that he was later to give to his 'Watteau Painting' (No.334), using white to bring a distant object near. In this case the distant object is based on East Cowes Castle, the subject of a number of sketches on blue paper done during Turner's visit in 1827 (T.B.CCXXVII (a); see Nos.303–6).

The critic of the *Literary Gazette* for 17 May 1828 recognised Turner's reference to his fellow artists, ancient and modern; referring to Turner's other exhibits that year (see No.321) he begins '– On land, as well as on water, Mr Turner is determined not merely to shine, but to blaze and dazzle. Watteau and Stothard, be quiet! Here is much more than you could match.' But he goes on to attack the picture as a 'sketch . . . With respect to the details in this gaudy experiment the less they are inspected the better for the reputation of the artist'. The *Athenaeum* for 21 May attacked it as 'the *ne plus ultra* of yellow, and gaudiness, and of corrupt art'. *The Times* for 6 May, however, after describing another of Turner's exhibits as 'extremely beautiful and powerful' said of Boccaccio 'that it displays equal genius and the same fault . . . it is like nothing in nature'.

323 The Morning after the Wreck *c.*1827–30
Oil on canvas, 18 × 24 (38 × 61)
National Museum of Wales, Cardiff

Included in the sale of M. T. Shaw at Christie's on 20 March 1880 as from the collection of John Pound, the son by her first marriage of Turner's housekeeper Mrs Booth, but the work of this title in his sale at Christie's on 25 March 1865 was given different measurements. In any case it seems to be a genuine work of the late 1820s, similar to some of the Cowes sketches and to 'Rocky Bay with Figures' (No.483).

324 Sailing Boat off Deal *c.*1827–30
Oil on millboard, 9 × 12 (23 × 30.5)
National Museum of Wales, Cardiff

Similar in technique and approach to the oil sketches on millboard found among the Turner Bequest at the British Museum (see No.469). This example came from the family of John Pound, the son of Turner's housekeeper Mrs Booth by her first marriage, and was sold at Christie's on 11 June 1909. The title is taken from that sale catalogue. In style this sketch seems to date from the late 1820s rather than from the later period of most of the British Museum sketches such as Nos.498–500.

9. Petworth 1828–37

George Wyndham, Third Earl of Egremont, was the most important of Turner's patrons. He formed a fine collection of works by contemporary British painters and sculptors and had bought a large number of Turner's paintings between 1802 and 1813, including a view of 'Petworth, Sussex, the Seat of the Earl of Egremont: Dewy Morning', exhibited at the Royal Academy in 1810 and still at Petworth. Egremont extended his hospitality to a number of artists and in the later 1820s and 1830s Turner spent a considerable amount of time at Petworth, even having his own studio there. Besides the oils and watercolours specifically associated with Petworth, these visits seem to have led to a renewed interest in historical and Biblical subjects coupled with a particular influence from the paintings of Rembrandt. See also p.192.

325 Petworth Park, Tillington Church in the Distance *c.*1828
Oil on canvas, 25⅜ × 57⅜ (64.5 × 145.5)
Tate Gallery (559)

326 The Lake, Petworth *c.*1828
Oil on canvas, 25½ × 55½ (65 × 141)
Tate Gallery (2701)

327 Chichester Canal *c.*1828
Oil on canvas, 25¾ × 53 (65.5 × 134.5)
Tate Gallery (560)

328 The Old Chain Pier, Brighton *c.*1828
Oil on canvas, 27¼ × 53¼ (69 × 135) (repr. on p.71)
Tate Gallery (2064)

329 A Ship Aground *c.*1828
Oil on canvas, 27½ × 53½ (70 × 136)
Tate Gallery (2065)

These works were painted in connection with the four more finished pictures designed to hang below the full-length seventeenth-century portraits in the panelled Grinling Gibbons room at Petworth. Evidence recently discovered by John Gage, but not yet published, shows that two of the finished pictures were *in situ* by 1828, a

year or so earlier than the group has hitherto been dated, and he has also shown that Lord Egremont had interests in both the Chain Pier at Brighton, which was opened in 1823, and Chichester Canal, from which he withdrew his money in 1826.

The finished pictures, still at Petworth but now hung more accessibly in another room, follow the first four with minor changes of detail, which also tends to be more clearly defined. Extra animals have been added in the foreground of 'Petworth Park', including a pair of fighting bucks, and there is a cricket match going on behind the deer on the left; the scene of the dogs rushing out to meet their master is omitted. Turner also introduced deer drinking into the right-hand side of 'The Lake, Petworth', and swans on the left. Similarly, he added the debris on the beach in the foreground of 'The Chain Pier, Brighton'. The least altered is 'Chichester Canal' but here, as in 'Petworth Park', the great arch of the sky, almost as tangible as the answering sweep of the foreground below, has been tamed and looses its weight in the composition. Nor, in 'Chichester Canal' and 'The Lake, Petworth', does the setting sun cut so markedly (and with optical correctness) into the horizon as in the sketches. In general it may be said that the final pictures represent a taming and a prettification of the original versions.

John Gage has suggested (1969, p.260, n.91) that the Tate sketches were originally painted for the setting at Petworth but turned out to be too large, but, although the finished version of 'The Lake' is appreciably shorter, the differences between the others are not very large and the final view of No.325 is if anything longer. It may therefore be that Lord Egremont, used to Turner's earlier style, found the sketches now at the Tate Gallery too freely painted for his taste.

The sketch of 'A Ship Aground' was not used at Petworth but seems to lie behind two paintings exhibited at the Royal Academy in 1831, 'Fort Vimieux' and, to a lesser extent, 'Life-boat and Manby Apparatus' (Nos.510 and 509). Here the setting sun adds to

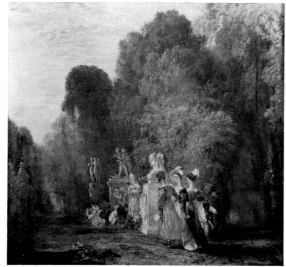

307

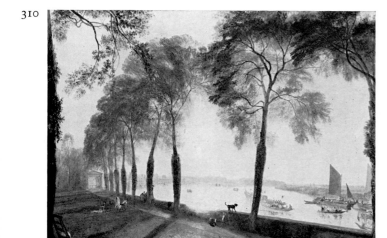

310

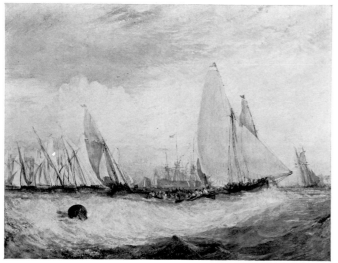

321

the melancholy desolation of the scene.

There are related compositions among the Petworth gouaches on blue paper but these were probably done independently, perhaps later (T.B.CCXLIV-2, 3 and 7 are especially close; see No.342).

330 Evening, Chichester Canal *c.*1825–8
Oil on canvas, $25\frac{1}{2} \times 49\frac{1}{2}$ (65×126)
Tate Gallery (5563)

This picture did not come to the Tate Gallery as part of the Turner Bequest but was presented in 1944 by Miss M. H. Turner, a descendant of the artist's next-of-kin who successfully disputed his will. The attribution has even been doubted but it is quite definitely in Turner's hand and seems to be the first idea for the composition of 'Chichester Canal' (No.327), seen at a slightly different angle, with the setting sun but without the ship and the distant glimpse of Chichester Cathedral that add important accents to the composition in the later versions. It is more thickly painted than the other sketches and the way in which the paint has been worked on the canvas when wet is closer to works like Nos.308, 315 and 483.

331 Jessica R.A.1830
Oil on canvas, $48 \times 36\frac{1}{4}$ (122×92)
Exh: R.A. 1830 (226)
H.M. Treasury and the National Trust, from Petworth House (91)

Exhibited in 1830 with a reference to Shakespeare's *Merchant of Venice*:

Shylock – Jessica, shut the window, I say.

There is probably an oblique reference to Rembrandt's Jewish subjects; in any case the composition of a girl seen half-length through an opening, her left hand extended to hold a feature at the edge of that opening, recalls Rembrandt's 'Lady with a Fan' in the Royal Collection (repr. illustrated souvenir, *Dutch Pictures 1450–1750*, Royal Academy 1952–3, p.7). Turner had already made a direct allusion to his model in the rather similar picture of 'Rembrandt's Daughter', exhibited in 1827 (Fogg Art Museum, Harvard University). But Rembrandt's near-monochrome is transformed into a blaze of colour, which, together with Turner's somewhat ill-drawn but by no means unattractive figure, seems to have aroused the universal condemnation of the critics. *The Morning Chronicle* for 3 May 1830 called it an 'abortion' and went on, 'If it resembles anything conceivable, and that is scarcely so, it is a lady jumping out of a mustard-pot', while the *Athenaeum* for 5 June claimed that 'A hazy old clotheswoman at a back window in Holywellstreet, would show a delicate and soft-eyed Venus, compared with this daub of a drab, libelling Shakespeare out of a foggy window of King's yellow'.

Despite these criticisms Lord Egremont purchased the picture the following year, as reported in the *Library of the Fine Arts* for April 1831. This was apparently as a replacement for the large landscape of 'Palestrina' which Turner began *con amore* for Lord Egremont as his first work in Rome in 1828 and also exhibited in 1830 (it was later bought by Elhanan Bicknell and is now in the Tate Gallery, 6283); John Gage suggests that Lord Egremont's taste stopped short of the new style revealed in such Italian landscapes as

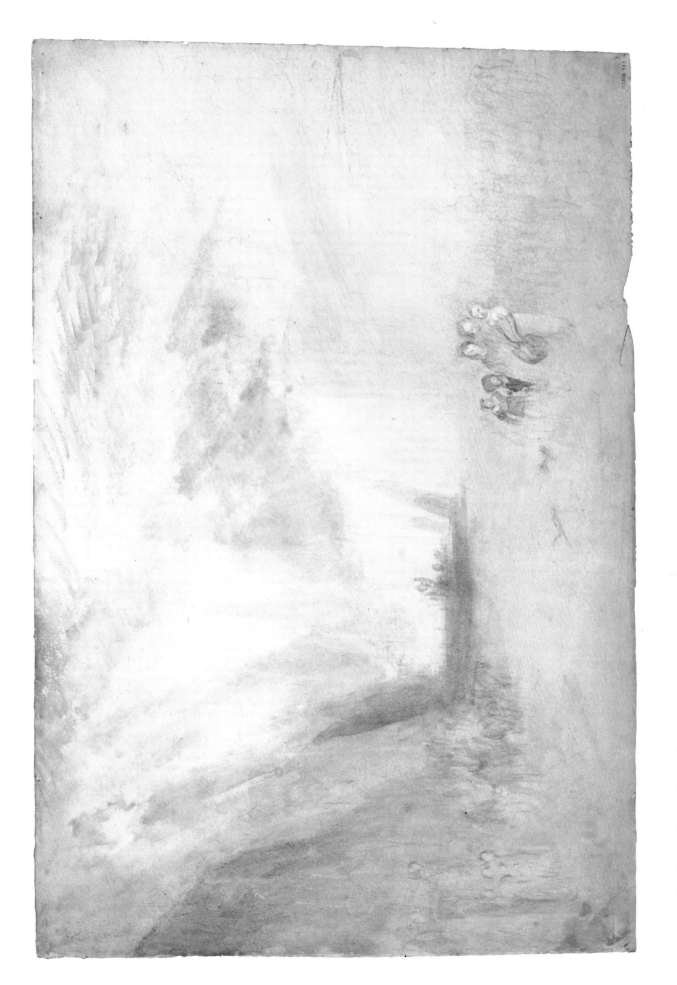

447 **The High Street, Oxford** *c.*1830–5 (entry on p.125)

482 **Ulysses deriding Polyphemus** 1829 (entry on p.133)

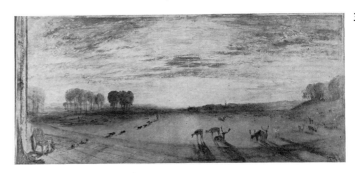

325

this (for similar works in the exhibition see Nos.485 and 486).

332 Pilate washing his Hands R.A.1830
Oil on canvas, 36 × 48 (91.5 × 122)
Exh: R.A. 1830 (7)
Tate Gallery (510)

Exhibited in 1830 with the text from *Matthew* XXVII, 24:

> And when Pilate saw he could prevail nothing, but that rather a tumult was made, he took water and washed his hands before the multitude, saying, I am innocent of the blood of this just person; see ye to it.

The first of three paintings of Biblical subjects that owe a lot to Rembrandt, already represented with works of this general character at the National Gallery from its opening in 1824; the others are 'Shadrach, Meshach and Abednego', exhibited in 1832 (see No.B39), and the unfinished 'Christ driving the Traders from the Temple', also of about this date (Tate Gallery 5474). The renewed interest in figures, which, though relatively small in scale, dominate the composition, their rich costumes and the types of the Jewish priests, as well as the dramatic use of light and the thick, heavily worked paint all point to Rembrandt, to whom Turner had already paid tribute in 'Rembrandt's Daughter', exhibited in 1827 (Fogg Art Museum, Harvard University). Turner uses the fall of light to pick out the tiny figures of Pilate and the statue of Dagon in the background, but unlike Rembrandt the picture glows with colour as well as light.

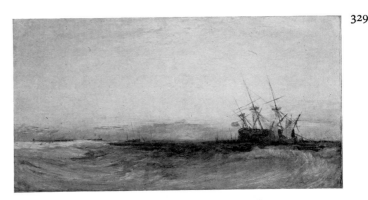

329

This picture and the similarly Rembrandtesque 'Jessica', so different from the landscapes shown the same year, provoked the virulence of the critics. The *Literary Gazette* for 8 May 1830 called it 'wretched and abortive' and followed this up the next week by quoting a wag 'saying, he fancied "a pilot washing his hands" was a fine marine subject'. *The Morning Chronicle* for 3 May more interestingly linked its attack with an early account of Turner's practice of completing his pictures on the Academy's Varnishing Days. Speaking of this picture and 'Orvieto' the critic wrote, 'We understand that when these pictures were sent to the Academy, it was difficult to define their subject; and that in the four or five days allowed (exclusively, and, therefore, with shameless partiality to A's [Associates] and R.A.'s to touch on their works, and injure as much as possible the underprivileged) they have been got up as we see them. They still partake of the character of conundrums.'

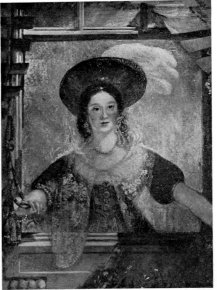

331

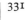

333 Lucy, Countess of Carlisle, and Dorothy Percy's Visit to their Father Lord Percy, when under Attainder upon the Supposition of his being concerned in the Gunpowder Plot R.A.1831
Oil on oak, 15¾ × 27¼ (40 × 69.5)
Exh: R.A. 1831 (263)
Tate Gallery (515)

This picture, like its companion 'Watteau Study by Fresnoy's Rules', is a tribute to another artist, in this case Van Dyck, the figures all being based on pictures by, or attributed to, that artist at Petworth. There is moreover a family connection between the subject of the picture and Petworth, which belonged to the Percy family from 1150 until the end of the seventeenth cen-

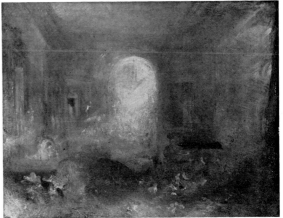

339

tury. Henry Percy, 9th Earl of Northumberland (1564–1632), known as the 'Wizard Earl' on account of his scientific and alchemical experiments, was suspected of complicity in Guy Fawkes' Gunpowder Plot in 1605 and was imprisoned in the Tower of London for sixteen years. On his release in 1621 he retired to Petworth. He is shown with his two daughters, and among the pictures on the right-hand wall are a view appropriately labelled 'Tower of London' and another of the Angel releasing St. Peter from prison.

This picture and its companion were painted on the panels of two matching doors, which one would like to think came from a cupboard at Petworth, used when Turner had run out of more orthodox supports. The framing members round each panel were retained as the inner frames which bear the old Turner Bequest labels.

Both pictures have unfortunately darkened irretrievably so it is particularly interesting that the *Library of the Fine Arts* for June 1831 singled out 'the flood of light pouring like water over the ledges of a cataract into Lord Percy's chamber, dispelling its sombre hue', an effect to be carried much further in 'Interior at Petworth' (No.339). *La Belle Assemblée* for the same month recognised that 'the artist has ingeniously adopted some of Vandyke's costumes. This production also, as well as the Watteau study by Fresnoy's rules ..., will attract notice as an extraordinary combination of colour'. *The Morning Chronicle*, 16 May, was less complimentary to Turner, whom it called 'The Yellow Admiral': 'It seems that the design has no reference to history, but is amongst Mr. T.'s *jeux d'esprit* and represents the present Percy, Duke of Northumberland, huddled up in an arm chair with the stomach-ache, on *Dolly* and the other daughters of corruption announcing to him the success of *Reform*' (the Reform Bill was finally passed the following year).

334   Watteau Study by Fresnoy's Rules R.A.1831
  Oil on oak, $15\frac{3}{4} \times 27\frac{1}{4}$ (40 × 69.5)
  Exh: R.A. 1831 (298)
  Tate Gallery (514)

Exhibited in 1831 with the following lines from du Fresnoy's *De Arte Graphica*:

  White, when it shines with unstained lustre clear,
  May bear an object back, or bring it near.

Turner illustrates this theory with a tribute to Watteau, including among the pictures in the background 'Les Plaisirs du Bal', in reverse and therefore probably from the engraving by Gerard Scotin although the picture was already in the Dulwich Gallery, and 'La Lorgneuse' which then belonged to Turner's friend Samuel Rogers. The companion painting (No.333) was similarly a tribute to Van Dyck.

As in the case of the companion picture contemporary critics were on the whole surprisingly complimentary, showing an appreciation of Turner's special effects of colour. Who but Turner, asked the *Library of the Fine Arts* for June 1831, could have painted this picture 'with its almost impossible effects produced on principles directly opposed to those generally adopted, his lights merging in depths, his depths thrown deeper by his lights, and this all in a mere sketch and apparently produced without effort?' The *Athenaeum* for 21 May called it 'of the wildest of this artist's colouring fancies'

but went on, 'What a trifle in the tone would destroy the beauty. We have not seen this picture commended, but to our taste it is full of delicacy and beauty, and is a rich gem.'

335   Death on a Pale Horse *c*.1830
  Oil on canvas, $23\frac{1}{2} \times 29\frac{3}{4}$ (60 × 75.5)
  Tate Gallery (5504)

The theme of the riders of the Apocalypse was a common one among the more imaginative of British neoclassical artists in the later eighteenth and early nineteenth centuries, for example Benjamin West, John Hamilton Mortimer, P. J. de Loutherbourg and William Blake. Turner, typically, transforms it into a vision of cloud and fire, a manifestation of the destructive power of nature. Lawrence Gowing suggests that it may have been inspired by the death of Turner's father in 1829 (1966, p.27), and it also reflects Turner's renewed interest in figure paintings about this time. The rubbing and scratching away of the wet paint to produce special textures parallels that in some of the Cowes sketches of 1827 (see Nos.315 and 318) and 'Rocky Bay with Figures' of *c*.1830 (No.483).

336   Music Party, Petworth *c*.1835   (repr. on p.72)
  Oil on canvas, $47\frac{3}{4} \times 35\frac{5}{8}$ (121 × 90.5)
  Tate Gallery (3550)

This painting develops on a large scale the interior scenes of life at Petworth of the body-colours on blue paper (Nos.343–362). As in the case of 'Interior at Petworth' (No.339) no actual room can be identified but the mood of relaxed social activity, with an element of dressing up, comports with contemporary accounts of life in Lord Egremont's informal circle. It is impossible to date these pictures at all precisely, but the relatively thick paint and virtuoso handling seem to be characteristic of a stage in Turner's development in the mid 1830s, partly as a result of his interest in Rembrandt (see Nos.331, 332 and 338).

337   Not exhibited

338   Dinner in a Great Room with Figures in Costume *c*.1835
  Oil on canvas, $35\frac{3}{4} \times 48$ (91 × 122)
  Tate Gallery (5502)

The title, evocative of the party-like splendour of life at Petworth, is Lawrence Gowing's. This particular version of the theme of the interior at Petworth is especially close to Rembrandt in its massing of light and shade, richness of effect and disposition of figures in an interior. The figure silhouetted against a shaft of light on the left is like that in the early Rembrandt formerly called 'The Philosopher', which seems to have passed through the London sale rooms twice in the 1790s and to have remained in this country until it finally entered the National Gallery in 1917 (3214; see Neil Maclaren, *National Gallery Catalogues: The Dutch School*, 1960, p.332). But Turner reinterpreted Rembrandt's relatively low-toned chiaroscuro in terms of colour which glows even in this dimly lit interior.

339 Interior at Petworth c.1837
Oil on canvas, 35¾×48 (91×122)
Tate Gallery (1988)

Although identified as Petworth when first listed in the National Gallery inventory in 1905 the picture depicts no recognisable room. It is however the culmination of a series of oil paintings of interiors associated with Petworth (see Nos.336 and 338) and is also a development of the theme of a number of the Petworth body-colours on blue paper (Nos.343–362). David Thomas, in an unpublished lecture, has suggested that this picture represents Turner's reaction to the news of his friend and patron Lord Egremont's death in 1837. The suggestion of a catafalque with coat-of-arms, surrounded by dogs, and the sculptures that possibly allude to Lord Egremont's collection of Antique and contemporary examples, support this. All is in a state of dissolution; above all from the power of light flooding in from the right. The heavy drying-crackle in the foreground, rare in Turner's work, indicates his haste. It is also fascinating in that, until recent restoration, it revealed a layer of bright, untempered red underlying much of the foreground. The strong greens are also impossible to explain from the point of view of representation and are used colouristically and expressionistically.

340 'Petworth' Sketchbook c.1830
Bound in grey boards, leather spine; one clasp
82 leaves, 13 drawn on in pencil or pen and brown ink, 4½×7¼ (11.5×18.4)
Watermarked: 1819
Inscr. on spine: 'Petworth'
Trustees of the British Museum (T.B.CCXLIII)

ff.77ᵛ–78ʳ Petworth Park, with the Spire of Tillington Church
Pencil

Contains only a few pen and ink studies of plants, and pencil sketches of Petworth Park and the surrounding country.
ff.77ᵛ–78ʳ are connected with the painting now at Petworth, an oil sketch for which is at the Tate Gallery (No.325).

THE PETWORTH DRAWINGS

116 drawings are listed by Finberg under the heading of 'Petworth Watercolours' in the Turner Bequest, CCXLIV; he dates them to about 1830. They are all executed in colour, predominantly bodycolour, on sheets of blue paper folded and torn in 5½×7½in rectangles. Turner used the same size and type of paper, and the same medium, for his series of drawings for the *French Rivers* tours, Seine and Loire; and for the series which seem to be connected with a project for similar tours on the Meuse and Moselle and perhaps in southern France. These continental subjects were developed out of material gathered during the 1820s, and particularly from journeys of 1826 and 1829. There are considerable variations in Turner's approach to the different geographical areas, notably in palette and in the use of a pen to point up detail, but it seems

probable that all the series were executed at about the same time. It would be consistent with Turner's methods of work too that all the Petworth studies were made within a short period, probably during one visit. He had made just such a sequence of intimate studies, on similar paper, but using a pen only, during his stay at East Cowes Castle in 1827 (see Nos.303–6).

Although many of the Petworth drawings are very slight, they were all begun in colour and there is no evidence that Turner made preparatory sketches in pencil and chalks as he did in the case of the Meuse/Moselle drawings or in pencil and pen as he did for the Loire and Seine series. The Petworth group is remarkable, in fact, for its feeling of spontaneity. Turner appears to have wandered freely round house and grounds, with a pad of ready-torn sheets of paper, noting scenes as he found them. The still lifes, of flowers in a vase (No.348) or of a console table flanked by Chinese vases (No.345) for instance, have every appearance of being records made on the spot. It may be that Turner drew some of his other subjects from memory – the after-dinner recital of a harpist (No.353) or a sermon in the Chapel (No.356) – but on the whole, the figure subjects also seem to be directly noted from what Turner saw, with recurrent characters, such as the lame man who can be seen lying on a sofa with his crutch in a number of the drawings. That Turner was not the only artist to enjoy the hospitality of Lord Egremont is shown by the several studies of painters at work, in one case a pair of them together, engaged on canvases side by side (No.359). Painters like George Jones and C. R. Leslie were regular guests and it may be that they are shown in some of these drawings.

In some of his careful drawings of particular rooms, Turner records the identity and position of pictures and objects with a care reminiscent of his Farnley interiors of a decade earlier. These were larger in format but similar in medium, and anticipated the beautiful effects of indoor light which Turner achieves in such Petworth studies as the 'Red Room' (No.347) and the 'Drawing Room' (No.361). But other Petworth drawings lead on to the dramatic, not domestic, oil paintings of the 1830s, in which the interior of the house becomes a great gilded cavern resonant with bursts of brilliant light (Nos.338 and 339). The study of the 'Gallery with Flaxman's St. Michael' (No.349) is seen in just such a theatrical way, and even the intimacy of a bedroom (No.344) takes on something of the same intensity.

341 Petworth: a Windmill at Sunset ?1828
Watercolour and bodycolour on blue paper, 5½×7⅞ (14×18.8)
Trustees of the British Museum (T.B.CCXLIV–1)

342 Petworth: Sunset across the Park ?1828
Bodycolour on blue paper, 5½×7½ (13.9×19)
Trustees of the British Museum (T.B.CCXLIV–2)

343 Petworth: Study of a Bed with Pink Satin Curtains ?1828
Watercolour and bodycolour on blue paper, 7¹¹⁄₁₆×5½ (19.4×14)
Trustees of the British Museum (T.B.CCXLIV–15)

344 **Petworth: A Bedroom with a Large Four-Poster Bed** ?1828
Watercolour and bodycolour on blue paper, $5\frac{3}{8} \times 7\frac{1}{2}$ (13.8 × 18.9)
Trustees of the British Museum (T.B.CCXLIV–17)

345 **Petworth: Part of the Wall of a Room, with Large Blue and White China Jars flanking a Gilt Console Table** ?1828
Watercolour and bodycolour on blue paper, $5\frac{3}{8} \times 7\frac{1}{2}$ (13.7 × 19)
Trustees of the British Museum (T.B.CCXLIV–19)

346 **Petworth: the Library, with a Painter seated before an Easel** ?1828
Watercolour and bodycolour on blue paper, $5\frac{7}{16} \times 7\frac{1}{2}$ (13.8 × 19)
Trustees of the British Museum (T.B.CCXLIV–20)

347 **Petworth: the Red Room** ?1828
Bodycolour on blue paper, $5\frac{3}{8} \times 7\frac{1}{2}$ (13.7 × 19)
Trustees of the British Museum (T.B.CCXLIV–21)
The two full-length portraits on either side of the door are those of Sir Robert Shirley and his wife in Eastern costume, by Van Dyck.

348 **Petworth: A Vase of Lilies, Dahlias and other Flowers** ?1828 (repr. on p.89)
Bodycolour on blue paper, $5\frac{3}{8} \times 7\frac{3}{8}$ (13.7 × 18.8)
Trustees of the British Museum (T.B.CCXLIV–23)

349 **Petworth: the Gallery, with Flaxman's 'St. Michael'** ?1828
Watercolour and bodycolour with pen and black ink and scraping-out on blue paper, $5\frac{5}{8} \times 7\frac{1}{2}$ (14.2 × 18.9)
Trustees of the British Museum (T.B.CCXLIV–25)
Flaxman's colossal marble sculpture of St. Michael was commissioned by Lord Egremont in 1819 and finished in 1826, when it was set up in the sculpture gallery at Petworth.

350 **Petworth: a group of Figures seated in an Interior** ?1828
Bodycolour, with some pen and brown ink on blue paper, $5\frac{9}{16} \times 7\frac{9}{16}$ (14.1 × 19.2)
Trustees of the British Museum (T.B.CCXLIV–26)

351 **Petworth: a Candlelit Interior with Figures seated at a Table** ?1828
Watercolour and bodycolour on blue paper, $5\frac{3}{8} \times 7\frac{1}{2}$ (13.8 × 19)
Trustees of the British Museum (T.B.CCXLIV–41)

352 **Petworth: A Woman in Black sitting with a Framed Painting on a Pink Sofa** ?1828
Watercolour and bodycolour, $5\frac{3}{8} \times 7\frac{9}{16}$ (13.8 × 19.2)
Trustees of the British Museum (T.B.CCXLIV–42)

353 **Petworth: Interior with Several Figures listening to a Woman in Black playing the Harp** ?1828
Watercolour and bodycolour on blue paper, $5\frac{1}{2} \times 7\frac{3}{8}$ (14 × 18.7)
Trustees of the British Museum (T.B.CCXLIV–43)
Another sketch of the same scene is CCXLIV–28.

354 **Petworth: the Pulpit in the Chapel** ?1828
Watercolour and bodycolour on blue paper, $5\frac{3}{8} \times 7\frac{3}{8}$ (13.7 × 18.7)
Trustees of the British Museum (T.B.CCXLIV–62)

355 **Petworth: the Chapel, with Pulpit and Organ** ?1828
Watercolour and bodycolour on blue paper, $5\frac{9}{16} \times 7\frac{3}{8}$ (14.1 × 18.8)
Trustees of the British Museum (T.B.CCXLIV–64)

356 **Petworth: Interior of the Chapel during a Sermon** ?1828
Watercolour and bodycolour on blue paper (discoloured), $5\frac{3}{8} \times 7\frac{1}{2}$ (13.8 × 19)
Trustees of the British Museum (T.B.CCXLIV–66)

357 **Petworth: a Group of Ladies conversing** ?1828
Bodycolour on blue paper, $5\frac{1}{2} \times 7\frac{1}{2}$ (13.9 × 19.1)
Trustees of the British Museum (T.B.CCXLIV–101)

358 **Petworth: an Artist painting in a Room with a Large Fanlight** ?1828
Bodycolour on blue paper, $5\frac{1}{2} \times 7\frac{1}{2}$ (14 × 18.9)
Trustees of the British Museum (T.B.CCXLIV–102)

359 **Petworth: Two Artists painting** ?1828
Bodycolour on blue paper, $5\frac{1}{2} \times 7\frac{3}{8}$ (13.9 × 18.8)
Trustees of the British Museum (T.B.CCXLIV–103)

360 **A Meet** ?1828
Bodycolour on blue paper, $7\frac{1}{2} \times 11$ (19.1 × 28)
Trustees of the British Museum (T.B.CCXLIV–104)
One of the Petworth series, this sketch occupies a sheet twice the usual size, folded vertically in the centre.

361 **Petworth: the Drawing Room** ?1828
Bodycolour on blue paper, $5\frac{3}{8} \times 7\frac{1}{2}$ (13.7 × 18.9)
Trustees of the British Museum (T.B.CCXLIV–108)
The large painting in the centre of the wall is Reynolds' 'Macbeth and the Witches' painted in 1789, and acquired by Lord Egremont in 1807 or shortly after. It is still at Petworth.

362 **Petworth: the Hall and Staircase** ?1828
Bodycolour on blue paper, $5\frac{1}{2} \times 7\frac{1}{2}$ (13.9 × 18.9)
Trustees of the British Museum (T.B.CCXLIV–109)

10. The French Rivers 1827–35

In 1833, 1834 and 1835 Charles Heath, promulgator of the *England and Wales* scheme (see p.121), published three elegant volumes under the title of *Turner's Annual Tour*. These consisted of a series of steel engravings by various hands after designs by Turner, accompanied by descriptive text in the form of a travel journal by Leitch Ritchie, a journalist whom Heath had employed for his *Picturesque Annual* and other publications. The first volume was *Wanderings by the Loire. . . with twenty-one engravings from Drawings by J. M. W. Turner, Esq. R.A.*, the second and third were *Wanderings by the Seine*, each with twenty plates. Twenty-one of the finished Loire drawings (including some never engraved) are in the Ashmolean Museum; nearly all the Seine designs, with many unpublished drawings and sketches, are in the Turner Bequest (CCLIX–CCLXII).

The illustrations are based on pencil sketches made in France over a period of several years; Turner seems to have used material obtained on tours of 1821, 1824, 1826, 1828 and possibly 1829. The final designs are on the small 5½ × 7½ in sheets of blue paper, and in the bodycolour, that Turner used for his Petworth interiors. Many of the preliminary studies are also on blue paper. Some of the outline sketches in pen and brown ink are very similar to the sketches made at East Cowes Castle in the summer of 1827 (see Nos.303–6). It seems likely, therefore, that Turner was at work on the project in 1827, and it would be characteristic of him to have completed the series rapidly. But as the first engravings did not appear till 1833, it may be that the finished drawings were not ready until 1831 or 1832. Slight differences of style are detectable, between the Loire and the Seine drawings for example, and this may indicate that they were executed at different dates.

The *Rivers of France* were intended as part of a larger work, *Great Rivers of Europe*, or *River Scenery of Europe*, which was announced by Heath in 1833. It would have included the Meuse and Moselle designs which Turner had begun to make after his journey along these rivers in 1826 (see No.372) and was presumably the motive for several of his tours in the 1830s, including another to the Meuse and Moselle in 1834 and one along the Danube probably in 1833. Turner seems to have collected material for the same project during his journey to Italy in 1828 (see No.377).

363 'Dieppe, Rouen and Paris' Sketchbook 1821
Bound in red morocco with gilt tooling
34 leaves all drawn on in pencil, one or two in black chalk, 4½ × 8½ (11.6 × 21.5)
Watermarked: 1819
Inscr. Finberg transcribes Turner's label on spine: '54. Rouen'
Trustees of the British Museum (T.B.CCLVIII)

f.10ᵛ, 11ʳ A Street in Rouen, looking towards the Cathedral; with Architectural Notes
Pencil
Inscr. lower left: 'Vegata . . .'

Dated by Finberg (1909, II, p.785) to about 1830, but subsequently placed earlier (1961, p.271), this book contains numerous views of Rouen showing the old spire of the Cathedral, destroyed in 1822. Many of the sketches here were used as bases for the *Rivers of France* designs. On ff.19ᵛ, 20ʳ and 34ʳ are notes of the compositions of paintings apparently by Claude and Poussin.

364 'Holland, Meuse and Cologne' Sketchbook
1825
Bound in grey boards with leather spine; one clasp
90 leaves, the majority drawn on in pencil, 4½ × 7½ (11.4 × 18.8)
Watermarked: 1819
Inscr. on spine: 'MEUSE'
Trustees of the British Museum (T.B.CCXV)

ff.66ᵛ–67ʳ View of Cologne from the River
Pencil

Includes sketches of Dover, the cliffs seen from the Channel, Boulogne, Rotterdam and Amsterdam, made on Turner's tour of August–September 1825.

365 'Rivers Meuse and Moselle' Sketchbook
1826
Bound in calf, one clasp
274 leaves, with marbled fly-leaf at each end
Nearly all pages drawn on in pencil, 4½ × 3 (11.7 × 7.7)
Watermarked: 1822
Trustees of the British Museum (T.B.CCXVI)

ff.53ᵛ–54ʳ Sketches at Dinant
Pencil

This small book is packed from cover to cover with tiny but often fine and detailed studies of the towns and changing scenery through which Turner passed on his tour of the rivers in the autumn of 1826. f.154ᵛ has a rough sketch of a diligence being dug out of a ditch between Ghent and Brussels – perhaps the vehicle in which he was travelling. The first nine leaves contain notes and sketch-maps of his itinerary. See also No.372.

366 'Loire, Tours, Orleans and Paris' Sketchbook ?1826
Bound in cardboard
46 leaves, all drawn on in pencil, 6 × 4 (15.3 × 10.2)
Inscr. on back cover: 'Loire Tours Orleans Paris' and inside front cover: '1826 23 Augt Colnaghis'
Trustees of the British Museum (T.B.CCXLIX)

f.35ᵛ Paris: the Pont au Change and Palais de Justice
Pencil
f.36ʳ Paris: the Louvre
Pencil

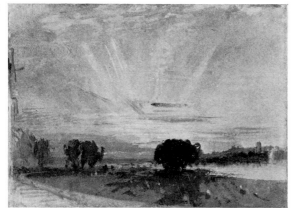

342

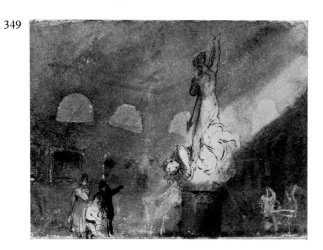

349

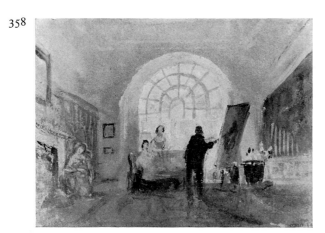

358

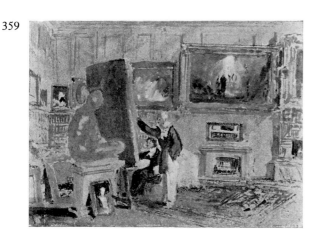

359

The book contains several sketches developed into illustrations for the *Loire* tour, 1833.

367 'Seine and Paris' Sketchbook 1829
Bound in yellow parchment
98 leaves, the majority drawn on in pencil
$7 \times 4\frac{1}{8}$ (10.8 × 17.4)
Trustees of the British Museum (T.B.CCLIV)

f.82ᵛ Five Studies of a Town near the Mouth of the Seine (?Honfleur)
Pencil
f.83ʳ Study of a Row of Buildings with a Church in the Centre
Pencil
Inscr. with brief notes

This book includes a number of slight sketches later worked up into *Rivers of France* subjects.

368 'Paris and Environs' Sketchbook ?1829
Bound in parchment
169 leaves, all drawn on in pencil, $7 \times 4\frac{1}{2}$
(17.5 × 11.5)
Bears the label of: 'Collard, Mᵈ Papetier, Rue Neuve des Petits-Champs' (Paris)
Trustees of the British Museum (T.B.CCLVII)

ff.83ᵛ-84ʳ Studies of the Palace of St. Cloud
Pencil
Inscr. with brief notes

Many of the sketches in this book were used for Turner's *French Rivers* series *Wanderings by the Seine* of 1835. The last page (f.169ᵛ) has a drawing of travellers waiting for a coach, apparently sitting round a fire.

369 'Guernsey' Sketchbook 1829
Bound in buff boards, leather spine, one clasp
92 leaves of white paper, the first six washed with grey on one side only (cf. 'Minstrelsy of the Scottish Border' Sketchbook, No.449);
almost all drawn on in pencil, $4\frac{1}{2} \times 7\frac{1}{4}$ (11.4 × 18.7)
Watermarked: 1828
Inscr. on spine: 'Guernsey'
Trustees of the British Museum (T.B.CCLII)

ff.47ᵛ-48ʳ St. Peter Port: the Harbour with Little Russel and Castle Cornet
Pencil

Finberg (1961, p.318) suggests that Turner concluded his tour to Paris of August 1829 by travelling down the Seine to Honfleur, thence to St. Malo and Guernsey. This sketchbook contains drawings made on the boat to Portsmouth from the Channel Islands with views of Tancarville, Caudebec, etc. The series of drawings of a ruined Abbey on ff.30ᵛ-36ᵛ show Netley Abbey, near Portsmouth, and were presumably made after Turner disembarked. ff.37ᵛ-38ʳ probably show shipping in Portsmouth harbour. The remainder of the drawings seem to have been made in the Channel Islands.

370 'Spa, Dinant and Namur' Sketchbook 1834
Bound in marbled boards, parchment spine
66 leaves, almost all drawn on in pencil, 6×4
(15.2 × 9.3)
Watermarked: 1810

Bears the label of 'P. J. Heyvaert Panwels,
Imprimateur, Papetier, Bruxelles'
Trustees of the British Museum (T.B.CCLXXXVII)

f.24ᵛ **View of a Town among Hills**
Pencil
Inscr. 'Jeal' (? – perhaps for Jalhay)
f.25ʳ **View along a Road**
Pencil

This sketchbook records part of Turner's tour through
Belgium and along the Rhine and Moselle to Cologne
and Coblenz, in July and August 1834.

Finberg suggests that f.24ᵛ shows Spa; but the inscription appears to be the name of the place represented. A drawing, apparently of the same view, in pen and
bodycolour on blue paper, is in the 'Meuse-Moselle'
series, T.B.CCXCII–66.

**371 'Givet, Mézières, Verdun, Metz,
Luxembourg and Trèves' Sketchbook** 1834
Bound in boards, leather spine, front edges and
back corners
68 leaves, the majority drawn on in pencil, 6½ × 4
(16.8 × 10)
Inscr. on back cover: '2'
Trustees of the British Museum (T.B.CCLXXXVIII)

ff.47ᵛ–48ʳ **Outline Sketch of a Group of
Buildings**
Pencil

A sketchbook used on the same tour as No.370.

Possibly a note made from a moving coach, the sketch
exhibited apparently shows a large ecclesiastical building.

372 Buildings by a Lake *c.*1828
Bodycolour on blue paper, 5½ × 7⅜ (13.9 × 18.7)
Trustees of the British Museum (T.B.CCXXI–R)
Turner's tour of the Rivers Meuse and Moselle between August and November 1826 is recorded in
the 'Rivers Meuse and Moselle' sketchbook (T.B.
CCXVI, No.365), the 'Huy and Dinant' sketchbook
(T.B.CCXVII), and the 'Trèves and Rhine' sketchbook
(T.B.CCXVIII). These contain a running visual 'diary'
of what he saw; there is also a long series of slight
studies in pencil, some with pen and white heightening,
on blue paper (T.B.CCXXIV) which may have been done
en route or may represent an intermediate stage towards the series of small studies, more or less finished,
in bodycolour on similar blue paper, which Turner
must have made after his return. Their resemblance in
format and technique to the *Rivers of France* bodycolour drawings (Nos.383–408) suggests that they were
executed at about the same time, though the fact that
few are ever as specific in detail as are many of the
French ones seems to indicate that Turner did not
originally have such a development in mind. In fact,
these drawings may have been made after the *French
Rivers* series when Turner was thinking of a further
series featuring other views. He revisited the Meuse and
Moselle in 1834 with this intention (see the sketchbooks
connected with that tour, Nos.370 and 371).

373 Sunset over a Ruined Castle *c.*1828
Bodycolour and black chalk on blue paper,
5½ × 7½ (14 × 18.9)
Trustees of the British Museum (T.B.CCXXI–J)
Perhaps a view of the castle at Beilstein: cf. pencil
sketches in the 'Meuse and Moselle' sketchbook (T.B.
CCXVI, ff.119–123).

374 Luxembourg *c.*1828
Bodycolour with pen and brown ink on blue
paper, sight 5⁵⁄₁₆ × 7⅜ (13.5 × 18.7)
Private collection
One of the bodycolour studies of Meuse and Moselle
subjects which were intended to constitute a sequel to
the *French Rivers*. The drawing belonged to Ruskin.

**375 A Fortress on the Sea with Low Cliffs under
Grey Cloud** *c.*1828
Bodycolour on blue paper, 5⅜ × 7½ (13.7 × 19.1)
Trustees of the British Museum (T.B.CCLIX–173)
Possibly at Wimereux; cf. the pencil and pen sketches
T.B.CCXXIV–1, 2, 3; f.1 is inscribed 'Viemirux'. There
is a slight sketch in pencil on the verso.

376 A Bridge over a River under a High Cliff
*c.*1828
Bodycolour on blue paper, 5½ × 7⅜ (13.9 × 18.8)
Trustees of the British Museum (T.B.CCLIX–159)
This drawing appears to represent the fortress overlooking the Meuse at Huy; it is based on the pencil
sketch on f.41ᵛ of the 'Meuse and Moselle' sketchbook
(T.B.CCXVI). There is a slight sketch in white chalk on
the verso.

377 The Lighthouse at Marseilles, from the Sea
?*c.*1828
Pencil and bodycolour, with scraping-out and
some pen on grey paper, 5½ × 7½ (14.1 × 19)
Trustees of the British Museum (T.B.CCLIX–139)
The lighthouse in this drawing seems to be the same as
that in CCXCII–74, a subject identified by Finberg as
belonging to the Meuse-Moselle-Rhine series of about
1834. The use of grey paper reinforces the view that the
drawing belongs to that series, as does the vivid colour;
but Turner drew the lighthouse and other buildings
round the harbour in the 'Lyons to Marseilles' sketchbook used on his way to Italy in 1828 (T.B.CCXXX–52ʳ,
53ʳ and ᵛ) and it may be that these bodycolour studies
were executed nearer to that date and to the date of the
French Rivers drawings.

378 ? A Village on the South Coast of France
?*c.*1828
Bodycolour with some pen on blue paper,
5⅝ × 7⅝ (14.2 × 19.2)
Trustees of the British Museum (T.B.CCLIX–140)

379 Crimson Buildings on Hills above a Lake
*c.*1828
Bodycolour on grey paper, 5⅜ × 7⁷⁄₁₆ (13.7 × 18.8)
Trustees of the British Museum (T.B.CCXCII–30)

380 A Fortress by a Calm Lake ?*c.*1828
Bodycolour on grey paper, 5½ × 7⁹⁄₁₆ (14.1 × 19.2)
Trustees of the British Museum (T.B.CCXCII–31)

381 Study of Grey and Blue Mountains *?c.*1828
Bodycolour on grey paper, $5\frac{1}{2} \times 7\frac{9}{16}$ (14×19.3)
Trustees of the British Museum (T.B.CCXCII–76)

382 Towers among Mountains: Daybreak
*?c.*1828
Bodycolour on blue paper, $5\frac{1}{2} \times 7\frac{1}{2}$ (13.9×19)
Trustees of the British Museum (T.B.CCXCII–72)

The views shown in these drawings have not been identified, but they probably belong to the group of studies made for a projected publication on southern or north-eastern France; see Nos.372 and 375.

THE RIVERS OF FRANCE SERIES

383 Angers *c.*1829
Pencil, pen and brown ink and white bodycolour on blue paper, $5\frac{5}{16} \times 7\frac{9}{16}$ (13.5×19.2)
Dr Charles Warren

This study is typical of the composition studies that Turner seems often to have made on the spot in France in addition to his more usual pencil sketches. It apparently shows the Château du Roi René at Angers. Turner made pencil studies at Angers in his 'Nantes, Angers and Saumur' sketchbook, probably of 1826 or 1827 (T.B.CCXLVIII–29^v, etc) and a coloured drawing in the *Loire* series is T.B.CCLIX–94. The drawings belonged to Ruskin and Finberg.

384 Amboise *c.*1829
Bodycolour on blue paper, $5\frac{3}{8} \times 7\frac{3}{8}$ (13.7×18.7)
Visitors of the Ashmolean Museum, Oxford
Engraved by W. R. Smith for *Turner's Annual Tour – the Loire*, 1833 (Rawlinson No.437).

This and Nos.385, 386 and 387 were among the Turner drawings presented to Oxford University by Ruskin in 1861; it has recently been shown that Ruskin had acquired his Loire drawings from the niece of Turner's friend Charles Stokes (see No.B142), who had bought them through Thomas Griffith in 1850 (see Luke Herrmann, 'Ruskin and Turner: A riddle resolved' in *Burlington Magazine*, CXII, 1970, pp. 696–9).

385 Chateau Hamelin *c.*1829
Bodycolour with some pen and red-brown colour on blue paper, $5\frac{7}{16} \times 7\frac{1}{2}$ (13.7×18.9)
Visitors of the Ashmolean Museum, Oxford
Engraved by R. Brandard for *Turner's Annual Tour – the Loire* 1833 (Rawlinson No.448).

386 Blois *c.*1829
Bodycolour with some pen and black ink on blue paper, $5\frac{5}{16} \times 7\frac{3}{16}$ (13.5×18.2)
Visitors of the Ashmolean Museum, Oxford
Engraved by R. Brandard for *Turner's Annual Tour – the Loire*, 1833 (Rawlinson No.435).

Ruskin described this and the 'Montjeu', also at Oxford (Herrmann 1968, No.40), as 'full of repentirs and entirely bad' but 'sent them with the rest [of his gift] – lest it should be thought that I had kept the two best – many people might think them so. They are instructive, as showing the ruin that comes on the greatest men when they change their minds wantonly'. It is difficult to understand why Ruskin was critical of this design.

387 The Canal of the Loire and Cher near Tours
*c.*1829
Bodycolour on blue paper, $4\frac{13}{16} \times 7\frac{1}{8}$ (12.2×18)
Visitors of the Ashmolean Museum, Oxford
Engraved by T. Jeavons for *Turner's Annual Tour – the Loire*, 1833 (Rawlinson No.439).

388 A Steamboat and Small Craft by a Quay, with a Sailing Ship Beyond *c.*1829
Pencil, pen and brown ink and grey wash and white bodycolour on blue paper, $5\frac{1}{2} \times 7\frac{1}{2}$ (14×19.1)
Trustees of the British Museum (T.B.CCLX–35)

389 Two Paddlesteamers and other Craft *c.*1829
Pencil, pen and brown ink and wash and white bodycolour on blue paper, $5\frac{1}{2} \times 7\frac{1}{2}$ (14×18.9)
Trustees of the British Museum (T.B.CCLX–36)

390 A Heap of Baskets by a Harbour; a Horse-Drawn Cart and Shipping Beyond
*c.*1829
Bodycolour on blue paper, $5\frac{1}{2} \times 7\frac{1}{2}$ (14×19)
Trustees of the British Museum (T.B.CCLIX–225)

391 Figures on a Beach *c.*1829
Black chalk and bodycolour on blue paper, $5\frac{1}{2} \times 7\frac{1}{2}$ (13.9×19)
Trustees of the British Museum (T.B.CCLIX–226)

392 Figures on a Beach near a Breakwater: Rainy Weather *c.*1829
Bodycolour on blue paper, $5\frac{7}{16} \times 7\frac{1}{2}$ (13.8×19)
Trustees of the British Museum (T.B.CCLIX–229)

393 Study of Figures on a Promenade by the Sea *c.*1829
Pen and black ink and wash and black and yellow chalk on blue paper, $5\frac{5}{16} \times 7\frac{5}{8}$ (13.5×19.4)
Trustees of the British Museum (T.B.CCLX–99)

394 A Group of Figures round a Woman in a Wheel-Chair pulled by two Boys *c.*1829
Black and white chalks on blue paper, $5 \times 7\frac{1}{2}$ (13.5×19.1)
Trustees of the British Museum (T.B.CCLX–100)

395 Figures on the Shore *c.*1829
Black and white chalks on blue paper, $5\frac{5}{8} \times 7\frac{5}{8}$ (14.2×19.3)
Trustees of the British Museum (T.B.CCLX–101)

396 Sunset: Rouen? *c.*1829 (repr. on p.90)
Bodycolour on blue paper, $5\frac{5}{16} \times 7\frac{1}{2}$ (13.5×18.9)
Trustees of the British Museum (T.B.CCLIX–101)

397 Harfleur *c.*1829
Bodycolour on blue paper, $5\frac{1}{2} \times 7\frac{1}{2}$ (13.9×19.1)
Trustees of the British Museum (T.B.CCLIX–102)
Engraved by J. Cousen for *Turner's Annual Tour – the Seine*, 1834 (Rawlinson No.457). Based on the rough pencil drawing of this view on f.5^v of the 'Tancarville and Lillebonne' sketchbook (T.B.CCLIII) dated by Finberg to about 1830 but possibly in use a few years earlier.

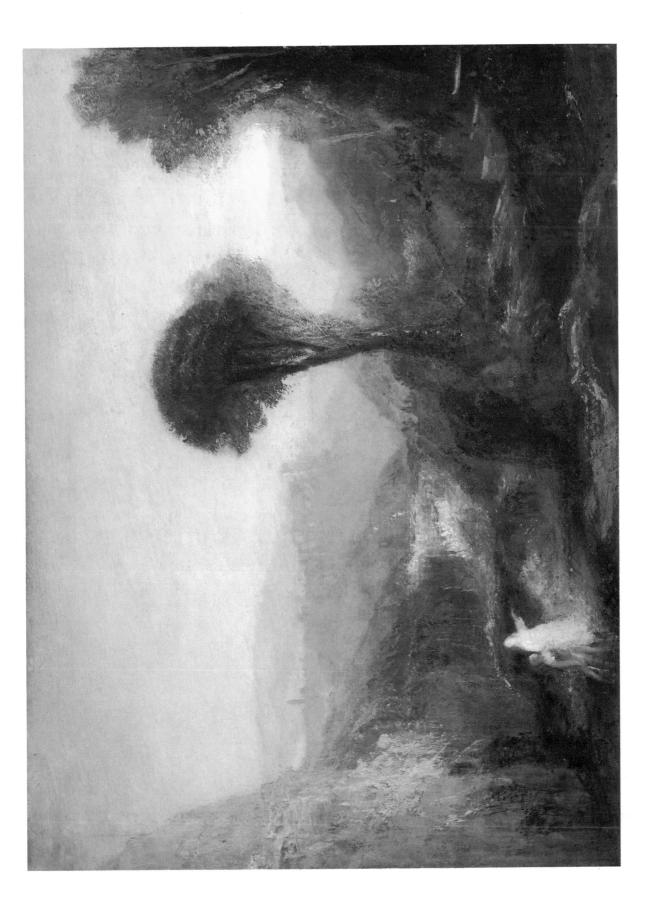

488 **Tivoli: Tobias and the Angel** *c.*1830–5 (entry on p.135)

494 **Yacht approaching the Coast** *c.*1835–40 (entry on p.136)

398 Quilleboeuf *c.*1829
  Bodycolour with some pen on blue paper, $5\frac{1}{2} \times 7\frac{7}{16}$
  (14 × 18.9)
  Trustees of the British Museum (T.B.CCLIX–103)
Engraved by Robert Brandard for *Turner's Annual Tour – the Seine*, 1834 (Rawlinson No.471).

  The central motif of this study was reproduced closely in the painting of the 'Mouth of the Seine, Quille-boeuf' shown at the R.A. in 1833 (No.491). Sketches are on ff.77^r and ^{v}, 79^v, of the 'Seine and Paris' sketchbook (No.367).

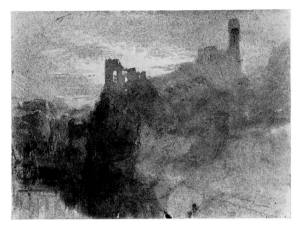

373

  Robert BRANDARD (1805–1862) after TURNER
399 Quilleboeuf 1834
  Engraving, proof, $3\frac{3}{4} \times 5\frac{7}{16}$ (9.6 × 13.8); plate
  $5\frac{15}{16} \times 8\frac{7}{8}$ (15 × 22.5)
  Trustees of the British Museum (1868-8-22-4184)
From the drawing in the Turner Bequest (No.398), for *Turner's Annual Tour – the Seine*, 1834 (Rawlinson 471).

400 Between Quilleboeuf and Villequier *c.*1829
  Watercolour, bodycolour and pen on blue paper,
  $5\frac{7}{16} \times 7\frac{1}{2}$ (13.8 × 19)
  Trustees of the British Museum (T.B.CCLIX–104)
Engraved by Robert Brandard for *Turner's Annual Tour – the Seine*, 1834 (Rawlinson No.470). A sketch showing steam boats on the Seine near Quilleboeuf is in the 'Seine and Paris' sketchbook (No.367), f.80^r.

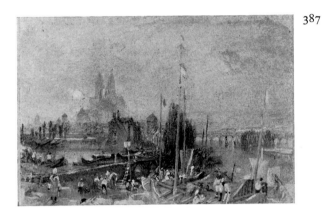

387

401 Rouen, looking up the Seine *c.*1829
  Bodycolour with some pen on blue paper,
  $5\frac{1}{2} \times 7\frac{9}{16}$ (14.1 × 19.2)
  Trustees of the British Museum (T.B.CCLIX–107)
Engraved by R. Brandard for *Turner's Annual Tour – the Seine*, 1834 (Rawlinson No.465) and by Himely in aquatint, date uncertain (Rawlinson No.832a).

402 Rouen, looking down the Seine *c.*1829
  Bodycolour on blue paper, $5\frac{1}{2} \times 7\frac{9}{16}$ (14 × 19.2)
  Trustees of the British Museum (T.B.CCLIX–108)
Engraved by R. Brandard for *Turner's Annual Tour – The Seine*, 1834 (Rawlinson No.466); and by Himely in aquatint, date uncertain (Rawlinson No.832b).

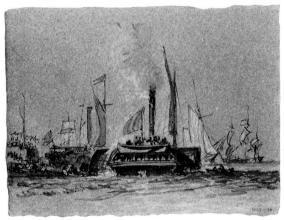

389

  The central tower of Rouen Cathedral was destroyed in 1822 and this drawing, with its companion view looking up the river (No.401), may have used sketches made before that event, perhaps those in the 'Dieppe, Rouen and Paris' sketchbook (No.363), ff.6^v–7^r, 22^v. Turner was concerned to extract the maximum dramatic effect from the height of the tower and therefore ignored its disappearance.

403 Vernon *c.*1829
  Bodycolour with some pen on blue paper,
  $5\frac{7}{16} \times 7\frac{5}{8}$ (13.8 × 19.4)
  Trustees of the British Museum (T.B.CCLIX–129)
Engraved by J. T. Willmore for *Turner's Annual Tour – The Seine*, 1835 (Rawlinson No.475).

404 View of the Seine between Mantes and Vernon *c.*1829
  Bodycolour with some pen on blue paper,
  $5\frac{9}{16} \times 7\frac{5}{8}$ (14.2 × 19.3)
  Trustees of the British Museum (T.B.CCLIX–114)

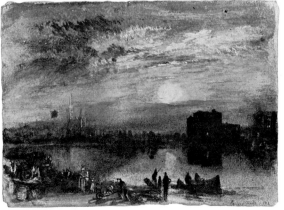

408

Engraved by Robert Brandard for *Turner's Annual Tour – the Seine*, 1835 (Rawlinson No.477).

405 Paris: View of the Seine from the Barrière de Passy, with the Louvre in the Distance *c.*1829
Bodycolour with some pen on blue paper, $5\frac{1}{2} \times 7\frac{1}{2}$ (14×19.1)
Trustees of the British Museum (T.B.CCLIX–117)
Engraved by J. T. Willmore for *Turner's Annual Tour – the Seine*, 1835 (Rawlinson No.485). A few rough studies of the Seine at Passy are in the 'Loire, Tours, Orléans, Paris' sketchbook (No.366), ff.38ᵛ–40ᵛ. A more detailed drawing corresponding to the final composition in some respects, including the Barrière itself on the left, is on f.156 of the 'Paris and Environs' sketchbook (No.368). It is also possible that Turner referred to the drawing he had made at Passy in his 'Paris, France, Savoy' sketchbook of 1819 (T.B.CLXXIII, f.14ʳ).

406 Paris: The Pont Neuf and the Ile de la Cité *c.*1829
Bodycolour on blue paper, $5\frac{1}{2} \times 7\frac{7}{16}$ (14.1×18.8)
Trustees of the British Museum (T.B.CCLIX–118)
Engraved by W. Miller for *Turner's Annual Tour – the Seine*, 1835 (Rawlinson No.486). Drawings of the view are in the 'Paris and Environs' sketchbook (No.368), ff.55ᵛ, 56ᵛ (half of the bridge shown on each page).

407 St. Germain en Laye *c.*1829
Bodycolour with some pen on blue paper, $5\frac{1}{2} \times 7\frac{9}{16}$ (14×19.2)
Trustees of the British Museum (T.B.CCLIX–122)
Engraved by J. B. Allen for *Turner's Annual Tour – the Seine*, 1835 (Rawlinson No.480). Three slightly noted views from St. Germain are on f.166ʳ of the 'Paris and Environs' sketchbook (No.368). A drawing on blue paper which gives the whole of this subject in panoramic format ($3\frac{3}{4} \times 11$) is T.B.CCLX–59; this was probably done in pencil on the spot, and worked up later with a pen and a little colour.

408 St. Denis, Moonlight 1829
Bodycolour on blue paper, $5\frac{7}{16} \times 7\frac{9}{16}$ (13.8×19.2)
Trustees of the British Museum (T.B.CCLIX–121)
Engraved by S. Fisher for *Turner's Annual Tour – the Seine*, 1835 (Rawlinson No.481). A pencil study of the church of St. Denis is on ff.152ᵛ–153ʳ of the 'Paris and Environs' sketchbook (No.368), and a general view corresponding to this one, with boats in the foreground, occurs on f.154ʳ.

409 View in the Gardens of Versailles *c.*1829
Bodycolour on blue paper, $5\frac{5}{8} \times 7\frac{1}{2}$ (14.2×19)
Trustees of the British Museum (T.B.CCLIX–46)
A number of pencil studies of the gardens at Versailles are in the 'Paris and Environs' sketchbook (No.368), ff.20, 33ʳ and ᵛ, 34ᵛ etc.

410 Extensive View with the Sea in the Distance *c.*1829
Pencil and bodycolour on blue paper, $12\frac{9}{16} \times 7\frac{1}{2}$ (31.9×18.9)
Trustees of the British Museum (T.B.CCLIX–49)

411 The Interior of a Church *c.*1829
Bodycolour on blue paper, $5\frac{9}{16} \times 7\frac{1}{2}$ (14.1×18.9)
Trustees of the British Museum (T.B.CCLIX–50)

412 Fishing Boats near a Jetty, with Dead Fish *c.*1833
Pencil and watercolour, vignette approx. $6\frac{7}{8} \times 5\frac{1}{2}$ (17.5×14) on sheet $7\frac{7}{8} \times 6$ (20×15.3)
Trustees of the British Museum (T.B.CCLXXX–4)
Not engraved, but close in general treatment to vignette designs for the *Rivers of France* and perhaps connected with that series (compare the study for 'Light Towers at La Hève' at the Lady Lever Art Gallery). See also No.413.

413 Fishing Boats, with Oars, a Pot over a Fire, and a Basket of Lobsters *c.*1833
Pencil and watercolour, vignette approx. $6 \times 5\frac{3}{4}$ (15.5×14.5); on sheet 8×6 (20.2×15.4)
Trustees of the British Museum (T.B.CCLXXX–3)
Not engraved. See No.412.

Thomas HIGHAM (1796–1844) after TURNER
414 Rouen Cathedral 1834
Engraving, proof, $3\frac{9}{16} \times 5\frac{9}{16}$ (9.9×14.2); plate $5\frac{15}{16} \times 9\frac{1}{16}$ (15.1×23.0)
Trustees of the British Museum (1868-8-22-4180)
From the drawing in the Turner Bequest (CCLIX–109), for *Turner's Annual Tour – the Seine*, 1834 (Rawlinson No.467). Detailed studies of the façade of the cathedral are on ff.9ʳ, 22ʳ of the 'Dieppe, Rouen and Paris' sketchbook (No.363), though they are not from such a close viewpoint as that of this composition.

William MILLER (1797–1882) after TURNER
415 Rouen from St. Catherine's Hill 1834
Engraving, proof, $3\frac{15}{16} \times 5\frac{1}{8}$ (10×13); plate $5\frac{15}{16} \times 8\frac{15}{16}$ (15×22.7)
Inscr. with names of artist and engraver
Trustees of the British Museum (1868-8-22-4182)
Rawlinson No.468. One of the loveliest of the *Seine* series illustrating *Turner's Annual Tour*, 1834. The drawing was owned by Ruskin; its subject derives from pencil sketches of Rouen from St Catherine's Hill in the 'Rouen' sketchbook, T.B.CCLV, which, as Finberg points out (1909 III, p.776) shows the cathedral with no central spire, and was therefore presumably used between 1822 and 1827 (perhaps on Turner's visit of 1826). The sketch on f.8ᵛ is closest to Turner's final composition, though several other studies were also probably referred to. See also the 'Dieppe, Rouen and Paris' sketchbook (No.363), f.30ʳ.

John Carr ARMYTAGE (1810–97) after TURNER
416 The Confluence of the Seine and the Marne 1835
Engraving, proof, $3\frac{7}{8} \times 5\frac{3}{8}$ (9.9×13.7); plate $6 \times 8\frac{15}{16}$ (15.2×22.7)
Inscr: 'Drawn by J. M. W. Turner R A' and 'Engraved by J. C. Armytage'
Trustees of the British Museum (1868-8-22-4202)
From the second of Turner's *Annual Tours* on the Seine, published in 1835. Rawlinson No.490. Drawings of the Seine and Marne occur in the 'Seine and Paris' sketchbook (No.367).

11. 'England and Wales' and Scotland 1826–38

Charles Heath's ambitious publication of *Picturesque Views in England and Wales* was the most elaborate and wide-ranging of all the illustrative schemes on which Turner embarked in the 1820s and 1830s, and the watercolours he made for it rank among the most wonderful objects of their kind ever produced. They occupied him between 1826 and 1838, and involved him in travelling to collect new material (see Nos.418 and 442) and experimenting with compositional ideas, sometimes in considerable depth (see Nos.443 to 447). In addition, as illustrator of Cadell's editions of Scott (see Nos.289–92 and 449–53), he visited Scotland in 1831 and 1834. The first of these tours included a trip to Staffa and Fingal's Cave which resulted in what may be seen as the first of the sea pictures in Turner's late style (No.490); and many of his most atmospheric shore and marine sketches belong to this period.

Turner was engaged to work on the *England and Wales* views by Charles Heath, the engraver, in 1826. The series came out in 24 parts between 1827 and 1838, when the scheme, having met with a poor response from the public, ended in Heath's bankruptcy. Turner himself bought up the unsold stock and plates at Heath's sale, for £3,000, the reserve price. The prints were sold at Christie's in 1873 and 1874.

The richness of invention in the ninety-six designs for the project covers almost every aspect of Turner's interest in landscape. The drawings themselves are highly finished, and immense care was obviously lavished on details as well as on general effects, and the colour scheme of each design, notwithstanding they were all to be published in black and white, is unique to itself. As Rawlinson says, 'every hour is represented – dawn, sunrise, midday, afternoon, sunset, twilight, moonrise, full moon. So is every phase of weather, every passing atmospheric effect.'

Robert WALLIS (1794–1878) after TURNER
417 Colchester 1827
Engraving, first published state, $6\frac{5}{8} \times 9$
(16.7×23.1); plate, $10\frac{1}{2} \times 11\frac{3}{4}$ (26.7×29.8)
Inscr: 'Robt Wallis 1827'
Trustees of the British Museum (1849-10-31-133)
The plate, Rawlinson No.213, was No.1 in Part II of *Picturesque Views in England and Wales*; the drawing is in the Courtauld Institute Galleries (Kitson, *Turner Watercolours from the collection of Stephen Courtauld*, 1974, No.8). Pencil sketches for it are in the 'Norfolk, Suffolk and Essex' sketchbook (No.418).

418 'Norfolk, Suffolk and Essex' Sketchbook
1824
Bound in grey boards with leather spine, one clasp
89 leaves, the majority drawn on in pencil, $4\frac{1}{2} \times 7\frac{1}{2}$ (11.5×18.7)
Watermarked: 1819
Inscr. on front cover: 'Essex'
Trustees of the British Museum (T.B.CCIX)

f.6^v **Colchester**
Pencil
f.7^r **Three Studies of the Skyline of a Coastal Town**
Pencil

f.6^v was used for the watercolour for the series of *Picturesque Views in England and Wales*, engraved in 1827 (Rawlinson No.213; No.417). Further studies for the design are on ff.7^v and 71^r.

419 Lancaster Sands – Lancashire *c.*1826
Watercolour, $10\frac{15}{16} \times 15\frac{15}{16}$ (27.8×40.4)
Exh: Moon, Boys and Graves Gallery 1833(42)
Trustees of the British Museum (1910-2-12-279)
Engraved by R. Brandard, 1828, for *Picturesque Views in England and Wales*, Part V, No.3 (Rawlinson No.227).

A watercolour of Lancaster Sands using similar elements, but more dramatic in atmosphere, was made in about 1818 and bought by Walter Fawkes (see No. 179). The *England and Wales* watercolour was lent to the 1833 exhibition by Thomas Tomkinson.

Robert BRANDARD (1805–1862) after TURNER
420 Lancaster Sands 1828
Engraving, first published state, $6\frac{1}{2} \times 9\frac{1}{4}$
(16.5×23.6); plate, $10\frac{1}{16} \times 12\frac{1}{16}$ (25.5×30.7)
Inscr: 'engd by R. Brandard from a Drawing by J M W Turner R.A. 1828'
Trustees of the British Museum (1889-7-24-137)
Rawlinson No.227; No.3 in Part V of *Picturesque Views in England and Wales*; from the drawing in the British Museum (No.419).

421 Richmond, Yorkshire *c.*1826
Watercolour, $10\frac{13}{16} \times 15\frac{5}{8}$ (27.5×39.7)
Exh: ?Moon, Boys and Graves Gallery 1833(4)
Trustees of the British Museum (1910-2-12-276)
Engraved by W. R. Smith, 1827, for *Picturesque Views in England and Wales*, Part II, No.3 (Rawlinson No. 215).

Turner made a series of drawings showing Richmond on its impressive site during his Yorkshire tour of 1816; one of these, T.B.CXLVIII–13^v, served as the basis for this view; but he treated the subject several times: twice for Whitaker's *History of Richmondshire* (Rawlinson Nos.169, 170) and again in the *England and Wales* series (Part VI No.4; now Fitzwilliam Museum; Rawlinson No.232). Turner had made his first drawings of Richmond in 1796 (T.B.XXXIV–26) and the Bequest includes a number of 'colour-beginnings' which seem to represent the town. Having given one view of Richmond to Cambridge, Ruskin showed this one at the Fine Art Society in 1878 and 1900 (No.24), with the comment 'I don't think anybody is likely to get [it] while I live'. A watercolour of 'Richmond Castle and Town – Lancashire' was lent to the 1833 exhibition by B. G. Windus.

422 Louth – Lincolnshire *c.*1827
Watercolour and scraping-out, $11\frac{1}{4} \times 16\frac{1}{2}$
(28.5×42)
Exh: Egyptian Hall, 1829; Moon, Boys and
Graves Gallery 1833(35)
Trustees of the British Museum (1910-2-12-278)
Engraved by W. Radclyffe, 1829, for *Picturesque Views
in England and Wales*, Part VII, No.1 (Rawlinson No.
233).

The background of this drawing is taken directly
from an architectural study in pencil on f.80 of the
'North of England' sketchbook of 1797 (T.B.XXXIV, No.
23). Ruskin, in his notes on his own collection, *Ruskin
on Pictures*, 1902 p.325, No.35) calls this 'Another
drawing of what he [Turner] clearly felt to be objectionable and painted, first as a part, and a very principal
part of the English scenery he had undertaken to illustrate [in the *England and Wales* series] . . . He dwells,
(I think, ironically) on the elaborate carving of the
church spire, with which the foreground interests are so
distantly and vaguely connected.'

Rawlinson (loc. cit.) disagrees with this: 'homely
subjects were by no means uncongenial to him . . . he
would probably have thoroughly enjoyed the sights and
sounds of a country fair . . . I have no doubt that the
contrast here between foreground and background was
intentional.'

'Louth' was originally owned by Thomas Griffith.
It was one of seventeen *England and Wales* watercolours completed by 1829 and shown in June of
that year by Charles Heath at an exhibition to promote
the enterprise held at the Egyptian Hall, Piccadilly.
In all, forty drawings by Turner were included.

423 Dunstanborough Castle – Northumberland
*c.*1828
Watercolour, $11\frac{1}{4} \times 16\frac{7}{16}$ (28.5×41.7)
Exh: Moon, Boys and Graves Gallery 1833(41)
City Art Gallery, Manchester
Engraved by R. Brandard for *Picturesque Views in
England and Wales*, 1829, Part VIII, No.2 (Rawlinson
No.238).

Derived from the drawing of Dunstanborough in the
'North of England' sketchbook of 1797 (No.23) which
was first used for an oil painting and a watercolour
and later became the basis of the *Liber Studiorum*
plate (R.14). This *England and Wales* watercolour
was lent to the 1833 exhibition by Thomas Tomkinson,
and later became one of the large number of *England
and Wales* subjects owned by H. A. J. Munro of Novar,
including 'Lancaster Sands' (No.419), 'Louth' (No.
422), 'Blenheim' (No.427), 'Ullswater' (No.428) and
'Richmond Terrace' (No.434).

424 Malvern Abbey and Gate – Worcestershire
*c.*1830
Watercolour with some scraping-out, $11\frac{3}{8} \times 15\frac{7}{8}$
(28.9×41.8)
Exh: Moon Boys and Graves Gallery 1833(14)
City Art Gallery, Manchester
Engraved by J. Horsburgh, 1832 for *Picturesque Views
in England and Wales*, Part XIII, No.2 (Rawlinson No.
258).

An earlier drawing of the same view (1794) is now in
America. Turner showed a view of the Gate, facing to-

wards the viewpoint of the *England and Wales* drawing,
at the R.A. in 1799 (336), now in the Whitworth Art
Gallery; this was based on a pencil study of about 1793
(T.B.XIII–D). Horsburgh's engraving in its final form
has a vivid flash of lightning striking the central
chimney from the dark cloud on the left. B. G. Windus
lent the watercolour to the 1833 exhibition.

425 Upnor Castle – Kent *c.*1831
Watercolour and bodycolour with some
scraping-out, $11\frac{1}{2} \times 17\frac{1}{4}$ (29.1×43.8)
Exh: Moon, Boys and Graves Gallery 1833(50)
Whitworth Art Gallery, Manchester (0.41.1924)
Engraved by J. B. Allen for *Picturesque Views in Eng-
land and Wales*, Part XVI, No.3, 1833 (Rawlinson 271).

Derived from the pencil sketch of the Medway at
Upnor on ff.87ᵛ and 88ʳ of the 'Medway' sketchbook,
T.B.CXCIX. A more detailed study of the Castle itself,
from a slightly different angle, is on f.23ᵛ of the same
book. The watercolour was lent to the 1833 exhibition
by Thomas Griffith.

426 Dudley – Worcestershire *c.*1832
Watercolour and bodycolour, $11\frac{3}{8} \times 16\frac{15}{16}$
(28.8×43)
Exh: Moon Boys and Graves Gallery 1833(77)
*Trustees of the Lady Lever Art Gallery,
Port Sunlight*
Engraved by R. Wallis for *Picturesque Views in England
and Wales*, Part XIX, No.2 (Rawlinson No.282).

Numerous small pencil sketches of architectural and
industrial details at Dudley occur in the 'Birmingham
and Coventry' sketchbook, T.B.CCXL, ff.39–50. The
'Kenilworth' sketchbook, T.B.CCXXXVIII (No.442)
was used on the same trip and includes several larger
views at Dudley, including one of the town and castle
from roughly the same viewpoint as in this watercolour,
but with a rural foreground of wooded banks.

The subject is one of the most striking of Turner's
records of the industrial scene – compare the views of
Shields (No.241) and Leeds (No.186). Rawlinson calls
it 'one of the most deeply poetical of Turner's works.
The contrast between the past and the present is so
profoundly felt, so impressively rendered. The quiet,
pathetic beauty of the once dominant, but now ruined
feudal castle is strikingly brought out by the forges and
the busy life of the nineteenth century below'. Charles
Heath lent the watercolour to the 1833 exhibition, so
presumably it was being engraved at that time.

427 Blenheim House and Park – Oxford *c.*1832
Watercolour with some scraping-out, $11\frac{3}{4} \times 18\frac{7}{16}$
(29.6×46.8)
Exh: Moon, Boys and Graves Gallery 1833(51)
City Museums and Art Gallery, Birmingham
Engraved by W. Radclyffe for *Picturesque Views in Eng-
land and Wales*, Part XVI, No.2, 1833 (Rawlinson No.
270).

Based on pencil drawings in the 'Kenilworth' sketchbook of *c.*1830 (T.B.XXXVIII, esp. 11ᵛ and 12ʳ). A
colour-beginning of the subject is T.B.CCLXIII–365, in
which the light coming through the arch of the bridge
and its reflection, in the form of a sun-like disc, is the
focus of the design. Thomas Griffith lent the watercolour to the 1833 exhibition.

428 Ullswater *c.*1833
Watercolour, 12$\frac{13}{16}$ × 17 (32.6 × 43.2)
Brian Pilkington, Esq.
Engraved by J. T. Willmore for *Picturesque Views in England and Wales*, 1835, Part XIX, No.4 (Rawlinson No.284). The engraving is No.429. The subject was probably suggested by Turner's visit to the lakes on his way to Scotland in 1831. He seems to have made several drawings of Ullswater, in the 'Minstrelsy of the Scottish Borders' sketchbook (No.449) ff.18^v–24^r.

James Tibbetts WILLMORE (1801–1863) after
TURNER

429 Ullswater, Cumberland 1835
Engraving, first published state, before all letters, 6$\frac{9}{16}$ × 9$\frac{5}{8}$ (16.6 × 24.4); plate, 9$\frac{5}{8}$ × 12$\frac{1}{8}$ (24.4 × 30.8)
Trustees of the British Museum (1850-1-12-34)
Rawlinson No.284; for *Picturesque Views in England and Wales*, Part XIX, No.4, from the watercolour No. 428. A progress proof in the British Museum (1894-2-26-103) bears a note by Turner instructing the engraver to alter his work on the foreground: 'Too much of stones all too equal as to size and work – They should be smaller and smaller from the front and less defined'; the relevant area in the print itself is marked 'Lighter'.

430 Llanthony Abbey *c.*1834
Watercolour and bodycolour, 11$\frac{13}{16}$ × 16$\frac{3}{4}$ (30 × 42.5)
Watermarked: 1833
Mr and Mrs Kurt F. Pantzer, Indianapolis
Engraved by J. T. Willmore for *Picturesque Views in England and Wales*, 1836, Part XX, No.3 (Rawlinson No. 287).

As Ruskin (who owned the drawing) pointed out, the composition is derived from the views of Llanthony made by Turner in 1794–5 (T.B.XXXVII–R etc.), based on the pencil sketch T.B.XII–F; see No.11.

431 Longships Lighthouse, Land's End *c.*1835
Watercolour, 11$\frac{1}{16}$ × 17 (28.1 × 43.2)
Lady Agnew
Engraved by W. R. Smith, 1836, for *Picturesque Views in England and Wales*, Part XX, No.4 (Rawlinson No. 288; No.432).

Turner visited Land's End in 1811 when making notes for the *Southern Coast* series (see the 'Ivy Bridge to Penzance' sketchbook, T.B.CXXV, ff.50, 51). The forms of the rocks and rough seas at that point on the coast seem to have continued to fascinate him; several 'colour-beginnings' dark in tone and perhaps dating from *c.*1817 are apparently based on his experience of this spot. The *Southern Coast* plate, however, does not give such prominence to the sea itself. This drawing has much in common with 'Lowestoft', of about the same date (B.M. 1958-7-12-441).

William Richard SMITH (1787–1839) after
TURNER

432 The Longships Lighthouse, Land's End 1836
Engraving, proof corrected by Turner, 6$\frac{7}{16}$ × 9$\frac{15}{16}$ (16.4 × 25.2); plate, 10 × 12$\frac{7}{8}$ (25.4 × 32.8)
Inscr. by Turner: 'I have touched it generaly [sic] but cannot carry on without the other treated Proofs. back, as to the Water you must put in Lines between to get rid of the line-like look it has leaving the lights [sketch] thus to answer to my Drawing amongst those you have too many of'.
Trustees of the British Museum (1894-2-26-109)
Rawlinson No.28; for No.4 in Part XX of the *Picturesque Views in England and Wales* (the drawing itself is No.431). Another proof of the plate, also in the British Museum, has a further note by Turner: 'Water wants filling in with work to take away the equal width through[out ?] with one line Etching and make the lights dashing and sharp'.

433 Mount St. Michael, Cornwall *c.*1836
Watercolour with some bodycolour,
sight 12$\frac{5}{8}$ × 17 (31.8 × 43.3)
University of Liverpool
Engraved by S. Fisher, 1838, for *Picturesque Views in England and Wales*, Part XXIV, No.4 (Rawlinson No. 304). Turner made several studies of St. Michaels' Mount in his 'Ivy Bridge to Penzance' sketchbook of 1811 (T.B.CXXV, ff.31–46); these were used for the *Southern Coast* subject engraved in 1814 (Rawlinson No.88), and may have been referred to again for this, one of the latest of the *England and Wales* designs.

434 Richmond Terrace, Surrey *c.*1836
Watercolour and bodycolour, 11$\frac{1}{2}$ × 11$\frac{3}{8}$ (28.5 × 44.1)
Walker Art Gallery, Liverpool
Engraved by J. T. Willmore, 1838, for *Picturesque Views in England and Wales*, Part XXIV, No.3 (Rawlinson No.303).

Compare this treatment of the subject with the larger watercolour of *c.*1825 and with the 'colour-beginnings' which also use the panorama from Richmond Hill (Nos.256 and 257). There is a tradition that the view was taken from Wick House, built for Sir Joshua Reynolds by Sir William Chambers; but it seems more probable that it was intended to show the garden of the 'Star and Garter' Inn which may be the building on the extreme left.

435 The Thames above Waterloo Bridge *c.*1830–5
Oil on canvas, 35$\frac{5}{8}$ × 47$\frac{5}{8}$ (90.5 × 121)
Tate Gallery (1992)
Datable for stylistic reasons to the early 1830s, it is just possible that this was projected as Turner's answer to Constable's picture of 'Waterloo Bridge from Whitehall Stairs, June 18th, 1817', exhibited at the Royal Academy in 1832 (repr. Basil Taylor, *Constable*, 1973, pl.154). The effect of smoke-belching industry contrasts with the sparkling clear atmosphere of the Constable, and a large twin-funnelled steam-boat replaces the royal yacht. The possibility of Turner setting out to rival this particular Constable is reinforced by an incident during the 1832 Varnishing Days, when Turner's 'Helvoetsluys', a relatively subdued picture, was hung next to Constable's painting. This seemed, as C. R. Leslie relates, 'as if painted with liquid gold and silver', but Turner dealt with the competition by adding 'a round daub of red lead, somewhat bigger than a shilling, on his grey sea', later shaping it into a buoy.

419

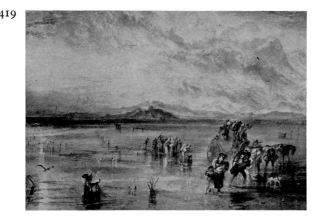

427

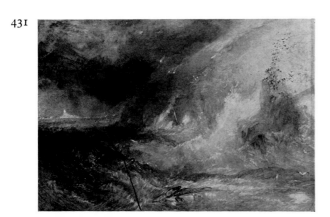

431

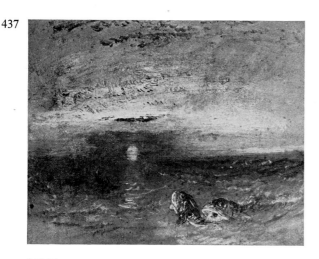

437

**436 Funeral of Sir Thomas Lawrence,
a Sketch from Memory** 1830
Watercolour and bodycolour, $22\frac{1}{16} \times 31\frac{1}{16}$
(56×76.8); mount $24\frac{1}{4} \times 32\frac{1}{2}$ (61.6×82.5)
Inscr. bottom left: 'Funeral of Sir Thoˢ Lawrence
PRA Janʸ 21 1830 SKETCH from MEMORY
IMWT
Exh: R.A. 1830 (493)
Trustees of the British Museum (T.B.CCLXIII–344)
The sheet was mounted, before the drawing had been
started, on another slightly larger sheet showing a mar-
gin all round of about $1\frac{1}{4}$ in on which are a number of
colour trials.

Turner had lost his father on 21 September 1829, and
an old friend, Harriet Wells, on 1 January 1830. His
fellow Academician George Dawe had also only
recently died, as he mentioned in a letter to George
Jones written on 22 January:

Dear Jones, – I delayed answering yours until the
chance of this finding you in Rome, to give you some
account of the dismal prospect of Academic affairs,
and of the last sad ceremonies paid yesterday to departed talent gone to that bourne from whence no
traveller returns. Alas, only two short months Sir
Thomas followed the coffin of Dawe to the same
place. We then were his pallbearers. Who will do the
like for me, or when, God only knows how soon; my
poor father's death proved a heavy blow upon me,
and has been followed by others of the same dark
kind. However, it is something to feel that gifted
talent can be acknowledged by the many who yesterday waded up to their knees in snow and muck to see
the funeral pomp swelled up by carriages of the
great ... (Quoted by Finberg, 1961, p.320).

437 Sunset at Sea with two Gurnets *c.*1835
Watercolour and bodycolour with some black
chalk on buff paper, $8\frac{5}{8} \times 11\frac{3}{16}$ (21.8×28.4)
Whitworth Art Gallery, Manchester (D.8. 1912)
Perhaps related to the two sea studies in bodycolour on
buff paper in the Bacon collection (Nos.438 and 439).
There may also be a connection with the two studies
of fish exhibited by Ruskin in 1878 (Nos.108–9) with a
note associating them with the 'Slaver' – i.e. 'Slavers
throwing overboard the Dead and Dying' (No.518)
shown at the R.A. in 1840. One of these studies (No.
B125) is of a Gurnard (an alternative spelling of Gur-
net); a similar drawing is in the Fogg Art Museum.

438 Sunset over a Beach ?*c.*1835
Bodycolour on coarse buff-grey paper, $8\frac{13}{16} \times 11\frac{5}{8}$
(22.4×29.3)
Sir Edmund Bacon, Bart.

439 Figures on the Shore ?*c.*1835
Bodycolour on coarse buff paper, $9\frac{1}{8} \times 11\frac{1}{2}$
(22.3×29.2)
Sir Edmund Bacon, Bart.
This drawing appears to have been executed at the same
time as 'Sunset over a Beach' (No.438) from the same
collection, which is similar in size, medium and paper.

440 A Misty Shore with Breakwater ?*c.*1835
Watercolour, $7\frac{9}{16} \times 11$ (19.2×28)
Trustees of the British Museum (T.B.CCLXIII–230)

441 Two Figures on the Sea Shore ?c.1835
Watercolour, 7⁹⁄₁₆ × 11 (19.2 × 28)
Trustees of the British Museum (T.B.CCLXIII–233)
From a series of very economical studies of sea-shore effects, some of which are on paper watermarked 1825 (e.g. CCLXIII–272).

442 'Kenilworth' Sketchbook 1828–1830
Bound in buff boards, with leather spine, one clasp
92 leaves the majority drawn on in pencil, 4½ × 7½ (11.2 × 19)
Watermarked: 1820
Trustees of the British Museum (T.B.CCXXXVIII)

f.1ᵛ The High Street, Oxford
Pencil
f.2ʳ Magdalen College, Oxford from the Bridge
Pencil

The book contains drawings of Virginia Water, Kenilworth, Dudley, Tamworth, Lichfield, etc., made on a tour of the Midlands on which Turner collected material for the *England and Wales* watercolours.

The view of the High Street, Oxford (f.1ᵛ) was used by Turner as the starting point for a series of 'colour-beginnings', experiments in broad effects of light; see Nos.443–447.

443 The High Street, Oxford c.1830–35
Watercolour, 13⅞ × 20¼ (35.2 × 51.4)
Trustees of the British Museum (T.B.CCLXIII–106)
One of a group of treatments of Oxford High Street made in the early 1830s (see Nos. 444–447). The introduction of figures into two of the studies (Nos.445 and 447) shows that these variations on a single subject are not experiments in a vacuum. They are almost certainly preliminary exercises in the development of an *England and Wales* composition which was never realised. This conjecture is supported by the fact that the motif is taken from a pencil study in the 'Kenilworth' sketchbook (No.442), used during the tour of the Midlands of 1830 which Turner undertook with the specific intention of collecting material for *England and Wales*. The theme is one which Turner had already explored in his painting of about 1810 (No.159), which was itself based on a considerably earlier drawing, T.B.CXX–F.

A number of other colour-beginnings in the Turner Bequest appear to have been made, like the 'Oxford' series, in connection with *England and Wales* subjects; many of them were not used for finished watercolours.

444 The High Street, Oxford c.1830–35
Watercolour, 12 × 19⅛ (30.4 × 48.4)
Trustees of the British Museum (T.B.CCLXIII–3)
See No.443. Here the design is blocked out boldly and simply in pale yellow and blue with an intensification of the tonal contrast to grey and white at one point of the composition; other versions show a more elaborate treatment of light.

445 The High Street, Oxford c.1830–35
Watercolour, 6⅜ × 19⅛ (16.2 × 48.6)
Trustees of the British Museum (T.B.CCLXIII–4)

446 The High Street, Oxford c.1830–35
Watercolour, 14⅝ × 21⅝ (37.2 × 54.7)
Trustees of the British Museum (T.B.CCLXIII–5)
See No.443. A treatment of the theme in a cooler range of colours – blue-grey, purple-grey, and muted yellow. A second tower, that of St. Martin and All Saints, is visible beyond that of St. Mary's.

447 The High Street, Oxford c.1830–35
(repr. on p.107)
Pencil and watercolour, 15¹⁄₁₆ × 22 (38.2 × 55.8)
Trustees of the British Museum (T.B.CCLXIII–362)
See No.443. This study is considerably more elaborate than the others in its treatment of atmosphere and in the detail of the figures.

448 'Marine Dabblers' Sketchbook 1830
Album, bound in mottled boards, with red tooled leather spine and corners and panel on front cover with 'ALBUM' in gilt letters
80 leaves of different coloured paper, the majority left blank; 21 drawn on in pencil with one slight sketch in bodycolour, 4½ × 3½ (11.2 × 9)
Trustees of the British Museum (T.B.CCXLI)

f.38ᵛ Studies of Figures on a Promenade
Pencil on pink paper
Inscr: '489 Sept 28 1830' and 'Wan, Ink' (?)
f.39ʳ Studies of Figures on the Shore
Pencil on cream paper
Inscr: 'Sun 15' [?] 'Girl Red P.B. Arm BB' 'Weedy depth' [?]

The sketchbook is named after an inscription on f.46ᵛ, which is difficult to read. Turner used the phrase 'Marine Dabblers' as the title of one of his *Liber Studiorum* plates (R.29) published in 1811; it has no connection with the present sketchbook, which contains a number of small pencil drawings of figures and boats by the sea and one bedroom scene (f.79ᵛ) which is rather similar in subject to the supposed 'Scene at a Play' (T.B.CCCXVIII–17). The resemblance is no doubt accidental.

449 'Minstrelsy of the Scottish Border' Sketchbook 1831
Bound in buff boards, leather spine; one clasp
92 leaves of white paper, the first eight (numbered at the end) washed with grey (c.f. 'Guernsey' Sketchbook, No.369); the majority of the leaves drawn on in pencil; ff.69–84 blank, 4½ × 7¼ (18.4 × 11.5)
Watermarked: 1828
Trustees of the British Museum (T.B.CCLXVI)

ff.14ᵛ–15ʳ Landscape with a view of Kendal
Pencil

The book was used on Turner's journey to Scotland where he toured in July to September 1831, collecting material for Cadell's edition of *Scott's Poetical Works* of 1834 and *Scott's Prose Works* of 1834–6. The sketches begin at Birkenhead, with views of Liverpool (ff.1–7); then Turner seems to have travelled via Preston, Kendal and the Lakes to Carlisle, thence to the Border. ff.14–18 have a series of drawings made in or near Kendal.

[125]

450 'Abbotsford' Sketchbook 1831
Bound in buff boards, leather spine; one clasp
92 leaves, the majority drawn on in pencil, $4\frac{1}{2} \times 7\frac{1}{4}$
(11.5 × 18.4)
Watermarked: 1828
Trustees of the British Museum (T.B.CCLXVII)

ff.68ᵛ–69ʳ The Interior of the Armoury at Abbotsford
Pencil

In addition to the series of sketches of Edinburgh, Kelso, Melrose, Dryburgh, Sedburgh and Smailholme which were used for Cadell's *Scott*, this book also contains a page of studies of Norham Castle (f.59ᵛ), which may well have rekindled Turner's interest in the theme, and been used as the basis for some of the later 'colour-beginnings' leading on to the final painting (see Nos. 649–50).

451 'Stirling and Edinburgh' Sketchbook 1831
Bound in buff boards, leather spine, one clasp
91 leaves almost all drawn on in pencil, $4\frac{1}{2} \times 7\frac{1}{4}$
(11.3 × 18.4)
Watermarked: 1828
Trustees of the British Museum (T.B.CCLXIX)

ff.78ᵛ–79ʳ View of Edinburgh from Calton Hill; with a small sketch of the Nelson Monument and other buildings on the hill
Pencil

Used on the tour of Scotland which Turner made preparatory to illustrating *Scott* for Cadell. As well as studies of Edinburgh and Stirling, the book contains a series of sketches of the falls of Clyde (ff.1–12) and some of Bothwell Castle (ff.26–30).

452 'Staffa' Sketchbook 1831
Bound in marbled boards, leather spine and corners
98 leaves mostly drawn on in pencil, $7\frac{1}{2} \times 4\frac{1}{2}$
(19 × 11.3)
Trustees of the British Museum (T.B.CCLXXIII)

ff.58ᵛ–59ʳ Studies of Groups of Figures in a Scottish Harbour
Pencil
Inscr. on f.58ᵛ: 'furniture'(?) and 'colts tyed together'

Used on the west coast of Scotland, the book includes a series of drawings of Staffa and Fingal's Cave, ff.18ᵛ to 22. The oil painting of 'Staffa, Fingal's Cave' was shown at the R.A. 1832 (No.490), and a vignette of the subject appeared in *Scott's Poetical Works*, 1834 (Rawlinson No.512).

453 'Inverness' Sketchbook 1831
Bound in marbled boards, leather spine
145 leaves, many blanks, the remainder drawn on in pencil, $6\frac{1}{2} \times 4$ (16.5 × 10.3)
Bears the label of 'D. Morrison. Bookseller, Inverness'
Trustees of the British Museum (T.B.CCLXXVII)

f.138ᵛ Buildings at Elgin (?)
Pencil

f.139ʳ Study of Elgin Cathedral
Pencil
Inscr. with numbers: '1' '2' '3'; and an illegible note

Contains drawings at Inverness, Elgin and elsewhere in the Highlands.

454 'Life Class' sketchbook No.1 ?c.1832
Bound in red morocco; one clasp
64 pages, almost all drawn on in pencil, $3\frac{1}{2} \times 4\frac{1}{2}$
(8.5 × 11)
Watermarked: 1831
Trustees of the British Museum (T.B.CCLXXIX(a))

f.7ʳ A Man talking to an Oysterwoman
Pencil
Inscr: 'The Bivalve Courtship'
Opposite on f.6ᵛ are rough diagrams and illegible inscriptions

Containing sketches of random subjects, including two sketches of a life drawing class (ff.20ᵛ, 52ʳ), and a series of studies from a female model in the class; also a few rough sketches of erotic subjects, and landscape and seaside views.

455 'Colour Studies' Sketchbook No.1 c.1835
Bound in leather, one clasp
54 leaves, with two marbled fly-leaves, all drawn on in pencil or watercolour, with some pen, 3×4
(7.7 × 10.2)
Trustees of the British Museum (T.B.CCXCI(b))

f.29ᵛ Two Figures watching a Sleeping Woman
Grey-brown wash
f.30ʳ A Couple on a Bed
Grey-brown wash

The watercolour landscape sketches on ff.51ᵛ, 52ᵛ are similar to Turner's studies for vignettes to Campbell's *Poems* on which he was engaged in about 1835 (see Nos.295–298).

The sketchbook contains a series of studies of nude figures, singly or in couples, in a bedroom. It has been associated with Turner's various visits to Petworth about 1830, and the series of bodycolour studies made there (Nos.343–362); but these bedroom scenes are presumably imaginary. Another small sketchbook, T.B.CCXCI(c), contains one watercolour sketch similar to the Petworth interiors (f.1), but it appears to be the first of a series of studies narrating an erotic adventure (ff.1–12ᵛ). There are further colour studies on similar themes throughout the book. Whether these drawings were made at Petworth or not, their preoccupation with the chiaroscuro of interiors chimes in with Turner's revived interest in Rembrandt during the early 1830s (see Nos.331–2, 338).

456 The Burning of the Houses of Parliament
1834
Watercolour and bodycolour, sight
$11\frac{1}{2} \times 17\frac{5}{16}$ (29.3 × 44)
Trustees of the British Museum
(T.B.CCCLXIV–373)
Turner was an eye-witness of the fire which destroyed

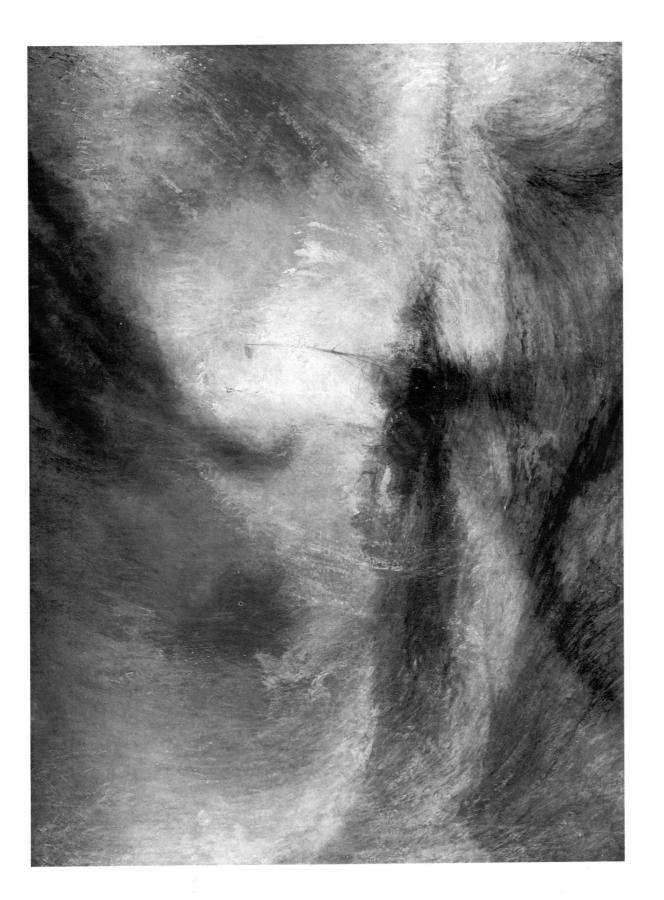

504 **Snow Storm – Steam Boat off a Harbour's Mouth** 1842 (entry on p.140)

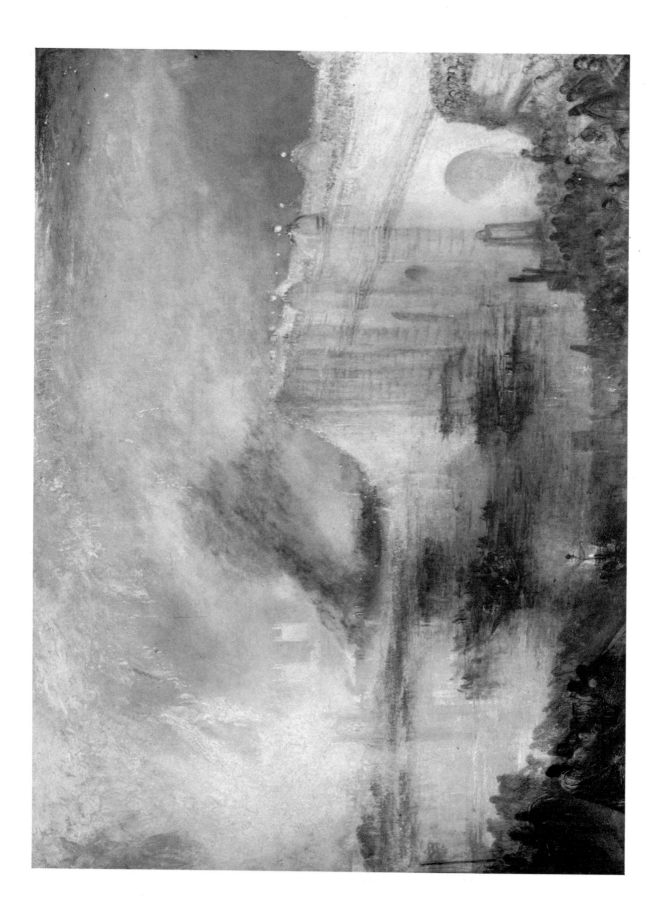

512 **The Burning of the House of Lords and Commons** 1835 (entry on p.142)

the old Houses of Parliament on the night of 16 October 1834, and he made a number of slight pencil sketches on the spot (T.B.CCLXXXIV). In addition, a sketchbook in the Turner Bequest (CCLXXXIII) contains nine watercolour studies of the scene (see Nos.457–460). It has been suggested that these too were executed on the spot, though it would perhaps be more consistent with Turner's normal practice if he had done them from memory, or on the basis of pencil outlines, immediately on returning home. The large, more finished watercolour was then worked up from this material, though it is not known whether Turner envisaged selling or exhibiting it. It remained in his studio. See also No.512.

A vignette showing the fire, seen under one of the arches of Westminster Bridge, was engraved by J. T. Willmore in 1835 for the *Keepsake* (Rawlinson No.332).

457   The Burning of the Houses of Parliament
1834
Watercolour, $9\frac{1}{8} \times 12\frac{3}{4}$ (23.2 × 32.4)
Trustees of the British Museum
(T.B.CCLXXXIII-2)

458   The Burning of the Houses of Parliament
1834
Watercolour, $9\frac{1}{8} \times 12\frac{3}{4}$ (23.2 × 32.4)
Trustees of the British Museum
(T.B.CCLXXXIII-4)

459   The Burning of the Houses of Parliament
1834
Watercolour $9\frac{1}{8} \times 12\frac{3}{4}$ (23.2 × 32.4)
Trustees of the British Museum
(T.B.CCLXXXIII-6)

460   The Burning of the Houses of Parliament
1834
Watercolour $9\frac{1}{8} \times 12\frac{3}{4}$ (23.2 × 32.4)
Trustees of the British Museum
(T.B.CCLXXXIII-7)

See No.456. Four colour studies from a sketchbook containing a sequence of nine similar drawings.

461   Study of a Stormy Sea (pink, blue, yellow and black) ?c.1840
Watercolour, 10×14 (25.4 × 35.5)
Trustees of the British Museum (T.B.CCCLXIV-145)

462   Sun among Red Clouds over the Sea ?c.1840
Watercolour, $10\frac{11}{16} \times 14\frac{11}{16}$ (27.2 × 37.4)
Trustees of the British Museum (T.B.CCCLXIV-143)

12. Rome and After 1828–35

Turner's second visit to Italy was very different from his first. He went straight to Rome and spent much of his time there painting in oils as well as watercolours. Moreover, besides the pictures he actually exhibited in Rome (see Nos.472–4), there was no hesitation in the flow of Italian subjects that he continued to exhibit after he returned to England; every year from 1829 to 1846 he exhibited at least one picture inspired by Italy, though in some years, and particularly after 1840, the stress was on Venice rather than Rome and the Campagna. In addition a large number of oils of Italian subjects, not exhibited during Turner's lifetime, can be dated to the ten or so years following this second visit.

463   'Genoa and Florence' Sketchbook 1828
Bound in white parchment
94 leaves, almost all drawn on in pencil, 6 × 4
(14.4 × 10)
Trustees of the British Museum (T.B.CCXXXIII)

ff.77ᵛ–78ʳ **Two views of Florence from near S. Miniato**
Pencil

Used on Turner's second journey to Italy, August–October 1828, from which he returned in January 1829. The book includes drawings of Genoa, Lucca, Florence, Pisa and Livorno.

The exhibited studies show Florence in much the same view that Turner chose for his three finished watercolours of Florence, one of which was engraved for the *Keepsake* in 1828 (see No.466) and must, therefore, have been done prior to this visit to Italy.

464   'Viterbo and Ronciglione' Sketchbook 1828
Bound in boards, leather spine
48 leaves, mostly drawn on in pencil, 5 × 7
(12.4 × 17.7)
Trustees of the British Museum (T.B.CCXXXVI)

f.24ᵛ **Three slight sketches of Landscapes**
Pencil
f.25ʳ **Six Landscape Compositions**
Pencil

The composition at the top right of f.25ᵛ seems to be related to the 'Southern Landscape with an Aqueduct and Waterfall' in the Turner Bequest (Tate Gallery 5506); that immediately below it is perhaps a development of the motif sketched on the opposite page (bottom drawing); and the composition bottom left is apparently a view of Orvieto, connected with the painting of 1828 (No.472).

465   'Rome, Turin and Milan' Sketchbook 1829
Bound in yellow parchment
62 leaves, nearly all drawn on in pencil, $5\frac{1}{2} \times 3\frac{1}{2}$
(19.1 × 14.5)
Trustees of the British Museum (T.B.CCXXXV)

[129]

f.5ᵛ **Castello Portalengo**
Pencil
Inscr. with the name of the town
f.6ʳ **Lodi**
Pencil
Inscr. with the name of the town

A note inside the cover indicating Turner's itinerary from Rome to Milan suggests that this book was in use on the journey back from Rome in January 1829. The drawings are all very rough – Ruskin described them as 'careless work'.

466   Arona *c.*1828
Watercolour, 11½ × 17 (29.2 × 43.1)
Brian Pilkington, Esq.
Engraved by W.R. Smith for the *Keepsake*, 1829, as 'Lago Maggiore' (Rawlinson No.321). One of three Italian subjects published in the *Keepsake* in 1828 and 1829; the other two are 'Florence from S. Miniato' (drawings now in the Herbert Art Gallery, Coventry and private collection, Scotland) and 'Lake Albano' (ex coll. J. Pierpont Morgan). The mood and technique of these watercolours are similar to those of the vignette designs for Rogers' *Italy*, which Turner had nearly finished when he left England for Rome in 1828 (see No.272). It is very probable that the *Keepsake* subjects were also done before he went abroad in that year.

467   Two Trees in a Landscape ?*c.*1828
Watercolour, 13⁹⁄₁₆ × 20⅛ (34.5 × 51)
Trustees of the British Museum (T.B.CCLXIII–29)
Finberg describes this economical sketch as 'an Italian Landscape' but it is difficult to say whether Turner had any particular location in mind.

The trees are similar to those in 'Coast Scene near Naples', provisionally dated to 1828 (No.470), but the background of this drawing, apparently showing a lake, does not correspond to that of the painting. There is perhaps a connection with the watercolour of 'Arona on Lake Maggiore' (No.466), where two trees, coloured contrastingly in very dark green (almost black) and yellow are seen against the waters of the lake. 'Arona' is also dateable to about 1828.

468   A Classical Landscape ?*c.*1828
Watercolour, 12³⁄₁₆ × 17¼ (31 × 43.8)
Trustees of the British Museum (T.B.CCLXIII–189)
Perhaps connected thematically with the 'Bay of Baiæ' of 1823 or 'Ulysses' of 1829 (Nos.237 and 482); compare also the 'Coast Scene near Naples' of about the same date (No.470), and the colour-beginning 'Two Trees in a Landscape' (No.467).

469   Landscape with Buildings *c.*1828
Oil on millboard, irregular, 12 × 18¾ (30.5 × 47.7)
Trustees of the British Museum (1972-U. 738)
This is one of a group of oil sketches on millboard found in the 1950s in a brown paper parcel among the Turner Bequest drawings at the British Museum. Two are distinct in style and the thickness of the millboard used, but the others form a fairly consistent group, though their sizes vary. In so far as they can be dated by stylistic criteria the majority would seem to have been painted in the 1830s or even the 1840s (see Nos.498–500). This

example, however, is so close in composition and colouring to some of the sketches thought to have been painted while Turner was in Rome in 1828 (see Nos. 475–80) that it is grouped with them.

470   Coast Scene near Naples ?1828
Oil on millboard, 16⅛ × 23½ (41 × 59.5)
Tate Gallery (5527)
One of a number of similar sketches on millboard, distinct in style, however, from those also from the Turner Bequest found at the British Museum (e.g. Nos. 469, 498–500). A number of them seem to show landscapes around Rome and Naples. Though very different from earlier sketches from nature like those done on the Thames *c.*1807–8 they have a directness and freshness which suggests that they may also have been done out-of-doors, though with formal compositions in mind from the outset. There is no secure evidence that Turner went to Naples on his second visit to Rome but it would have been easy for him to do so and this group of sketches has usually been dated to this visit. However they could have been done on the 1819 visit; see also under No.471.

471   Hill Town on the Edge of the Campagna
?1828
Oil on millboard, 16⅛ × 23⅜ (41 × 59.5)
Tate Gallery (5526)
Another of the group of sketches discussed under No.470. In this case there are fairly close parallels with watercolours and drawings definitely done when Turner went to Italy in 1819, for instance 'Roman Campagna: Morning' and 'The Tiber' (T.B.CLXXXVII–34 and T.B.CLXXXIX–24; repr. Thomas Ashby, *Turner's Vision of Rome*, 1925, pls.6 and 1; the former also repr. Reynolds 1969, pl.93), but he could of course have painted similar views on both visits.

472   View of Orvieto, painted in Rome 1828
Oil on canvas, 36 × 48½ (91.5 × 123)
Exh: Rome 1828–9; R.A. 1830 (30)
Tate Gallery (511)
Turner went to Rome for the second time in 1828, leaving England in August and arriving in October; he stayed until January 1829 and was back in England in February. Sir Charles Eastlake told Thornbury (1862, I, p.221) that they both stayed at 12 Piazza Mignanelli and that Turner 'painted there the "View of Orvieto", the "Regulus", and the "Medea" [Nos.474 and 473]. Those pictures were exhibited in Rome in some rooms which Turner subsequently occupied at the Quattro Fontane. The foreign artists who went to see them could make nothing of them'.

Turner advertised that he was to exhibit 'due Paessaggi' for a week at the Palazzo Trulli in the *Diario di Roma* for 17 December 1828. These John Gage identifies (1968, p.679) as 'Orvieto' and 'Regulus', though it is known that 'Medea' was on view on 16 December (Finberg 1961, p.311). In a letter written in February 1829 Eastlake confirmed that Turner exhibited these three works, as well as beginning 'eight or ten pictures', presumably including 'Palestrina' (see under No.331), three further works on identical canvases tacked to the stretchers with the same tacks, 'Venus reclining', 'Outline of the Venus de' Medici', and 'Southern Landscape' (Tate Gallery 5498, 5509 and 5510), 'Italian Landscape with a Road in the Foreground' (Tate Gallery 5473), and perhaps the composition sketches on similar but not identical coarse canvas mentioned under Nos.475–80. Turner himself reported his progress in a letter to Sir Francis Chantrey of 6 November 1828: 'I have confined myself to the painting department . . . and having finished *one*, am about the second, and getting on with Lord E.s' [Palestrina'], which I began the very first touch at Rome; but as folk here talked that I would show them *not*, I finished a small three feet four to stop their gabbling'; this last was presumably 'Orvieto'.

Eastlake's account in Thornbury goes on, 'When those same works were packed to be sent to England, I advised him to have the cover covered with waxed cloth, as the pictures without it might be exposed to wet. Turner thanked me, and said the advice was important; "for", he added, "if any wet gets to them, they will be destroyed". This indicates his practice of preparing his pictures with a kind of tempera, a method which, before the surface was varnished, was not waterproof [in fact analysis has failed to show that Turner used anything like tempera, though he did quite often use watercolour on his oils]. The pictures referred to were, in fact, not finished; nor could any of his exhibited pictures be said to be finished till he had worked on them when they were on the walls of the Royal Academy'. This is supported by the review of 'Orvieto' in *The Morning Chronicle* for 3 May 1830 quoted under 'Pilate washing his Hands' (see No.332), though in fact 'Orvieto' is much more thinly painted, and apparently much less gone over, than 'Pilate'. Although Turner had hoped that his Rome paintings would reach London in time for the Royal Academy exhibition in 1829 there were shipping delays and 'Orvieto' and 'Palestrina' were not exhibited until 1830, 'Medea' until 1831 and 'Regulus' until 1837.

473 Vision of Medea 1828

Oil on canvas, $68\frac{3}{8} \times 98$ (173.5×241)
Exh: Rome 1828–9; R.A. 1831 (178)
Tate Gallery (513)

While on his way to Italy in 1828 Turner wrote from Paris to his friend Charles Eastlake, who was already in Rome, asking 'that the best of all possible grounds and canvass size 8 feet $2\frac{1}{2}$ by 4 feet $11\frac{1}{4}$ Inches to be if possible ready for me, 2 canvasses if possible'. This was partly so that he could begin straight away on a picture for Lord Egremont, 'Palestrina' (see under No.331); the second canvas could have been for 'Medea' though the height is a bit greater. This was one of the three pictures Eastlake said Turner exhibited at Rome (see also Nos.472 and 474), telling Thornbury that 'Turner's economy and ingenuity were apparant in his mode of framing those pictures. He nailed a rope around the edges of each, and painted it with yellow ochre in tempera' (Thornbury 1862, I, p.221). The present reconstruction is by Lawrence Gowing.

Lord Broughton, who was taken by the sculptor Thomas Campbell to see Turner's exhibits on 16 December, noted in his diary that 'The chief of these strange compositions, called the "Vision of Medea", was a glaring extravagant daub, which might mistaken for a joke – and a bad joke too. Mr Campbell told us

that the Romans who had seen these pictures were filled with wonder and pity' (Finberg 1961, p.311). The *Moderne Kunstchronik*, published in 1834 by J. A. Koch in collaboration with other German artists who were in Rome at the time, was equally scathing, perhaps in jealousy of the 'large and vulgar crowd which had gathered to see the exhibition of the world-famous painter, Turner. . . . The pictures were surrounded with ship's cable instead of gilt frames. . . . The composition purporting to show the Vision of Medea was remarkable enough. Suffice it to say that whether you turned the picture on its side, or upside down, you could still recognise as much in it' (Gage 1969, pp.104–5).

At the Royal Academy in 1831 the picture was exhibited with the following lines attributed to Turner's 'MS Fallacies of Hope':
Or Medea, who in the full tide of witchery
Had lured the dragon, gained her Jason's love,
Had filled the spell-bound bowl with Æson's life,
Yet dashed it to the ground, and raised the poisonous snake
High in the jaundiced sky to writhe its murderous coil,
Infuriate in the wreck of hope, withdrew
And in the fired palace her twin offspring threw.

The critic of the *Athenaeum* for 14 May started off from these lines for his attack on the picture: 'The painting is of a piece with the poetry. Here we have, indeed, the Sister Arts – and precious sisters they are! Mr. Turner, doubtless, smeared the lines off with his brush, after a strong fit of yellow insanity . . . The snakes, and the flowers, and the spirits, and the sun, and the sky, and the trees, are all in an agony of ochre!' The artist had achieved 'a gambouge phrenzy worthy of the Bedlam lines. . . . "Jaundiced sky!" – "a good phrase – a good phrase"!' But other critics, though deploring the main figures, found something to praise, albeit sometimes rather grudgingly. 'Colour! colour! colour!' exclaimed the *Literary Gazette* for 7 May; 'Still there is something so enchanting in the prismatic effect which Mr. Turner has produced, that we soon lose sight of the extravagance, in contemplating the magical results of his combinations'. For *La Belle Assemblée* for June 1831, 'as a combination of colour, the work is truly wonderful'.

In some ways, despite the glow of colour that so astounded Turner's contemporaries, the picture looks back to his grand machines of the early 1800s. The use of a coarse Italian canvas is accompanied by something of a return to Titian, found even more in the large 'Venus reclining', similarly painted in Rome on an identical piece of canvas, which is based on Titian's 'Venus of Urbino' (Tate Gallery 5498). Comparing these pictures with the near-contemporary 'Orvieto' and 'Caligula's Palace' (Nos.472 and 485) makes it clear how much Turner adapted his style and technique to the kind of subject he was attempting.

474 Regulus 1828

Oil on canvas, $35\frac{3}{4} \times 48\frac{3}{4}$ (91×124)
Exh: Rome 1828–9; British Institution 1837 (120)
Tate Gallery (519)

One of the paintings, like 'Orvieto' (see No.472), known to have been painted and exhibited in Rome in 1828, but considerably re-worked before being exhibited again in 1837. The young Sir John Gilbert (1817–97), having a picture opposite Turner's in the British Institution, observed Turner at work on it. 'He was absorbed in his work, did not look about him, but kept on scumbling a lot of white into his picture – nearly all over it. . . . The picture was a mass of red and yellow of all varieties. Every object was in this fiery state. He had a large palette, nothing on it but a huge lump of flake-white; he had two or three biggish hog tools to work with, and with these he was driving the white into all the hollows, and every part of the surface. This was the only work he did, and it was the finishing stroke. The sun, as I have said, was in the centre; from it were drawn – ruled – lines to mark the rays; these lines were rather strongly marked, I suppose to guide his eye. The picture gradually became wonderfully effective, just the effect of brilliant sunlight absorbing everything and throwing a misty haze over every object. Standing sideway of the canvas, I saw that the sun was a lump of white standing out like the boss on a shield' (Gage 1969, p.169). A small oil by Thomas Fearnley shows the scene (repr. Gage 1969, pl.30).

The composition is a Claudian seaport of the kind sketched by Turner at probably much the same time as he first worked on this picture (see No.479) and the colour also resembles the rather unusual colour of these sketches. The absence, among the scene of activity, of any figure actually identifiable as Regulus has been fascinatingly explained by John Gage (p.143): Regulus, having deliberately failed to negotiate an exchange of prisoners with the Carthaginians, returned from Rome to Carthage and was punished by having his eye-lids cut off and being exposed to the sun, which blinded him. The spectator stands in the position of Regulus, with the sun shining out of the picture full in his face.

All the same, the *Literary Gazette* for 4 February 1837 wasted some space in speculating on the whereabouts of the protagonist, despite recognising that the 'sun absolutely dazzles the eyes'. 'Nevertheless', wrote the critic, 'who could have painted such a picture but Mr. Turner? What hand but his could have created such perfect harmony? Who is there so profoundly versed in the arrangement and management of colours?'. The *Spectator* for 11 February made an interesting comparison with Claude: 'Turner is just the reverse of Claude; instead of the repose of beauty – the soft severity and mellow light of an Italian scene – here all is glare, turbulence, and uneasiness. The only way to be reconciled to the picture is to look at it from as great a distance as the width of the gallery will allow of, and then you see nothing but a burst of sunlight. This is scene-painting – and very fine it is in its way.'

475 Sketch for 'Ulysses deriding Polyphemus' ?1828
Oil on canvas, 23⅝ × 35⅛ (60 × 89)
Tate Gallery (2958)

476 Lake Nemi ?1828
Oil on canvas, 23¾ × 39¼ (60.5 × 99.5)
Tate Gallery (3027)

477 Tivoli, the Cascatelle ?1828
Oil on canvas, 23⅞ × 30⅝ (60.5 × 77.5)
Tate Gallery (3388)

478 Archway with Trees by the Sea ?1828
Oil on canvas, 23⅝ × 34½ (60 × 87.5)
Tate Gallery (3381)

479 Claudian Harbour Scene ?1828
Oil on canvas, 23⅝ × 36⅜ (60 × 92.5)
Tate Gallery (3382)

480 Scene on the Banks of a River ?1828
Oil on canvas, 23¾ × 35⅛ (60.5 × 89)
Tate Gallery (3385)

The first two of these oil sketches were originally on one large canvas with five others (Tate Gallery 2959, 2990–2, 3026); the compositions were separated in about 1914. The others come from nine further examples similar in style, technique and type of canvas (Tate Gallery 3380–8) which are not recorded as having been originally joined. The 1856 Schedule of the Turner Bequest does, however, list four 'Roll[s] containing 4 subjects', only two of which are accounted for by the Cowes sketches, one of which in fact contained five compositions (see Nos.311–19); the other two rolls could have been that mentioned above together with one containing the other sketches. In addition the second group of Italian sketches shares with the first the peculiarity of having been tacked to some sort of stretcher or support from the front, Turner having gone over the tacks with paint in the process of painting each composition. This suggests that in both cases a large piece of canvas was remounted on a relatively small support each time Turner wanted to paint a new sketch.

Those landscapes that can be identified are Italian and the first sketch was used for the large picture exhibited at the Royal Academy in 1829 (No.482). It seems likely that they were done in Italy during Turner's second visit in 1828–9, the use of large rolls of canvas being presumably for ease of transport as seems to have been the case with the Cowes sketches. However, the canvas is not identical with that of the pictures that were exhibited by Turner in Rome (see Nos.472–4), nor did those pictures reach London, having been sent by sea, until after the opening of the 1829 Academy exhibition, but Turner would not have needed the 'Polyphemus' sketch directly in front of him to paint the large picture.

Unlike the Cowes sketches, which seem to have been the direct result of specific experiences even if they were not painted on the spot, these works are essays in composition; even those based on actual landscapes are already of places known to Turner from his travels in Italy in 1819 if not from pictures by other artists: both Lake Nemi and Tivoli (for which see Nos.B35–6) had been painted by Wilson. They are studies in broad areas of strongly contrasted tones of flatly applied colour, occasionally enlivened, as in the case of 'Lake Nemi', by a flurry of heavy impasto. The subjects range from recognisable Italian landscapes, through the 'Polyphemus' sketch which uses landscape motives based on what Turner could have seen in Italy, to the Claudian sea-port which depends entirely on his knowledge of the work of another artist. Differing in size one from the other, and not adhering to any of the standard sizes usually used by Turner, these are works that can definitely be described as sketches rather than 'unfinished' paintings which could have been carried further. For a work very similar in composition and, it

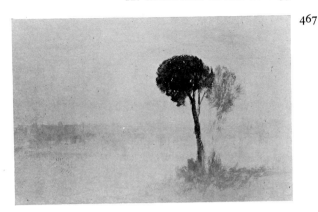
467

would seem, date, but of quite different purpose see 'Rocky Bay with Figures' (No.483).

481 Not exhibited

482 Ulysses deriding Polyphemus – Homer's Odyssey R.A.1829   (repr. on p.108)
Oil on canvas, $52\frac{1}{4} \times 80$ (132.5 × 203)
Inscr. on flag of ship: 'Ο Δ Υ Σ Σ Ε'
Exh: R.A. 1829 (42)
Trustees of the National Gallery, London (508)

The subject is from Book IX of the *Odyssey* and had been first sketched by Turner about 1807 in the 'Wey, Guildford' sketchbook, though there is no connection in composition (T.B.XCVIII–5). This picture is based on one of the sketches on coarse canvas almost certainly painted in Italy in 1828–9 (No.475), though the hollowed-out arches of rock, probably based on those around the Bay of Naples, are only found in another of the sketches (Tate Gallery 2959).

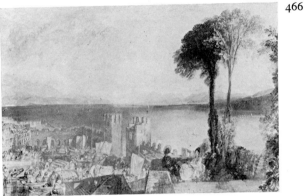
466

Ruskin, who called this 'the *central picture* in Turner's career', noted Turner's fidelity to Pope's translation of the text in the portrayal of the morning light, though his suggestion that the sun-god Apollo is formless because 'he *is* the sun' is countered by Thornbury's statement that 'thanks to sugar of lead, Phoebus has vanished' (1862, I, p.315). John Gage has also pointed out Turner's fidelity over such things as Ulysses' ship being in 'the shallows clear' and the way in which Polyphemus almost forms part of the 'lone mountain's monstrous growth', but he suggests that Turner went further by using the mythological subject to illustrate a picture about the forces of nature (1969, pp.128–32). The smoke rising from the mountain gives it a distinctly volcanic appearance and Polyphemus' fellow Cyclops were associated with thunder and lightning, which had themselves been associated with volcanic activity in the later eighteenth century. The Nereids playing around Ulysses' ship are not mentioned by Homer and seem to have been introduced as embodying the idea of phosphorescence, as in Erasmus Darwin's *The Botanic Garden* of 1791. By now, Gage summarises, Turner had moved beyond the mere personifying of natural causes that he had found in Thomson and Akenside to something 'far closer to the more purely scientific mythography of Shelley' (p.145).

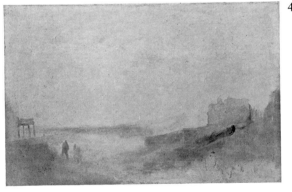
469

Gage (pp.95–6) also suggests that the heightened colouring, particularly in the sky, was partly influenced by Italian fourteenth and fifteenth-century frescoes and temperas, to which Turner seems to have paid particular attention on his second visit to Italy, perhaps reflecting the growing interest in this period of his friends Samuel Rogers, Thomas Phillips and William Young Ottley (see the 'Roman and French' notebook of 1828, T.B.CCXXXVII–38ᵛ and 39, for Turner's notes on the frescoes in the Campo Santo at Pisa). Indeed the *Morning Herald* for 5 May 1829 held that Turner's bright colouring, which had 'for some time been getting worse and worse', had in this picture 'reached the perfection of un-natural tawdriness. In fact, it may be taken as a specimen of *colouring run mad* – positive vermilion – positive indigo, and all the most glaring tints of green, yellow, and purple contend for mastery of the canvas, with all the vehement contrasts of a kaleidoscope or Persian carpet'. The *Literary Gazette*

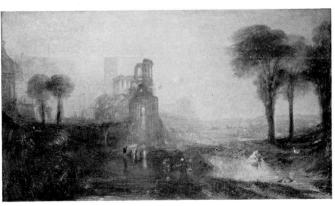
485

for 9 May protested that 'Although the Grecian hero has just put out the eye of the furious Cyclops, that is really no reason why Mr. Turner should put out both the eyes of us, harmless critics. . . . Justice, however, compels us to acknowledge, that although Mr Turner thus continues to delight in violating nature and defying common sense, yet that, considering this performance as a gorgeous vision of the imagination, as a splendid dream of practical fancy, it is highly captivating'. Other critics too felt that the painter's excesses were justified by his poetical feeling. Ruskin's perhaps over-subjective view was that 'The somewhat gloomy and deeply coloured tones of the lower crimson clouds, and of the stormy blue bars underneath them, are always given by Turner to skies which rise over any scene of death, or one connected with any dreadful memories', and in *Modern Painters* he lists the picture among works in which the sky is 'the colour of blood' (Vol.IV, 1856, Library Edition VI, p.381).

483 Rocky Bay with Figures *c*.1830
Oil on canvas, 36 × 49 (91.5 × 124.5)
Tate Gallery (1989)

In composition this is a variation on the theme of a number of the sketches on coarse canvas probably painted in Rome in 1828 (see No.475 and Tate Gallery 2959, 3380), and also the finished 'Ulysses deriding Polyphemus' exhibited in 1829. But it is very different in technique from the sketches, the paint being worked over, partly with the handle of the brush or even the fingers, to produce infinite gradations of tone; the colouring is also much subtler. The sky is as finished in its more delicate style as that of 'Ulysses deriding Polyphemus' and this may be the beginning of another work for exhibition, in Turner's standard four-foot by three-foot size; indeed MacColl suggested that it was possibly another episode in the story of Ulysses (1920, p.30). It is also related, in reverse, to one of the unpublished *Liber Studiorum* plates, 'Glaucus and Scylla' (R.73), but the figures in the painting are different and greater in number and there is a suggestion of long, low ships across the water on the right.

484 The Vision of Jacob's Ladder *c*.1830
Oil on canvas, 48½ × 74 (123 × 188)
Tate Gallery (5507)

Listed in the Schedule of the Turner Bequest, No.266, merely as 'Scriptural Subject 6′2½″ × 4′0″', but certainly the Vision of Jacob's Ladder, *Genesis* XXVIII, 10–12, though Jacob is accompanied by his family and is being addressed by an angel rather than by the Lord God. Martin Davies (*National Gallery Catalogues: The British School*, 1946, p.162) describes this as a very early work, but in fact it seems to have been worked on over a considerable period. The basic forms, and particularly the craggy hill in the centre, are close to such paintings as 'The Goddess of Discord choosing the Apple of Contention in the Garden of the Hesperides' and 'Fall of the Rhine at Schaffhausen', both exhibited in 1806 (Tate Gallery 477 and Museum of Fine Arts, Boston) but the impressionistic technique and the way in which the whole picture is illuminated by the apparition suggest a much later date, probably close to the 'Vision of Medea', which also reflects a return to earlier ideas and Venetian painting (see

No.473). The general effect owes much to Titian but the flicked-in forms of the angels are still closer to Tintoretto.

This painting not only shared the general neglect of most of the works kept in Turner's studio but was even turned to the wall and used as an impromptu palette. The dabs of paint were only removed when the picture was recently restored at the Tate Gallery.

485 Caligula's Palace and Bridge R.A.1831
Oil on canvas, 54 × 97 (137 × 246.5)
Exh: R.A. 1831 (162)
Tate Gallery (512)

Exhibited in 1831 with the following lines attributed to Turner's *Fallacies of Hope* (here quoted from Turner's own list of his 1831 exhibits, now in the Tate Gallery archive):

> What now remains of all the mighty Bridge
> Which made the Lucrine Lake an inner pool,
> Caligula, but massy fragments left,
> As monuments of doubt and ruind hopes
> Yet gleaming in the Morning's ray, doth tell
> How Baia's shore was loved in times gone by?

Here Turner returns to the theme of 'Bay of Baiæ' (No.237), the decay of past glories. Caligula's bridge crossed the three and a half Roman miles from Baiae to Puteoli and was described by Oliver Goldsmith as 'the most notorious instance of his fruitless profusion'. Although the bridge was, in fact, a bridge of boats Turner followed popular accounts in showing it as a solid structure (see Gage 1974, p.47).

Unlike 'Vision of Medea' this picture seems to have aroused universal praise. 'In this picture "the fit hath gone off"' said the *Athenaeum* for 14 May 1831; 'Here we have the poetry of nature lavished upon us with a courteous hand'. *La Belle Assemblée* described it, in its June number, as 'one of the most magnificent and extraordinary productions of the day; . . . it is poetry itself. The air-tint – the distances – are magical: for brilliancy and depth, and richness, and power, it can hardly be surpassed.' For *The Times* of 6 May it was 'one of the most beautiful and magnificent landscapes that ever mind conceived or pencil drew.' The *Library of the Fine Arts* for June 1831, anticipating Ruskin's criticisms of these packed Italian landscapes as 'nonsense pictures', described it more positively as 'a composition, any one portion of which is in itself a picture, and would make the fortune of another artist'.

As luck had it Turner's picture hung next to Constable's 'Salisbury Cathedral from the Meadows' (Lord Ashton of Hyde). 'Fire and water', the *Literary Gazette* for 14th May exclaimed; 'Exaggerated, however, as both these works are, – the one all heat, the other all humidity, – who will deny that they both exhibit, each in its way, some of the highest qualities of art? None but the envious or ignorant.' Apparently Constable, who was on the Hanging Committee that year, had moved Turner's picture and replaced it with his own, for which Turner teased him unmercifully at a dinner at General Phipps' in Mount Street, to the great amusement of the party, mainly artists (the story is David Roberts', given in Thornbury 1862, II, p.56, and dated to this year by Finberg 1961, p.327).

The picture was engraved in 1842 by E. Goodall, whose son told W. G. Rawlinson (II, 1913, pp.336–7)

that Turner, deciding that the composition required
more figures, added them on the picture himself, first
with white chalk, and then, when Goodall was unable
to follow these slight sketches, in watercolour. According to Thornbury, who however asserts that the figures
were introduced, with Turner's assent, by Goodall,
they were the children playing with goats in the foreground (1862, I, p.319). Recent restoration, however,
failed to determine that any of the figures as they now
are were painted in watercolour; perhaps Turner went
over them later in oil.

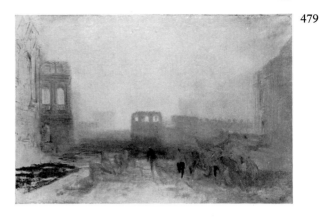

479

486 Christ and the Woman of Samaria c.1830
    Oil on canvas, 57¼ × 93½ (145.5 × 237.5)
    Tate Gallery (1875)

A large Italianate landscape of the kind exhibited by
Turner from 'Bay of Baiae' onwards, but in this case
perhaps not carried quite to the degree of finish he
deemed necessary for an exhibited work of this
character. It is probably the 'Scriptural subject . . .
7′10″ × 4′10‴' listed as No.251 in the Schedule of the
Turner Bequest and seems to show Christ and the
Woman of Samaria by Jacob's Well (*John* IV, 6–7), set
in a landscape with an Italian hill town similar to but
not the same as Tivoli (see No.477). The composition,
with the hill town on the left and the avenue of trees on
the right, is particularly close to 'Palestrina', begun in
Rome in 1828 as a companion to Lord Egremont's
Claude of 'Jacob and Laban' and exhibited at the Royal
Academy in 1830 (Tate Gallery 6283). The composition, like that of 'Orvieto', is considerably more re-
strained than the earlier 'Bay of Baiæ' or such later
examples as 'Childe Harold's Pilgrimage: Italy' (R.A.
1832; Tate Gallery 516). Turner's second visit to Rome
in 1828 may have produced a return to classical discipline, though to date this picture c.1830 on such grounds
is perhaps rather foolhardy.

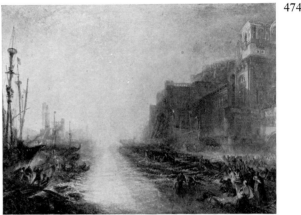

474

491

487 The Arch of Constantine, Rome c.1830–5
    Oil on canvas, 36 × 48 (91 × 122)
    Tate Gallery (2066)

488 Tivoli: Tobias and the Angel c.1830–5
    Oil on canvas, 35⅝ × 47⅝ (90.5 × 121)
    Tate Gallery (2067)   (repr. on p.117)

These two Italian scenes, carried to the same degree of
near-completion, probably arose out of Turner's second
visit to Rome, developing compositions of the kind
found among the sketches on coarse canvas of, probably,
1828 (see Nos.475–80). The heavy impasto and rich
colouring seem to parallel the treatment of the various
interior scenes associated with Petworth and thought to
date from the mid-1830s, but the dating is very tentative (MacColl, 1920, p.34, dated them both 1840 or
later). Tivoli, a recurrent subject among Turner's
Italian landscapes, ultimately derived from Wilson (see
No.B36), is here made the setting for a Biblical subject
in the same way as happened in 'Christ and the Woman
of Samaria' (No.486).

489 Not exhibited

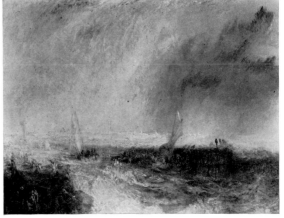

506

13. Late Sea Pictures 1830–45

Turner had always been preoccupied with the sea but in his later years he seems to have become increasingly interested in it as one of the most powerful embodiments of the forces of nature. A whole series of oils of stormy seas in the Turner Bequest reflects this interest, which also provided the theme of a considerable proportion of his exhibited works.

490 Staffa, Fingal's Cave R.A.1832
Oil on canvas, 36 × 48 (91.5 × 122)
Inscr. bottom centre right: 'J M W Turner RA'
Exh: R.A. 1832 (453)
The Lord Astor of Hever

Exhibited with the following lines from Sir Walter Scott's *Lord of the Isles*, Canto IV:
— nor of a theme less solemn tells
That mightly surge that ebbs and swells,
And still, between each awful pause,
From the high vault an answer draws.

Turner was invited by Scott to visit Abbotsford in the late summer of 1831 in connection with a project to illustrate his poems and took the opportunity to visit the Western Isles; he arrived at Staffa in 'a strong wind and head sea', as he wrote later to James Lenox. This picture was the result and is one of the first in which Turner's uniformity of treatment enforces the feeling of the union of all nature's elements against the puny devices of man; the cliffs and the sea on the left are run together in continuous strokes of paint.

The painting was well received at the Royal Academy, though the *Athenaeum* for 15 June remarked that 'The grandeur of the original, and the awe it impresses on the beholder, may be caught, perhaps, by a painter, but cannot be improved or exalted. Nature, in the original scene, has done her best, and Turner cannot surpass her'. For *Fraser's Magazine*, July 1832, 'All is in unison in this fine picture, and impresses us with the sublimity of vastness and solitude. When it pleases him to do so, there is no one who can exhibit a greater mastery in these simple, but most powerful effects, swaying the phenomena of nature to his will, and eliciting from its uncombined elements alone that variety and depth of expression which others appear to be either regardless or unconscious of'. The *Morning Herald* for 7 May remarked on the novelty of the steamboat: 'Mr. Turner's love of yellow, red and blue, is conspicuous in all his works, but in his picture of "Staffa, Fingal's Cave", &c., the effect produced by those colours, when kept subordinate, is truly poetic; he has even flung a charm around that uncouth object yclept a "steam boat", and the black off-spring of its vivid fires'. This was the first Turner to go to America, being bought by James Lenox for £500 in 1845.

491 Mouth of the Seine, Quille-Bœuf R.A.1833
Oil on canvas, 36 × 48½ (91.5 × 123)
Exh: R.A. 1833 (462)
Fundaçao Calouste Gulbenkian, Lisbon

The 1833 Royal Academy catalogue contained the following explanatory note: 'This estuary is so dangerous from its quicksands, that any vessel taking the ground is liable to be sanded and overwhelmed by the rising tide, which rushes in in one wave.' This note is indicative of Turner's interest in the hazards of seafaring, which were, of course, of particular interest to one who did so much travelling under the conditions of the early nineteenth century. The composition is based on the body-colour on blue paper, painted c.1829 (No.398). The treatment of sea and sky, making due allowance for the fact that this is a picture that Turner sent in for exhibition, is also close to one of the unexhibited oils of stormy seas, 'Rough Sea with Wreckage', and may give a clue to the date of these works (see No.492).

For *The Spectator*, 11 May 1833, this picture was 'one of those daring triumphs of genius which Turner alone achieves. On the one side is the cold grey sea; on the other the yellow sands, and a ruined abbey on the shore, steeped in a flood of golden light. It is a resplendid work of art'. The *New Monthly Magazine* for May–August called it 'a specimen . . . of magical red and of magical yellow'. The *Athenaeum*, 25 May, pointed out 'the descent of a cloud of water-fowl' as 'finely managed'. Only the *Morning Chronicle* was critical, with the usual comments about 'yellow fever, and . . . a suspicion of the jaundice', 'brimstone and cayenne'.

492 Rough Sea with Wreckage c.1830–5
Oil on canvas, 36¼ × 48¼ (92 × 122.5)
Tate Gallery (1980)

One of a number of paintings of stormy seas in the Turner Bequest. These are in varying degrees of finish, but it is possible to place them provisionally in rough chronological order. This example, with its relatively solidly modelled clouds and waves making a disciplined composition notwithstanding the energy of the forces involved, can be tentatively dated to the early 1830s. It can in particular be related to 'Mouth of the Seine, Quille-Boeuf', exhibited in 1833 (No.491).

493 Hastings c.1830–5
Oil on canvas, 35½ × 48 (91 × 122)
Tate Gallery (1986)

A variation of the theme of 'The Old Chain Pier, Brighton' but more worked up in sea and sky, paralleling the development seen in 'Staffa, Fingal's Cave', exhibited in 1832, in the subservience of solid forms to the forces of nature (see No.490).

494 Yacht approaching the Coast c.1835–40
Oil on canvas, 40¼ × 56 (102 × 142)
Tate Gallery (4662)   (repr. on p.118)

The most glowing and colourful of Turner's sea pictures, with an audacious use of pure reds unmatched in any other picture. The fragmented surface is unified by the overall vortex which radiates from and embodies the main source of light in the picture. The rather unusual size is a reversion to that of 'Dorchester Mead' and 'Ploughing up Turnips, Slough', two pictures of 1809–10, and was also used for 'Stormy Sea with

513 **Keelmen heaving in Coals by Night** 1835 (entry on p.143)

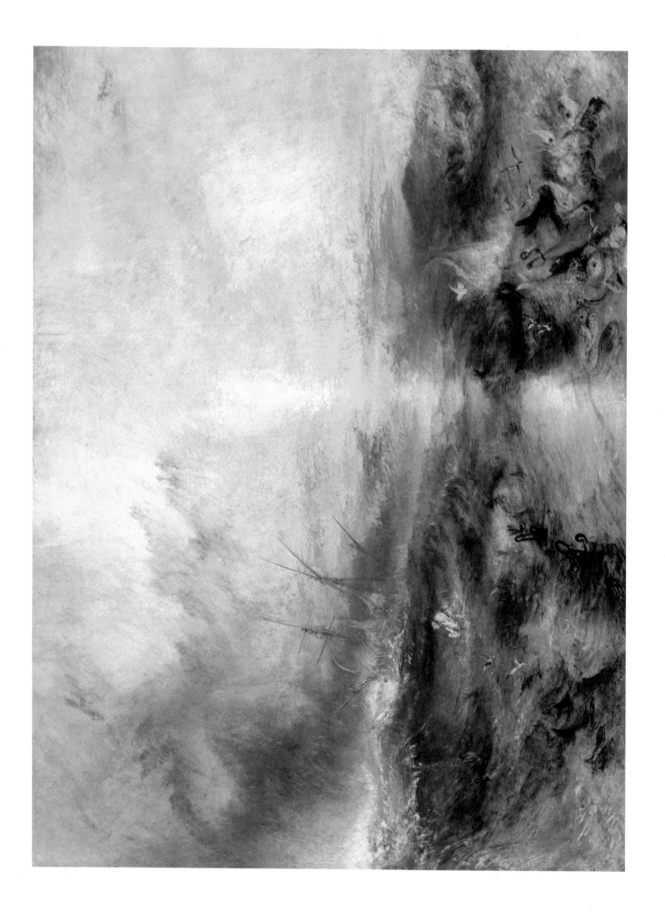

518 **Slavers throwing overboard the Dead and Dying** 1840 (entry on p.144)

Blazing Wreck', to which this picture is perhaps the counterpart, light against dark.

495 Stormy Sea with Blazing Wreck *c.*1835–40
Oil on canvas, 39⅛ × 55¾ (99.5 × 141.5)
Tate Gallery (4658)

One of Turner's rare night scenes, perhaps to be seen, in view of its unusually large size for this kind of subject, as a companion to the glowingly daylight scene of 'Yacht approaching the Coast' (No.494). The figures on the shore and the skeletal fragments of the wrecked ship are not dissimilar to those in 'Wreckers – Coast of Northumberland', exhibited in 1834 (private collection, U.S.A.), but the drama of the great wave crashing over the wreck in the centre is much greater.

496 Fire at Sea *c.*1835
Oil on canvas, 67½ × 86¾ (171.5 × 220.5)
Tate Gallery (558)

Despite its relatively 'unfinished' state this was given an inventory number immediately on entering the National Gallery in 1856, like the works exhibited in Turner's lifetime. There are three sketches of a ship on fire in the 'Fire at Sea' sketchbook, dated by Finberg *c.*1834 (T.B.CCLXXXII–3, 4 and 5) and the painting probably also dates from about this time; Turner's interest in fire subjects may well have been re-awakened by the burning of the Houses of Parliament in October 1834 (see No.512). It is on the large scale of 'The Shipwreck' of thirty years earlier (No.82) and displays both the continuity and the development of Turner's style. The most extraordinary thing about this picture is that the blazing ship is not actually shown, being merely an implied presence beyond the right-hand edge of the picture from which falls a rain of sparks.

497 Margate Harbour *c.*1835
Oil on canvas, 18 × 24 (46 × 61)
Walker Art Gallery, Liverpool

Stylistically akin to works of the mid-1830s. Almost certainly one of the works in the sale of John Pound, son of Turner's housekeeper Mrs Booth by her first husband, at Christie's on 25 March 1865. If so, this would strengthen the traditional association with Margate. Mrs Booth lived there from 1827 until 1846, when she moved to a house in Cheyne Walk, Chelsea, taken by Turner in her name; Turner seems to have stayed at Margate even before her second husband died in 1833 or 1834 (see Lindsay 1966, pp.175, 196–7). The picture may at some time have had the more specific title of 'Emigrants embarking at Margate', usually given to another picture at Liverpool, possibly also from the Pound collection but more doubtfully by Turner (see *The Emma Holt Bequest, Sudley*, 1971, pp.72–3, No.312, and pp.77–9, No.311).

498 Ship in a Storm *c.*1835–45
Oil on millboard, irregular,
11⅞ × 18¾ (30.2 × 47.6)
Trustees of the British Museum (1972–U. 739)

499 Two Figures on a Beach with a Boat
*c.*1835–45
Oil on millboard, irregular,
9⅝ × 13¹¹⁄₁₆ (24.4 × 34.7)
Trustees of the British Museum (1972–U. 747)

500 Sunset seen from a Beach *c.*1835–45
Oil on millboard, irregular,
9¹⁸⁄₁₆ × 11⅞ (24.9 × 30.2)
Trustees of the British Museum (1974–U. 848)

Three more of the sketches found at the British Museum but apparently painted considerably later than 'Landscape with Buildings' (see No.469). 'Ship in a Storm' is close in composition to 'Snow Storm – Steam-Boat off a Harbour's Mouth', exhibited in 1842 (No.504), while the 'Sunset' is an equivalent in oils of very late watercolours such as those in the 'Ambleteuse and Wimereux' sketchbook of 1845 (T.B.CCCLVII). However, compositional resemblances help very little in dating Turner's late works and comparison between works in different media is equally fruitless.

More important is the glimpse of Turner painting oil sketches in yet another way, not as 'colour beginnings' perhaps to be completed for exhibition, nor quite as try-outs of compositions to be used elsewhere (though this could apply to No.469), but more as self-sufficient, 'private' compositions like many of the late watercolours. The technique, though close to that of many of Turner's watercolours, fully exploits the oil medium, the 'Two Figures on a Beach' being largely painted with the palette knife.

501 Stormy Sea with Dolphins *c.*1835–40
Oil on canvas, 35¾ × 48 (91 × 122)
Tate Gallery (4664)

Most of Turner's pictures of stormy seas are, relatively speaking, without colour but this picture is vibrant with reds and oranges, perhaps the reflections of an unseen ship ablaze. It also shows the introduction of strong colour into a seascape characteristic of 'Slavers', exhibited in 1840 (see No.518).

502 Seascape with Storm coming on *c.*1840
Oil on canvas, 36 × 47⅞ (91.5 × 121.5)
Tate Gallery (4445)

The centrifugal composition, with the strongest contrast of light and dark in the centre, was developed in such works as 'Snow Storm: Steam-Boat off a Harbour's Mouth', exhibited at the Royal Academy in 1842 (see No.504). In fact a picture such as the present example could well have been taken into the Royal Academy and worked up on the Varnishing Days into something like the 'Snow Storm'.

503 Seascape with Distant Coast *c.*1840
Oil on canvas, 36 × 48 (91.5 × 122)
Tate Gallery (5516)

First cleaned in 1973. This revealed that it is particularly close in style and handling to 'Seascape with Storm coming on' (No.502), though the composition is rather more amorphous; presumably Turner had not carried it quite so far.

The significance of the letters painted along the top towards the right is unclear. They were done before the main painting was fully dry, that is in Turner's studio, and seem to read 'M [above a small 'c'] MNNsTTs'. The nearest parallel is the set of letters inscribed in wet paint down the left-hand edge of 'Forum Romanum', which are equally inexplicable (see No.238).

504   Snow Storm – Steam Boat off a Harbour's Mouth making Signals in Shallow Water, and going by the Lead. The Author was in this Storm on the Night the Ariel left Harwich R.A.1842   (repr. on p.127)
Oil on canvas, 36×48 (91.5×122)
Exh: R.A. 1842 (182)
Tate Gallery (530)

One of the most extreme paintings exhibited by Turner in his own lifetime, and the culmination of his demonstrations of the puniness of man's creations in the face of the forces of nature. The whole composition is swept up in the vortex, and even the horizon slopes to accentuate the feeling of participation in the storm. The picture may recall a particularly bad storm in January 1842 though it has not been possible to tie down the exact incident. However, the Rev. William Kingsley told Ruskin of a conversation with Turner in which he stressed the truth of the incident and his interest in recording the experience: 'I did not paint it to be understood, but I wished to show what such a scene was like; I got the sailors to lash me to the mast to observe it; I was lashed for four hours and I did not expect to escape, but I felt bound to record it if I did. But no one had any business to like the picture.'

However, Ruskin records Turner's hurt reaction to the criticism that it was nothing but a mass of 'Soapsuds and whitewash': 'Turner was passing the evening at my father's house on the day this criticism came out: and after dinner, sitting in his arm-chair by the fire, I heard him muttering to himself at intervals, "Soapsuds and whitewash! What would they have? I wonder what they think the sea's like? I wish they'd been in it".' The *Athenaeum*'s review on 14 May was typical of this abuse: 'This gentleman has, on former occasions, chosen to paint with cream, or chocolate, yolk of egg, or currant jelly, – here he uses his whole array of kitchen stuff. Where the steam-boat is – where the harbour begins, or where it ends – which are the signals, and which the author in the *Ariel* . . . are matters past our finding out.' Or, as the *Art Union* for 1 June observed, 'Through the driving snow there are just perceptible portions of a steam-boat labouring on a rolling sea; but before any further account of the vessel can be given, it will be necessary to wait until the storm is cleared off a little. The sooner the better.'

505   Rough Sea *c.*1840-5
Oil on canvas, 36×48 (91.5×122)
Tate Gallery (5479)

Probably the boldest of all the unexhibited oils of stormy seas in the Turner Bequest; it is tempting to place this last in the series. Here the swirling composition is interrupted by the dark form thrusting in from the left so that it impinges on the light glowing out of the centre of the picture, a heightened contrast of tones typical of Turner.

506   Ostend R.A.1844
Oil on canvas, 36½×48½ (93×123)
Exh: R.A. 1844 (11)
Thos. Agnew & Sons Ltd

Bought by H. A. J. Munro of Novar, perhaps in 1844 at the R.A.; in any case he owned it by 1847 when it was recorded as hanging in his London house, 113 Grosvenor Square, by the *Art Union Journal*. Bell relates that this picture was later bought by Cornelius Vanderbilt, without any provenance, as a view of Boulogne Harbour. It was the American painter, Thomas Moran (1837-1926), an ardent admirer of Turner's work, who identified it as the 'Ostend' exhibited in 1844.

At the Academy, most critics concentrated on 'Rain, Steam and Speed' (National Gallery 538) but the *Spectator* for 11 May considered that ' "Ostend" and "Port Ruysdael" are two magnificent sea-pieces, without exaggeration; and in these scenes the general effect is all sufficient . . .'.

Ruskin in *Modern Painters* thought 'Ostend' 'somewhat forced and affected', and he mistakenly reported the year of its exhibition as 1843. In fact this is the only time it has been shown in public since 1844.

507   Sunrise with Sea Monsters *c.*1845
Oil on canvas, 36×48 (91.5×122)
Tate Gallery (1990)

Nearer to the 'Whalers' pictures of 1845 and 1846 (see No.524) than to the 'Slavers' of 1840 (No.518) and therefore probably to be dated *c.*1845. There is a drawing of a fairly similar composition in the 'Whalers' sketchbook (T.B.CCCLIII–21; see also No.633) and the group of sea monsters is also related to Turner's various studies of fish such as that in the Victoria and Albert Museum (No.B127; see also Nos.269 and 271). John Gage has suggested that Turner's interest in the fantastic and monstrous aspects of fish was further suggested by the Rev. Thomas Gisbourne's *Walks in a Forest*, published in 1795 but quoted by Turner in connection with his 'Dawn of Christianity', exhibited in 1841 (No.519); see also No.B108.

508

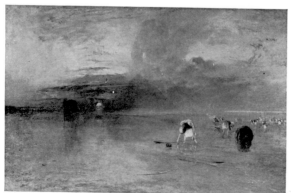

510

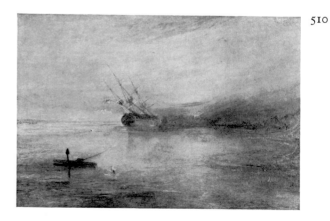

14. Exhibited Oil Paintings 1830–50

Despite Turner's increasing isolation from the art of his contemporaries he continued to exhibit regularly at the Royal Academy. The works shown at the Academy, some of which are also included in Sections 13, 15 and 16, reflect a great range of interests, from historical subjects to the industrial scene of his own day, from political moralising to aesthetic theory. Only in his last years was there any falling off in the number and originality of his exhibits, and this seems to have been due to ill-health; in 1850, the last year in which he exhibited, he roused up enough energy to produce four works on a unified theme, Dido and Aeneas at Carthage, that summed up a lifetime of aspirations as a painter of history.

508 Calais Sands, Low Water, Poissards collecting Bait R.A.1830
Oil on canvas, 27 × 41½ (68.5 × 105.5)
Exh: R.A. 1830 (304)
Bury Public Library, Art Gallery and Museum

A later reinterpretation of the theme of 'Blythe-Sand' (No.155) with the elegiac mood also found in 'A Ship Aground' (No.329) and 'The Evening Star' (National Gallery, London, 1991). Turner had visited Calais a number of times, the latest being in the late summer of 1829 on the way to Paris, and the 'Meuse and Moselle' sketchbook includes a drawing related to the figures and inscribed 'Fisher women looking for bait' (CCXVI–227). The 'poissards' of the final title recall Turner's use of this made up word in the title of 'Calais Pier' (No.75). John Gage (exhibition catalogue, *La Peinture Romantique Anglaise et Les Préraphaélites*, Petit Palais, Paris, 1972, no.264) suggests that the picture is also in part a tribute, and a challenge, to the memory of Bonington, who had died in 1828 and the contents of whose studio, including a number of beach scenes at Calais, had been sold in London in June 1829.

The painting was well received and even the *Morning Chronicle* for 3 May 1830, which attacked Turner's 1830 exhibits for their lack of finish and for 'taking an unpardonable liberty with the public', allowed that 'Calais Sands' was 'perhaps the only one excusable in its slightness, – it is literally nothing in labour, but extraordinary in art'. Even so it was not sold at the time, but it was later among the eight pictures bought for £500 each by the Birmingham steel-pen manufacturer turned picture-dealer Joseph Gillott, who retained it in his own collection.

509 Life-Boat and Manby Apparatus going off to a Stranded Vessel making Signal (Blue Lights) of Distress R.A.1831
Oil on canvas, 36 × 48 (91.5 × 122)
Exh: R.A. 1831 (73)
Victoria and Albert Museum

Probably painted for John Nash and certainly in the sale of his pictures in 1835, when it was bought by Tiffin probably on behalf of John Sheepshanks, who gave it to the Victoria and Albert Museum in 1857.

When sold in 1835 it was entitled 'Blue Lights off Yarmouth', an identification that is probably correct as Great Yarmouth, Norfolk, was the home of George William Manby whose apparatus is the subject of the picture. This consisted of a mortar that fired a stone on the end of a length of rope to provide a lifeline to a ship in distress, and for this and other services to life-saving Manby was elected as a Fellow of the Royal Society in 1831.

Turner had passed Yarmouth on his way to Scotland in 1822 and had first visited it properly two years later (see T.B.CCIX). More closely related however is the 'colour beginning' of 'Firing Rockets at Yarmouth' (?) at the British Museum (T.B.CCCLXIV–134; see Graham Reynolds, 'Turner at East Cowes Castle' in *Victoria and Albert Museum Yearbook*, I, 1969, pp.75–8, repr. pl.13).

This picture is the first of a splendid series in which a ship is seen at the mercy of the waves, man's efforts, blue lights, smoke or whatever, being contrasted to the forces of nature. It was well received at the Royal Academy. *La Belle Assemblée* for June 1831 called it 'a fine picture, full of nature and truth, and more in his manner of the olden time, than any thing we have seen of late', not that the work looks very conservative to modern eyes. For the *Library of the Fine Arts*, June 1831, it was 'a magnificent picture, warm and all life'.

510 Fort Vimieux R.A.1831
Oil on canvas, 27¾ × 42 (70.5 × 106.5)
Exh: R.A. 1831 (406)
Private Collection

The 1831 Royal Academy catalogue gave no title as such but the following long description: '"In this arduous service (of reconnoissance) on the French coast, 1805, one of our cruisers took the ground, and had to sustain the attack of the flying artillery along shore, the batteries, and the fort of Vimieux, which fired heated shot, until she could warp off at the rising tide, which set in with all the appearance of a stormy night." – *Naval Anecdotes*'. Turner was not alone at the exhibition in showing a picture recalling the heroic days of the Napoleonic wars, but the real inspiration in this case probably came from the unused Petworth sketch of 'A Ship Aground' (No.329).

Unlike the figure compositions in the same exhibition this painting seems to have been generally admired. The *Library of the Fine Arts* for June 1831 described how 'the firing of red-hot shot, the sun of a bloody hue "low, deep, and wan", the forlorn and frightened gull, the ball hissing in the water, and the stranded ship, present a vivid picture of the event, while the imagination of the *ensemble* is grand and stupendous. When will Mr Turner show symptoms of decay? . . . his genius is still green as when we first saw it in the boyhood of our life'.

Nevertheless the picture does not seem to have been sold until about 1845 when it was bought by Charles Meigh, probably for £500 (Finberg 1961, p.409). At his sale in 1850 it went for £693 to the first American collector of Turner's work, James Lenox, who had

514

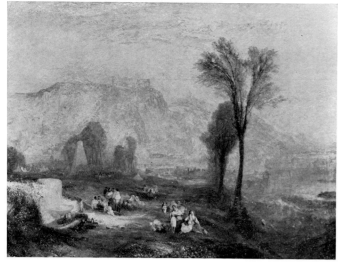

516

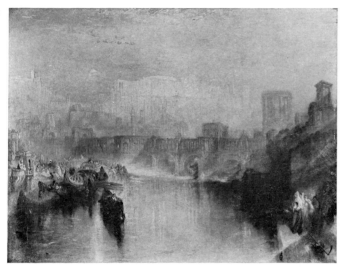

517

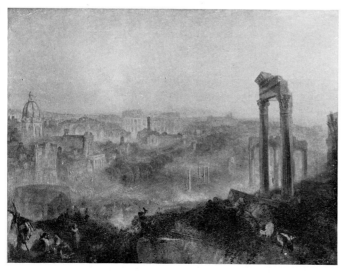

already bought 'Staffa, Fingal's Cave' (No.490). It returned to this country in 1956 and was then acquired by the present owner.

511 Not exhibited

512 **The Burning of the House of Lords and Commons, 16th of October, 1834** B.I.1835
Oil on canvas, $36\frac{1}{4} \times 48\frac{1}{2}$ (92 × 123)
Exh: British Institution 1835 (58) (repr. on p. 128)
Philadelphia Museum of Art (John H. McFadden Collection)

One of the two oil paintings of this subject exhibited in 1835; the other, taken from a more distant viewpoint down river, was exhibited at the Royal Academy and is now in the Cleveland Museum of Art. For the watercolours done at the time and subsequently see Nos. 456–60.

This is one of the paintings for which there are eye-witness accounts of Turner's activity on the Varnishing Days before the opening of the exhibition to the public. 'The picture sent in was a mere dab of several colours and "without form and void", like chaos before the creation,' wrote E. V. Rippingille (see Finberg 1961, pp.351–2, for a fuller version); 'for the three hours I was there – and I understood it had been the same since he began in the morning – he never ceased to work, or even once looked or turned from the wall on which his picture was hung. A small box of colours, a few very small brushes, and a vial or two, were at his feet. . . . In one part of the mysterious proceedings Turner, who worked almost entirely with his palette knife, was observed to be rolling and spreading a half-transparent stuff over his picture, the size of a finger in length and thickness. As Callcott was looking on I ventured to say to him "What is that he is plastering his picture with ?" to which inquiry it was replied "I should be sorry to be the man to ask him." . . . Presently the work was finished: Turner gathered his tools together, put them into and shut up the box, and then, with his face still turned to the wall, and at the same distance from it, went sidelong off, without speaking a word to anybody. . . . Maclise, who stood near, remarked, "There, that's masterly, he does not stop to look at his work; he *knows* it is done, and he is off" !'

The *Spectator* for 7 February 1835 made allusion to this activity of Turner's: 'And the execution of the picture is curious: to look at it close, it appears a confused mass of daubs and streaks of colour; yet we are told the painter worked at it within a few inches of the canvas for hours together, without stepping back to see the effect. Turner seems to paint slovenlily [sic] – daubing, as one would say; yet what other painter preserves equal clearness of colour ? Not that we like this scene-painting manner; we should prefer being able to look at a picture near as well as at a distance; but such a one as this we are content to look at in any way the artist chooses – with all its faults.' The *Spectator* went on to point out that the picture stood out from its neighbours through its 'purity, transparency, and harmony of colouring', not through its 'quantity or intensity'. It praised the various effects of light, with the qualification that 'There is an effect of daylight in the picture, however, which is not counterbalanced by the gas-lamp in the foreground', and that the figures were too bad for one to distinguish whether they were 'Christians or Pagans, fine ladies or coalheavers'. *The Times* for 10 February also asserted that 'The sky is painted in much too light a tint, and is more applicable to a morning than a night scene', and the *Athenaeum* for 14 February called the picture 'a splendid impossibility' for the same reason; 'truth is sacrificed for effect, which, however, is in parts of the picture, magnificent'. However, the *Literary Gazette* for 14 February pointed out that Turner had achieved his effects 'not by any striking opposition of light and dark', but by 'the contrast of warm and cold, of the blazing flame and of the early morning'. Turner was later to use a similar contrast for emotional effect in 'The Fighting Temeraire' (National Gallery, London, 524). The *Literary Gazette* summed up the picture as manifesting 'quite as much of vision and poetry as of nature'. A later issue, on 25 April, noted that the picture had been bought by C. Hall, and by 1852 it belonged to Charles Birch of Edgbaston.

513 Keelmen heaving in Coals by Night R.A.1835
Oil on canvas, 36¼ × 48¼ (92 × 122.5)
Exh: R.A. 1835 (24)   (repr. on p.137)
National Gallery of Art, Washington (Widener Collection)

According to Henry McConnell, the picture's first owner, it was 'painted at my special suggestion' (letter of 28 May 1861 to John Taylor, who seems to have bought the picture from McConnell in 1849). McConnel bought the painting of Venice exhibited at the Royal Academy the previous year (almost certainly the 'Venice: Dogana and San Giorgio Maggiore' also in Washington; repr. Rothenstein and Butlin 1964, pl.98) and it is probable that a deliberate contrast was planned between the two pictures. The Venetian picture, in Turner's standard three-foot, four-foot format, shows a clear light and calm activity at a far remove from the smoky haze and industrial bustle of 'Keelmen', in which Turner contrasted moonlight and man-made fires just as he had in his very first exhibited oil painting. The scene is on the Tyne, which had already been shown with its rising smoke in two watercolours of 'Shields, on the River Tyne' and 'Newcastle-on-Tyne' engraved for the *Rivers of England* in 1823 (T.B.CCVIII–V and K; see No.241).

'Keelmen' met with much the same criticism as 'The Burning of the House of Lords and Commons': it was too light. 'The full moon', wrote the *Spectator* for 9 May 1835, 'pours a flood of silver radiance that fills the scene, excepting the dusky hue of colliers, with the light and smoke of the beacons on the riverside. The aerial brilliancy of the effect is surprising. The tone seems too like daylight; but a year or two hence it will be as bright and true a night scene as ever – or rather *never* was painted'. The *Literary Gazette* of the same date thought the treatment inappropriate: 'And such a night! – a flood of glorious moonlight wasted upon dingy coal-whippers, instead of conducting lovers to the appointed bower'. But as usual there was a feeling that Turner had brought it off: 'At the first glance, the word "extravagant" rose to our lips,' reported the *Athenaeum* for 23 May, 'but as we lingered before the scene, other feelings triumphed, and we could not help pronouncing it a striking, if not wondrous performance.' The same day *The Times* called it 'One of those masterly

productions by which the artist contrives to convey very striking effects with just so much of adherence to nature as prevents one from saying they are merely fanciful'.

514 The Bright Stone of Honour (Ehrenbreitstein) and the Tomb of Marceau, from Byron's 'Childe Harold'
R.A.1835
Oil on canvas, 36¼ × 48½ (92 × 123)
Exh: R.A. 1835 (74)
Private Collection

Exhibited with the following text from *Childe Harold* Canto III, alluding to the death of the French Revolutionary General Marceau at the siege of Ehrenbreitstein in 1796:

By Coblentz, on a rise of gentle ground,
There is a small and simple pyramid,
Crowning the summit of the verdant mound:
Beneath its base are heroes' ashes hid,
Our enemy's – but let that not forbid
Honour to Marceau——
——He was freedom's champion!
Here Ehrenbrietstein, with her shattered wall,
Yet shews of what he was.

The *Spectator* for 9 May 1835 called the picture 'a splendid tribute of genius to one of the champions of freedom' and the picture was generally praised. For the *Athenaeum*, 23 May, 'Imagination and reality strive for mastery in this noble picture: there is an aerial splendour about it, such as the poetic love, and at the same time such a truthful representation of the real scene, as satisfies those who conceive that a landscape should be laid down with the accuracy of a district survey.' Only the *Morning Herald* for 2 May and the *Examiner* for 10 May dissented in blanket attacks on all his works at the 1835 exhibition. The picture was not sold until 1844, when the collector Elhanan Bicknell bought it together with five others.

Turner had visited Ehrenbreitstein on his tour of the Rhine in 1819 and again in 1834 when he was planning a series of engravings of German rivers to follow the *Rivers of France*. A large sheet of paper in the British Museum, folded into 16 sections, bears a number of related drawings (T.B.CCCXLIV–I to 16, especially 1, 3 and 6). Turner painted several watercolours of Ehrenbreitstein in the 1840s.

515 Rome from Mount Aventine R.A.1836
Oil on canvas, 36 × 49 (91.5 × 124.5)
Exh: R.A. 1836 (144)
The Earl of Rosebery

Until 1902, when Armstrong's catalogue was published, there was considerable confusion between this picture and 'Modern Rome – Campo Vaccino' (No.517). Both were bought at the Royal Academy by H. A. J. Munro of Novar but the titles became transposed, both in the catalogue of the R.A. Winter Exhibition in 1896 and by Bell in 1901.

This was one of the three pictures exhibited in 1836 (with 'Juliet and her Nurse' and 'Mercury and Argus') which were so viciously attacked by the Rev. John Eagles (1783–1855) in *Blackwood's Edinburgh Magazine* for October 1836. It was this attack that caused Ruskin, in a state of 'black anger' to take up his pen in Turner's defence and to write 'A Reply to Blackwood's Criticism of Turner', the seed which later blossomed into *Modern Painters* (5 vols. 1843–60). Ruskin was advised by his father to seek Turner's permission to publish his reply and made a copy in his 'best hand' which he sent to the painter. Turner replied by advising against publication, saying 'I never move in these matters, they are of no import save mischief and the meal tub . . .' Turner, however, asked Ruskin's leave to send the manuscript on 'to the possessor of the picture of Juliet' (also Munro of Novar). See Nos.B143–5.

In fact, Eagles' strictures on 'Rome from Mount Aventine', though not nearly so intemperately phrased as those on Turner's other two exhibits, were pretty damning: '. . . . a most unpleasant mixture, whereon white gamboge and raw sienna are, with childish execution, daubed together'. However, during the Academy exhibition itself, the picture was on the whole well received. The *Athenaeum*, 14 May, called it 'a gorgeous picture, full of air and sunshine, though sadly unfinished in its execution' while the *Morning Post*, 3 May, wrote 'This is one of those amazing pictures by which Mr. Turner dazzles the imagination and confounds all criticism. It is beyond praise.'

516 Ancient Rome; Agrippina landing with the Ashes of Germanicus. The Triumphal Bridge and Palace of the Caesars restored
R.A.1839
Oil on canvas, 36 × 48 (91.5 × 122)
Exh: R.A. 1839 (66)
Tate Gallery (523)

Exhibited in 1839 with the following lines:
———The clear stream,
Aye, – the yellow Tiber glimmers to her beam,
Even while the sun is setting.

Germanicus Julius Caesar was the nephew and adopted son of the Emperor Tiberius and, by his wife Agrippina, the father of the future Emperor Caligula and Nero's mother, the younger Agrippina. He died in Antioch, the cause being rumoured to be poison or the magical arts. In his verses Turner is presumably alluding to this incident as a stage in the decline of Rome. The picture is a pair to 'Modern Rome – Campo Vaccino' (No.517).

The subject had been treated before by such neoclassical artists as Benjamin West, but Turner treats it as an architectural fantasy in the style of Joseph Gandy and Harvey Lonsdale Elmes. The massive building on the summit of the hill is very close in spirit to the latter's designs for St. George's Hall, Liverpool, which won the competition for that building in the same year as this picture was exhibited. The bridge recalls that in 'Caligula's Palace' of eight years before (No.485).

517 Modern Rome – Campo Vaccino R.A.1839
Oil on canvas, 35½ × 48 (90 × 122)
Inscr. on a large stone in the centre foreground:
'PONT [IFEX ?] MAX'
Exh: R.A. 1839 (70)
The Earl of Rosebery

Exhibited in 1839 with the following quotation from Byron:
The moon is up, and yet is is not night,
The sun as yet divides the day with her.

A companion to 'Ancient Rome; Agrippina Landing

with the Ashes of Germanicus' (No.516). This pair, following the 'Ancient Italy' and 'Modern Italy' exhibited in 1838, reflect the impact on Turner of Thomson's poem *Liberty* of which Part III (published in 1735) is devoted to tracing the establishment of Liberty in Rome and its subsequent loss after the death of Brutus.

At the Academy the two pictures received mixed opinions. The most favourable were in the *Art Union* for 15 May and the *Spectator* for 11 May. 'Ancient Rome' the *Art Union* called 'Another of Turner's gorgeous works – a reckless example of colour, but admirable in conception, and brilliant in execution . . . As usual, he has introduced "a story" . . . and has summoned his fancy to restore the ancient glories of the eternal city'. 'Modern Rome' was 'A fine and forcible contrast . . . The glory has departed. The eternal city, with its splendours – its stupendous temples, and its great men – all have become a mockery and a scorn. The plough has gone over its grandeurs, and weeds have grown in its high places.' The *Spectator* wrote that 'Turner is as gorgeous and mysterious as ever; and while we regret and condemn his extravagances, it is impossible not to admire the wondrous power of his art in representing an atmosphere of light. *Ancient Rome* . . . is a blaze of orange-golden sunshine, reflected from piles of architecture that must be of marble to be so steeped in the hues of light; and *Modern Rome – Campo Vaccino* . . ., of which we see just enough to know what it is meant for, is also immersed in a flood of radiance, with a stream of silvery light from the new-risen moon glancing across the scene.' But the *Athenaeum*, 11 May, considered both 'Ancient Rome' and 'Modern Rome' to be in Turner's 'maddest manner' and Thackeray, writing under the name of Michael Angelo Titmarsh in *Fraser's Magazine*, June 1839, after praising 'The Fighting Temeraire', admitted that Turner's 'other performances are for the most part quite incomprehensible to me.' As usual *Blackwood's Magazine*, July–December 1839, was particularly harsh in its strictures: 'We have Ancient and Modern Rome, both alike in the same washy-flashy splashes of reds, blues and whites, that, in their distraction and confusion, represent nothing in heaven and earth, and least of all that which they profess to represent, the co-existant influence of sun and moon. It is too painful; and we stay our hand in disgust and sorrow.'

518 Slavers throwing overboard the Dead and Dying – Typhon coming on R.A.1840
Oil on canvas, 35¾ × 48 (91 × 122) (repr. on p.138)
Exh: R.A. 1840 (203)
Museum of Fine Arts, Boston

Exhibited in 1840 with the following lines from the *Fallacies of Hope*:
Aloft all hands, strike the top-masts and belay;
Yon angry setting sun and fierce-edged clouds
Declare the Typhon's coming.
Before it sweep your decks, throw overboard
The dead and dying – n'er heed their chains.
Hope, Hope, fallacious Hope!
Where is thy market now?

Several sources seem to lie behind this subject. 'Summer' in Thomson's *Seasons* includes an account of a typhoon. T. Clarkson's *History of the Abolition of the*

Slave Trade, of which a second edition had just been published in 1839, gave the story of the slave-ship *Zong* in 1783, in which slaves dying of an epidemic were thrown overboard so that insurance, available for loss 'at sea' but not from disease, could be claimed. Topicality was also ensured by the publication in 1839 of the *Life of William Wilberforce* (who had died in 1833) by his sons, and of his *Correspondence* in 1840, and by the fact that Prince Albert was the President of the Anti-Slavery League. See Nos.B108–9.

This picture was the most advanced of Turner's pictures to be exhibited up to this time. So full of colour in comparison to his 'grey' sea-pieces such as Nos.502 and 503, it probably stemmed from such 'unfinished' oils as the 'Stormy Sea' (No.501) though the latter is even more boldly painted.

The critics were, not altogether surprisingly, overwhelmed by the picture's extravagance. The young Thackeray, in 'A Pictorial Rhapsody by Michael Angelo Titmarsh' in *Fraser's Magazine*, June 1840, wrote that it 'is the most tremendous piece of colour that ever was seen . . . Is the picture sublime or ridiculous? Indeed I don't know which. Rocks of gamboge are marked down upon the canvass; flakes of white laid on with a trowel; Bladders of vermillion madly spirited here and there . . . The sun glows down upon a horrible sea of emerald and purple . . . If Wilberforce's statue downstairs [by Samuel Joseph, No.1100 in the exhibition] were to be confronted with this picture, the stony old gentleman would spring off his chair and fly away in terror!'. The *Art Union* for 15 May, after observing that even 'in his wildest caprices there is so much evidence of genius of the very highest order', exclaimed 'Who will not grieve at the talent wasted upon the gross outrage on nature' in this picture, 'the leading object in which is a long black leg, surrounded by a shoal of rainbow-hued "John Dorys", seen more clearly through the ocean surface than flies in amber'. For the *Athenaeum*, 16 May, it was 'a passionate extravagance of marigold sky, and pomegranate-coloured sea, and fish dressed as gay as garden flowers in pink and green, with one shapeless dusky-brown leg thrown up from this parti-coloured chaos to keep the promise of the title.' Today, on the other hand, one revels in the bravura handling and richness of colour.

In 1844 the picture was given to Ruskin as a New Year's present by his father but after some years he found the subject 'too painful to live with' and sold it; bought in at Christie's in 1869 it was sold in America in 1872. Meanwhile, in the first volume of *Modern Painters*, 1843, Ruskin had written, 'But, beyond dispute, the noblest sea that Turner has painted, and, if so, the noblest certainly ever painted by man, is that of the Slave Ship. . . . Purple and blue, the lurid shadows of the hollow breakers are cast upon the mist of night, which gathers cold and low, advancing like the shadow of death upon the guilty ship as it labours amidst the lightning of the sea, its thin masts written upon the sky in lines of blood, girded with condemnation in that fearful hue which signs the sky with horror, and mixes its flaming flood with the sunlight, and, cast far along the desolate heave of the sepulchral waves, incardines the multitudinous sea. I believe, if I were reduced to rest Turner's immortality upon any single work, I should choose this. Its daring conception, ideal

in the highest sense of the word, is based on the purest truth, and wrought out with the concentrated knowledge of a life; . . . and the whole picture dedicated to the most sublime of subjects and impressions (completing thus the perfect system of all truth, which we have shown to be formed by Turner's works) – the power, majesty, and deathfulness of the open, deep, illimitable sea!'

519 Dawn of Christianity (Flight into Egypt)
R.A.1841
Oil on canvas, 31 × 31 (78.5 × 78.5)
Exh: R.A. 1841 (532)
Ulster Museum, Belfast

Exhibited in 1841 with the quotation, '"That star has risen" – Rev. T. Gisborne's Walks in a Forest' (No. B108). Possibly a companion picture to 'Glaucus and Scylla', also painted on a square canvas of the same size though less definitely intended to be seen as a circular composition; this was exhibited the same year and is now in the Kimbell Art Foundation, Fort Worth, Texas. Both were bought by B. G. Windus at the Academy. However, the composition and treatment are much closer to 'Bacchus and Ariadne', exhibited the year before (Tate Gallery 525). Both show a return to Titian and the Venetians, the figures in 'Bacchus and Ariadne' having been directly copied from the picture of the same subject which had entered the National Gallery in 1826 and of which Turner had a copy.

Turner experimented with variously shaped compositions on square canvases in a number of exhibits from 1840 to 1846 as well as some unexhibited paintings of the same period (see Nos.521–3 and 525–6). The format, perhaps developed from his vignette watercolours such as Nos.272–298, was particularly suitable for his funnel-like, vortex compositions, but created a problem over how to fill the corners. He seems usually to have begun by painting up to the edges, but close examination shows that he often modified the shape as he went along, completing them when they were already in their final circular or octagonal frames. However, in this case Turner, working out his composition on a discarded canvas (Tate Gallery 5508), had envisaged the circular format from an early stage.

The press, while delighting in Turner's Venetian subjects at the 1841 exhibition, were united in their condemnation of the 'other wonderful fruits of a diseased eye and a reckless hand', as the *Athenaeum* for 5 June put it. To the *Art Union*, 15 May, this picture was 'another example of a great man's folly. It is far more like the dawn of creation – when "earth was without form and void" – before "the Spirit of God moved upon the face of the waters".'

520 Not exhibited

521 Peace - Burial at Sea R.A.1842
Oil on canvas, 34¼ × 34⅛ (87 × 86.5)
Exh: R.A. 1842 (338)
Tate Gallery (528)

Exhibited with the following lines from the *Fallacies of Hope*:

The midnight torch gleamed o'er the steamer's side
And Merit's corse was yielded to the tide.

The painting is a memorial to Turner's friend and

erstwhile rival Sir David Wilkie who died on board the *Oriental* on the way back from the Middle East on 1 June 1841; he was buried at sea off Gibraltar at 8.30 the same evening. Turner's picture was done in friendly rivalry with George Jones, who did a drawing of the burial as seen on deck (see No.B40). Jones reported that Clarkson Stanfield objected to the darkness of the sails; 'I only wish I had any colour to make them blacker,' replied Turner, who may also have been alluding to Wilkie's marked use of black in his later pictures.

At the Academy the painting was paired with 'War. The Exile and the Rock Limpet', a picture of Napoleon on St. Helena (Tate Gallery 529) and complementary in colour, being dominated by reds. Such pairings of works of contrasted colour were also to be a feature of Turner's Academy contributions in 1843 and 1845 (see Nos.522-3 and 526).

As usual the critics, after praising, in most instances, Turner's Venetian exhibits, vented their fury on his more imaginative works. 'He is as successful as ever in caricaturing himself, in two round blotches of *rouge et noir*', wrote the *Spectator* for 7 May 1842. The *Athenaeum*, 14 May, felt embarrassed that foreign visitors should see such works and concluded, 'We will not endure the music of Berlioz, nor abide Hoffmann's fantasy-pieces' – interesting comparisons – 'Yet the former is orderly, and the latter are commonplace, compared with these outbreaks'. Both *Ainsworth's Magazine*, June 1842, and the *Art Union*, 1 June, came out with the old suggestion that they would look as well turned upside down.

Surprisingly even Ruskin, though finally spurred on to write the first volume of *Modern Painters* by the hostility of the critics in 1842, had little to say about 'Peace' (though a considerable amount about 'War') and dismissed it as 'Spoiled by Turner's endeavour to give funereal and unnatural blackness to the sails'.

522 Shade and Darkness – the Evening of the Deluge R.A.1843
Oil on canvas, 31 × 30¾ (78.5 × 78)
Exh: R.A. 1843 (363)
Tate Gallery (531)

523 Light and Colour (Goethe's Theory) – the Morning after the Deluge – Moses writing the Book of Genesis R.A. 1843
Oil on canvas, 31 × 31 (78.5 × 78.5)
Exh: R.A. 1843 (385)
Tate Gallery (532)

The two pictures were exhibited in 1843 with two sets of verse attributed to the *Fallacies of Hope*:

The moon put forth her sign of woe unheeded;
But disobedience slept; the dark'ning Deluge closed
   around,
And the last token came: the giant framework floated,
The roused birds forsook their nightly shelters
   screaming,
And the beasts waded to the ark.
and
The Ark stood firm on Ararat; th' returning sun
Exhaled earth's humid bubbles, and emulous of light,
Reflected her lost forms, each in prismatic guise
Hope's harbinger, ephemeral as the summer fly
Which rises, flits, expands, and dies.

The allusion to Goethe's *Farbenlehre*, of which Turner owned and annotated an English translation (No.B120), parallels his allusion to Du Fresnoy in 'Watteau Painting' twelve years earlier (No.334). It refers to Goethe's theory of a colour-circle divided into 'plus' and 'minus' colours: the former, reds, yellows and greens, were associated by Goethe with gaiety, warmth and happiness, while the latter, blues, blue-greens and purples, were seen as productive of 'restless, susceptible, anxious impressions'. But the verses given to 'Light and Colour', which demonstrates the 'plus' colours, make it as pessimistic as 'Shade and Darkness'. Turner translated the rainbow of the Covenant into scientifically induced prismatic bubbles, each one an ephemeral harbinger of hope, born to die. In addition the Biblical concordance between Noah's Covenant and that of Moses, which is expressed by the strange conceit of showing Moses writing the Book of Genesis apparently on the Tables of the Law, with the Brazen Serpent, foreshadowing the Crucifixion, before him, must be seen in the light of Turner's constant use of the serpent as a symbol of evil (see Gage 1969, pp.185-7, for a fuller development of this theory).

The critics were universal in their condemnation of these pictures, though the *Spectator* for 13 May 1843 found them intelligible as illustrations 'of Goethe's Theory of Light and Colour . . . but further we cannot follow the painter. There may be some sublime meaning in all this . . . but . . . we see in these two octagon-shaped daubs only two brilliant problems – chromatic harmonies of cool and warm colours'. The *Athenaeum* for 17 June as usual regretted 'Mr. Turner's flagrant abuse of his genius' but admitted that 'there is a poetical idea dimly descried through the prismatic chaos, which arrests the attention and excites the fancy'.

524 Whalers (Boiling Blubber) entangled in Flaw Ice, endeavouring to extricate Themselves R.A.1846
Oil on canvas, 35⅞ × 47¼ (90 × 120)
Exh: R.A. 1846 (494)
Tate Gallery (547)

Turner exhibited four pictures of 'Whalers', two in 1845 and two in 1846; one of those exhibited in 1845 is now in the Metropolitan Museum, New York, while the others are in the Tate Gallery. All save this example were given references to 'Beale's Voyages', Thomas Beale's *The Natural History of the Sperm Whale*, published in 1839. Though generally similar in character and probably worked up on the basis of unfinished sea-pieces such as Nos.502-3, they are contrasted in colour and hence mood, and were probably seen as deliberate variations on a theme. There are composition sketches, related to the oils in general terms, in the 'Whalers' sketchbook (T.B.CCCLIII-6 to 14; see No. 633). See also No.B117.

Turner's whaling pictures were fairly well received though the *Art Union* for June 1846 thought them the result of an 'eccentric movement in search of material... We are indebted, however, to "Beale's Voyage" . . . for having saved us from the infliction of passages from the "Fallacies of Hope".' Of 'Whalers (Boiling Blubber)' it wrote, 'There is a charming association of colour here – the emerald green tells with exceeding freshness; but it

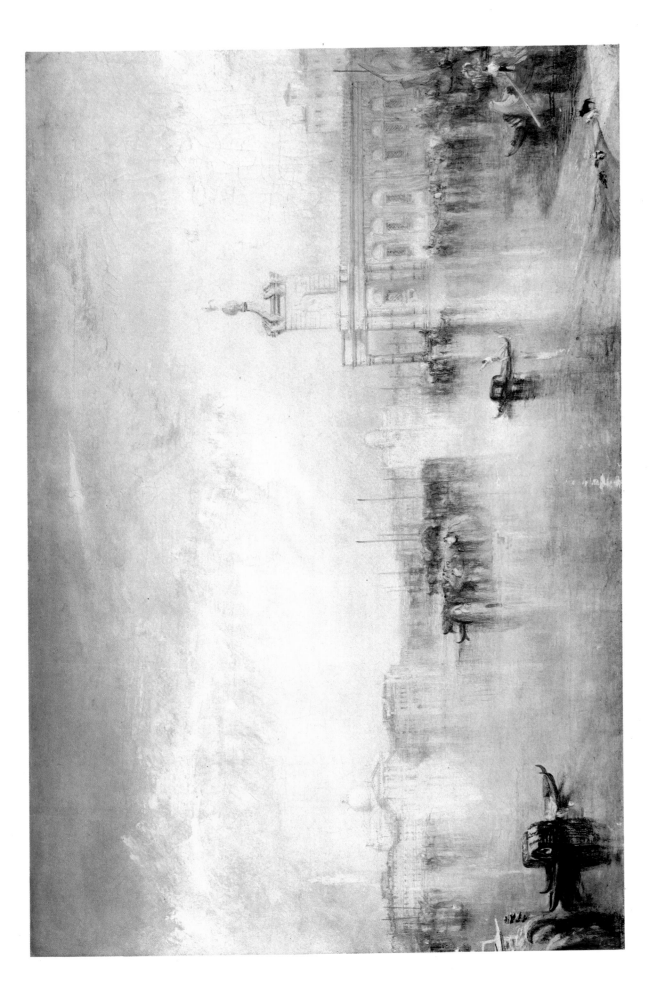

532 **The Dogano, San Giorgio, Citella, from the Steps of the Europa** 1842 (entry on p.152)

555 Venice: the Grand Canal with the Salute 1840 (entry on p.156)

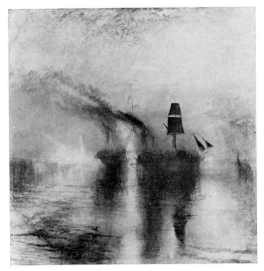

521

would be impossible to define anything in the composition save the rigging of the ship.' To the *Athenaeum*, 9 May, it presented 'something more tangible' than usual; 'one *can* make forms out of those masses of beautiful, though almost chaotic colours. The sea-green hue of the ice, the flicker of the sunbeam on the waves, the boiling of the blubber, and the tall forms of the ice-bound vessels, make up an interesting picture, dressed in Turner's magic glow'.

525 Not exhibited

526 **The Angel standing in the Sun** R.A.1846
    Oil on canvas, 31 × 31 (78.5 × 78.5)
    Exh: R.A. 1846 (411)
    Tate Gallery (550)

Painted as the companion to 'Undine giving the ring to Masaniello, fisherman of Naples', also exhibited at the Royal Academy in 1846 (384). This had no accompanying text in the catalogue but 'The Angel standing in the Sun' was accompanied by the following passage from the *Book of Revelation* XIX, 17–18:

> And I saw an angel standing in the sun; and he cried with a loud voice, saying to all the fowls that fly in the midst of heaven, Come and gather yourselves together unto the supper of the great God;
> That ye may eat the flesh of kings, and the flesh of captains and the flesh of mighty men, and the flesh of horses, and of them that sit on them, both free and bond, both small and great.

and also by a quotation from Samuel Roger's *Voyage of Columbus*, where, significantly, it has the subtitle 'The Flight of an Angel of Darkness':

> The morning march that flashes to the sun;
> The feast of vultures when the day is done.

It appears then that here even the beneficent power of the sun has been transformed into something terrible, indissolubly linked with its opposite, the 'Angel of Darkness'. The relevance of the Neapolitan revolutionary Masaniello is difficult to determine, but he is probably about to be enticed into the sea by the water-nymph, who, surrounded in a typically Turneresque phosphorescent bubble, embodies another piece of pessimistic symbolism based on the forces of nature.

The two pictures provoked the usual lament from the *Athenaeum* for 9 May 1846: 'That there is art in them, consummate art, in reconciling to the eye such effusions of all the strongest and most opposing colours of the palette, we freely admit: but we as freely declare our regret, that over such aberrations of talent no controlling influence exerts its genial restraint'. The *Spectator* for the same date found more, though qualified, praise, calling them 'tours de force that show how nearly the gross materials of the palette can be made to emulate the source of light – of the figures we can only say that Turner seems to have taken leave of form altogether'.

527 **The Hero of a Hundred Fights** R.A.1847
    Oil on canvas, 35¾ × 47¾ (91 × 121)
    Exh: R.A. 1847 (180)
    Tate Gallery (551)

Exhibited in 1847 with the following explanation, attributed rather oddly to the *Fallacies of Hope*: 'An idea suggested by the German invocation upon casting the bell: in England called tapping the furnace.' The

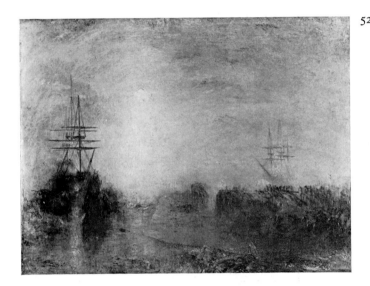

524

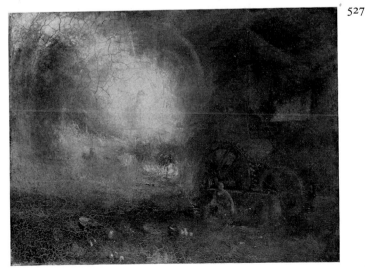

527

scene is the casting of M. C. Wyatt's bronze equestrian statue of the Duke of Wellington which had occurred in September 1845, but was superimposed by Turner on a much earlier picture of an interior with large pieces of machinery, akin to though not identical with the drawing of the interior of a belfry in the 'Swans' sketchbook of c.1798 (T.B.XLII-60 and 61). The original painting must have been done in the first decade of the century. When Turner came to rework it he left much of the original untouched, adding the great burst of light on the left and highlighting the still-life in the foreground.

This was Turner's only exhibit in 1847, but the following year he was even more hard-pressed, exhibiting nothing at all; in 1849 he sent in two early pictures, 'Venus and Adonis' (No.78) and 'The Wreck Buoy' which he repainted all over (Walker Art Gallery, Liverpool; repr. Rothenstein and Butlin 1960, pl.126). One suspects that most of the work on 'The Hero of a Hundred Fights' was done on the Varnishing Days. That he was there is known from his having touched in a portion of the rainbow of Maclise's 'Sacrifice of Noah' (see No.B64) which hung next to it, causing Ruskin to complain in a letter to Clarkson Stanfield, commiserating with him over the poor position of one of his exhibits, that 'They have served Turner worse, however; there is nothing in his picture but even colour, and they must needs put Maclise's rainbow side by side with it – which takes part – and a very awkward and conclusive part too in its best melody'. The *Literary Gazette* for 8 May 1847 thought the opposite however, saying that the Turner was 'painted up to such a blaze as to extinguish Noah's rainbow. It is a marvellous piece of colouring. If Turner had been Phaeton, he must have succeeded in driving the chariot of the sun'. Other reviews were less favourable. 'Fantastical absurdity' and 'dazzling obscurity', exclaimed the *Spectator* on 8 May, adding, on 19 June, that 'As a "vision", it is a burlesque on poetic licence.' 'Full of fine passages of chromatic arrangement,' said the *Athenaeum* for 8 May, 'it has so little foundation in fact that the sense is merely bewildered at the unsparing hand with which the painter has spread forth the glories of his palette.' Amazingly no one seems to have noticed the stylistic dichotomy between the original painting and the superimposed glow that so dazzled them.

528 Mercury sent to Admonish Æneas R.A.1850
Oil on canvas, $35\frac{1}{2} \times 47\frac{1}{2}$ (90.5 × 121)
Exh: R.A. 1850 (174)
Tate Gallery (553)

Although Turner did not die until 19 December 1851, this was the last year in which he exhibited. As if to make amends for the thin showing of the previous three years he sent in a group of four pictures devoted to Aeneas' stay at Carthage, tempted by love for Dido to resist the destiny that called him to Italy. All were accompanied by verses from the *Fallacies of Hope*, those for this picture being:

Beneath the morning mist,
Mercury waited to tell him of his neglected fleet.
Of the other three pictures 'Æneas relating his story to Dido' is said to have perished nearly sixty years ago, while 'The Visit to the Tomb' and 'The Departure of the Fleet' are at the Tate Gallery. All the compositions follow much the same pattern with figures crowded on

steep banks on either side of a brightly illuminated centre in which the sun is drawn, as it were, to the surface of the picture to dominate the whole scene. They may well have been worked up over delicate, watercolour-like lay-ins of the character of 'Sunrise with a Ship between Headlands' and 'Norham Castle'. The colours on the whole lack Turner's usual exquisite balance and are unnaturally hot and foxy, though this example escapes this defect.

Indeed, the *Athenaeum* for 18 May 1850 picked out 'Mercury sent to admonish Æneas' as 'exquisite for delicacy and refinement'. The group as a whole were characterised as 'full of combinations of forms of richest fancy and of colours of most dazzling hue', though 'they must be approached no nearer than to the spot at which the general effect can be judged of. . . . They must be looked on as great pictorial *schemes*, abounding in rich stores of Nature and deductions from Art, – great poetical ideas, in fact, the principles of which the student will do well to investigate. The practise which spurns at the expression of details it will be prudent for him to avoid.' The *Spectator* for 4 May was less complimentary, talking of 'a splendid perplexity, respecting which the name would convey no information to the reader; with a companion equally brilliant to the eye and dark to the understanding' and saying of the *Fallacies of Hope*, 'the said fallacy being, any hope of understanding what the picture means'.

526

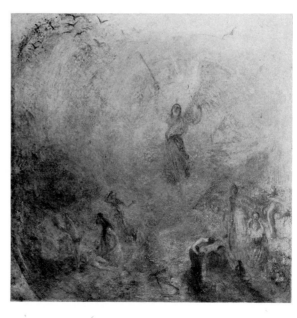

15. Venice 1833-45

Although Turner had visited Venice on his way to Rome in 1819 he did not exhibit any oil paintings of the city until 1833, when he sent two examples to the Royal Academy, No.529 and the now untraced 'Ducal Palace, Venice'. To explain his sudden interest, so long after his visit to Venice of 1819, some scholars have suggested another visit in 1832, but the evidence points to Turner not having returned until the summer of 1833, after the Royal Academy exhibition (Hardy George, 'Turner in Venice' in *Art Bulletin* LIII, 1971, pp.84-7). Only after artistic pressures had led him to embark on Venetian subjects did Turner feel the urge to return. He continued to exhibit Venetian subjects from 1834 to 1837 and again from 1840 (the year of his last visit) to 1846. Those shown here mainly follow the small two-foot by three-foot format, but in the 1830s there were also examples in his standard three-foot, four-foot size. Whereas most of his time during his first visit to Venice in 1819 seems to have been taken up with sketching in pencil, he produced only a few pencil drawings in 1833; in 1840 most of his works were in watercolour. A discussion of these watercolours and their dating is on p.154.

529 Bridge of Sighs, Ducal Palace and Custom-House, Venice: Canaletti Painting R.A.1833
Oil on mahogany, 20¼ × 32½ (51 × 82.5)
Exh: R.A. 1833 (109)
Tate Gallery (370)

The title shows that this was in part a tribute to the most renowned of painters of Venetian *vedute*. Canaletto himself is shown painting away at a picture in a heavy gilt frame on the left, although Turner, of all artists, would have been aware of the unlikelihood of such an event. The picture may also, as Graham Reynolds has suggested (1969, pp.158-60), have been in part inspired by the Venetian scenes of Bonington, whose death in 1828 had been followed by a large sale of his works in London in 1829. But the immediate cause seems to have been friendly rivalry with one of his followers, William Clarkson Stanfield (1793-1867), who exhibited 'Venice from the Dogana' the same year. According to the *Morning Chronicle* for 6 June 1833 Turner did his picture, 'it is said, in two or three days, on hearing that Mr. Stanfield was employed on a similar subject – not in the way of rivalry of course, for he is the last to admit anything of the kind, but generously, we will suppose, to give him a lesson in atmosphere and poetry.' The same story was repeated by Allan Cunningham and *Arnold's Magazine* for November 1833–April 1834. Stanfield's picture was, in fact, bought by his patron Lord Lansdowne, who had an important collection of Bonington's works, so the two possible causes for Turner's taking up Venetian subjects would have been interrelated.

The critics readily accepted Turner as the winner in this contest. For *Arnold's Magazine* 'the juxtaposition brought out more glaringly the defects of Stanfield, and illustrated more strongly the fine powers of Turner. For, viewed from whatever distance, Turner's work displayed a brilliancy, breadth, and power, killing every other work in the exhibition', though an anecdote by George Jones, whose 'Ghent' hung next to the Turner, suggests that Jones won another contest that occurred at that exhibition. Turner first put down Jones' bright colours by increasing his own but Jones then added 'a great deal more white' to his sky, making the Turner 'look much too blue'. The *Morning Chronicle* went on with its review of the Turner to say that 'It is beautiful and replete in the greys on the left, &c, with his magical powers, so often disgraced in other pieces, and frittered away for pence in his little drawings.' Here we have a continuing theme of later criticisms, which praised Turner's Venetian works while attacking his 'extravagances'. The *Athenaeum*, 11 May, thought that Turner had worsted Canaletto as well, describing Turner's picture as 'more his own than he seems aware of: he imagines he has painted it in the Canaletti style: the style is his, and worth Canaletti's ten times over.'

The picture was bought at the Academy by Robert Vernon, a typical example of the new manufacturing class from which many of Turner's later patrons were to come, as opposed to the aristocracy who bought his early works. Vernon, who had already bought a sea-piece the previous year, was building up a collection of contemporary British painting which he gave to the National Gallery in 1847, by which time it included four Turners (see also No.532).

530 Venice, the Bridge of Sighs R.A.1840
Oil on canvas, 24 × 36 (61 × 91.5)
Exh: R.A.1840 (55)
Tate Gallery (527)

Exhibited in 1840 with the following lines from Byron's *Childe Harold's Pilgrimage*:

I stood upon a bridge, a palace and
A prison on each hand.

The quotation shows that Turner saw even the beauties of Venice as a sham, concealing the grim realities on which her now departed glories had depended.

This is an unusually close-up, architectural view, matched only by the vast unfinished picture of the Rialto of *c*.1820 mentioned under No.236.

Most of the critics of the 1840 Academy exhibitions were so shattered by Turner's other contributions that they failed to mention the two Venetian scenes, this picture and the 'Venice from the Canale della Giudecca, Chiesa di S Maria della Salute, &c' (Victoria and Albert Museum). Even the *Spectator*, which did notice them, could not forbear to include them in the general condemnation: all were 'mere freaks of chromomania', the Venetian pictures being included with their 'sundry patches of white and nankeen, with a bundle of gayer colours, . . . intended to represent buildings and vessels.'

531 Giudecca, La Donna della Salute and San Giorgio R.A.1841
Oil on canvas, 24 × 36 (61 × 91.5)
Exh: R.A. 1841 (66)
Mr William Wood Prince

The view is taken from the Canal di Fusina with the Giudecca on the right. The picture was bought at the Academy by Elhanan Bicknell and was well received by the critics, together with Turner's other Venetian subject, 'Ducal Palace, Dogana, with Part of San Giorgio, Venice' (Oberlin College, Ohio). The *Athenaeum* for 5 June praised them as 'so much less extravagant than his late Turnerisms . . . In these Venetian pictures it would be hard to exceed. The clearness of air and water – the latter taking every passing reflection with a pellucid softness beyond the reach of meaner pencil. The architecture, too, is more carefully made out than has lately been the case with Mr. Turner, and both pictures are kept alive by groups of southern figures, which, seen from a certain remoteness, give a beauty and not a blemish to the scenes they animate.' For the *Spectator*, 8 May, both pictures were 'gorgeous creations conveying a poetical idea of the actual scene steeped in an atmosphere of light and colour.'

532 The Dogano, San Giorgio, Citella, from the Steps of the Europa R.A.1842 (repr. on p.147)
Oil on canvas, $24\frac{1}{2} \times 36\frac{1}{2}$ (62×92.5)
Exh: R.A. 1842 (52)
Tate Gallery (372)

Turner seems to have stayed at the Hotel Europa on some if not all of his visits to Venice. There are many drawings and watercolours made from the hotel, including views of fireworks taken from the roof or an upper room (see Nos.557 and 562). Exceptionally among Turner's later oil paintings this picture seems to be in part taken from a drawing of the Dogana and the Zitella (the 'Citella' of Turner's title) in the 'Milan to Venice' sketchbook, made on Turner's first visit in 1819 (T.B. CLXXV–40, repr. Finberg *Venice* 1930, pl.2; see No. 208). However, the view is such a well-known one that recourse to a drawing may not have been necessary. A similar view but omitting San Giorgio on the left appears in the watercolour entitled 'The New Moon' in the collection of D. G. Ells. This probably dates from about 1840 but, *pace* Finberg (*ibid*, pp.140, 161, repr. in colour pl.24), is unlikely to have been used as a basis for the oil as the viewpoint is slightly different.

This picture and the other Venetian oil exhibited in 1842, 'Campo Santo, Venice' (Toledo Museum of Art) were, on the whole, highly praised by the critics. For the *Spectator*, 7 May, they were 'two lovely views of Venice, gorgeous in hue and atmospheric in tone.' For the *Athenaeum* of the same date they were 'among the loveliest, because least exaggerated pictures, which this magician (for such he is, in right of his command over the spirits of Air, Fire, and Water) has recently given us. Fairer dreams never floated past poets' eye; and the aspect of the City of Waters is hardly one iota idealised. As pieces of effect, too, these works are curious; close at hand, a splashed palette – an arm's length distant, a clear and delicate shadowing forth of a scene made up of crowded and minute objects!' The *Art Union* for 1 June was rather more critical. 'Venice was surely built to be painted by Canaletti and Turner . . . The Venetian pictures are now among the best this artist paints, but the present specimens are of a decayed brilliancy; we mean, they are by no means comparable with others he has within a few years exhibited. A great error in Mr. Turner's smooth water pictures is, that the reflection of

colours in the water are painted as strongly as the substances themselves, a treatment which diminishes the value of objects.' The picture was purchased at the Academy by Robert Vernon and given to the National Gallery with three other Turners in 1847 (see No.529). Placed on view as a token of the whole of Vernon's collection of contemporary painting, it was the first Turner to be shown there.

533 Dogana, and Madonna della Salute, Venice
R.A.1843
Oil on canvas, $24\frac{3}{4} \times 36\frac{5}{8}$ (63×93)
Inscr. bottom right: 'J M W T'
Exh: R.A. 1843 (144); Society of Artists, Birmingham 1843 (54)
National Gallery of Art, Washington (*given in memory of Governor Alvan T. Fuller by the Fuller Foundation 1961*)

Apparently bought at the Academy by Edwin Bullock of Handsworth. One of the three Venetian pictures on view with Nos.534 and 535, all characterised by the *Spectator* for 13 May as 'beaming with sunlight and gorgeous colour, and full of atmosphere; though, as usual, all forms and local hues are lost in the blaze of effect.'

534 The Sun of Venice going to Sea R.A.1843
Oil on canvas, $24\frac{1}{4} \times 36\frac{1}{4}$ (61.5×92)
Inscr. on the sail, damaged and retouched:
'Sol de VENEZA . . .'
Exh: R.A. 1843 (129)
Tate Gallery (535)

The pessimism that lies behind Turner's views of Venice is here made apparent by the verses from the *Fallacies of Hope* published in the Royal Academy catalogue:

Fair shines the morn, and soft the zephyrs blow,
Venezia's fisher spreads his painted sail so gay,
Nor heeds the demon that in grim repose
Expects his evening prey.

Based in part on Thomas Gray's 'The Bard' these lines appear slightly differently in different copies of the catalogue, as Ruskin explained in a footnote to his notes on the Turners shown at Marlborough House in 1856: 'Turner seems to have revised his own additions to Gray, in the catalogues, as he did his pictures on the walls, with much discomfiture to the printer and the public. He wanted afterwards to make the first lines of this legend rhyme with each other; and to read:

Fair shines the moon, the Zephyr [west wind] blows a gale
Venetia's fisher spreads his painted sail.

The two readings got confused, and, if I remember right, some of the catalogues read "soft the Zephyr blows a gale" and "spreads his painted sail so gay" – to the great admiration of the collectors of the Sibylline leaves of the "Fallacies of Hope".' John Gage suggests that Turner was also influenced, both in his verbal imagery and in the underlying pessimism, by the section on Venice in Shelley's 'Lines written among the Euganean Hills'; this section was included in S. C. Hall's anthology *The Book of Gems*, 1838, a copy of which Turner owned.

The picture was one of Ruskin's favourites. In his diary he wrote, under 29 April 1844, 'Yesterday, when

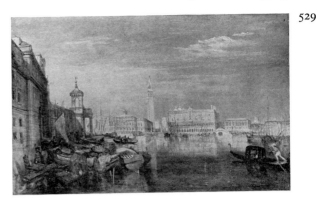
529

I called with my father on Turner, he was kinder than I ever remember. He shook hands most cordially with my father, wanted us to have a glass of wine, asked us to go upstairs into the gallery. When there, I went immediately in search of the "Sol di Venezia", saying it was my favourite. "I thought", said Turner, "it was the 'St. Benedetto'" [No.535]. It was flattering that he remembered that I had told him this. I said the worst of his pictures was one could never see enough of them. "That's part of their quality," said Turner.' A year later, as Ruskin wrote in a letter to his father of 14 September 1845, he was delighted to see 'a fishing boat with its *painted* sail full to the wind, the most gorgeous orange and red, in everything, form, colour & feeling, the very counterpart of the Sol di Venezia'.

The critics of the 1843 Academy exhibition were less enthusiastic, being rather put off by the verses that give the picture its hidden note of doom. 'His style of dealing with quotations', wrote the *Athenaeum* for 17 June, 'is as unscrupulous as his style of treating nature and her attributes of form and colour', while the *Art Union* for June 1843 suggested that Turner's 'wretched verses may have had some deliterious influence on the painter's mind – may have cast a spell over a great genius. Oh! that he would go back to nature!' The critic went on, 'The most celebrated painters have been said to be "before their time", but the world has always, at some time, or other, come up with them. The author of the "Sun of Venice" is far out of sight; he leaves the world to turn round without him: at least in those of his works, of the light of which we have no glimmering, he cannot hope to be even overtaken by distant posterity; such extravagances all sensible people must condemn; nor

is the winter of *our* discontent

Made glorious summer by this "Sun of Venice"'.

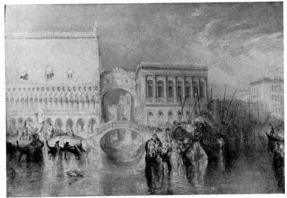
530

535 St. Benedetto, looking towards Fusina

R.A.1843
Oil on canvas, $24\frac{1}{2} \times 36\frac{1}{2}$ (61.5 × 92)
Exh: R.A. 1843 (554)
Tate Gallery (534)

The title is partly imaginary, there being no church of San Benedetto visible in this view looking west along the Canal della Giudecca towards Fusina. There is a watercolour, probably of 1840, of a similar view in the Turner Bequest (T.B.CCCXV–13).

This picture vied with 'The Sun of Venice' for first place in Ruskin's estimation. In his notes on the Turners shown at Marlborough House in 1856 he wrote, 'Take it all in all, I think this is the best Venetian picture of Turner's which he has left to us.'

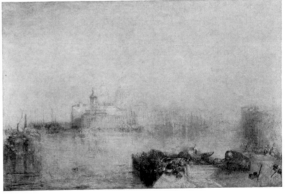
533

536 Venice with the Salute *c.*1840–5
Oil on canvas, $24\frac{1}{2} \times 36\frac{1}{2}$ (62 × 92.5)
Tate Gallery (5487)

537 View in Venice *c.*1840–5
Oil on canvas, $24\frac{1}{2} \times 36\frac{1}{2}$ (62 × 92.5)
Tate Gallery (5488)

Turner exhibited no fewer than eighteen small Venetian scenes of this size at the Royal Academy between 1840 and 1846 (and one rather larger example). These two pictures from the Turner Bequest, only recently revealed by cleaning, are presumably lay-ins for further works for exhibition; luckily for us, in view of the rather turgid effect of most of the later exhibits, they

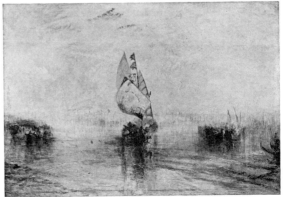
534

550

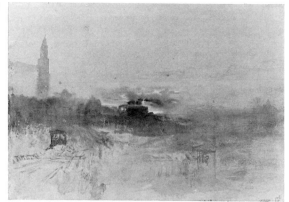

554

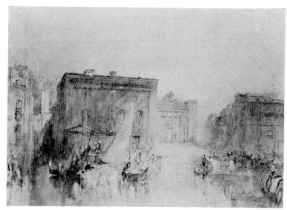

559

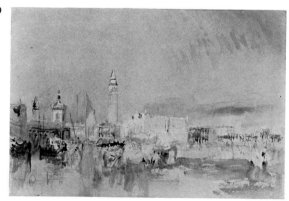

563

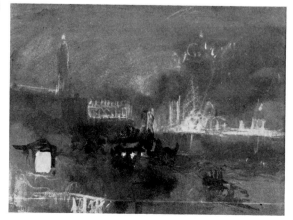

were not carried any further. The first seems to show the Madonna della Salute seen along the Grand Canal from near the present Accademia bridge; another view of the Salute, from the opposite direction, was one of the 1844 exhibits (Tate Gallery 539). It has not been possible to identify the other view.

538 Festive Lagoon Scene, Venice c.1840-5
Oil on canvas, $35\frac{3}{4} \times 47\frac{3}{4}$ (91 × 121)
Tate Gallery (4660)

An unfinished Venetian scene in Turner's standard three-foot, four-foot size, used for some exhibited examples in 1834 and 1835 but not in the 1840s, the probable date of this picture. It is typical of a number of Turner's later works in the way in which the spectator is drawn into the picture between serried rows of staring faces, running the gauntlet, as it were, of the frenzied inhabitants of Turner's imaginative world.

539   Not exhibited

THE LATE VENETIAN DRAWINGS

Turner's Bequest includes a large number of watercolour drawings of Venetian subjects which must be connected with either of his two last visits to the city, in 1833 and 1840. (When Finberg wrote his *In Venice with Turner* the date of the earlier visit was thought to have been 1835.) The problem of deciding to which of the two dates particular drawings belong has not yet been solved, although various suggestions have been made, none conclusive. The drawings can be arranged, as is so often the case in Turner's output, into groups which seem to belong together and appear to have been executed at one time; for the most part their grouping is based on size and type of paper, but stylistic arguments have also been used to distinguish one batch from another.

The groups which are easiest to distinguish are those on grey or brown paper; these also make use of bodycolour as well as, or instead of, watercolour. Twenty-one drawings on grey paper are T.B.CCCXVII; they appear to belong to a series which includes views on the Rhine and in the Tyrol (see No.582). A further ten, on brown paper and executed entirely in bodycolour, are T.B.CCCXVIII. Of the pure watercolours, five (T.B. CCCXVI–II to 15) are on cream-tinted, rough paper, but the remainder are on smooth white Whatman or similar paper. Twenty-one of them are from the roll sketchbook T.B.CCCXV, which is watermarked 1834 and must, therefore, have been used on the 1840 visit; and the rest, some thirty-seven drawings, are loose sheets listed in the *Inventory* under T.B.CCCXVI. At least twenty-eight other watercolours of Venice, dating from either 1833 or 1840, are in public and private collections in Great Britain.

The roll sketchbook provides some stylistic evidence on which to attempt the dating of the rest of the Venetian views. Many of the loose sheets can be associated with it; but it has become generally accepted that one particular series, depicting a violent thunderstorm, dates from the earlier visit. The Vaughan 'Storm in the Piazzetta' (Edinburgh), the Ruskin

'Storm at Sunset' (Fitzwilliam) and the Quilter-Sale 'Storm' now in the British Museum belong to this group, as does the 'Dogana and S. Giorgio Maggiore in a Storm' (No.551). The colour in these drawings is perhaps fuller and richer than that of the roll sketchbook, where Turner employs the lightest and most vaporous washes, probably applied later to a slight pencil outline made on the spot, but sometimes apparently directly from nature without underdrawing. But there is no evidence beyond slight stylistic differentiations to separate the two groups.

On the same ground, that heavier colour seems more appropriate to the earlier date (and particularly in view of Turner's work in bodycolour on the *French Rivers* drawings about 1830) the bodycolour drawings on grey and brown paper have also been assigned to 1833, but one of them, showing the Campanile of St. Mark's with scaffolding round it, probably dates from 1840 (see Nos.558 and 559). It may be possible to associate one of these bodycolour studies, that of 'San Stefano' (T.B.CCCXVII–32), with a drawing in the 'Rotterdam and Venice' sketchbook of 1840; such a connection would suggest that all the drawings in bodycolour on grey paper belong to 1840, or perhaps later, since Turner may well have worked up these subjects after returning home. The extraordinary series of sketches on brown paper (Nos.562–566), much freer than those on grey, would then also seem to fit into the pattern at a fairly late stage. Certainly, comparison between their use of bodycolour and that of the Petworth and *French Rivers* drawings makes it difficult to believe that such radically different approaches to the medium could have appeared concurrently. Oddly enough, the nearest approach to Turner's use of bodycolour in these brown paper sketches is to be found in his 'Academical' sketchbook of 1798 (No.44), where some of the studies of Caernarvon Castle on a brownish ground achieve almost the same freedom as the scenes in a Venetian theatre forty years later (Nos.564–566).

One of the brown paper sketches is a view by moonlight of the roof of the Hotel Europa from Turner's bedroom (No.562). The same view, in daylight, appears among the watercolours (No.557), and owing to the presence of figures this drawing has been associated with the roof-top view of Venice in the painting 'Juliet and her Nurse' shown at the Royal Academy in 1836 (repr. Rothenstein and Butlin, 1964, pl.102). There is in fact no precise connection between the two designs. The drawing is also related to a smaller view from the Hotel Europa (T.B.CCCLXIV–43), one of a series in slightly smaller format which appear for stylistic reasons to date from 1840. The daylight view with figures strongly resembles in palette and technique several of the watercolours usually assigned to 1840, in particular the 'Riva degli Schiavoni with a Fishing-Boat' (No.556) and both of these have affinities with the small view of 'S. Giorgio Maggiore' (No.547) which belongs to the same group as T.B.CCCLXIV–43.

It is, therefore, possible that all the late Venice drawings were made either in 1840 or immediately afterwards, and that date has been given to them in this catalogue. It is not contended, however, that such a simple grouping is wholly supported by evidence and the problem must remain unresolved.

540   'Venice' Sketchbook 1833
Bound in cardboard
100 leaves, the majority drawn on in pencil, $8 \times 4\frac{1}{4}$ (20.2 × 11)
Trustees of the British Museum (T.B.CCCXIV)

ff.38ᵛ–39ʳ   Two rapid sketches of S. Maria della Salute from the Giudecca
Pencil

Dated by Finberg to about 1839 but very possibly a book in use on Turner's 1833 visit to Venice. Its contents are devoted wholly to sketches of Venetian architecture, some of considerable detail.
ff.38ᵛ–39ʳ are among the freest notes in the book.

541   'Venice and Botzen' Sketchbook 1840
70 leaves, almost all drawn on in pencil, $6\frac{3}{4} \times 4\frac{3}{4}$ (17.1 × 12.6)
Inscr. inside front cover: 'Venice'
Trustees of the British Museum (T.B.CCCXIII)

f.2ᵛ   Venice: St. Mark's seen from a Balustraded Parapet with Statues
Pencil
f.3ʳ   Two views of the Grand Canal near the Dogana
Pencil
Bound in grey boards

The forceful freedom of the sketches in this book suggests a fairly late date; and George (1971, p.86) argues that the views of the Campanile show it as it was in 1840.

542   A Serene Evening on a Lake? ?1840
Pencil and watercolour, $13\frac{3}{4} \times 20\frac{1}{4}$ (34.9 × 51.4)
Trustees of the British Museum (T.B.CCLXIII–44)
The delicate colouring of this exquisite study is strongly reminiscent of the watercolours known to belong to Turner's first visit to Venice (Nos.212–214) and the preparation of the paper with pale washes of blue and yellow has much in common with the 'colour-beginnings' in the 'Como and Venice' sketchbook (No.209). There is, however, no more specific evidence for giving the sheet so early a date, and Finberg placed it among 'colour-beginnings' of the 1820s. The freedom of the pencilled-in boat and buildings suggests an even later date, as does the pencil scribble in the top right corner of the sheet which may read as an 'M', perhaps identifying a location, like the 'L' on many late drawings of Lucerne. Nevertheless, the pencil details seem to suggest that the scene is intended to be Venice.

543   Venice: Distant View of the Entrance to the Grand Canal 1840
Watercolour on off-white paper, $9\frac{1}{16} \times 11\frac{15}{16}$ (23 × 30.3)
Trustees of the British Museum (T.B.CCCXVI–13)

544   Venice: the Salute, the Dogana and the Grand Canal: Sunset 1840
Watercolour, $8\frac{5}{8} \times 12\frac{11}{16}$ (22 × 32.3)
Trustees of the British Museum (T.B.CCCXV–17)

545   Venice: the Dogana and S. Maria della Salute 1840
Pencil and watercolour, $9\frac{5}{8} \times 11\frac{15}{16}$ (24.5 × 30.3)
Trustees of the British Museum (T.B.CCCXVI–1)

546   Venice: the Giudecca, with the Salute to the Left, S. Giorgio Maggiore at the Right 1840
Watercolour, $9\frac{5}{8} \times 8\frac{3}{16}$ (24.5 × 20.8)
Trustees of the British Museum (T.B. CCCXVI–8)

547   Venice: S. Giorgio Maggiore 1840
Pencil and watercolour and bodycolour, $7\frac{1}{2} \times 11\frac{1}{16}$ (19 × 28.1)
Trustees of the British Museum (T.B.CCCXVI–28)

548   Venice: the Salute, the Campanile of St. Mark's and S. Giorgio Maggiore 1840
Pencil and watercolour with pen and red ink, $9\frac{1}{2} \times 11\frac{15}{16}$ (24.1 × 30.3)
Trustees of the British Museum (T.B.CCCXVI–19)

549   Venice: looking down the Grand Canal towards the Casa Corner and the Salute 1840
Pencil and watercolour, $8\frac{11}{16} \times 12\frac{3}{4}$ (22.1 × 32.3)
Inscr. bottom left: 'B A I D I' (?)
Trustees of the British Museum (T.B.CCCXV–6)

550   Venice: Sunset 1840
Watercolour, $7\frac{3}{4} \times 11$ (19.6 × 28)
Trustees of the British Museum (T.B.CCCLXIV–106)
Presumably looking from the Dogana towards the Campanile of St. Mark's on the left, the Doge's Palace centre, and S. Giorgio Maggiore at the extreme right.

551   Venice: the Dogana and S. Giorgio Maggiore in a Storm 1840
Watercolour, $8\frac{5}{8} \times 12\frac{5}{8}$ (22 × 32)
Private Collection
Probably the drawing catalogued by Finberg (*Venice* 1930, p.159) as 'The Approaching Storm', and dated by him to *c*.1835. The subject and treatment have affinities with the Sale drawing (British Museum 1915-3-13-50) and the Ruskin 'Storm at Sunset' (Fitzwilliam Museum No.590); all three may record the same storm as perhaps may the 'Storm in the Piazzetta' in the National Gallery of Scotland (repr. Finberg, *Venice*, 1930, pl.xix).

552   Venice: the Grand Canal 1840
Watercolour and pen, $8\frac{7}{16} \times 12\frac{3}{8}$ (21.5 × 31.5)
Visitors of the Ashmolean Museum, Oxford
Given by Ruskin to Oxford University in 1861. Like the 'Venice: Calm at Sunrise', which Ruskin included in his gift of twenty-five Turner drawings to Cambridge University shortly after the gift to Oxford, this and the two other Venetian watercolours in the Ashmolean Museum seem to date from Turner's final visit to Venice in 1840 and are similar in type and size to the series in the Turner Bequest. It has been supposed that they were extracted from the roll sketchbook T.B.CCCXV, but Turner probably made use of numerous books of the same type, which were broken up and dispersed among friends and patrons, or left among the many miscellaneous Venetian drawings in his studio (T.B.CCCXVI).

553   Venice: the Riva degli Schiavoni 1840
Watercolour with pen and some scraping-out, $8\frac{9}{16} \times 12\frac{1}{2}$ (21.8 × 31.8)
Visitors of the Ashmolean Museum, Oxford
Given by Ruskin to Oxford University in 1861.

554   Venice: the Accademia 1840
Pencil and watercolour with pen and grey, blue and red colour, $8\frac{1}{2} \times 12\frac{7}{16}$ (21.6 × 31.6)
Visitors of the Ashmolean Museum, Oxford
Given by Ruskin to Oxford University in 1861.

555   Venice: the Grand Canal with the Salute 1840   (repr. on p.148)
Watercolour with some bodycolour and scraping-out over traces of pencil, $8\frac{5}{8} \times 12\frac{1}{2}$ (21.8 × 31.8)
Private Collection
This drawing, which is perhaps more highly finished than the majority of the Venetian views of 1840, is known to have been in the collection of Turner's agent, Thomas Griffith.

556   Venice: the Riva degli Schiavoni, with a Fishing Boat 1840
Watercolour, $8\frac{11}{16} \times 12\frac{9}{16}$ (22.1 × 32.1)
Trustees of the British Museum (T.B.CCCXV–9)
Close in palette and technique to the 'View from the Roof of the Hotel Europa' (No.557). The subject is perhaps connected with the pencil sketches of the Riva and S. Giorgio Maggiore on f.86ʳ and ᵛ of the 'Rotterdam to Venice' sketchbook (T.B.CCCXX).

557   Venice: View from the Roof of the Hotel Europa 1840
Pencil and watercolour, $9\frac{5}{8} \times 12$ (24.5 × 30.5)
Trustees of the British Museum (T.B.CCCXVI–36)
This drawing has been supposed to reflect a connection with 'Juliet and her Nurse', shown at the R.A. in 1836 (repr. Rothenstein and Butlin, 1964, pl.102). A smaller drawing of the same view, without figures, is T.B. CCCLXIV–43, and a similar view by moonlight in bodycolour on brown paper is No.562. In palette and technique the present drawing closely resembles the 'Riva degli Schiavoni with a Fishing Boat' (No.556) which may be related to a sketch in the 'Rotterdam to Venice' sketchbook of 1840.

558   Venice: the Campanile of St. Mark's with the Pilastri Acritani, from the Porta della Carta 1840
Pencil and watercolour and bodycolour on grey paper, $11\frac{1}{8} \times 7\frac{1}{2}$ (28.2 × 19)
Trustees of the British Museum (T.B.CCCXVII–19)
The bodycolour drawings of Venice on grey paper (see also Nos.559–561) have been dated to 1833 on the ground that Turner was using bodycolour extensively at that period. There appear, however, to be connections between some of these drawings and the 'Rotterdam and Venice' sketchbook of 1840 (T.B.CCCXX); e.g. the bodycolour study of 'S. Stefano', T.B.CCCXVII–32, is apparently based on a sketch on f.91ᵛ of that book. The present drawing shows the Campanile of St. Mark's with scaffolding round it, and it has been pointed out that, while it is known that scaffolding was

there in 1840, 'it is unlikely that the scaffolding put up in 1830 was still there in 1832–35', i.e. during Turner's 1833 visit (George, 1971, p.85, note 6). It therefore seems rather more probable that this and the other drawings like it belong to 1840.

559 Venice: the Dogana, Campanile of St. Mark's and Doge's Palace 1840
Pencil, watercolour and bodycolour on grey paper, $7\frac{9}{16} \times 11\frac{1}{16}$ (19.2 × 28.1)
Inscr. bottom left: '8V'
Trustees of the British Museum (T.B.CCCXVII–20)
The evidence provided by the inscription that Turner was numbering a series of Venice views suggests his practice of about 1840 (cf. the Lucerne series with 'L' numbers, e.g. CCCLXIV–182, 183, etc.). The colour of these Venice studies on grey paper is often identical with that of white-paper watercolours generally agreed to date from 1840. Although the Campanile of St. Mark's was covered with scaffolding in 1840, but probably not in 1833, it seems likely that in most cases Turner omitted the scaffolding and indicated in his drawings what he knew to be the architecture beneath it (see, however, No.558).

The technique of this series of drawings on grey paper is similar to that of the views on the Rhine and at Botzen, on paper of the same type and size, CCCLXIV–292 to 301 (see No.582).

560 Venice: Interior of a Bedroom 1840
Watercolour and bodycolour on grey paper, $8\frac{15}{16} \times 11\frac{13}{16}$ (22.7 × 30)
Inscr. on verso: 'J.M.W.T. Bedroom at Venice' and 'F' (?)
Trustees of the British Museum (T.B.CCCXVII–34)

561 Venice: the Entrance to the Grand Canal with the Campanile and Doge's Palace 1840
Pencil, watercolour and bodycolour with some coloured chalk on grey paper, $7\frac{7}{16} \times 11$ (18.9 × 28)
Trustees of the British Museum (T.B.CCCXVII–5)

562 Venice: the Campanile of St. Mark's from the Roof of the Hotel Europa; Moonlight 1840
Watercolour and bodycolour on brown paper, $9\frac{3}{8} \times 12\frac{1}{8}$ (23.8 × 30.7)
Trustees of the British Museum (T.B.CCCXVIII–5)
A similar view is T.B.CCCXVI–36 (No.557).

563 Venice: a Display of Fireworks seen from the Zattere 1840
Watercolour and bodycolour with white chalk on brown paper, $8\frac{7}{8} \times 11\frac{11}{16}$ (22.5 × 29.7)
Inscr. on verso: '12' (?)
Trustees of the British Museum (T.B.CCCXVIII–10)

564 Venice: a Scene from a Play? 1840
Watercolour and bodycolour on brown paper, $9 \times 11\frac{9}{16}$ (22.9 × 29.3)
Inscr. on verso: '16' (?)
Trustees of the British Museum (T.B.CCXVIII–12)
Finberg calls this drawing 'Interior of a Church with Figures', but it seems more likely that it belongs to the series of scenes at a play (see No.565).

565 Venice: Two Women at a Window, below which stand Two Men 1840
Watercolour and bodycolour with white chalk on brown paper, $9\frac{5}{16} \times 12\frac{5}{16}$ (23.6 × 31.3)
Inscr. on verso: '26' (?)
Trustees of the British Museum (T.B.CCCXVIII–20)
Finberg conjectures that the subject is a scene from a play, possibly *The Merchant of Venice*. The interior of a theatre, which appears unquestionably in CCLXVIII–18 and less certainly in CCCXVIII–4 (No.566), both executed on the same brown paper as is this drawing, suggest that Turner may well have recorded his impressions of a play in this series. f.17 of this group appears to show a theatrical scene – Finberg suggests the murder of Desdemona by Othello; but the nudity of the figure on the bed is perhaps not consistent with such an interpretation. f.12 (No.564), may also record a scene from a play; and f.22, described as a 'Canal Scene', with its illuminated archway, may possibly show some place of entertainment connected with the theatre, or with the firework display shown in f.10 (No.563).

In 1837 Turner showed at the Academy an oil painting called 'Scene – a Street in Venice' with a brief quotation from *The Merchant of Venice* (Huntington Library and Art Museum, San Marino).

566 Venice: an Open-Air Theatre? 1840
Watercolour and bodycolour on brown paper, $8\frac{7}{8} \times 11\frac{1}{2}$ (22.6 × 29.2)
Inscr. on verso: '1' (?)
Trustees of the British Museum (T.B.CCCXVIII–4)

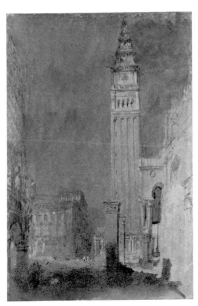

558

16. The Alps and Central Europe 1836–45

In the late summer of 1836 Turner went to the Continent with H. A. J. Munro of Novar, a Scottish landowner and amateur artist. They travelled through France and Switzerland to the Val d'Aosta. This journey with an old friend and patron may have led to Turner's renewed interest in mountain subjects for oil paintings. Turner also visited the Alps more than once in the early 1840s, usually travelling via Germany which also supplied him with subjects for finished pictures. In 1842 and 1843 he invited commissions for finished watercolours of Swiss subjects through the dealer Thomas Griffith, a new and not altogether successful way of appealing to a wider public; see p.161.

**567 Snow-Storm, Avalanche, and Inundation –
a Scene in the Upper Part of Val D'Aout,
Piedmont** R.A.1837
Oil on canvas, 36 × 48¼ (91.5 × 122.5)
Exh: R.A. 1837 (480);
British Institution 1841 (104)
*Art Institute of Chicago (Frederick T. Haskell
Collection)*

Turner revisited the Alps in the summer of 1836 in company with his friend and patron H. A. J. Munro of Novar, who subsequently bought this picture; one of the places they visited was the Val d'Aosta. In this picture Turner returned to both the scene and the dominant vortex of 'Hannibal crossing the Alps' of twenty-five years earlier (see No.88). Here the application of paint is much more uniform, furthering the impression that all the elements in the painting, whether solid or vaporous, are united in the cataclysmic force of nature. Only the figures stand apart from this overall treatment, small puny victims of the irresistible storm.

Blackwood's Magazine, never the most appreciative of Turner's critics, spent most of its review in the July–December number attacking Turner's other contributions to the 1837 exhibition, but dismissed this work as 'an excuse for as much white as he pleases . . . Has any accident befallen Mr. Turner's eyes? Have they been put out by his own colours?'. The *Spectator* for 6 May on the other hand termed it 'extraordinary for colour and effect'.

This picture was exhibited again at the British Institution in 1841 together with 'Rockets and Blue Lights (close at hand) to warn Steam-Boats of Shoal Water', previously exhibited at the Royal Academy the year before (Clark Art Institute, Williamstown, Mass.; repr. Rothenstein and Butlin 1964, pl.113). Both were savagely attacked in the *Athenaeum* for 6 February 1841: 'We have heard of a caricature current in Rome, in which a painter was seen charging a pistol with gamboge, carmine, and ultramarine, his easel standing for target . . . In his Snow-Storm . . . he [Turner] has loaded his weapon of offence with such pigments as the Quakers love, and shot a round of drab, dove-colour, and dirty white, with only a patch of hot, southern red, in the foreground, to heighten, as it were, the horrors of a snow scene by a few *probable* touches of fire and sunshine. To speak of these works as pictures, would be an

abuse of language.' Other reviewers mixed praise with the usual complaints of extravagance. For the *Spectator*, 6 February, it was 'a wondrous arrangement of tints, and one can make out something like a chaos of elements; but the scene wants alpine grandeur'. For the *Art Union*, 15 February, both pictures were 'Wonderful, as examples of colour – prodigious as eccentric flights of genius. They would be equally effective, equally pleasing, and equally comprehensible if turned upside-down; indeed we are not quite sure that one of them has not actually been reversed.'

568 Mountain Scene, perhaps the Val d'Aosta
c.1835–40   (repr. on p.165)
Oil on canvas, 36 × 48 (91.5 × 122)
National Gallery of Victoria, Melbourne

This picture, which, like the 'Landscape' from the Louvre (see No.620), was formerly in the Groult collection in Paris, is one of the small group that 'got away' from the Turner Bequest. Some can be traced back to the descendants of Turner's housekeeper (see No.623) but no early history is known in this case. The title is, therefore, based on supposition but there is a strong possibility that this picture and the two smaller oils in the Turner Bequest (Nos.569 and 570) were the result of the same visit to the Alps that produced 'Snow-Storm, Avalanche, and Inundation – a Scene in the Upper Part of the Val d'Aout, Piedmont', exhibited in 1837 (No.567). In fact this picture may well be an 'unfinished' beginning of a companion work. On the other hand, it is just possible that the composition, like several other 'unfinished' oils of this character, was derived from a *Liber Studiorum* subject. There is some resemblance, particularly in the fairly sharply differentiated foreground, to 'Ben Arthur', R.69, published on 1 June 1819 and classified as 'M' for Mountainous.

The picture may have been that referred to in a letter by Camille Pissarro written in June 1894 to his son Lucien, describing an exhibition of English pictures then being held in Paris, which included 'two Turners belonging to Groult, which are quite beautiful'. At that time Groult owned only two genuine Turners, the Louvre 'Landscape' and this picture, although he was soon to acquire 'Ancient Italy – Ovid banished from Rome' (private collection, Portugal).

569 Mountain Landscape with Hut c.1835–40
Oil on canvas, 28 × 38 (71 × 96.5)
Tate Gallery (5476)
570 Mountain Landscape c.1835–40
Oil on canvas, 28 × 38 (71 × 96.5)
Tate Gallery (5486)

These two landscapes, never before exhibited and cleaned specially for the exhibition, probably date from about the same time as the larger oil from Melbourne (see No.568).

571 Not exhibited
572 Not exhibited
573 Not exhibited

574 Heidelberg *c.*1840–5
Oil on canvas, 52 × 79½ (132 × 201)
Tate Gallery (518)

A large finished picture of the kind normally exhibited by Turner, but for some reason this particular work does not seem to have been shown at the Academy or anywhere else during his lifetime. The German subject and general composition are similar to the 'Opening of the Walhalla, 1842', exhibited in 1843 (Tate Gallery 533), there being the same rather hectic air of festivity.

In this case the costumes suggest that Turner was alluding to the short-lived court of the 'Winter Queen', Elizabeth sister of Charles I, who married Frederick Elector Palatine but who spent most of her life in exile after the failure of his attempt to hold the crown of Bohemia.

There are a number of sketches of Heidelberg, Frederick's original capital, in the 'Spires and Heidelberg' sketchbook and the 'Heidelberg up to Salzburg' sketchbook of 1840 (T.B.CCXCVII and CCXCVIII; see No.577 and also Nos.586–8). Turner has restored the castle, which was partly destroyed by the French in 1689.

575 'Dresden' Sketchbook ?1833
Bound in marbled boards
40 leaves, the majority drawn on in pencil, 6¼ × 4 (15.9 × 9.8)
Trustees of the British Museum (T.B.CCCI)

ff.3ᵛ–4ʳ Two views of Dresden
Pencil

Other studies of Dresden occur in the 'Dresden and Berlin' sketchbook (No.576). The inside cover contains German phrases written in Turner's and other hands. Finberg qualified the title of this sketchbook with a question-mark but there is no doubt that it was used in Dresden.

576 'Dresden and Berlin' Sketchbook ?1833
Bound in marbled boards, leather spine and corners
59 leaves, all drawn on in pencil, 6½ × 3½ (16.1 × 8.7)
Inscr. inside front cover: '1813'
Trustees of the British Museum (T.B.CCCVII)

f.6ᵛ–6ʳ Studies of Paintings in the Royal Gallery, Dresden
Pencil
Inscr: with colour notes, and, top right: 'Sporer Strasse' f.8ʳ left

Called simply 'Dresden' by Finberg, this sketchbook is renamed 'Dresden and Berlin' here to distinguish it from the 'Dresden' sketchbook, T.B.CCCI. The first two leaves are taken up with German phrases and their translations; it seems likely that this book was in use at the same time as Turner's other Dresden sketchbook (No.575), which also contains German phrases. Both books seem to belong to the 1833 tour which took Turner from Berlin to Vienna and on to Venice. ff.20–31 seem to have been used in Berlin.

Ff.6ʳ–7ᵛ contain rough pencil sketches of the paintings in the Dresden Gallery, including Raphael's 'Sis-

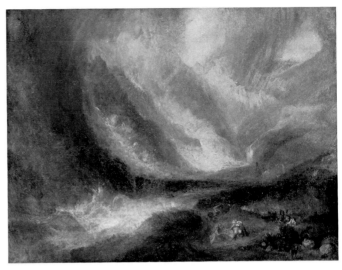

567

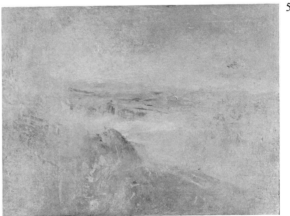

570

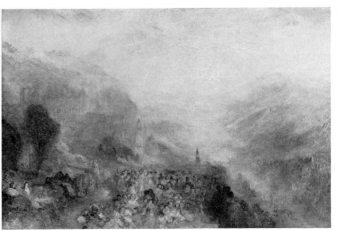

574

tine Madonna', Correggio's 'Mary Magdalen reading' and Aert van Gelder's 'Presentation of Christ'. The exhibited pages show studies after Correggio's 'Madonna of St George', 'Madonna of St Francis' and 'Madonna of St Sebastian', with a sketch of a 'Fête Champêtre' by Watteau. There is also a thumbnail sketch of a street in Dresden.

577 'Heidelberg up to Salzburg' Sketchbook
?c.1835
Bound in marbled boards
98 leaves, almost all drawn on in pencil, $6\frac{1}{2} \times 4$ (16.3 × 10.1)
Inscr. inside front cover: 'Heidelberg up to Salzburg'
Trustees of the British Museum (T.B.CCXVIII)

ff.16ᵛ–17ʳ **Two views in Heidelberg**
Pencil

Sketches made on a journey from Heidelberg through Ludwigsburg, Cannstadt, Kirchheim, and Ulm, presumably to Augsberg, and thence to Munich, Wasserburg and Salzburg. Many of the drawings are the briefest notes made from a moving carriage, with names scribbled on them. The book was opened at random, no sequence being followed. The most extensive series in any one place is the group of views of Munich, ff.55–60, 71ᵛ, and 82ʳ. It is not certain in which year Turner made this journey.

578 'Rhine, Frankfurt, Nuremberg and Prague' Sketchbook ?1835
Bound in marbled boards, cloth spine and corners
102 leaves, nearly all drawn on in pencil, $7\frac{1}{2} \times 4\frac{1}{2}$ (19 × 11.5)
Trustees of the British Museum (T.B.CCCIV)

f.79ʳ **Extensive view of Prague**
Pencil
f.78ᵛ **Rough sketches made in Prague, showing the city and the river**
Pencil

The book contains sketches made principally on the Rhine, at Frankfurt-am-Main, Nuremberg and Prague.
   f.79ʳ shows Prague with the Cathedral of St. Veit on the hill, and the Nicolauskirche in the foreground. One of a long series of sketches of Prague, including panoramas from many points and views of the Rathaus, Brucketurm, Cathedral, etc. ff.65–102.

579 'Val d'Aosta' Sketchbook c.1834–6
Bound in buff boards, leather spine
92 leaves (f.30 missing) all drawn on in pencil, $4\frac{1}{2} \times 7\frac{1}{4}$ (11.3 × 18.5)
Watermarked: 1828
Inscr. on front cover: 'Vale D'Aouste'; and on back cover: 'Stratford-upon-Avon' and '5 Leaves after France and Italy' (transcribed by Finberg, now illegible)
Trustees of the British Museum (T.B.CCXCIII)

ff.52ᵛ–53ʳ **Views of Lausanne**
Pencil

Contains material sketched in Switzerland on a tour

with H. A. J. Munro of Novar in the summer of 1836. In spite of the inscription recorded by Finberg there appear to be no Italian subjects in the book. Among the sketches made at Stratford at the back is a study of the Shakespeare monument used for an illustration to *Scott's Prose Works*, 1834 (Rawlinson No.524).

580 'Rotterdam' Sketchbook ?1840
Bound in marbled boards, leather spine
57 leaves, the majority drawn on in pencil, $6 \times 3\frac{3}{4}$ (15.3 × 9.5)
Trustees of the British Museum (T.B.CCCXXI)

f.14ᵛ **View of Brill in the Rain**
Pencil, with another view of rain over the land sketched below it
f.15ʳ **Two slight sketches of Boats**
Pencil

Bachrach dates this sketchbook and the 'Rotterdam and Rhine' sketchbook (T.B.CCCXXII) to Autumn 1841, presumably following Finberg's suggestion (1961, p.384) that Turner was then in Holland. Finberg (1909, II, pp.1033–5) gives a general date of 1837–41 for these books. Holland was frequently the starting and finishing-point for Turner's numerous Continental tours during this period. The 'Rotterdam to Venice' sketchbook (T.B.CCCXX) must have been in use in 1840, the only year after 1833 in which Turner seems to have visited Venice. The sketch of Rotterdam with the churches of St. Dominicus (built about 1836 according to Bachrach) and St. Lawrence on f.2ʳ of that book seems to belong to the same visit as do those of similar views in the 'Rotterdam' sketchbook, ff.1ᵛ, 2ᵛ and it may be, therefore, that this book belongs to the same year as the last Venetian journey, i.e. 1840.

581 Snow-Covered Mountains ?1836
Watercolour, $9\frac{5}{8} \times 12\frac{1}{16}$ (24.8 × 30.6)
Trustees of the British Museum (T.B.CCCLXIV–93)
Although very different in colouring this view may be the same as that in the Fitzwilliam drawing (No.1612) known as 'Monte Rosa from the Val d'Aosta'. Another drawing called 'Monte Rosa' is at Edinburgh (Vaughan Bequest, 887) but the identification of the mountain has been questioned. This drawing may be one of those which resulted from Turner's tour of the Alps in 1836 with H. A. J. Munro of Novar.

582 Mainz ?1840
Pencil, watercolour and bodycolour with pen and blue and red colour on blue paper, $7\frac{5}{8} \times 11\frac{1}{8}$ (19.3 × 28.2)
Trustees of the British Museum (T.B.CCCLXIV–293)
One of a sequence of views, apparently on the Rhine and at Botzen, which corresponds closely in type with a group made in Venice probably in 1840 (CCCXVII–1 to 5; see Nos. 559 and 561) which are listed by Finberg with numerous other subjects on grey paper (T.B. CCCXVII–6 to 34).

583 Oberwesel 1840
Watercolour and bodycolour with scraping-out, $13\frac{5}{8} \times 20\frac{3}{4}$ (34.5 × 53)
Inscr. bottom right: 'IMWT. 1840'
Private Collection

Engraved by J. T. Willmore, 1842, for Finden's *Royal Gallery of British Art*, in which prints of 'Lake Nemi' (B.M.1958-7-12-444) and the 'Fighting Temeraire' also appeared (Rawlinson 660). The hot colour and extensive scraping-out of this drawing are characteristic of the flamboyant manner of Turner's finished watercolours at the end of the 1830s. It immediately precedes the softer, broader style of the late Swiss watercolours, which some of his regular patrons found unacceptable because of their extreme fluidity and atmospheric 'disintegration', a development clearly foreshadowed in the surface 'sparkle' of 'Oberwesel'. It is possible that Turner's almost excessive use of scattered lights at this period is a reflection of the late mannerism of Constable (d.1837).

A number of pencil sketches of Oberwesel occur in the 'Trèves to Cochem' sketchbook of 1834 (T.B.CCXC, ff.76ʳ etc.) and in the 'Brussels up to Mannheim' sketchbook of about 1840 (T.B.CCXCVI, f.62ᵛ etc.), but none seems to correspond with the subject of this watercolour.

584 Passau *c.*1840
Pencil and watercolour, $8\frac{5}{16} \times 10\frac{15}{16}$ (21.2 × 27.8)
Trustees of the British Museum (T.B.CCCXL–3)
The subject was tentatively identified as Grenoble by Finberg, who on the strength of that hypothesis called the sketchbook (T.B.CCXL) 'Grenoble?'. It is clear, however, that the town represented is that which appears in the 'Coburg, Bamberg and Venice' sketchbook (T.B.CCCX, ff.55, 56). Many drawings in both CCCXL and CCCX can be identified as showing sites on the Danube near Ratisbon, including the 'Walhalla', completed in 1840.

585 Fribourg *c.*1841
Pencil and watercolour with pen and red and grey colour, $9\frac{3}{16} \times 13\frac{3}{16}$ (23.3 × 33.5)
Trustees of the British Museum (T.B.CCCXXXV–19)
The economical style of this drawing, which relies on a combination of very broad, delicately coloured washes and work with a pen dipped in red colour, is typical of a large group of views made in roll sketchbooks (soft covered books which could be rolled up; see No.618) along the Rhine and the Neckar and in Switzerland in about 1840–1. Many of the Venetian subjects (see e.g. Nos.553, 554) use the same technique, but in these drawings Turner is conspicuously reticent in his use of colour, very often creating effects which are almost monochrome.

586 Heidelberg by Moonlight *c.*1841
Watercolour with some pencil and pen, $9\frac{5}{16} \times 11\frac{7}{8}$ (23.7 × 30.1)
Trustees of the British Museum (T.B.CCCLXIV–325)

587 Heidelberg *c.*1835–40
Pencil and watercolour, $19\frac{1}{16} \times 27\frac{1}{4}$ (48.4 × 69.3)
Watermarked: 1794
Inscr. bottom centre with various numerals; and top left with further numerals and '10 Mar 41'
Trustees of the British Museum (T.B.CCCLXV–34)
A preparatory study for No.588.

588 Heidelberg, Sunset *c.*1835–40
Pencil, watercolour and bodycolour, $14\frac{5}{16} \times 21\frac{3}{8}$ (36.4 × 54.2)
City Art Gallery, Manchester
The composition is close to that of a view of Heidelberg of about 1842 in the Vaughan Bequest, National Gallery of Scotland; but in details of style and colouring both this and the preliminary study (No.587) seem to be earlier in date, say about 1835. The inscription on the study suggests that it was made in 1841 and that the finished watercolour was therefore executed at about that time; but it may be susceptible of a different interpretation. An extremely rough pencil sketch of the town from this viewpoint is on f.16ʳ of the 'Heidelberg up to Salzburg' sketchbook; more detailed studies of groups of buildings are on ff.14, 15ᵛ and elsewhere in the same book. The 'Berne, Heidelberg and Rhine' sketchbook (T.B.CCCXXVI) contains a series of views of the town from the opposite bank of the Neckar (ff.39 and 42) which probably formed the immediate basis of the composition.

17. The Great Swiss Watercolours 1840–46

In the early 1840s Turner seems to have been content to return year after year to the same familiar spots – the lakes of Switzerland, especially Lake Lucerne, became an almost obsessive preoccupation. Their scenery stimulated him to produce quantities of brilliant colour sketches and finished watercolours of a type quite different from the successful works of his earlier years. But his idea that they would prove equally popular was miscalculated. In his series of studies of the Rigi Turner records one dramatic landmark in many different lights, as he had done before with Fonthill and Ehrenbreitstein; but here he brings his contemplation of nature to a level of elegiac grandeur which is the culminating utterance of his life as a landscape painter.

In his 'Epilogue' to the Fine Art Society Exhibitions of 1878 and 1900, Ruskin recounted at length the circumstances under which Turner's two late series of Swiss watercolours came into being:

In the years 1840 and 1841, Turner had been, I believe, for the greater part of his summers in Switzerland, and . . . had filled, for his own pleasure, many note-books with sketches . . . [One of these, Dazio Grande] with fourteen others, was placed by Turner in the hands of Mr Griffith of Norwood, in the winter

582

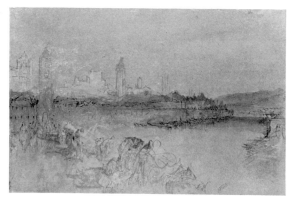

583

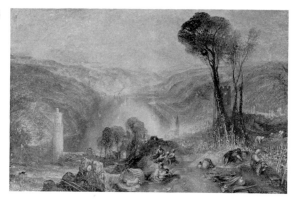

585

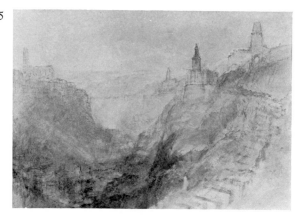

590

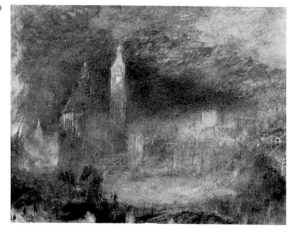

of 1841–2, as giving some clue to, or idea of, drawings which he proposed to make from them, if any buyers of such productions could by Mr Griffith's zeal be found.

There were, therefore, in all, fifteen sketches, of which Turner offered the choice to his public; but he proposed only to make *ten* drawings. And of these ten, he made anticipatorily four, to manifest what their quality would be, and honestly 'show his hand' (as Raphael to Dürer) at his sixty-five years of age, – whether it shook or not, or had otherwise lost its cunning.

Four thus exemplary drawings I say he made for specimens, or *signs*, as it were, for his re-opened shop, namely:

1 The Pass of Splügen [see No.604].
2 Mont Righi, seen from Lucerne, in the morning, dark against dawn [No.599].
3 Mont Righi, seen from Lucerne, at evening, red with the last rays of sunset [No.603].
4 Lake Lucerne (the Bay of Uri) from above Brunnen, with exquisite blue and rose mists and 'mackerel' sky on the right.

And why he should not have made all the ten, to his own mind, at once, who shall say? . . . why . . . of these direct impressions from the nature which he had so long loved, should he have asked anybody to choose which he should realise? So it was, however; partly, it seems, in uncertainty whether anybody would care to have them at all . . . .

One day, then, early in 1842, Turner brought the four drawings above-named, and the fifteen sketches in a roll in his pocket, to Mr Griffith (in Waterloo Place, where the sale-room was).

I have no reason to doubt the substantial accuracy of Mr Griffith's report of the first conversation. Says Mr Turner to Mr Griffith, 'What do you think you can get for such things as these?'

Says Mr Griffith to Mr Turner: 'Well, perhaps, commission included, eighty guineas each.'

Says Mr Turner to Mr Griffith: 'Ain't they worth more?'

Says Mr Griffith to Mr Turner: (after looking curiously into the execution which, you will please note, is rather what some people might call hazy) 'They're a little different from your usual style' – (Turner silent, Griffith does not push the point) – 'but – but – yes, they are *worth* more, but I could not *get* more.' . . .

So the bargain was made that if Mr Griffith could sell ten drawings – the four signs, to wit, and six others – for eighty guineas each, Turner would make six others from such of the fifteen sketches as the purchasers chose, and Griffith should have ten per cent, *out* of the eight hundred total (Turner had expected a thousand, I believe).

So then Mr Griffith thinks over the likely persons to get commissions from, out of all England for ten drawings by Turner! and these not quite in his usual style, too, and he sixty-five years old . . .

He sent to Mr Munro of Novar, Turner's old companion in travel; he sent to Mr Windus of Tottenham; he sent to Mr Bicknell of Herne Hill; he sent to my father and me.

Mr Windus of Tottenham came first, and at once

said 'the style was changed, he did not quite like it . . . He would not have any of these drawings.' I, as Fors would have it, came next . . . The Splügen Pass I saw in an instant to be the noblest Alpine drawing Turner had ever till then made; and the red Rhigi, such a piece of colour as had never come *my* way before. I wrote to my Father, saying I would fain have that Splügen Pass, if he were home in time to see it, and gave me leave . . . .

Mr Bicknell of Herne Hill bought the blue Rhigi, No.2 . . .

Then Mr Munro of Novar, and bought the Lucerne Lake, No.4 (and the red Rhigi?) and both Mr Munro and Mr Bicknell chose a sketch to be 'realized' – Mr Bicknell, another Lucerne Lake; and Mr Munro, a Zürich, with white sunshine in distance.

So . . . Three out of the four pattern drawings he had shown were really bought – 'And not *that*' said Turner, shaking his fist at the Pass of Splügen; but said no more! . . .

Munro of Novar came again . . . and made up his mind, and bought the Pass of Splügen . . . .

. . . only nine drawings could be got orders for, and there poor Mr Griffith was. Turner growled; but said at last he would do the nine, i.e. the five more to be realized.

He set to work in the spring of 1842; after three or four weeks, he came to Mr Griffith, and said, in growls, at intervals, 'The drawings were well forward, and he had after all put the tenth in hand, out of those no one would have; he thought it would turn out as well as any of them; if Griffith liked to have it for his commission he might.' Griffith agreed, and Turner went home content, and finished the ten drawings for seven hundred and twenty guineas, cash clear . . . .

Four or five years ago – Mr Vokins knows when, he came out to me saying he wanted a first-rate Turner drawing, had I one to spare?

'Well,' I said, 'I have none to spare, yet I have a reason for letting *one* first-rate one go, if you give me a price.'

'What will you take?'

'A thousand pounds.'

Mr Vokins wrote me the cheque in Denmark Hill drawing-room, . . . and took the Lucerne . . . .

I wished to get *dead* Turner, for one drawing, his own original price for the whole ten, and thus did. Of the remaining eight drawings, this is the brief history.

Mr Munro some years afterwards would have allowed me to have the Splügen Pass, for four hundred pounds, through White of Maddox Street; my father would then have let me take it for that, but I myself thought it hard on him and me, and would not, thinking it would too much pain my father. It remained long in the possession of Mr Munro's nephew; so also the Novar Lucerne Lake, and Zürich. But of that, and of the red Righi, there were at first vicissitudes that are too long to tell; only when the ten drawings were finished, and at Waterloo Place, their possession was distributed thus:

1	Splügen [see No.604]	Munro of Novar
2	Blue Rhigi [No.601]	Mr Bicknell
3	Red Righi [No.603]	Munro of Novar
4	Lucerne Lake	Munro of Novar
5	Lucerne Lake [No.608]	Mr Bicknell
6	Lucerne Town [No.607]	J R
7	Coblentz	J R
8	Constance	Mr Griffith
9	Dark Righi	Munro of Novar
10	Zürich [No.605]	Munro of Novar

Mr Griffith soon afterwards let me have the Constance for eighty guineas and the day I bought that drawing home to Denmark Hill was one of the happiest in my life.

Turner had never made any drawings like these before, and never made any like them again. But he offered in the next year (1843), to do ten more on the same terms. But now – only five commissions could be got. My father allowed me to give two: Munro of Novar took three. Nobody could take any more. Turner was angry; and partly ill, drawing near the end, you perceive. He did the five, but it was lucky there were no more to do.

The five were:

1	Küssnacht [No.609]	Munro of Novar
2	Zug [No.606]	Munro of Novar
3	(I forget at this moment Munro's third.) I think it was the Zürich by Moonlight, level over the rippling Limmat; a noble drawing, but not up to the mark of the rest.	
4	Goldau [No.611]	J R
5	St Gothard [No.612]	J R

Turner did not, however, altogether cease to make watercolours of Swiss views for sale to patrons. A few subjects were executed for Ruskin, Munro and Windus between 1843 and c.1846; see for example Nos.614–616.

589 Lake of Brientz *c.*1841
Watercolour and bodycolour, $9\frac{1}{8} \times 11\frac{5}{16}$
(23.1 × 28.8)
Sir Edmund Bacon, Bart.
From Ruskin's collection.

590 A Conflagration, Lausanne *c.*1841
Watercolour and bodycolour, $9\frac{1}{2} \times 12$
(23.8 × 30.5)
Whitworth Art Gallery, Manchester (D.6.1912)
The measurements correspond with those of Lot 66 of the J. E. Taylor sale Christie's 5 July 1912, which is described in the catalogue as 'Lausanne: a View of the Town and Cathedral: Evening Light', and this drawing may possibly be identified with that. The sheet is probably a page from one of the broken-up roll sketchbooks of Swiss subjects, T.B.CCXXXII, etc.

591 Spiez on the Lake of Thun *c.*1842
Watercolour, $9\frac{7}{8} \times 13\frac{7}{8}$ (24.5 × 35.2)
Mrs C.G. Keith
The subject was known in the nineteenth century as 'Lake Garda'. When the watercolour was shown at Agnew's in 1967 (No.79) it was pointed out that although frequently stated to have belonged to Charles Swinburne, the drawing in fact comes from the collection of John Leigh Clare, in whose sale it appeared, Christie's, 28 March 1868(97). It was subsequently owned by W. G. Rawlinson.

594

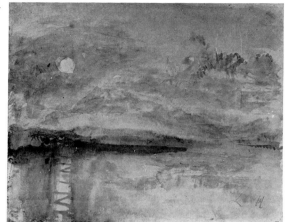

598

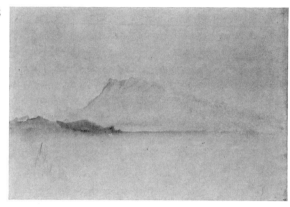

599

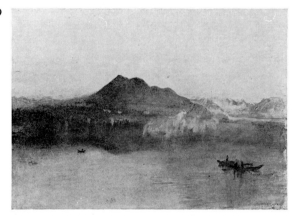

601

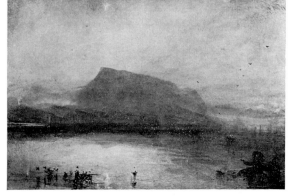

592   Evening: Cloud on Mount Rigi, seen from Zug *c.*1841
Watercolour, $8\frac{9}{16} \times 10\frac{9}{16}$ (21.8 × 26.8)
Visitors of the Ashmolean Museum, Oxford
One of the drawings belonging to Ruskin, which he presented to the Ruskin School, Oxford. The Rigi, a distinctively formed rock facing Lucerne across the lake, had a particular fascination for Turner, who, during his visits to Switzerland of 1840 and 1841, made studies of it over and over again in different lights and climatic conditions. He seems hardly ever to have drawn it in pencil, though there are a few rough notes of it in sketchbooks such as the 'Between Lucerne and Thun' Sketchbook (T.B.CCCXXIX); and sometimes the colour sketches are washed in over a slight outline. They often approach an extreme of delicacy hardly to be paralleled in Turner's output (see No.597). It is an indication of the interest which the Rigi had for him that three of the ten subjects proposed to Griffith in 1841 (see p.163) showed it (see Nos.601 and 603). See also the 'Lucerne' sketchbook, No.618.

593   The Rigi: Last Rays *c.*1841
Watercolour, $9\frac{1}{2} \times 11\frac{3}{4}$ (24.1 × 29.8)
Trustees of the British Museum
(T.B.CCCLXIV–219)

594   The Rigi: Pink, with a Full Moon *c.*1841
Watercolour, $10\frac{7}{8} \times 13\frac{5}{8}$ (27.6 × 34.5)
Inscr. bottom right: 'L11' (?)
Trustees of the British Museum (T.B.CCCLXIV–192)
Many drawings of this date are marked by Turner with 'L' (for Lucerne) and a serial number.

595   The Rigi: with Full Moon and the Spires of Lucerne Cathedral *c.*1841   (repr. on p.166)
Watercolour, $9\frac{3}{16} \times 12\frac{5}{16}$ (23.3 × 31.1)
Trustees of the British Museum (T.B.CCCLXIV–221)

596   The Rigi: with Lucerne in the Foreground *c.*1841
Watercolour with pen, $9\frac{9}{16} \times 11\frac{13}{16}$ (24.3 × 30)
Trustees of the British Museum (T.B.CCLXIV–220)

597   The Rigi: Pale Grey and Yellow *c.*1841
Watercolour, $9\frac{13}{16} \times 14\frac{9}{16}$ (24.9 × 37)
Inscr. bottom centre: 'Stadtz'; bottom right: 'L 18'
Trustees of the British Museum (T.B.CCCLXIV–196)
'Stadtz' may mean Stanz, or Stans, a town on the southern side of Lake Lucerne.

598   The Rigi: Yellow and Pink *c.*1841
Watercolour with pencil, $9\frac{13}{16} \times 14\frac{9}{16}$ (24.9 × 37)
Inscr. bottom right: 'L 9'
Trustees of the British Museum (T.B.CCCLXIV–175)

599   The Rigi: Blue, with Sun rising behind it *c.*1841
Watercolour, $9\frac{1}{16} \times 12\frac{11}{16}$ (23 × 32.2)
Inscr. on verso: 'J. A. Munro Esq. 31'
Trustees of the British Museum (T.B.CCCLXIV–279)
The inscription on the back of this drawing, which is really a completed watercolour in itself, indicates that it was the design submitted to Griffith as a 'sample'

568 **Mountain Scene, perhaps the Val d'Aosta** *c*.1835–40 (entry on p.158)

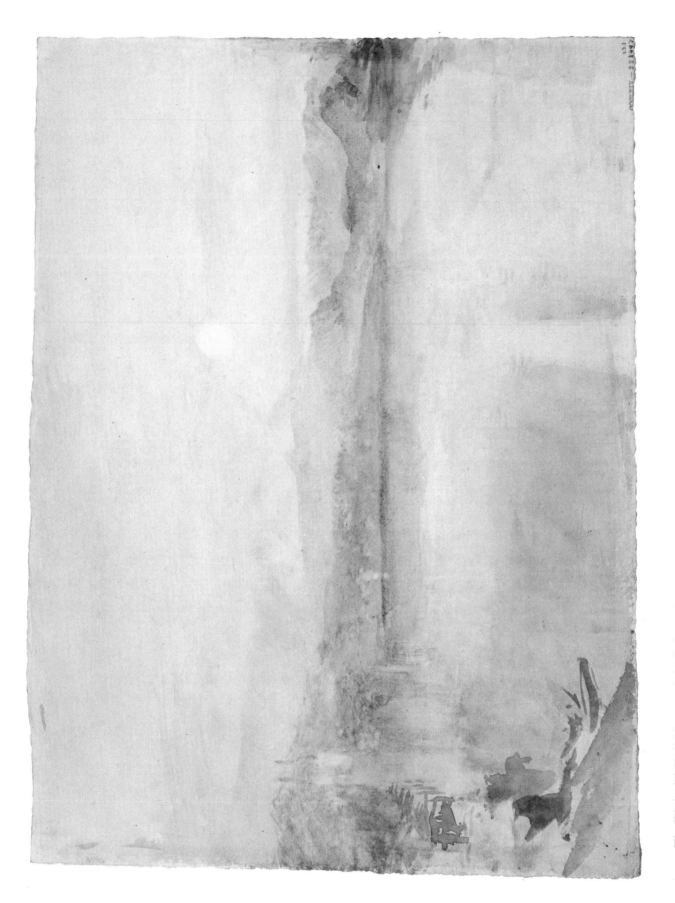

595 **The Rigi with Full Moon and the Spires of Lucerne Cathedral** *c*.1841 (entry on p.164)

composition from which the 'Blue Rigi' (No.601) was developed.

600 Study for the 'Blue Rigi' *c.*1841
Watercolour with some pencil, $8\frac{11}{16} \times 10\frac{5}{8}$ (22 × 27)
Inscr. bottom right: 'L' (for Lucerne)
Trustees of the British Museum (T.B.CCCLXIV–327)

601 The Blue Rigi: Lake of Lucerne, Sunrise
1842
Watercolour, $11\frac{11}{16} \times 17\frac{3}{4}$ (29.7 × 45)
Private Collection
The second of the set of ten Swiss views made for Griffith in 1842, of which Ruskin said 'Turner had never made any drawings like these before, and never made any like them again'; the 'Red Rigi' (No.603) was the third. The 'specimen' drawing from which this watercolour was developed is No.599. The 'Blue Rigi' was bought by Elhanan Bicknell of Herne Hill.

602 Study for the 'Red Rigi' *c.*1841
Watercolour, $9 \times 11\frac{15}{16}$ (22.8 × 30.3)
Trustees of the British Museum (T.B.CCCLXIV–275)

603 The Red Rigi 1842
Watercolour, 12×18 (30.5 × 45.8)
National Gallery of Victoria, Melbourne
One of the ten Swiss drawings of 1842; No.3 in Ruskin's list. It was bought by Munro of Novar, and subsequently owned by Ruskin, J. E. Taylor and R. A. Tatton. The preparatory watercolour is in the Turner Bequest (No.602), and another study was shown at Agnew's exhibition, *Turner*, 1967 (85).

604 Splügen *c.*1841
Pencil and watercolour, $9\frac{9}{16} \times 12$ (24.2 × 30.5)
Trustees of the British Museum (T.B.CCCLXIV–277)
'Splügen' was No.1 in Ruskin's list of the ten Swiss watercolours of 1842; it was bought by Munro and is now in a private collection in America (repr. Agnew, *Turner*, 1967, No.86). This drawing is a fully worked-out watercolour in its own right, and served as the basis for Munro's version of the subject, in which the scale of the rock on the left is considerably enlarged.

Another view up the valley towards Splügen is T.B. CCCXXXVI–11, but it has neither the tower on the rock nor the straight road which are characteristic of this design. The drawings of Splügen in the 'Como and Splügen' sketchbook (T.B.CCCXXXVIII, inside cover and f.16) are even further removed from the present watercolour.

605 Zürich *c.*1842
Watercolour over traces of pencil, $9\frac{9}{16} \times 11\frac{7}{8}$
(24.2 × 30.2)
Trustees of the British Museum (T.B.CCCLXIV–291)
Used as the basis of the drawing bought by Munro in 1842 and now B.M.1958-7-12-445. Another view over Zürich, predominantly yellow rather than blue, is T.B. CCCLXIV–289.

606 Arth, from the Lake of Zug *c.*1842
Pencil and watercolour with some pen, $8\frac{15}{16} \times 11\frac{3}{8}$
(22.7 × 28.9)
Inscr. on verso: 'Arth – Lake of Zug. No.9';

'X 810' and 'Mr Munro'
Trustees of the British Museum (T.B.CCCLXIV–280)
This is apparently the 'specimen' drawing for the view of the Lake of Zug which Turner made for Munro in 1843, No. 2 in Ruskin's second list. The drawing was subsequently owned by Ruskin himself, and later by Sir Donald Currie; it is now in the Metropolitan Museum, New York.

607 Lucerne from the Walls 1842
Watercolour with scraping-out, $11\frac{5}{8} \times 17\frac{15}{16}$
(29.5 × 45.5)
Lady Lever Art Gallery, Port Sunlight
Listed by Ruskin as No.6 of the ten Swiss views made in 1842, and the first that he himself bought. It was the drawing he sold to the dealer Vokins for £1,000 as 'I wished to get *dead* Turner, for one drawing, his own original price for the whole ten, and thus did'. The preparatory watercolour of the subject is in the Turner Bequest, CCCLXIV–290. Several rough pencil sketches of parts of Lucerne and its walls are in the 'Lucerne and Berne' sketchbook, T.B.CCCXXVIII–3ᵛ, 4, etc.

608 Brunnen 1842
Watercolour, $11\frac{7}{8} \times 18\frac{1}{4}$ (30.2 × 46.4)
Private Collection
Listed by Ruskin as No.5 of the ten Swiss views made in 1842 and called by him 'Lucerne Lake'. The drawing was bought by Elhanan Bicknell.

609 Küssnacht and William Tell's Chapel on
Lake Lucerne *c.*1841
Pencil and watercolour with pen and scratching-out, $9 \times 11\frac{7}{16}$ (22.9 × 29.1)
Trustees of the British Museum (T.B.CCCLXIV–208)
The subject was used for one of the series of Swiss views made in 1843 for H. A. J. Munro, and now at Manchester City Art Gallery.

610 Goldau with the Lake of Zug in the Distance
*c.*1842
Pencil and watercolour with pen, $9 \times 11\frac{3}{8}$
(22.8 × 28.8)
Inscr. on verso: 'Goldau – Rigi – and the Lake of Zug'
Trustees of the British Museum (T.B.CCCLXIV–281)
An elaborate study preliminary to the 'Goldau' (No. 611), one of the five Swiss subjects made in 1843 and bought by Munro and Ruskin. The view was noted in rough sketches on f.11ʳ&ᵛ of the 'Lake of Zug and Goldau' sketchbook, 1841 (T.B.CCCXXXI).

611 Goldau 1843
Watercolour, $12 \times 18\frac{1}{2}$ (30.5 × 47)
Private Collection
Drawn for Ruskin, who considered it 'on the whole the mightiest drawing of his final time', together with 'The Lake of Zug – early morning', executed for Munro (now Metropolitan Museum of Art, New York). The preliminary watercolour sketch is No.610; it has none of the brilliant red colouring of this more elaborate version. Ruskin wrote: 'He was very definitely in the habit of indicating the association of any subject with circumstances of death, especially the death of multitudes, by placing it under one of his most deeply

607

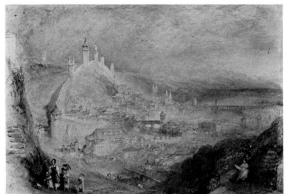

611

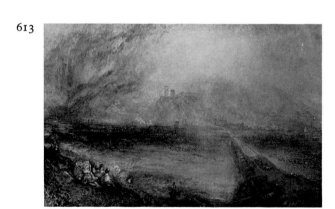

613

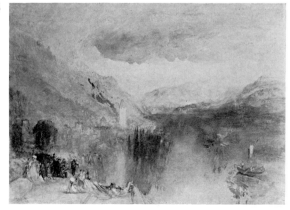

616

crimsoned sunset skies . . . . . The sky of this Goldau is in its scarlet and crimson, the deepest in tone of all that I know in Turner's drawings.'

612 The Pass of Faido, St. Gothard 1843
Watercolour, $12 \times 18\frac{1}{2}$ (30.5 × 47)
Private Collection
One of the five watercolours executed in 1843 and bought by Ruskin and Munro (see also Nos.606 and 611); No.5 in Ruskin's list. The preparatory water-colour on which it is based is T.B.CCCLXIV-209.

613 Bellinzona from the Road to Locarno 1843
Watercolour, $11\frac{1}{2} \times 17\frac{18}{16}$ (29.3 × 45.6)
Aberdeen Art Gallery
Executed, according to Ruskin, for Munro of Novar in 1843, the watercolour is closely based on T.B.CCCXXXII -25 which is inscribed on the verso 'Bellinzona. No.12' and 'Mr Munro'.

614 The Pass of St. Gothard; the First Bridge above Altdorf *c.*1843
Pencil and watercolour and pen, $9\frac{5}{16} \times 11\frac{5}{8}$ (23.7 × 29.5)
Inscr. on verso: 'Altdorf'
Trustees of the British Museum (T.B.CCCLXIV-283)
According to Finberg, this drawing was the basis for a watercolour executed for Ruskin in 1845. The *Inventory* records 'a name (?John Ruskin) which has since been rubbed out' on the back of the drawing. In addition to the watercolour of 1843 (No.612), Ruskin owned several late views of the St. Gothard; he gave three to the University of Cambridge in 1861 (their Nos.586 587, 588) but these were all roll-sketchbook leaves like the present drawing.

615 Pallanza, Lago Maggiore *c.*1845
Watercolour, $14\frac{1}{2} \times 21\frac{1}{4}$ (37 × 54)
Private Collection
A watercolour study of Pallanza is in the Turner Be-quest, CCCLXIV-326.

616 The Lake of Geneva *c.*1846
Watercolour $14\frac{1}{2} \times 21\frac{1}{4}$ (36.8 × 54)
Watermarked: 1846
Mr and Mrs Kurt F. Pantzer, Indianapolis
The catalogue of the Pantzer collection (No.46) says that this watercolour is a companion to the 'Lake of Thun' in the Taft Museum, Cincinnati, and gives 1840 as the probable date; but the recently discovered watermark provides evidence that this is in fact one of the latest of all Turner's finished watercolours. It is even freer in handling than the group usually dated to about 1845, which includes 'Bellinzona' and 'Pallanza' (Nos.613, 615), and is in many ways close to some of the rough sketches of Swiss subjects which may have been made at this date. The subject was probably taken from material gathered during Turner's visit to Geneva in the summer of 1841, which occasioned a number of pencil sketches of the Lake in the 'Rhine, Flushing and Lausanne' sketchbook (T.B.CCCXXX) and watercolour views of the city in the 'Fribourg, Lausanne and Geneva' sketchbook (T.B.CCCXXXII); there is also a crudely-stitched folder of torn paper, T.B.CCCXLIV-271 to 289, which contains rough

sketches apparently of Lake Geneva. However, no obvious source for the composition of the Pantzer watercolour is among these studies.

617 **'Lake of Zug and Goldau' Sketchbook** 1842
Paper covered notebook with printed Almanack for 1842 on back cover
32 leaves of pencil sketches, 7 × 3 (17.4 × 7.5)
Trustees of the British Museum (T.B.CCCXXXI)

ff.20ᵛ–21ʳ **Views of various towns**
Pencil

618 **'Lucerne' Sketchbook** 1844
Paper covers

24 leaves, the majority drawn on in watercolour with some pencil (ff.4–9 blank), 9 × 12¾ (22.9 × 32.7)
Watermarked: 1844
Trustees of the British Museum (T.B.CCCXLV)

f.12ᵛ **The Rigi at Sunset, with Lucerne Cathedral**
Watercolour

The majority of the studies in this roll sketchbook seem to be of the Lake of Lucerne; the Rigi appears on ff.13ᵛ, 15ᵛ, 16ᵛ, 17ᵛ, 18ᵛ, 20ᵛ, 24ᵛ.

18. Last Works 1835–50

Many of Turner's late unfinished oils seem to imitate his late watercolours in their washes of delicate colour over a white ground. Most of these oils remained in his studio and entered the national collection as part of the Turner Bequest, but a surprising number seem to have escaped–surprising in view of their remoteness from what was considered acceptable in the art-market of the mid-nineteenth century. For a discussion of how such works left Turner's studio see under No.620. Another slight peculiarity about this group of oils is the number that are based on earlier *Liber Studiorum* subjects; see Nos.620–23, 650 and ?568.

619 **Monte Rosa** *c.*1835–40
Oil on canvas, 36 × 48 (91.5 × 122)
Mr and Mrs Paul Mellon, Upperville, Virginia
The mountain is seen from Lake Maggiore near Stresa and Pallanza, which Turner could have visited on his way to Venice in 1840 or from Bellinzona in 1841. It may therefore be a bit later than 'Mountain Scene, perhaps the Val d'Aosta' (see No.568) but is similar in status, a 'colour beginning' in oils. On the other hand Turner could have been working from memories of earlier journeys through North Italy, as on the way to Venice in 1819 and 1833.

The early history of this picture, which belonged to Sir Donald Currie by the 1890s, is unknown. For a discussion of how such works escaped being in the Turner Bequest, see under the Louvre landscape, No.620.

620 **Landscape with a River and a Bay in the Distance** *c.*1835–40
Oil on canvas, 37 × 48½ (94 × 123)
Musée du Louvre, Paris
Without any reasonable doubt to be identified with the picture enthusiastically described by Edmond de Goncourt in his *Journal* when he spent 'Un après-midi devant les tableaux anglais de Groult'. This may also be one of the Turners mentioned by Camille Pissarro, in a letter to his son written in June 1894, as being in an exhibition in Paris: '. . . an exhibition of the English School is being held; some superb Reynolds, several very beautiful Gainsboroughs, two Turners belonging to Groult which are quite beautiful . . .'. Camille Groult (died 1907) also owned the 'Mountain Scene' at Melbourne (No.568).

How such pictures left Turner's studio is unknown. Two of the series (see No.623) were sold at Christie's in 1865 from the collection of John Pound, the son by her first marriage of Mrs Sophia Caroline Booth, Turner's mistress and housekeeper in Chelsea. Turner had presumably given these pictures either to her or to her son, but none of the others in the series can be traced back to the Booth/Pound collection (see Michael Kitson, 'Un nouveau Turner au Musée du Louvre' in *La Revue du Louvre* XIX, 1969, p.254). There remains the possibility that they were among the pictures that were rejected from the Turner Bequest by the executors in 1856 on the grounds that they were not genuine. Against this suggestion must be weighed the fact that these exclusions were made by Sir Charles Eastlake, a friend of Turner's who knew his work well, and that he accepted as part of the Bequest a number of canvases which were still less 'finished' than those in this series (see Michael Kitson, 'Nouvelles Précisions sur le "Paysage" de Turner du Musée du Louvre' in *ibid* XXI, 1971, p.90). They may simply have remained as a parcel of unstretched canvases, perhaps rolled up together, and have been stolen from Turner's studio by Mrs Booth or by someone else; Stefan Slabczynski, of the Tate Gallery, who cleaned this picture for the Louvre, reported that it had formerly been rolled, as have been others of this group of works. A letter written by Effie Ruskin to her mother on 24 August 1852, telling her that Ruskin had renounced the executorship of Turner's Will as he was sickened by all the dispute over it, continued '. . . Certain it is that already Turner's lawyer has *stolen* a bag of drawings', which makes it sound as if the studio was open to pilfering of this kind.

This picture belongs to a series of canvases, probably painted about 1835 or shortly afterwards, which are all connected – some more closely than others – with engravings published in the *Liber Studiorum* many years before. In this case, the 'Junction of the Severn and the Wye' (R.28), published in June 1811, and classified as 'E.P.' for Epic, Elegant or Elevated Pastoral, served as the basis, although Chepstow Castle has been omitted from the picture and the composition has in general been very much simplified. Turner's purpose in painting this series (none of which was sold or exhibited during his lifetime) is unclear, but Evelyn Joll suggests that, having made up his mind to leave his pictures to the nation, Turner might have wished to include a cross-section of examples of his late style in his bequest, and that this series formed part of a project which (like the *Liber Studiorum*) he never completed. For further examples of the reworking of *Liber Studiorum* subjects see Nos.621, 622, 623, 650 and ?568; not included in the exhibition are 'The Rape of Europa' after the frontispiece, R.I (Taft Museum, Cincinnati), and 'Walton Bridges' after 'The Bridge in Middle Distance', R.13 (Henry S. Morgan, New York).

621   Falls of the Clyde *c.*1835–40
Oil on canvas, 35 × 47 (89 × 119.5)
Trustees of the Lady Lever Art Gallery, Port Sunlight

One of the group of late 'unfinished' oils based on *Liber Studiorum* subjects, in this case R.18, published 29 March 1809 and classified as 'E.P.' (?Epic Pastoral). Turner had already treated the subject in a watercolour exhibited in 1802 with the sub-title 'Noon' and a reference to Akenside's *Hymn to the Naiads* (Walker Art Gallery, Liverpool). Akenside saw the Naiads as allegorical deities, symbolising the interaction of sun and running water in 'giving motion to the air, and exciting summer breezes'. This late painting was, in its prismatic colouring, much more effective as an allegory about the forces of nature than the early versions (see Gage 1969, pp.144–5, and exhibition catalogue, *Landscape in Britain*, Tate Gallery, 1973–4, No.218).

Turner's use of watercolour on this canvas can be seen in the little droplets where the oil paint has rejected total assimilation. The paint surface also shows vertical cracking from rolling, typical of most if not all of this group of 'unfinished' oils that have escaped the Turner Bequest. For the possible early history of these works see No.620. The first known owner of this picture was the Rev. Thomas Prater in 1871.

622   Sunrise, a Castle on a Bay: 'Solitude'
*c.*1835–40
Oil on canvas, 35¾ × 48 (91 × 122)
Tate Gallery (1985)

Another development of a *Liber Studiorum* composition, 'Solitude', R.53, published 12 May 1814 and classified as 'E.P.' (?Epic Pastoral). The *Liber Studiorum* design is as usual much more detailed and includes the Magdalen, reclining in meditation under the group of trees on the left.

623   Dream of Italy: Woman with Tambourine
*c.*1835–40
Oil on canvas, 34¾ × 46½ (88.5 × 118)
Mrs M. D. Fergusson

Derived closely from the *Liber Studiorum* composition 'The Woman and Tambourine', R.3, published June 1807 and classified as 'E.P.' (?Epic Pastoral) like the other designs used for similar late oils; for a discussion of the group as a whole see No.620.

This is one of the two oils of this size that can be traced to the sale of John Pound, son of Turner's housekeeper Mrs Booth by her first marriage, at Christie's on 25 March 1865; the other was the 'Walton Bridges', sometimes known as 'Italy', in the collection of Henry S. Morgan, New York.

624   River Landscape with Hills behind
*c.*1835–40
Oil on canvas, 36¼ × 48¼ (92 × 122.5)
Walker Art Gallery, Liverpool

Similar in style to other late, thinly painted 'unfinished' oils from the Turner Bequest and elsewhere. Unlike many of this group it is not, however, based on a *Liber Studiorum* design, but Michael Kitson suggests that, like the Louvre and Port Sunlight pictures (Nos.620 and 621) it shows a view generalised from some place in the British Isles ('Nouvelles Précisions sur le "Paysage" de Turner du Musée du Louvre' in *La Revue du Louvre* XXI, 1971, pp.89–93). The painting was probably bought by Robert Durning Holt in the late 1870s but its earlier history is unknown (see Kitson *ibid*, p.90).

625   Sunrise, with a Boat between Headlands
*c.*1835–40
Oil on canvas, 36 × 48 (91.5 × 122)
Tate Gallery (2002)

This is one of the unfinished oil paintings in which Turner approaches closest to his late watercolour style. It appears to be an independent composition, unrelated to any other work, though in many respects it is similar to the oils derived from the *Liber Studiorum* subjects, particularly to 'Norham Castle' (No.650).

626   Yarmouth Roads *c.*1842   (repr. on p.183)
Pencil and watercolour with scraping-out,
9¼ × 13¾ (23.5 × 35)
Trustees of the Lady Lever Art Gallery, Port Sunlight (WHL4716)

The motif of the steamship in a vortex of sea and sky is close to that of the 'Snowstorm: Steam Boat off a Harbour's Mouth' (No.504) exhibited in 1842; though here the tonality is altogether more sombre.

627   Sunset over the Sea   ?*c.*1842
Watercolour, 10 × 15⁹⁄₁₆ (25.4 × 39.5)
Trustees of the British Museum (T.B.CCCLXIV–232)

628   Eu 1845
Pencil and watercolour with some pen and red, brown and mauve colour, 9¹⁄₁₆ × 12¹⁸⁄₁₆ (23 × 32.5)
Trustees of the British Museum (T.B.CCCLIX–13)

Turner visited Eu, Tréport and Dieppe in September 1845 (see No.632).

629   Eu Cathedral 1845
Pencil and watercolour, 9¹⁄₁₆ × 12⅞ (23.1 × 32.7)
Inscr. bottom right: 'E. pine saw mill'(?), 'E P of W Argenteuil'(?)
Trustees of the British Museum (T.B.CCCLIX–16)

Compare with CCCXXXIV-16 (No.630). There is a slight pencil sketch of figures in a square on the verso.

630 A Large Church with a Square beyond 1845
Pencil and watercolour, $9\frac{1}{16} \times 12\frac{7}{8}$ (23.1 × 32.6)
Inscr. top centre: 'all White'
Trustees of the British Museum (T.B.CCCXXXIV-16)
Grouped by Finberg with the 'Lausanne' sketchbook and dated by him to about 1841; the book contains principally views in Lausanne and Berne, but this is apparently a view of Eu Cathedral, taken from a viewpoint very similar to that of CCCLIX-16, made in 1845 (No.629). It seems likely that the two drawings were made at the same time, and indeed probably belonged to the same roll sketchbook.

631 Interior of a Church (Eu Cathedral?) 1845
Pencil and watercolour, $12\frac{7}{8} \times 9\frac{1}{16}$ (32.6 × 23.1)
Trustees of the British Museum (CCCLIX-10)
A similar interior is CCCLIX-7; both are assigned by Finberg to the 'Eu and Tréport' sketchbook, used during Turner's visit to the coast of Picardy in September 1845.

632 'Dieppe' Sketchbook 1845
Paper covers
22 leaves, all drawn on in pencil and watercolour, 9×13 (23 × 32.9)
Watermarked: 1844
Trustees of the British Museum (T.B.CCCLX)

f.23ᵛ: **A brilliantly lit Interior with Figures**
Pencil and watercolour

A roll sketchbook, used on a tour to Dieppe and the coast of Picardy in 1845. The drawing shown is perhaps related in subject to the sketch on f.22ᵛ of figures round a banqueting table with lighted candelabra, and that of an interior with arches and figures, f.21ᵛ. A further drawing which seems to belong to the group (f.20ᵛ) shows a gaslit room with large paintings round the walls; the function represented may have been a Royal Academy Dinner. There is a story (quoted by Finberg, 1961, p.411) that while Turner was at Eu, on this tour, Louis Philippe 'sent to desire his company to dinner (they had been well known to one another in England). Turner strove to apologise – pleaded his want of dress – but this was overruled; his usual costume was the dress-coat of the period, and he was assured that he only required a white neck-cloth, and that the King must not be denied . . . [Turner's landlady] easily provided a white neck-cloth by cutting up some of her linen, and Turner declared that he spent one of the pleasantest evenings in chat with his old Twickenham acquaintance.' It is just possible that the interiors in the 'Dieppe' sketchbook record Turner's dinner with Louis Philippe.

633 Whalers Boiling Blubber *c.*1845
Watercolour and bodycolour and coloured chalks, $8\frac{11}{16} \times 13\frac{1}{8}$ (22.1 × 33.2)
Trustees of the British Museum (T.B.CCCLIII-7)
Connected with the series of paintings representing the activities of whalers which Turner showed at the R.A. in 1845 (50, 77) and 1846 (237, 494) of which the last was 'Whalers (boiling blubber) entangled in flaw ice,

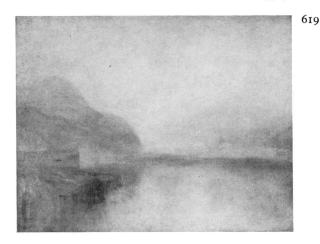
619

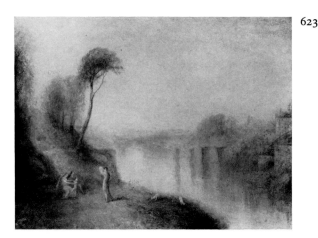
623

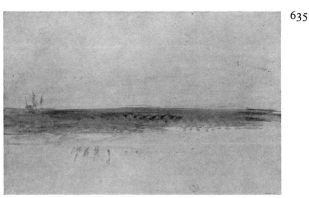
635

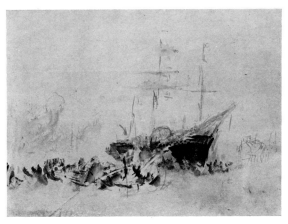
636

endeavouring to extricate themselves' (No.524). This sheet is one of the twenty used leaves of the 'Whalers' sketchbook, which contains a series of studies in the unusual medium of combined coloured chalks and watercolour, some on a grey prepared ground. Another whaling study, very loosely drawn with a little watercolour and inscribed 'He breaks away' is in the Fitzwilliam Museum (PD.116.1950). It probably came from the 'Ambleteuse and Wimereux' sketchbook, T.B.CCCLVII, which contains an impressive watercolour sketch of a floundering whale (repr. Butlin, 1962, pl.31). Whether Turner actually saw the animal during his channel crossing in 1845 is not certain; he had obviously been interested in whales and whaling before that journey.

634 A Rainstorm and Sunshine over the Sea
*c.*1843
Watercolour, $11\frac{3}{4} \times 17\frac{3}{16}$ (29×43.7)
Trustees of the British Museum (T.B.CCCLXV–20)
A similar drawing is T.B.CCCLXV–19.

635 A Sailing Ship at Sea, seen from the Shore
*c.*1843
Watercolour, $11\frac{1}{16} \times 17\frac{1}{2}$ (28.1×44.4)
Trustees of the British Museum (T.B.CCCLXV–21)
One of a series of extremely free atmospheric studies, some of which are on paper watermarked 1837; but one (11) bears the watermark '1842' and it is likely that the whole group were executed, together, after that date, probably in England.

636 A Sailing Ship surrounded by Small Boats
*c.*1845
Watercolour, $9\frac{1}{4} \times 12\frac{3}{8}$ (23.5×31.5)
Trustees of the British Museum (T.B.CCCLXIV–138)
A complex scene economically noted in red and black: the subject is probably some ceremonial occasion; or it may be connected with the series of whaling subjects on which Turner was engaged in 1845–6 (see Nos.524 and 633).

637 Red and Blue Sunset Sky ?*c.*1845
Watercolour, sight $9\frac{9}{16} \times 14\frac{1}{16}$ (24.3×35.7)
Sir Edmund Bacon, Bart.

638 Adieu Fontainebleau ?*c.*1845
Watercolour, $8\frac{5}{8} \times 11\frac{1}{2}$ (21.9×29.1)
Inscr: 'Adieu Fontainebleau'
Trustees of the British Museum (T.B.CCLXXX–29)
One of thirteen loose sheets in the covers of a Rowney sketchbook watermarked 1825. Finberg places the series with the studies for vignettes (T.B.CCLXXX) but it seems more probable that these extremely free and obscure sketches date from the last years of Turner's active life. They include three, apparently of the same view, which are inscribed with a word which may read 'Coblenz'; most of the others also bear practically illegible inscriptions in Turner's hand. Only No.37, which includes a pencil sketch of a figure with outflung arms, seems to have any possible relation to the vignettes. It is inscribed 'N' (as are many of the group) 'give [?] to the Lady (study)'.

19. Retrospect: Norham Castle 1798–1840

Turner first saw Norham Castle during his tour of the North of England in 1797, and the sketchbook he used on that journey (T.B.XXXIV, No.23) contains a single pencil outline sketch of the castle on its cliff above the river. In the foreground are noted the small house, moored boats and sailing boat which became features of the two large watercolours he made of the scene. One of these watercolours was shown at the Royal Academy in 1798, and the other was probably done a little later, perhaps as a result of the colour studies which Turner made of the subject, exploring different ranges of rich, predominately dark, tone. The Royal Academy drawing was entitled 'Norham Castle–Summer's Morn', and, although the identification is uncertain, may have been that shown here, No.640.

The colour studies, unusual and highly dramatic in their experiments with tonality, betray Turner's special interest in this particular view–an interest which was to remain with him through the whole of his active life. On his next visit to Norham, which he passed on his way to Scotland in 1801, he made not one but a whole series of pencil studies of the Castle, from different viewpoints, including one (No.641) which duplicates

the view in the 'North of England' sketchbook. This time, however, the foreground incident is simplified, and the line of the Castle against the sky noted in a single clear outline, more sharply focussed than in the earlier drawing: Turner was evidently thinking of the bold *contre-jour* effect which he had made the leading feature of his watercolours.

He did not take up the subject for any new purpose, however, until about 1815, when he redesigned it, apparently from the 1801 drawing, for use in a plate in his *Liber Studiorum* (No.642). This was executed, of course, in pen and brown wash, preparatory to the mezzotint. It retains all the features of the earlier versions, but the composition is tightened into a compact design of superimposed light and dark planes, the sail of the boat glowing against the black cliff, and the Castle, moved to the centre of the scene, in stark silhouette against the sky.

The new, concentrated form of the 'Norham Castle' design lent itself perfectly to the format of Turner's series of views illustrating the *Rivers of England*, undertaken about 1822–4. But a striking change occurs: the subject, previously conceived in sombre colours – in the

Liber plate it is, of course, in brown monochrome – emerges now in brilliant, shimmering colour (No.645). It has even been argued that this watercolour of 'Norham' marks the precise moment at which Turner began to apply colour prismatically–i.e. in juxtaposed touches of pure red, blue and yellow. At the same time its overall colour plan is bold: the central mass of misty blue flanked by areas of paler blue, pink and gold. This scheme occurs in a 'colour-beginning' (No.644) which may perhaps be dated immediately prior to the *Rivers* drawing, although in composition, with the tower set off-centre, it harks back to the first series of views. The hut in the foreground, enlarged and seen end-on, retains its gable, and is not the rather Italianate building of the *Liber* and *Rivers* designs; it is merely suggested as a pentagonal form on a surface articulated simply in blocks of flat colour.

In 1831 Turner made fresh sketches at Norham, to which he must have referred when drawing the Scott illustration of 'Norham by Moonlight' (No.648). This is the only view not to show the Castle against a low sun. In another 'colour-beginning' which probably belongs to a slightly later date (No.649) the sun itself is visible, and seems to break open the landscape, making a bold path of pale gold along the course of the river which now runs from front to back of the scene. On either side, the cliffs are a mere haze of pale apricot and mauve. This colour-scheme, and the presentation of the sun, are characteristic of 'colour-beginnings' that Turner was making in the late twenties and early thirties; and it seems to lead directly to his final and grandest account of 'Norham Castle'.

This is the oil painting which was probably done about 1835–40 (No.650). The pale colour-scheme, conditioned by diffused light radiating through mist from a low sun, is developed from the *Rivers* watercolour and the later 'colour-beginning'; the forms of the landscape are still further fragmented–even the tower of the Castle, so important in the other designs, is lost to view here, and we can make out only the low wall with its square perforations, a minimised indication of the architectural structure. Turner has dissolved his subject in sunlight, but he has not created an abstraction: the cow in the river, which he has retained from his earliest treatment of the view, reminds us that he is painting the real world and that here, as always, he understood light and colour as the means by which we perceive nature; it is as natural forces that they are capable of moving us most profoundly.

639 Norham Castle *c.*1798
Pencil and watercolour, $26\frac{1}{16} \times 33\frac{1}{16}$ (66.3 × 84)
Trustees of the British Museum (T.B.L–B)
Derived from the pencil drawing in the 'North of England' sketchbook (No.23). Like T.B.L–C, this study is built up in layers of delicate washes – cream, pink and pale blue underneath darker local colour. Much use is made of wiping-out lights. The experimental process of applying watercolour in thin glazes is characteristic of Turner's technical preoccupations during the closing years of the century, and reflects the new attitudes to picture construction, tonality and lighting which he was acquiring from his work in oil from 1796 onwards.

640 Norham Castle *c.*1798
Pencil and watercolour, sight $20 \times 28\frac{15}{16}$
(50.9×73.5)
Inscr. bottom left: 'Turner'
Private Collection
Another version of the subject is now in a private collection, U.K. It is not certain which of the two finished watercolours was that exhibited as 'Norham Castle on the Tweed, Summer's Morn' with a quotation from Thompson's *Seasons* at the R.A. 1798 (43); Finberg (1961, p.460) says that this was the Lascelles drawing subsequently owned by Laundy Walters; but in his *Liber* catalogue he states that the drawing owned by Lord Lascelles was *not* the Walters drawing but the Thwaites drawing, catalogued here. The subject is based on a pencil drawing in the 'North of England' sketchbook, f.57^r, and this watercolour may have been executed after the two large-scale colour studies, T.B. L–B and C (see No.639).

641 'Helmsley' Sketchbook 1801
Bound in calf, with one clasp
97 leaves of white paper (several having been cut out) and four fly-leaves of grey paper: the majority drawn on in pencil, some with watercolour, $6\frac{1}{2} \times 4\frac{1}{2}$ (16.3 × 11.3)
Inscr. on label on spine: '70 Helmsley to Newcastle Northumber^d Tweed'
Trustees of the British Museum (T.B.LIII)

ff.44^v and 45^r **Norham Castle**
Pencil

This book includes views of Durham and Peel Castles, Whitby and Newcastle. It was used en route to Edinburgh in 1801; on ff.91^v and 92^r there is a pencil sketch of Edinburgh from a distance.

ff.44^v and 45^r show almost the slightest of ten sketches of Norham (ff.42^v to 50^r), the starting point for the series of later variations, in particular the *Liber Studiorum* design and the *Rivers of England* illustration (Nos.642, 645).

642 Norham Castle *c.*1815
Pen and brown ink, grey and brown washes
$7\frac{1}{2} \times 10\frac{5}{8}$ (19 × 27)
Trustees of the British Museum (T.B.CXVIII–D)
The finished drawing for the *Liber Studiorum* plate (No.643), which is inscribed 'the drawing in possession of the late Lord Lascells'; derived from the sketches in T.B.XXXIV f.57^r and LIII ff.44^v and 45^r. This design is in fact much modified from that composition and was to form the basis of the *Rivers of England* drawing (No. 645).

Turner published the drawing as 'P' for Pastoral; but it would perhaps have been more appropriately grouped with such plates as the 'River Wye' (R.48), published as 'Epic Pastoral'.

Charles TURNER (1774–1857) and J. M. W. TURNER

643 Norham Castle on the Tweed 1815
Etching and mezzotint, third published state,
$7 \times 10\frac{1}{4}$ (17.8 × 26.2); plate $8\frac{1}{4} \times 11\frac{1}{2}$ (20.9 × 29.2)
Inscr. above: 'P' (for Pastoral); and with title:
'The drawing in the possession of the late Lord

Lascells', 'Publish'd Jan 1, 1816. by I.M.W. Turner, Queen Ann Street West'; and below: 'Drawn Etched by I.M.W. Turner; Engraved by C. Turner' and in MS ' "Day set on Norham's Castled Steep", Marmion Cant. I. stz.1 –'
Royal Academy of Arts

Turner's monochrome drawing for this plate is No.642. The plate, R.57, appeared in Part XII of the *Liber Studiorum*. For the Lascelles drawing see No.640.

644 Norham Castle ?*c.*1817
Watercolour, $11\frac{15}{16} \times 19\frac{3}{16}$ (30.4 × 48.8)
Trustees of the British Museum (T.B.CCLXIII–22)
The range of heavy colours employed in this 'colour-beginning' suggests a date similar to that of the 'colour-beginnings' of Tivoli, T.B.CXCVI–U and CXCVII–A (Nos.183 and 182). The design seems to represent a halfway stage between the early watercolours (Nos.639 and 640) and the *Rivers of England* design of about 1822, which was also to draw on the composition of the *Liber Studiorum* plate of the subject (No.643). Compare this study with the later version, T.B.CCLXIII–72 (No.649).

There is a watercolour of a lake among low hills on the verso.

645 Norham Castle on the River Tweed *c.*1822
Watercolour, $6\frac{1}{8} \times 8\frac{1}{2}$ (15.6 × 21.6)
Trustees of the British Museum (T.B.CCVIII–O)
Engraved in mezzotint by C. Turner, 1824, for *The Rivers of England* Part II pl.1 (Rawlinson No.756). The subject is a modification, smaller in format, of the design (T.B.CXVIII–D) for the *Liber Studiorum* plate mezzotinted by C. Turner in 1816 (No.643). Cooke's accounts show that he paid Turner eight guineas for the loan of the drawing in 1822. It has been argued, by Finley (1973, pp.386ff.), that this watercolour marks the beginning of Turner's application of prismatic colour theory in his work.

Charles TURNER (1774–1857) after J. M. W. TURNER
646 Norham Castle on the River Tweed 1824
Mezzotint, 1st published state, $6\frac{1}{16} \times 8\frac{9}{16}$ (15.4 × 21); plate $7\frac{1}{2} \times 10$ (19.1 × 25.8)
Inscr: 'Drawn by J.M.W. Turner, R.A.'; with title and: 'Engraved on Steel by Chas. Turner; Engraver in Ordinary to His Majesty'; and: 'Rivers of England: Plate 6, London, Published Jany.1, 1824; by W.B.Cooke, 9 Soho Square.'
Trustees of the British Museum (1850-1-14-124)
Rawlinson No.756. See the drawing on which this mezzotint was based, No.645.

Percy HEATH (fl.1827–30) after TURNER
647 Norham Castle 1827
Engraving, proof, $4 \times 6\frac{11}{16}$ (10.2 × 17)
Inscr. with title and: 'Engraved by Percy Heath 1827'
Trustees of the British Museum (1919-6-14-2)
Rawlinson No.317. It is not known for what purpose this plate was engraved. Turner's drawing for the *Rivers of England* series (No.645) was evidently the original for it; and Rawlinson records a tradition that it was intended for the *Literary Souvenir*, an illustrated annual for which five other of Turner's designs were used, including the large 'Richmond Hill' watercolour (No.257; Rawlinson No.314).

William MILLER (1797–1882) after TURNER
648 Norham Castle – Moonrise 1834
Engraving, first published state $3\frac{3}{8} \times 5\frac{1}{2}$ (8.6 × 14); plate $5\frac{3}{4} \times 8\frac{3}{8}$ (14.7 × 21.3)
Inscr. with names of artist and engraver and: 'Edinburgh, Published 1834, by Robert Cadell; and Hodgson, Boys & Graves, London'
Trustees of the British Museum (1868-8-22-3064)
Rawlinson No.522; the plate illustrates *The Provincial Antiquities of Scotland* in Cadell's edition of *Scott's Prose Works*, 1834–6. The finished watercolour from which it derives was in Munro's collection and later in America. Rawlinson considered the print 'perhaps the most beautiful of Turner's many engraved renderings of Norham Castle.'

649 Norham Castle ?*c.*1835
Watercolour, $12 \times 19\frac{3}{16}$ (30.5 × 48.7)
Trustees of the British Museum (T.B.CCLXIII–72)
Retaining the general outline of the castle as in the *Rivers of England* and *Liber* versions, this 'colour-beginning' is nevertheless the closest of the 'Norham' designs to the painting probably executed in the late 1830s (No.650), and, it may be, immediately precedes it in time.

Finberg suggested that Tamworth Castle was the subject of this 'colour-beginning' but its affinities with the Norham series leave little doubt of its starting point.

650 Norham Castle, Sunrise *c.*1835–40
Oil on canvas, $35\frac{3}{4} \times 48$ (91 × 122) (repr. on p.184)
Tate Gallery (1981)
This is one of the group of unfinished oils based on a plate in the *Liber Studiorum*, R.57 (see Nos.620–23) and like these can be roughly, and tentatively, dated *c.*1835–40. It could however be still later and marks the extreme of Turner's development from the topographical watercolour of *c.*1798 (No.640).

Life and Times

BOYHOOD AND APPRENTICESHIP

Joseph Mallord William Turner was born on 23 April 1775 above his father's barber shop in Covent Garden. His father, William Turner, was an uneducated man (see his letters in Lindsay, *Turner*, 1966, p.21), a 'chatty old fellow', who remained close to his son until the end. From Sandycombe Lodge at Twickenham (see No.B128), where he tended the garden, he would walk the eleven miles into London (see Farington, 24 May 1813). Turner's mother is far more mysterious: an 'ungovernable temper' led to madness; she was admitted as a curable patient to Bethlem Hospital on 26 December 1801, transferred to the Incurable List within a few weeks and died, probably in the same hospital, on 15 April 1804 (information from Miss P. Allderidge). Bethlem was undoubtedly chosen on account of Turner's former patron, Dr Thomas Monro, who was physician there (see Nos.B19 and 27), but Monro also ran a private asylum, with a far milder regime (see K. Jones, *A History of the Mental Health Services*, 1972, pp.75–7, 84, 111–12), and in a pamphlet he wrote that at Bethlem, 'the number of the objects to whom the charity is extended, and the comparative feebleness of the means for their relief, preclude the possibility of that nice discrimination, that minute and watchful attention to individual comfort, and those various indulgences that mitigate the sufferings of disease, and the severity of indispensable restraint, which can only be gained from the anxious kindness of domestic affection, or commanded by the power of wealth' (*Observations of Dr Thomas Monro upon the Evidence taken before the Commission of the House of Commons for regulating Madhouses*, 1816). Turner never seems to have referred to his mother after her death.

B1 J. M. W. TURNER
Self-Portrait *c.*1798   (repr. as frontis.)
Oil on canvas, 29¼ × 23 (74.5 × 58.8)
Tate Gallery (458)

B2 James Wykeham ARCHER (1823–1904)
Turner's Birthplace, 21 Maiden Lane, Covent Garden 1852
Watercolour, 14 × 8⅝ (35.5 × 22)
Trustees of the British Museum (1874-3-14-329)

B3 James Wykeham ARCHER
The Room where Turner was born 1852
Watercolour, 8¹¹⁄₁₆ × 13¹³⁄₁₆ (22.2 × 35.1)
Trustees of the British Museum (1874-3-14-328)

B4 **Memorial Tablet to Turner's Parents** 1832
St. Paul's, Covent Garden (photograph)
The awkwardness and the innaccuracy of the inscription (William Turner died in 1829, not 1830), and the coarseness of the carving, suggest that Turner was responsible for all of it. A mason's fee of 7s 6d paid by a churchwarden was never recovered (T. Miller, *Turner and Girtin's Picturesque Tours*, 1854, pp.xi, xxxix).

B5 **Two Medical Prescriptions for William Turner** *c.*1829
C. W. M. Turner, Esq.

B6 J. M. W. TURNER
Portrait of his Mother, Mary Anne Turner (?) *c.*1794
Trustees of the British Museum (T.B.XX–35) (photograph)

Turner's family gave him his first opportunities to travel out of London: about 1786 he went to his maternal uncle at Brentford, where he went to school, and coloured some of the plates in Boswell's *Antiquities*; in 1789 he was at the same uncle's house at Sunningwell, near Oxford (see No.1); and in 1791 he went to see his father's old friend, John Narraway in Bristol, where he sketched (see Nos. 3–4) and copied engravings, had his first experience of travelling in Wales and left a self-portrait, which Narraway's niece recalled that Turner was reluctant to paint, saying 'it is no use taking such a little figure as mine, it will do my drawings an injury, people will say such a little fellow as this can never draw'. (*Portfolio*, 1880, pp.69–71; Finberg 1961, p.27).

B7 H. BOSWELL
Picturesque Views of the Antiquities of England and Wales 1786
Hounslow Library Services
Some 100 of the 200 plates coloured by hand seem to have been done by Turner.

B8 J. M. W. TURNER
Sketchbook *c.*1791
6¼ × 8 (15.5 × 20.5)
Inscribed: 'left at Mr Nureaways [sic] Bristol about 1790 or 1791'
Princeton University Art Museum
The book contains a copy from a plate in the 1754 edition of Kirby's *Perspective* (see No.B55)

B9 J. M. W. TURNER
Self-Portrait *c.*1791–3
Watercolour touched with white, 3¾ × 2¾ (9.5 × 7)
Trustees of the National Portrait Gallery

Turner's beginnings in watercolour emerged from his employment as an architectural draughtsman and a colourist of prints; and they included a brief period as a drawing-master. Edward Dayes, in the earliest memoir of Turner (*c.*1803), stated that he taught himself 'without the assistance of a master', by copying from drawings and pictures. At some stage Turner was a pupil of Thomas Malton Jnr (see *Notes and Queries*, 2nd ser.v, p.475; Gage 1969, pp.22–3), and much work around 1790 bears the stamp of an architectural background, as well as a close affinity to Dayes. As a teacher of watercolour about 1794–7 Turner used similar methods, presenting pupils with his own models, as B17, to copy.

B10   Thomas MALTON Jnr (1748–1804)
Sir Charles Asgill's Villa at Richmond 1791
Pen and Watercolour, $14 \times 19\frac{1}{4}$ (35.5×50.6)
Visitors of the Ashmolean Museum, Oxford

B11   Thomas MALTON Jnr
Picturesque Tour through London and Westminster 1792
Royal Academy of Arts

B12   John SOANE (1753–1837)
Sketches in Architecture 1793
Royal Institute of British Architects
Turner owned a copy of this book.

B13   Thomas KIRK (1777–1845) and
J. M. W. TURNER
Officer of the Third Regiment of Foot Guards *c.*1791
Watercolour over etched outline $10\frac{7}{8} \times 6\frac{5}{8}$ (27.7×16.9)
Inscr. on verso: 'Coloured for Colnaghi by Mr. J.M.W. Turner when a Boy
Mr. Colnaghi gave this print to me as a great curiosity J.T. Smith'
Trustees of the British Museum (1890-8-6-2)
The outline was etched by Thomas Kirk after a design by Edward Dayes (1763–1804), draughtsman to the Duke of York, C. in C. of the Army, from 1791. Turner was probably employed directly by Colnaghi himself in this work.

B14   Edward DAYES (1763–1804)
Buckingham House, St. James's Park 1790
Pencil and watercolour, $15\frac{1}{2} \times 25\frac{1}{2}$ (31.8×64.8)
Inscr. lower right with signature and date.
Victoria and Albert Museum (1756–1871)
This watercolour may be connected with the 'drawing' of a 'View in St. James's Park' shown at the Society of Artists, 1791 (63).

In addition to his work as a picturesque and antiquarian topographer (see No.B15) Dayes made a series of views in London during the 1780s and early 1790s which are architectural records in the same vein as those of Malton (see No.B10). These views include figures, usually on a fairly large scale; the present drawing is, however, unusually crowded, and the building which is its ostensible subject has become merely a background. It seems likely that Dayes was imitating here the formula of Rowlandson's highly successful 'Vauxhall Gardens', shown at the Royal Academy in 1798 (503), and now in the Victoria and Albert Museum. Turner had this tradition of 'social topography' in mind when he composed his view of the 'Pantheon, Oxford Street' (No.7)

B15   Edward DAYES (1760–1804)
Interior of the Ruins of Tintern Abbey *c.*1792
Pen and black ink with grey, blue and coloured washes $15\frac{1}{4} \times 10\frac{13}{16}$ (38.7×27.5)
Inscr: 'Tintern Abbey, drawn by M^r. Thos Girtin Including the S. Trancept & part of the Choir'
Mrs P.F. Stritzl

This drawing is typical of the views Dayes was making in the early 1790s, which both Turner and Girtin imitated. Some examples of Dayes' work in this style are in the Turner Bequest, CCCLXXI; there are also many specimens of Dayes imitations, presumably mostly by Turner, but some may possibly be by Girtin. A copy of this drawing, attributed to Girtin, was sold at Sotheby's 24 June 1971 (71). The inscription on the old mount of the present drawing ascribing it to Girtin must for stylistic reasons be incorrect. An example of Dayes' more 'public' style is No.B14.

B16   J. M. W. TURNER
Inside of Tintern Abbey, Monmouthshire R.A.1794
Pencil and watercolour $12\frac{5}{8} \times 9\frac{7}{8}$ (32×24.8)
Exh: R.A.1794 (402)
Victoria and Albert Museum (1683–1871)
There is another version of this subject in the Turner Bequest, XXIII–A; it appears to have been left unfinished, so the present drawing is more likely to be that shown at the R.A. in 1794. Similar views of Tintern, but showing the Transept instead of the choir, are in the British Museum (1958-7-12-400) and the Ashmolean Museum (Herrmann 91).

The composition of these watercolours is Turner's own, based on a pencil study made at Tintern in about 1792 (T.B. XII–E); but it alludes clearly to the contemporary fashion for such picturesque antiquarian views, as practised by Thomas Malton, Thomas Hearne, and Edward Dayes (compare No.B15). Similar low-viewpoint architectural drawings were made by Thomas Girtin at about the same date.

B17   J. M. W. TURNER
Bridge, with Coach and Horses *c.*1796
Watercolour, $8\frac{7}{8} \times 11$ (22.7×28)
Inscr. on verso: 'W.T.' and 'Mr Turner's Drawing' (twice)
Trustees of the British Museum (T.B.XXXII, D)

B18   William BLAKE of Newhouse (1757–1827)
Mountain Landscape with Cattle *c.*1797
Watercolour, $7\frac{3}{4} \times 11\frac{3}{4}$ (19.7×29.8)
Trustees of the British Museum (1962-11-10-1)
Turner seems to have met Blake about 1792, and Blake was ordering work from him in 1797 (T.B.XXXIV-67). The style of this drawing is close to some of Turner's work about 1795 (e.g. T.B.XXVII-1). See also No.36

Dr Thomas Monro (1759–1833) was the most important of Turner's early patrons. They probably met in 1792, when Turner was sketching near Fetcham, Surrey, where Monro had a cottage. The doctor was a collector and imitator of Gainsborough's drawings, and he owned a large number of drawings and prints by Dutch and English artists. Between 1794 and 1797 he employed Turner and Thomas Girtin (see No.B43) at his house in the Adelphi, a few doors away from the Society of Arts, to make more developed copies from outlines by J. R. Cozens, Hearne and other artists:

> They went at 6 and stayed till ten. Girtin drew the outlines and Turner washed in the effects . . . Dr Monro allowed Turner 3s 6d each night. Girtin did not say what he had. (Farington, 11 Nov. 1798).

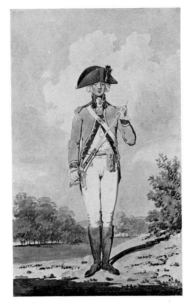

B13

Turner and Monro made portraits of each other (Monro's drawing of Turner (Kurt Pantzer Coll.) is reproduced in Finberg, 1961, pl.2), and Turner told Farington in 1798 that Monro had been 'a material friend to him'. Monro was almost certainly responsible for advising on the treatment of Turner's mother three years later.

B19 J. M. W. TURNER
Portrait of Dr Monro c.1796
Pencil, 8×6 (20.3 $\times$ 15.2)
Dr F. J. G. Jefferiss

B20 J. M. W. TURNER
St. Mary's Church, Hadley 1793
Watercolour, $10\frac{1}{2} \times 14$ (26.7 $\times$ 35.6)
G. K. Monro, Esq.
The house in the background was owned by Dr Thomas Monro's brother James (d.1806), who was buried in the church with their father (d.1791). This is the first dated document of Turner's contact with Monro.

B21 Thomas MONRO (1759–1833)
Landscape with an Inn and Cart
Stump and wash, $7\frac{7}{8} \times 6\frac{1}{4}$ (20 $\times$ 15.5)
Dr F. J. G. Jefferiss

B22 SOCIETY OF ARTS
Minutes of the Committee of Polite Arts
27 March 1793
Royal Society of Arts
The subject of Turner's prize drawing was 'Lodge Farm, Near Hambledon, Surrey'. His Greater Silver Palette is reproduced in *The Connoisseur*, LXV, 1923, p.79.

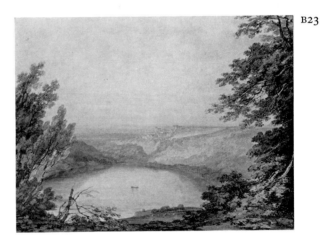

B23

B23 J. M. W. TURNER after J. R. COZENS (1752–1797)
Lake Nemi c.1796
Pencil and watercolour, $16\frac{1}{2} \times 21\frac{3}{4}$ (41.9 $\times$ 55.2)
Inscr. on verso: 'Nemi with Gensano'
Manning Galleries Ltd

B24 J. M. W. TURNER after J. R. COZENS
A Valley near Innsbruck c.1796
Pencil and watercolour, $6\frac{1}{4} \times 9\frac{1}{3}$ (16 $\times$ 23.3)
Private Collection
Based on a sketch on p.6 of J. R. Cozens' 'Hamilton Palace' sketchbook, No.1 (see B25).

B25 John Robert COZENS
Sketchbook 1782
Bound in leather. Contains thirty-two leaves of sketches in pencil and grey wash $7\frac{1}{4} \times 9\frac{3}{4}$ (17.8 $\times$ 23.8)
Leger Galleries Ltd

f.6ʳ A Valley near Innsbruck
Pencil and grey wash
Inscr. upper left: 'Near Inspruck June 6'

The first of seven sketchbooks from the collection of William Beckford used by Cozens during a visit to Italy in 1782 and 1783, known as the 'Hamilton Palace' Sketchbooks.
   Turner's copy of the drawing on f.6ʳ is No.B.24. It is not known how or when Beckford acquired the sketch-

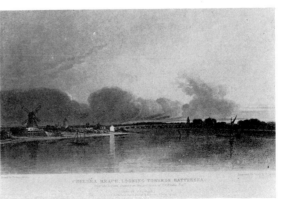

B43

books; they seem to have been in Cozen's possession until the onset of his illness in about 1792. Monro is known to have used them, however, as models for his protégés to copy.

B26   Thomas HEARNE (1744–1817)
Derwentwater
Watercolour, 8⅛ × 12 (20.6 × 30.5)
Tate Gallery (T.999)
Monro felt that Hearne was 'superior to everybody in drawing' and owned many works by him (Farington, 14 December 1795).

B27   John VARLEY (1778–1842)
Portrait of Dr Thomas Monro 1812
Pencil, 12½ × 8½ (31.7 × 21.6)
Inscr: 'Dr Monro the First Collector of Turner & Girtin's Drawings, Done with the Graphic Telescope April 12 1812. John Varley 1812'
Victoria and Albert Museum (1179–1927)
The graphic telescope, invented by Cornelius Varley, was a mechanical device for making drawings from nature.

OLD MASTERS AND CONTEMPORARIES

B28   Richard EARLOM (1743–1822)
Liber Veritatis: or a Collection of two hundred prints after the original designs by Claude le Lorrain 1777
Royal Academy of Arts

B29   W. F. WELLS (1762–1836) and J. LAPORTE (1761–1839)
A Collection of Prints Illustrative of English Scenery, from the Drawings & Sketches of Gainsborough 1802–5
Gainsborough House Society, Sudbury
W. F. Wells (see p.191) was the friend in whose house the *Liber Studiorum* was devised in 1806 (see p.61).

B30   C. TURNER (1773–1857) after
J. M. W. TURNER
The Farmyard with the Cock (R.17)
Etching and Mezzotint, proof before all letters, 7⅛ × 10⅜ (18 × 26.2); plate 8¼ × 11½ (21.1 × 29.4)
Royal Academy of Arts
R.17. Issued in part 4 of the *Liber Studiorum*, 29 March 1809; categorised as P for Pastoral.
On Turner's wish in the *Liber Studiorum*, to 'clarify the various styles of landscape', see p.61. His model for this project was Claude's *Liber Veritatis* engraved by Earlom for Boydell in the 1770s. The collection was also a repertory of the styles of those Old Masters whose landscapes Turner especially admired.

B31   Jean AUDRAN (1667–1756) after N. POUSSIN (1594–1665)
Winter (the Deluge)
Engraving, plate 24¼ × 17⅞ (61.5 × 45.5)
Courtauld Institute of Art
Turner saw this picture in the Louvre in 1802 and

made notes on it in his 'Louvre' sketchbook; see No.91. Poussin's 'Deluge' was the subject of several analyses by Turner, who, in a lecture of 1812, said of it: 'He has buried the whole picture under the deep-toned lurid interval of approaching horror, gloom, defying definition, yet looking alluvial; calling upon those mysterious memories which appear wholly to depend upon the association of ideas' (see Ziff in *Burlington Magazine*, CV, 1963, pp.315–6, 319–20).

B32   REMBRANDT van Rijn (1606–1669)
The Three Trees
Etching, 8⁷⁄₁₆ × 11 (21.4 × 28)
Castle Museum, Norwich
Of Rembrandt Turner said in a lecture of 1811:
He threw a mysterious doubt over the meanest piece of Common; nay, more, his forms, if they can be called so, are the most objectionable that could be chosen, namely, the Three Trees and the Mill, but over each he has thrown that veil of matchless colour, that lucid interval of Morning dawn and dewy light on which the Eye dwells so completely enthrall'd, and it seeks not for its liberty, but, as it were, thinks it a sacrilege to pierce the mystic shell of colour in search of form.
   See Nos.331–2, and Gage, *Turner: Rain, Steam and Speed*, 1972, ch.2.

B33   M. ROTA (1520–1583) after TITIAN (?1477–1576)
St. Peter Martyr
Engraving, 15⁵⁄₁₆ × 10⁹⁄₁₆ (38.9 × 26.8)
Trustees of the British Museum (1874-8-8-1941)
The 'St. Peter Martyr' was an historical landscape which especially fascinated Turner (see Nos.77 and 78). As late as 1819 in Venice he made a study from it (T.B.CLXXVI-40a) to test the validity of Reynolds' remarks on the generalisation of its foreground vegetation (*Discourse* XI); and in 1828 he painted a 'Vision of Medea' (No.473) in a very similar vein.

B34   James FITTLER (1758–1835) after
Philip James de LOUTHERBOURG (1740–1812)
The Battle of the Nile
Engraving, 20⅜ × 30⅜ (51.7 × 77.1)
National Maritime Museum
After the painting of 1800 in the Tate Gallery. Turner's version of this subject (now lost) was exhibited in 1799. For Loutherbourg's effect on the young Turner, see Nos.19 and 47.

B35   Richard WILSON (1714–1782) or Studio
Tivoli: The Cascatelle
Oil, 29 × 38 (73.7 × 96.5)
Tate Gallery (5538)
This painting, a version of the Wilson at Dulwich (W. G. Constable, *Richard Wilson*, 1953, pl. 117a), has hitherto been catalogued as a copy by Turner, since it was among his works at his death.

B36   J. M. W. TURNER after Richard WILSON
Tivoli: Temple of the Sibyl and the Roman Campagna
Oil on canvas 29 × 38 (73.5 × 96.5).
Tate Gallery (5512).

This was listed in the 1851 inventory of the Turner Bequest as No.298 with the marginal note 'copy from Wilson' and is indeed a copy of a Wilson that exists in a number of versions at Cardiff, Philadelphia, the Tate Gallery and elsewhere (the Tate version and one in a private collection repr. W. G. Constable, *Richard Wilson*, 1953, pls. 115a and 116b); the composition was also engraved in reverse by W. Byrne in 1765. Turner omits both the large tree and the figures that appear in varied forms in the Wilsons, thus making his copy more of a direct transcript of the view, though he does retain the large rocks that also seem to have been introduced into the foreground by Wilson.

Turner's admiration for Wilson is well documented. For instance, in his sixth lecture as Professor of Perspective (see p.181) in 1812 he spoke of 'the aerial mediums of Claude, the glowing expanse of Cuyp [and] the exquisite feeling of Wilson' (Gage 1969, p.201). There is another oil copy after Wilson at the Tate Gallery (5490), and there are several drawings after Wilson at the British Museum including those labelled by Turner himself 'Studies from Pictures. Copies of Wilson' (T.B.XXXVII). For an oil painting apparently by Wilson or his studio but included in the Turner Bequest as a copy by Turner see No.B35; other paintings by Wilson were included in the Turner sale at Christie's of 25 July 1874 (see Gage, p.243 n.94).

B37   Richard WILSON
Castel of S. Angelo
Pencil and black chalk on grey paper,
$9\frac{1}{2} \times 15\frac{1}{2}$ (24.1 × 39.4)
Tate Gallery (2438)

See p.86 for Turner's adoption of Wilson's methods in this type of drawing.

B38   George JONES (1786–1869)
The Burning Fiery Furnace R.A. 1832
Oil on panel, $35\frac{1}{2} \times 27\frac{1}{2}$ (89.5 × 69.8)
Exh: R.A. 1832 (256)
Tate Gallery (389)

B39   J. M. W. TURNER
The Burning Fiery Furnace R.A. 1832
Oil on panel, $35\frac{1}{2} \times 27\frac{1}{2}$ (89.5 × 69.8)
Exh: R.A. 1832 (355)
Tate Gallery (517)

B40   George JONES
The Burial of Sir David Wilkie 1842
Watercolour, $14\frac{1}{2} \times 10\frac{1}{2}$ (36.8 × 26.7)
Brinsley Ford, Esq.

See Nos.B38–9 and 521.

Sometimes Turner's subjects were the result of a direct stimulus from his friends and contemporaries. In 1832 he had asked Jones exactly what subject he intended to exhibit at the Royal Academy, and the size, and immediately proposed to paint a version himself in friendly competition (see Finberg, 1961, p.335). A decade later the story was repeated in their two memorial paintings for Wilkie, Jones' version of which is only known from No.B40.

B41   George Henry PHILLIPS (*fl*.1819–1841) after
Frances DANBY (1793–1861)
The Enchanted Island 1841
Mezzotint $8\frac{5}{8} \times 13\frac{3}{8}$ (22 × 34.1); plate $12\frac{1}{16} \times 15\frac{15}{16}$
(30.7 × 40.5)
Inscr. below: 'ENCHANTED ISLAND, Engraved by G. H. Phillips from a Picture painted by F. Danby A.R.A. in the possession of John Gibbons Esq.ʳ to whom this Plate is Inscribed. London, published Mar. 18, 1841, by Colnaghi & Puckle, Printsellers to Her Majesty, 23 Cockspur Street, Charing Cross'
Trustees of the British Museum (1862–10–11–249)

B42   J. M. W. TURNER
Queen Mab's Cave B.I. 1846
Oil, 26 × 48 (91.5 × 121.9)
Exh: British Institution 1846 (57)
Tate Gallery (548)

Danby's painting of this subject had been exhibited in 1825 (see F. Greenacre, *The Bristol School of Artists*, 1973, No.19), but it was almost certainly the print, re-issued when Danby was coming to prominence again in London after a long absence abroad, which stimulated Turner, who praised Danby as a 'poetical' painter in these years, to make his own version of the subject, No.B42.

B43   Thomas LUPTON (1791–1873) after
Thomas GIRTIN (1775–1802)
Chelsea Reach, Looking Towards Battersea
1823
Mezzotint $5\frac{1}{4} \times 8\frac{7}{8}$ (13.3 × 22.5); plate $6\frac{7}{8} \times 9\frac{15}{16}$
(16.7 × 25.2)
Inscr. below: 'Drawn by Thomas Girtin' and 'Engraved on Steel by T. Lupton.' with title and 'From the original Drawing, in the possession of B. G. Windus Esq.ʳ.', 'Gems of Art, Plate 7', and 'London, Published Aug. 1, 1823; by W. B. Cooke, 9 Soho Square.'
Trustees of the British Museum

Lupton was working for Turner a good deal in the 1820s, and another engraving of the subject by S. W. Reynolds was also published by Cooke in 1823. The owner of Girtin's watercolour (usually known as 'The White House at Chelsea'), B. G. Windus, was becoming an important collector of Turner at this time. The watercolour is now in the Tate Gallery; another version, once in the collection of Turner's Plymouth friend, A. B. Johns, is now in the Bacon collection.

B44   J. M. W. TURNER
Valley with Mountains *c*.1841
Pencil and white chalk, $4\frac{1}{4} \times 5\frac{3}{4}$ (10.6 × 14.7)
Inscr: 'Girtin's White House'
Trustees of the British Museum (T.B.CCCXLII–66ᵛ)

For Turner's continuing pre-occupation with white objects in a landscape, see Gage in *Burlington Magazine*, CVII, 1965, pp.75–6.

B47

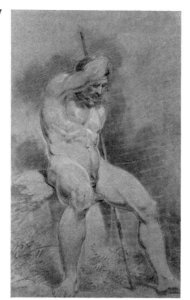

B54(c)

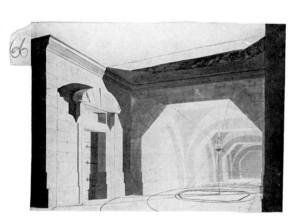

B54(d)

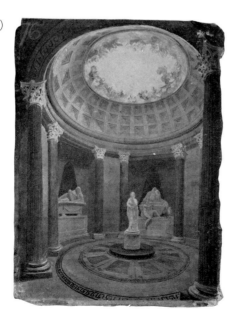

THE ROYAL ACADEMY

B45 Mauritius LOWE (1746–1793)
Mythological Subject with Six Figures
Pencil, pen and grey wash,
13¹³⁄₁₆ × 19⅜ (35.0 × 49.2)
Levens Hall Collection
Turner was recommended as a probationer at the Royal Academy Schools by the portraitist J. F. Rigaud and admitted as a student in December 1789. His interest in the Sublime style of History Painting may have been fostered by Lowe, who seems to have encouraged him to become a painter. Lowe, a pupil of Cipriani and a follower of Fuseli, had painted a large composition on the theme of the Deluge in 1783. (For this picture, see J. Northcote, *Memoirs of Sir Joshua Reynolds*, 1813, pp.294–6; and for Lowe's sponsorship of Turner, B. Falk, *Turner the Painter*, 1938, pp.25–6).

B46 **Cast of the Torso Belvedere**
Royal Academy of Arts
Turner is known to have presented a cast of the Torso Belvedere to the Royal Academy in 1842.

B47 J. M. W. TURNER
Seated Academy Study
Black, white and red chalk on brown paper,
18⅜ × 11⅜ (46.5 × 28.5)
Trustees of the British Museum (T.B.XVIII–C)

B48 J. M. W. TURNER
Standing Academy Study 1792–9
Black and white chalk on blue paper,
19½ × 11¾ (49.5 × 29.8)
Trustees of the British Museum (T.B.XVIII–I)

B49 William HOGARTH (1697–1764)
The Analysis of Beauty 1753, Pl.I
Royal Academy of Arts
Turner took over the 'Beard of Hudibras' in this plate in a poem (T.B.CX–Ia) and he adopted a characteristically academic dictum of Hogarth's: 'I know of no such thing as genius; genius is nothing but labour and diligence' (see R. Paulson, *Hogarth, his Life, Art and Times*, 1917, II, p.141; cf. Gage, 1969, p.225 n.2).

B50 **Hogarth's Palette**
Royal Academy of Arts
Presented by Turner to the Academy in 1831; the gift was provoked by Constable's presentation of Reynolds' palette in 1830. Constable wrote to C. R. Leslie in September: 'Turner has bought Hogarth's palette & means to give it to the Academy – he has got poor Eastlake "in secret" to enquire if the Academy *Paid* for the silver plate and glass case in which is the palette of Sir Joshua...' (R. B. Beckett, *John Constable's Correspondence*, III, 1965, p.47).

B51 William ETTY (1787–1849)
A Female Nude standing against a Statue of the Venus Pudica
Black, sanguine and white chalk on brown paper,
22¼ × 15¼ (56.3 × 38.8)
Courtauld Institute (Witt Collection)
Turner was devoted to the basic academic study of the

nude. He had worked as a student in the Cast Academy from 1789–92, and in the Life Class between 1792 and 1799. Farington reported that as early as December 1802, soon after he had become a full Academician, Turner was 'very urgent' to become a Visitor, although he became one only in 1812, holding the post for eight years in all up to 1838. He was Inspector of the Cast Collection at the Academy in 1820, 1829 and 1838. In the Life Class Turner interpreted the neo-classical idea of comparing living and sculptural form by posing the model in the attitude of a statue, a cast of which was placed by its side. Etty's study seems to belong to one of these occasions (see A. Gilchrist, *Life of William Etty*, II, 1855 p.59). Eastlake also noted Turner's novel idea of placing the Life Model on a white sheet to induce reflections, and 'infuse new life into the practice of the students' (*Report of the Commission . . . on the Royal Academy*, 1863, p.65).

B52 Royal Academy Catalogues: Address Lists
1801, 1802
Royal Academy of Arts

Turner was elected a full Academician on 12 February 1802 and henceforth his style changed from William Turner to Joseph Mallord William Turner, R.A.

Turner was elected Professor of Perspective at the Academy in December 1807, and gave his first lecture in 1811. He continued more or less regularly until 1828, and finally resigned the office in December 1837. The lectures had involved intense preparation, and the first series were generally well received, not least for the superb diagrams and the unfinished paintings which Turner sometimes showed at them. But in the 1820s they became more abstract, and attendance dwindled to nothing (see Gage 1969, pp.106–8, 128).

B53 J. M. W. TURNER
MS of Lecture IV on 'Light, Shade and Reflexes' 1818
C. W. M. Turner, Esq.

B54 J. M. W. TURNER
Perspective Diagrams
Trustees of the British Museum

a) T.B.CXCV–50
Pencil, pen and watercolour,
$19 \times 23\frac{3}{4}$ (48.2 × 60.3)

b) Interior of a Prison
Pencil, watercolour and body colour, $18\frac{3}{4} \times 27$ (47.7 × 68.8)
T.B.CXCV–120

c) Interior of a Prison
Pencil, pen and watercolour, $14\frac{1}{4} \times 20$ (36.8 × 50.8)
T.B.CXCV–121

b and c, together with CXCVI–128, are based on the 'Carcere Obscura', pl.2 in *Prima Parte di Architettura e Prospettive inventate ed incise da Gio. Batta. Piranesi . . .* 1743

d) Interior of Brocklesby Mausoleum
Watercolour, 25 × 19 (63.5 × 48.2)
T.B.CXCV–130
This seems to illustrate Lecture IV, 1818 (No.B50, f.12n)

e) Colour Diagram No.1 *c*.1825
Watercolour, $21\frac{1}{2} \times 29\frac{1}{2}$ (54 × 74.3)
T.B.CXCV–178

f) Colour Diagram No.2 *c*.1825
Watercolour, $21\frac{1}{2} \times 29\frac{1}{2}$ (54 × 74.3)
T.B.CXCV–179
For the texts relating to (e), the colours of light, and (f), the colours of pigments, see Gage, 1969, pp.209–12.

B55 Joshua KIRBY (1716–1774)
Dr Brooke Taylor's Method of Perspective
1768
C. W. M. Turner, Esq.
Turner's own copy, from the library of a descendant of Kirby, Henry Scott Trimmer.

B56 Moses HARRIS (*fl.*1770)
The Natural System of Colours 2nd ed. 1811
Victoria and Albert Museum
Thomas Phillips' copy, with his annotations.

B57 Thomas PHILLIPS (1770–1845)
Lectures on the History and Principles of Painting 1833
British Library
Phillips was a close friend of Turner in the 1820s, and was almost certainly the source of Turner's knowledge of Harris' diagram, adapted in one of his perspective diagrams (No.B54f; see Gage 1969, p.115f.).

B58 Collection of Perspective Treatises
comprising:
Viator, *De Artificiali Perspectiva*, 1505
G. Troili, *Paradossi per Pratticare la Perspettiva senza saperla*, 1683
H. Lautensack, *Des Cirkels und Richtscheyts, auch der Perspectiva und Proportion der Menschen und Rosse*, 1564
P. Accolti, *Lo Inganno de gl'occhi, Prospettiva Pratica*, 1625
British Library
Turner's mention of all these treatises in the 'Perspective' sketchbook (T.B.CVIII) suggests that this collection, which bears the earliest Museum Stamp and was probably acquired as a single volume, was the copy he used in the British Museum. (See also British Library 536 M.21: D. Barbaro, *Della Perspettiva*, 1568; L. Sirigatti, *La Pratica di Prospettiva*, 1625; J. F. Niceron, *La Perspective Curieuse ou Magie Artificielle*, 1638).

B59 L. C. WYON (1826–1891) after
D. MACLISE (1806–1870)
Turner Medal (Obverse) 1859
Bronze, diam. $2\frac{1}{8}$ (5.5)
Trustees of the British Museum

B60 Daniel MACLISE
Design for the Turner Medal (Reverse) 1859
Pencil, $6\frac{1}{2}$ (16.5) diam.
Royal Academy of Arts
In the first codicil to his will in August 1832 (See B152). Turner left £60 'for a Professor in Landscape to be read [*sic*] in the Royal Academy elected from the Royal

Academicians or a Medal called Turner's Medal equal to the Gold Medal now given by the Academy say £20 for the best Landscape every 2d year'. The idea of a Professorship of Landscape, which Turner had been proposing since about 1811, never came to anything, but in 1856 the Academy decided to institute a Medal, and in 1858 Maclise was invited to design it (see Arts Council, *Daniel Maclise*, 1972, No.125). The first award was made in 1857 to N. O. Lupton for 'An English Landscape': Henry Holiday recalled that it was not studied from nature, was 'loudly hissed' and 'felt to be an insult to the school'. No award was made at the second competition in 1859, nor again until 1863. (See H. Holiday, *Reminiscences of my Life*, 1914, pp.42, 45f; *Illustrated London News*, 14 April 1860, 27 February 1864; information from Chris Mullen).

In the 1830s and 1840s Turner painted a good proportion of his pictures on the walls of the Royal Academy itself, during the days called 'Varnishing Days', which had been formally instituted in 1809. T. S. Cooper recalled that about 1846 'Some of his work was, as usual, only just rubbed in, and it was a common practice of his, when he saw how his pictures were placed, to paint first a little on one, then on another, and so on till all were finished to his satisfaction' (*My Life*, 1890, II, pp.2–3). After the failure of the lectures in 1828, Turner may have felt that these days were the most suitable occasion for his teaching: certainly many young students took them as such (Gage, 1969, Ch. 10).

B61 S. W. PARROTT (1813–c.1878)
Turner on Varnishing Day c.1846
Oil on panel, 9⅞ × 9 (25 × 22.9)
University of Reading (Guild of St. George and Ruskin Collection)

B62 J. E. MILLAIS (1829–1896)
Varnishing Morning at the Royal Academy
1850
Pen and Ink, 7 × 8 (17.8 × 20.3)
Mrs Warwick Tompkin
Drawn by Millais from memory immediately after returning from the first Varnishing Day. Turner stands on a box in the background. (See exh. cat., *Millais*, 1967, No.256).

B63 Sir Edwin LANDSEER (1802–1873)
Turner at the Academy c.1840
Two oil offsets on paper, approx. 6 × 5⅞ (15.1 × 15) and approx. 7 × 4⅞ (17.6 × 12.2)
One inscr: 'Sketched at the R.A. on my Palette W. M. Turner R.A. 184–0 EL'
Dr. H. Judith Milledge
In an album of the collector William Wells of Redleaf.

B64 Daniel MACLISE (1806–1870)
Noah's Sacrifice 1847
Oil on canvas, 81 × 100 (205.8 × 254)
Leeds City Arts Gallery (photograph)
Parts of the rainbow and the sheep were painted on by Turner. See also No.527.

Turner's attitude towards the institutional aspect of the art-establishment of his day was, in the main, one of conscientious devotion; he saw it as a guarantee of the interests of artists against an often hostile or indifferent public. In 1827–8 he was engaged in preventing the Academy from damaging what he saw as its long-term interests by the sale of Stock, and, outside the Academy, he was a long-serving official of the Artists' General Benevolent Institution, which had been founded in 1814, 'for the relief of Decayed Artists of the United Kingdom whose works have been known and esteemed by the public; and for affording assistance to their widows and orphans'. Turner was Chairman of the Directors and Treasurer in 1815 and a Trustee in 1818. His resignation as Chairman and Treasurer in 1829 may have been related to a growing pre-occupation with his own Charitable Institution, 'Turner's Gift . . . for the Maintainance and support of Poor and Decayed Male Artists', mentioned in his will of 1831, which was to be 'governed guided managed and directed by such rules regulations directions restrictions and management generally as other Public Charitable Institutions resembling this my present one . . .' Turner remained nominally a Trustee of the A.G.B.I. until 1839, but repeated attempts to persuade him to resume the Chair as late as 1845 proved fruitless.

B65 **Royal Academy, Minutes of the General Assembly** 9 February 1828
Royal Academy of Arts
B66 J. M. W. TURNER to George JONES
Letter dated 5 April 1828
Alan Cole, Esq.
Turner expected the matter of Stock, raised in the General Assembly on 9 February, to be discussed on 5 April, but it was not.

B67 **Artists' General Benevolent Institution, Minutes of the Stewards' Meeting**
4 June 1816
Artists' General Benevolent Institution
B68 **Artists' General Benevolent Institution, Minutes of a Special Directors' Meeting**
15 July 1829
Artists' General Benevolent Institution

Turner joined the Academy Club on becoming an Associate in 1799, and, although the presentation of silver was no more than what was expected of an Academician, this, and Farington's account of the expedition to Eel Pye Island in 1819, serve to remind us of a sociable side to Turner's nature which is too easily overlooked (see Finberg 1961, p.259f). Turner was also an original and active member of the Athenæum Club from 1824.

B69 **One of a set of Twelve Silver Dessert Spoons Presented by Turner to the Academy on his Election in 1802**
Royal Academy of Arts

B70 Joseph FARINGTON (1747–1821)
Diary 7 July 1819
Her Majesty The Queen

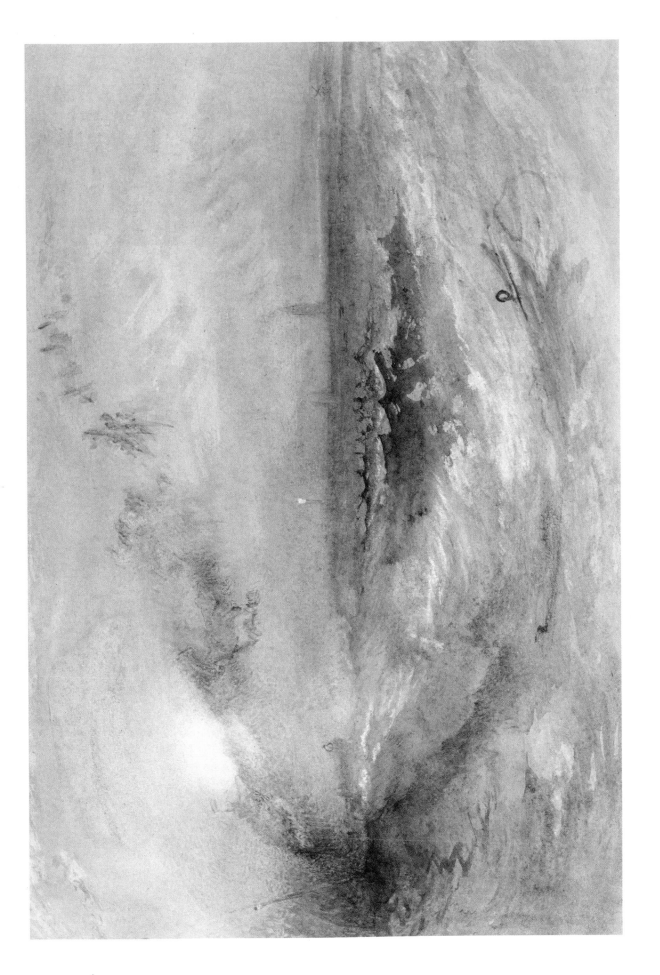

626 **Yarmouth Roads** c.1842 (entry on p.170)

650 **Norham Castle, Sunrise** c.1835-40 (entry on p.174)

TURNER'S GALLERY

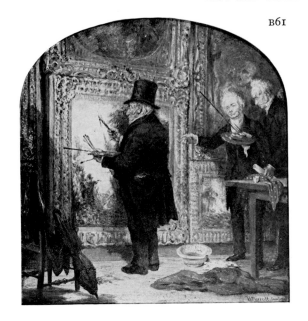

B71 Catalogue of Turner's Gallery 1810
Card, 5¼ × 3½ (13.3 × 8.9)
Private Collection
The poetic caption to 'The Fall of an Avalanche' (No.87) is the first that can be definitely attributed to Turner. (See H. Finberg, *Burlington Magazine*, XCIII, 1951, pp.383–6.)

B72 Card advertising Turner's Gallery 1814
British Library (Add MS 50118, f.41)
Turner's first private gallery in Queen Ann St West was opened in 1804 and finally closed in 1816. (See Finberg 1961, p.212.)

B73 J. M. W. TURNER
Plans and Sketches for a Second Gallery
Trustees of the British Museum (photographs)
From the 'Tabley' sketchbook No.3, T.B.C.V. ff.43 etc.

B74 George JONES
Lady Visitors in Turner's Gallery *c.*1852
Oil on Millboard, 5⅝ × 8⅞ (14.4 × 22.6)
Visitors of the Ashmolean Museum, Oxford

B75 George JONES
Turner lying in State in his Gallery,
29 December 1851 *c.*1852
Oil on Millboard, 5⅝ × 8⅞ (14.4 × 22.6)
Visitors of the Ashmolean Museum, Oxford

George Jones was an executor of Turner's will, and helped to draw up the Inventory of his work. Recognisable in these paintings are: 'Dido Building Carthage, (T.B.498), 'Hero and Leander' (T.B.521), 'Regulus' (No. 474), 'Snowstorm: Steamboat off a Harbour's Mouth' (No.504), 'Richmond Hill' (No.167), 'The Battle of Trafalgar' (No.84), 'Frosty Morning' (No.161), and 'Hannibal' (No.88). In 1848 Lucy Brightwell noticed 'The Slave Ship' (?No.518, perhaps returned from Ruskin for cleaning), 'Steam Tug' (?'Fighting Temeraire' T.B.524), 'Ship on Fire' (?No.496), '2 Whaling pictures (all white)' (cf. No.524), 'mad pictures Napoleon' ('War', cf. No.521), 'Wellington' (No.527), '& Apocalypse' (No.526) 'Crome-like sea-piece', '2 Venice &c'. (Norwich Record Office MS 69; M. Pidgeley).

B76 J. M. W. TURNER to Thomas GRIFFITH
Letter dated 1 February 1844
British Library (Add. MS 50119 f.131)
A letter complaining to his dealer of the poor condition of many works: 'the large pictures I am rather fond of tho' it is a pity they are subject to neglect and dirt', and hoping to find an assistant to help with their cleaning. (See Finberg 1961 p.397.)

B77 Turner's Paintbox, Palette, Colours, Ship
Models
Tate Gallery
See N. W. Hanson, 'Some Painting Materials of J. M. W. Turner', *Studies in Conservation*, 1954

B78 Turner's Watercolour Box and Palette
Royal Academy of Arts
See W. T. Whitley, 'Relics of Turner', *The Connoisseur* LXXXVIII, 1931, p.198.

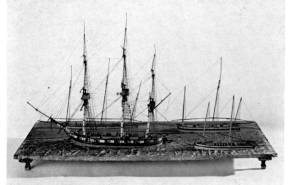

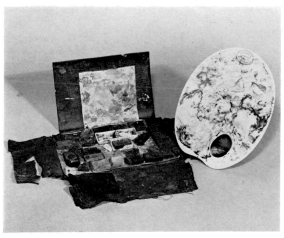

B79 John Joseph RUSKIN to John RUSKIN
Letter dated 19 February 1852
Ruskin Galleries, Bembridge School

An account of the dilapidation of Turner's Gallery and its contents at the artist's death (see J. Ruskin, *Works*, Library Edition, XIII, pp.xxvii–xxviii). Turner's second gallery seems to have been begun in 1819 and opened in 1822. Its top-lighting, diffused through blinds, and its dull red walls, made it one of the best appointed exhibition rooms in London. In the 1840s Turner would place visitors in a darkened room downstairs to make their eyes more sensitive to the dazzling light above (R. S. Owen, *The Life of R. Owen*, 1894, I, p.263), but it was in the same decade that gallery and contents suffered increasingly from neglect. (See R. Wornum, *The Turner Gallery*, 1872, pp.xiii–xiv; Gage, 1969, chapter 9.)

TRAVEL

Turner's first major tour was a journey of some three weeks through South Wales in July and August 1792. He seems to have followed an itinerary similar to that in Pennant's *Tour*, which he quoted in some sketchbooks of 1799 (T.B.XLV, XLVI). Very exceptionally, he kept a detailed diary and made his drawings on separate sheets, rather than in a sketchbook. The diary shows Turner to have been concerned with the social and historical, as well as the picturesque aspects of the Welsh scene, and the accounts of the weather show a sensitivity of vision which was not to be seen in watercolours and paintings until many years later (for an edition of the diary, see J. Gage (ed.) *Collected Correspondence of J. M. W. Turner* (forthcoming).

B80 J. M. W. TURNER
Diary of a Tour in Wales 1792
Pierpont Morgan Library, New York
B81 J. M. W. TURNER
Valle Crucis Abbey and Elisig's Pillar 1792
Pencil, 8¾ × 11 (21.4 × 28)
Trustees of the British Museum (T.B.XXI-H)

This drawing, with its Latin inscription, is referred to in the diary.

B82 Thomas PENNANT
A Tour in Wales, 1775 1781
British Library

Turner's first stimulus to the study of classical sites in Italy seems to have come from Sir Richard Colt Hoare, whom Turner met about 1796, who provided him with the model for his first classical subject-picture, the still thoroughly Wilsonian 'Lake Avernus' (No.46), and who probably sent Turner a copy of his privately printed *Hints*. But when Turner came to choose and evaluate Italian sites for use in pictures like the 'Bay of Baiae' (No.237), he drew on the ampler arguments of Eustace, who sought to interpret Classical history in modern terms. (See Gage in *Art Quarterly*, XXXVII, 1974, pp.37–48).

B83 Sir Richard Colt HOARE (1758–1838)
Lake Avernus c.1786
Pen and Wash, 14¾ × 21 (37.5 × 53.4)
The National Trust, from Stourhead

B84 H. R. C. [Richard Colt HOARE]
Hints to Travellers in Italy 1815
C. W. M. Turner, Esq.
Turner's own copy.

B85 J. C. EUSTACE
A Classical Tour of Italy 3rd ed. 1817
British Library

Although Turner painted many Italian subjects in the first two decades of the 19th century, he did not visit Italy until the late summer of 1819 (see p.86). Evidence of the seriousness with which he prepared himself for this important journey is provided by Nos. B.84, 85 and 86.

B86 M. REICHARD
Itinerary of Italy 1818
Trustees of the British Museum (T.B.CCCLXVII)
Annotated by Turner.

B87 James HAKEWILL (1778–1843)
Picturesque Tour in Italy 1818–20
British Library

James Hakewill, an architect, commissioned Turner to illustrate his *Picturesque Tour* after he had rejected drawings by John Varley, Copley Fielding and others as unsatisfactory. Turner made eighteen watercolours from pencil drawings which Hakewill had made on the spot with the aid of a camera lucida; the latter are now in the British School at Rome.

Rawlinson (vol. I, p.78) records that these sketches were sold at Christie's in 1889 and 'showed considerable powers of draughtsmanship as well as of composition; in many instances they were little modified by Turner'. A receipt dated 15 June 1818 shows that the publisher, John Murray, paid Turner 200 guineas for ten of his watercolours (see Finberg, 1961, p.253). The eighteen engraved plates are Rawlinson Nos.144 to 161.

B88 K. Brulart DE SILLERY, Comtesse de Genlis
Manuel du Voyageur 1829
C. W. M. Turner, Esq.

A popular phrase-book of English, French and Italian, annotated by Turner.

Turner had been interested in learning French as early as c.1799 (T.B.XLIV-G, XLVI), and he maintained an interest in later life (T.B.CLIX f.23ᵛ, 1817). Phrases in Dutch, German and Italian are scattered through later sketchbooks (e.g. CLIX, CLXXXVIII, CCXCVIII, CCCI, CCCVI, CCCVII).

B89 J. M. W. TURNER to James HOLWORTHY
Letter dated 7 January 1826
British Library (Add. MS 50118, ff.72–3)

The letter includes an account of the crossing of the Mont Cenis in January of 1820, on Turner's return from his first visit to Italy. The incident became the subject of the watercolour B90.

B90 J. M. W. TURNER
Snowstorm, Mont Cenis 1820
Watercolour $11\frac{1}{2} \times 15\frac{3}{4}$ (29.2 × 40)
Inscr: 'I. M. W. Turner' and 'Passage of Mt Cenis
15 Jan. 1820' b.r.
*City Museums and Art Gallery, Birmingham (by
courtesy of Mrs Dorian Williamson)*
Engraved by S. Fisher, 1833. The drawing belonged to
Walter Fawkes. The 'Return from Italy' sketchbook
(T.B.CXCII) contains pencil studies relating to Turner's
crossing of the Alps in January 1820, especially f2ᵛ
which includes the notes: 'Men clearing away snow for
the carriage. Women and Children begging – the sky
pink – the [?] light and the [?] cast shadows rather
warm – Trees are all cover [sic] with snow the trees in
the distance, and wood [?] getting darker'. The incident
was described by Turner in B89. Compare this subject
with the much larger 'Messieurs les Voyageurs . . . in
a snow drift upon Mount Tarrar' of 1829 (No.B91).

B91 J. M. W. TURNER
**Messieurs les Voyageurs on their return
from Italy par la diligence in a snow drift
upon Mount Tarrar, 22nd of January 1829**
R.A.1829
Watercolour, $21\frac{3}{8} \times 29\frac{1}{8}$ (54.5 × 74.7)
Trustees of the British Museum, Lloyd Bequest
(1958–7–12–431)
(Photograph)
Also described by Turner in a letter (see Gage, *Turner:
Rain, Steam and Speed*, 1972, pp.38–40) on Turner's
return from his second visit to Italy.

B92 **Map of the Duchy of Nassau** published by
J. Scholz, Wiesbaden
Trustees of the British Museum (T.B.CCCXLIV–425)
With pencil sketches by Turner of Bad Ems and
Wiesbaden, which Turner seems to have visited in
1817 and again about 1834 (T.B.CLIX, CCXCI(a)).

B93 **Carte Itineraire de la Bretagne** Paris
Published by Dezauche, an 8 [1800]
Trustees of the British Museum
(T.B.CCCXLIV–426)
With pencil sketches by Turner in the margins. Turner
was in Brittany in the late 1820s or early 1830s (T.B.
CCXLVI).

ENGRAVING

B94 Not exhibited

B95 **Interior View of Part of the New Premises
built for W. B. McQueen in 1832 at
184 Tottenham Court Road**
Watercolour, 17 × 28 (43 × 71)
P. N. McQueen, Esq.
This view shows one of the new iron rolling presses for
printing engraved plates. The more rigid and precise
construction, which began to replace that of the old
wooden presses from about 1810, made possible the
greater pressures necessary for the printing of the very

fine work in steel engravings.
The printer W. H. McQueen seems to have worked
first for Turner on Scott's *Provincial Antiquities* of 1819
(see No.204), and from this time he was a major printer
of the artist's engraved work, including fifteen plates of
Rogers' *Poems* (see No.B96), and the plate for the *Literary Souvenir* (B98).

B96 Samuel ROGERS
Poems 1834
British Library
For Turner's illustrations to this book see Nos.278–84.

B97 **Mezzotinted Steel Plates for 'Rivers of
England'** 1823–7
a) More Park (Rawlinson No.754) See No.240
b) Norham Castle (Rawlinson No.756) See
Nos.645 and 646
c) Dartmouth (Rawlinson No.759)
d) Stangate Creek (Rawlinson No.766)
Thomas Ross & Son
The engraver Thomas Lupton executed the first
mezzotint on steel in 1820 (see No.B43). The general
use of hardened steel as an engraving medium for book
illustration was encouraged by the activities of the bank-
note engraver Jacob Perkins in 1819. While fine lines
on copper could begin to break down after as little as 75
or 100 impressions, steel could go to 30,000 with little
sign of wear. See I. Bain, 'Thomas Ross & Son', *Journal
of the Printing Historical Society*, 2, 1966.

B98 a) **Steel Plate by E. Finden for 'Bolton
Abbey'** (Rawlinson No.315)
b) **The Literary Souvenir** 1826
Iain Bain, Esq.
A small plate of this size could take as much as thirteen
weeks to prepare. The greater part of the work was
etched with acid: on fine work particularly, the etcher's
needle, clearing lines through an acid resist, was a good
deal easier to handle than an engraver's burin cutting
directly into the hard metal.

B99 **Etching and Engraving Tools of Sir Frank
Short** 1857–1945
Victoria and Albert Museum
Sir Frank Short was an assiduous copyist of Turner's
Liber plates and engraved a number of subjects which
Turner had prepared but which remained uncom-
pleted when the impetus for the series failed.

B100 W. B. COOKE (1778–1855) after
J. M. W. TURNER
Lyme Regis 1814 (Rawlinson No.94)
Five proofs for Cooke's *Southern Coast* (see
No.168)
Trustees of the British Museum
An example of the sustained and careful attention
Turner gave to the progress of his engraved works. On
one proof Cooke has written:
> On receiving this proof, Turner expressed himself
> highly gratified – he took a piece of *white chalk* and a
> piece of *black*, giving me the option as to which he
> should touch it with. I chose the white; he then
> threw the black chalk at some distance from him.
> When done, I requested he would touch another

proof *in black*. 'No', said he, 'you have had your choice and must abide by it'.

B101 Charles TURNER (1773–1857) after J. M. W. TURNER

A Shipwreck 1806

Mezzotint, $23\frac{1}{8} \times 32$ (58.6 × 81.3); coloured by hand, probably not by Turner

Inscr: 'J. M. W. Turner Esqr R.A. pinx^t., C. Turner sculp.' and 'London Published Jany. 1. 1807. by C. Turner. No.50, Warren Street, Fitzroy Square'; 'A SHIPWRECK with Boats endeavouring to save the Crew'; 'this print is with permission engraved from the original Picture in the possession of Sir John Leicester Bar^t, to whom it his [sic] humbly Dedicated by his most ob^t. h^{ble} Servt. C. Turner.'

Trustees of the British Museum (1940–6–1–14)

Turner's painting, exhibited in 1805 (No.82) was so successful that the engraver, Charles Turner (no relation to the artist), proposed to publish a large mezzotint of the subject in an edition of 50. The resulting print (Rawlinson No.751), which was sold at 2 guineas an impression (4 guineas for proofs), was subscribed to by many of Turner's patrons and other members of the nobility and gentry, and by numerous artists, especially the younger generation. It was the first time that one of his paintings (as opposed to topographical watercolours) had been published, and considerably enhanced and spread Turner's reputation. The print may also have prompted the choice of a mezzotinter when Turner began his *Liber Studiorum* in this year. Turner reserved the right to colour late impressions himself.

B102 J. C. STADLER (fl.1780–1820) after TURNER

Ashburnham *c.* 1818

Aquatint, coloured by hand $16\frac{7}{8} \times 22\frac{7}{8}$ (42.8 × 58.1)

Inscr. below left: 'J. M. W. Turner R.A.', and right: 'I. C. Stadler sculpt', and centre: 'ASHBURNHAM'

Trustees of the British Museum (1856–10–11–102)

One of a set of four aquatints made in about 1818 by Stadler after subjects commissioned by John Fuller of Rosehill; Rawlinson Nos.822–825 (this is 823). These prints were among the very few coloured reproductions of Turner's work issued during his lifetime.

B103 A. SENEFELDER (1771–1834)

A Complete Course of Lithography 1819

C. W. M. Turner, Esq.

Turner's copy.

B104 J. M. W. TURNER

'Brighton and Arundel' Sketchbook *c.*1824

Trustees of the British Museum (T.B.CCX)

Contains several notes on lithography, some of them from B103 (see also T.B.CCXI–20, 22).

B105 James Duffield HARDING (1798–1863) after TURNER

Leeds 1823

Lithograph $11\frac{7}{8} \times 17$ (30.1 × 43.2)

Inscr. left: 'J. M. W. Turner. R.A. del'; 'J. D. Harding lithog' on right, and 'LEEDS' from a Drawing in the possession of J. Allnut Esqr.

London. Pubd. by Rodwell and Martin, New Bond Street. 1823. Printed by C. Hullmandel' below.

Trustees of the British Museum (1878–5–11–455)

From the watercolour dated 1816 (No.186). Rawlinson records that the print (Rawlinson No.833) was said to have been made for a new edition of Whitaker's *Loidis and Elmete* (a history of Leeds) first published in 1816, but there appears to be no evidence for this assertion.

About 1820 Turner was in close touch with Sir John Fleming Leicester, an early amateur of Lithography, and Charles Stokes, its early historian (see No.B142). McQueen in 1822–3 found the newly developed method of engraving 'extremely unprofitable'; and certainly Turner only allowed very few of his drawings to be reproduced by it. But as late as 1831 we find him frequenting the *conversazione* of C. J. Hullmandel, the printer of B105, where he seems to have met the chemist Faraday (E. W. Cooke, *Diary*, 18 Jan 1831 (Cooke Family Papers); Bence Jones, *Life and Letters of Faraday*, I, 1870, pp.419–20; information from M. Pidgeley: on Hullmandel in general: M. Twyman, *Lithography 1800–1850*, 1970).

TURNER'S MIND

B106 James THOMSON

'Hymn to Liberty'

in *The British Poets including Translations, in One Hundred Volumes*, Vol. XLIV, Chiswick 1822

Royal Academy of Arts

Turner first quoted from Thomson's *Seasons* in the Academy catalogue of 1798; his interest in *Liberty* dates from a rather later period, when he was much concerned with the theme of 'Ancient and Modern Italy Compared'. (See A. Livermore, 'Turner's Unknown Verse-Book', *Connoisseur Year Book*, 1957, pp.78–86, and Nos.516 and 517).

B107 J. M. W. TURNER

MS List of Academy Exhibits 1840

Harvard University, Houghton Library (Lowell Autographs)

B108 Thomas GISBORNE

Walks in a Forest

Illustrated by Sawrey Gilpin 1799

British Library

B109 Thomas BEALE

The Natural History of the Sperm Whale 1839

British Library

The 'Slavers' of 1840 (No.518) offers us a remarkable example of the richness and complexity of Turner's mental world, and of the synthesising power of his imagination. The immediate occasion for the picture was perhaps the increasing anti-slavery agitation of 1839–40, marked by the re-publication of Thomas Clarkson's *History of the Abolition of the African Slave-Trade* (which gave Turner his theme of the throwing overboard of slaves to secure the insurance) and the founding of T. F. Buxton's *Society for the Extinction of the Slave Trade and for the Civilisation of Africa*, in

1839. At the anniversary meeting of the Society in June 1840 Buxton alluded to the slave ship as 'a pestilence . . . upon the waters': 'the very shark knew the slave ship to be a bark of blood, and expected from it his daily sustenance' (*The Times*, 2 June 1840). He (and Turner) were drawing on a passage in Thomson's *Summer*, which perhaps also suggested to Turner the subject of the Typhoon. But the dense imagery of his picture, as well as the caption from the 'Fallacies of Hope' (a poem which had made its first appearance in 1812 (No.88), but which was probably never more than *ad hoc* passages to accompany specific pictures), reflect Turner's far wider-ranging curiosity on the subject of fish and sea-storms, as well as on slavery in these years. The emphasis on the predatory fish and the angry sky seems close to Gisborne, whom Turner quoted in the caption to No.519 the following year, and to Beale, whose *Natural History* he may have met around 1840 in the company of the whaling-entrepreneur Elhanan Bicknell, and whom he quoted in captions of 1845. Gisborne's *Walks*, modelled on Thomson, included in *Summer* a vigorous attack on slavery:

> See in the sable myriads of the West
> The smother'd flame of hate and vengeance fann'd
> By sighs of annual multitudes new brought
> Across the waves to misery and chains
> Burst with Etnaean rage. Behold yon isle [S. Domingo],
> Her smoking ruins mark, her crimson fields:
> Writhing in agony see every wretch
> Who bears your colour: hear their dying yells
> Proclaim to every circumjacent shore,
> An Empire raised by blood in blood shall fall.

Summer also includes an account of the migrations of shoals of herring, 'When ocean glitters like a field of gems'. Beale for his part had discussed the enormous sea-squids which attack men and which are so prominent in Turner's picture, and the typhoon after which 'the sun rose, appearing to spring out of the ocean, of a crimson hue; wild and tattered seemed the cloud which hung around him, gilded from his effulgence'. *Slavers* is the focus of an astonishingly wide range of reading.

B110 Mark AKENSIDE
'Hymn to the Naiads' in R. Anderson,
A Complete Edition of the Poets of Great Britain,
Vol.IX
C. W. M. Turner, Esq.
Turner quoted this poem in the caption to his 'Falls of the Clyde' in 1802 (cf.No.621). For his interest in Akenside's poetic ideas see J. Ziff, 'J. M. W. Turner on Poetry and Painting', *Studies in Romanticism*, III, 1964.

B111 Lord BYRON
Childe Harold's Pilgrimage: A Romaunt in Four Cantos 1819
British Library
Turner quoted 'Childe Harold' in captions to pictures several times between 1818 ('The Field of Waterloo', Tate Gallery) and 1844 ('Approach to Venice', Washington, National Gallery). In 1832, he exhibited 'Childe Harold's Pilgrimage – Italy' (Tate Gallery). See also Nos.514 and 517.

B112 Michelangelo BUONAROTTI (1574–1564)
Rime 1817
Royal Academy of Arts
Presented by Turner to the Royal Academy in 1846, perhaps to commemorate his service as Deputy President. He had looked enthusiastically at Michelangelo's work in Rome in 1819 and again in 1828 (T.B.CLXXX 1a; Finberg 1961, pp.309–10).

B113 J. M. W. TURNER
Notebook with Poems *c.*1806–10
C. W. M. Turner, Esq.
Turner's sketchbooks from about 1799 (T.B.XLIX) carry many drafts of poems, but this is the only surviving one given over to them entirely. (See J. Lindsay, *The Sunset Ship: Poems by J. M. W. Turner*, 1966.)

B114 J. M. W. TURNER
'Devonshire Coast No. 1' Sketchbook 1811
Trustees of the British Museum (T.B.CXXIII)
This book contains Turner's longest poem, which he intended should be published with his *Southern Coast* engravings (See No.168). But it was rejected by the publisher Cooke, who commissioned a journalist, William Combe, to write prose captions to the plates instead (see Gage, 1969, p.257). The poem ranged over many topics connected with the sea and with English history, and has many passages of patriotic enthusiasm for the coastal defences against Napoleon.

B115 J. M. W. TURNER
MS List of Academy Exhibits 1833
Tate Gallery
The caption to 'Mouth of the Seine' (No.491) is witness to the trouble Turner took even in prose composition.

B116 **Transactions of the Geological Society**
Vols. I–II, 1811–14
Geological Society of London
Turner owned these two volumes, which include articles on themes used in two later paintings: N. Nugent, 'An Account of "The Sulpher" or "Souffriere" of the Island of Monserrat' (Vol.I, pp.185–90; cf. No.163); J. Macculloch, 'On Staffa' (Vol.II, pp. 501–9; cf. No.490). When Turner later met Macculloch the geologist remarked on his 'clear, intelligent, piercing intellect' (Thornbury, 2nd ed. p.236). One of the closest of Turner's later friends, Charles Stokes (see No.B142), was Secretary and later Vice-President of the Geological Society of London.

B117 J. RICHARDSON
The Zoology of the Voyage of H.M.S. 'Erebus' and 'Terror' Part V, 'Fishes', 1845.
Zoological Society of London
Turner owned a copy of this report, whose plates supplied him with occasional images (cf. No.507) and the title of one of his whaling subjects of 1846: 'Hurrah! for the whaler Erebus! another fish!' (Tate Gallery 546).

B118 Joseph PRIESTLEY
History and Present State of Knowledge Relating to Vision, Light and Colours 1772
British Library

[189]

Turner took a list of the early authorities on Perspective from this book (Vol.1, pp.91–2, T.B.CIII–4a), which also gave him ideas about the phosphorescence of water and of fish.

B119 George FIELD
Chromatography 1835
Royal Academy of Arts

Turner was a subscriber to this book, although he told Field 'You have not told us too much', and later said that his ideas were fallacious. This copy was presented to the Academy by Turner's close friend, George Jones.

B120 J. W. VON GOETHE, translated by
C. L. EASTLAKE (1793–1865)
Theory of Colours 1840
C. W. M. Turner, Esq.

B121 [Sir David BREWSTER]
Review of Goethe's 'Theory', *Edinburgh
Review*, Vol.LXXII, 1840–1
National Library of Scotland

Turner's heavily annotated copy of Goethe's treatise, which had been translated by his friend Charles Lock Eastlake, shows his close engagement with the argument, which gave rise to a pair of paintings in 1843 (Nos.522–523). Eastlake may have shown the book to him, or he may have learned of it through Brewster's review, since he was an assiduous reader of the *Edinburgh Review* at the close of his life (Thornbury, 2nd ed. p.352). Brewster dismissed Goethe's arguments in terms very likely to appeal to Turner, who took a far less favourable view of the book than did Eastlake. 'Poets and painters', wrote Brewster, 'have, generally speaking, very imperfect conceptions of the force of mathematical and physical evidence. The predominance of the imagination over the judgement indisposes them for patient and profound thought. The slightest resemblances, the most fortuitous associations, are linked together as cause and effect: and even words unburdened with meaning and sentences unfreighted with thought, suggest to their fancy ideas and propositions blazing with all the lustre of truth. We are convinced indeed, that many individuals of high genius and learning are absolute sceptics regarding many of those parts of physics which so not afford the evidence of ocular or experimental demonstration' (p.124; for Turner's general treatment of Goethe, see Gage 1969, ch.11).

B122 Mary SOMERVILLE
**'On the Magnetising Powers of the More
Refrangible Solar Rays'** *Philosophical
Transactions of the Royal Society*, 1829, Vol.11
Royal Society

These experiments on the magnetising effects of the violet end of the spectrum were discussed by Turner with the photographer Mayall some years later (Gage 1969, pp.120f.). He seems to have had some direct contact with Mary Somerville around 1830, and owned her *Mechanism of the Heavens* of 1831.

B123 **Turner's Fishing Rods**
Royal Academy of Arts
Given by Mrs Booth to the dealer Vokins.

B124 W. SAY (1768–1834) after J. M. W. TURNER
Near Blair Atholl 1811 (R.30)
Etching and mezzotint, $7\frac{1}{8} \times 10\frac{7}{16}$ (18.1 × 26.5); plate $8\frac{1}{4} \times 11\frac{9}{16}$ (21 × 29.3)
Royal Academy of Arts

Issued in Part 8 of the *Liber Studiorum*, published 1 June 1811.

B125 J. M. W. TURNER
Study of a Gurnard c.1840
Watercolour and Body Colour, $7\frac{1}{2} \times 11$ (19 × 28)
Victoria and Albert Museum

(see also Nos. 269 and 271)

B126 Isaac WALTON
The Compleat Angler 1836, Vol.II
Illustrated by T. Stothard, W. Delamotte, J. Inskipp etc.
British Library

Turner describes a fishing-expedition in Wales as early as 1792 (No.B80), and he was a passionate angler all his life. But pastimes were not simply relaxation for him: as he wrote in his copy of Opie's *Lectures* about 1808, 'Every glance is a glance for study', and in 1821 the architect Cockerell, spending an evening with Turner, noted that he was 'gazing at everything & in truth always studying' (diary in the collection of Mrs Creighton). Turner's obsession with the effects of light on water is one that relates directly to his fishing, where the sun was to be kept in the face of the angler; and the delight in the opalescence of fish has its root in the same recreation. The elemental power of water, and the fragility of the may-fly and of bubbles, were themes presented to Turner in Walton's *Angler*, an edition of which was in his travelling library (Thornbury, 2nd ed. p.364): see Nos.473, 522–3 and 526.

B127 J. M. W. TURNER
The Farnley Book of Birds 1810
Nicholas Horton-Fawkes, Esq.

Turner is said to have shot most of the seventeen birds painted in this album, which was originally compiled as a series of illustrations to a scrapbook of ornithology. (See A. J. Finberg, 'Turner at Farnley Hall', *The Studio*, LV, 1912, pp.89–96.)

B128 W. B. COOKE (1778–1855) after
W. HAVELL (1782–1857)
Sandycombe Lodge 1814
From *Picturesque Views on the River Thames*
Victoria and Albert Museum

Turner bought land at Twickenham in 1807 and began building Solus Lodge (later Sandycombe Lodge) there in 1810, ostensibly to be close to the site of Reynolds' house at Richmond. He planted willows, dug a pond and stocked it with fish. Turner's father tended the garden, and it was because of his declining health that the house was sold in 1826. It was designed by Turner. (Thornbury, 2nd ed. pp.116–20; A. Livermore, 'Sandycombe Lodge', *Country Life*, 6 July 1951.)

B129 Not exhibited

FRIENDS AND PATRONS

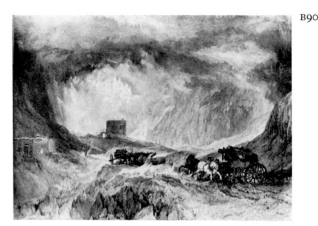

William Frederick Wells (*c.*1762–1836) was a drawing-master and watercolourist, a founder-member of the Watercolour Society in 1804. He had been introduced to Turner about 1792 and they remained close friends until Wells' death. It was at Wells' instigation that Turner began the *Liber Studiorum* (see Nos.99–112), and Wells' enthusiasm for Gainsborough (see No.B29) communicated itself to that publication. Turner was also the intimate of Wells' family, notably his daughter Clara, with whom he corresponded long after her father's death. (See J. M. Wheeler, 'W. F. Wells', *Old Water Colour Society's Club Annual*, XLVI, 1971.)

B130   W. F. WELLS (1762–1836)
The Dawn: Ruined Castle Above a River
1807
Watercolour, 20 × 28⅞ (50.9 × 71.5)
Victoria and Albert Museum

B131   J. M. W. TURNER
The Interior of a Cottage *c.*1806
Pen and black ink and watercolour, oil paint and gum on paper 10 13/16 × 14¾ (27.5 × 37.5)
Inscription on verso '103. Interior of a cottage, Kent'
Trustees of the British Museum (T.B.XCV (a)–C)

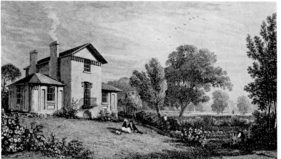

This subject may represent Wells's home at Knockholt, Kent, where Turner frequently stayed. Another cottage interior executed in precisely similar media (T.B.XCV(a)–A) is inscribed 'Wells' Kitchen, Knockholt' on the verso.

B132   **Turner's Annual Tours** 3 vols, 1832–4
Graham Pollard, Esq.
Turner's presentation copies to Wells. See p.113.

B133   J. M. W. TURNER to Clara WHEELER (née Wells)
Letter of 19 March 1829
The British Library (Add.MS 50119, f.3)
See *British Museum Quarterly*, XXII, 1960, pl.xxii.

Walter Ramsden Fawkes (1769–1825) of Farnley Hall, near Leeds, was the first of Turner's patrons to become a close personal friend. They met about 1798, and Fawkes was the most prominent buyer of the watercolours arising from Turner's first Continental Tour in 1802 (See Nos.65, 67–9). He also bought the entire set of Rhineland drawings done on the second tour in 1817 (see Nos.195–199). Turner was a frequent visitor to Farnley until Walter Fawkes' death in 1825; thereafter he never visited the place, although he remained on intimate terms with Hawksworth Fawkes throughout his life.

B134   John VARLEY (1778–1842)
Walter Fawkes *c.*1812
Pencil, 13 × 9 (33 × 22.8)
Victoria and Albert Museum (1158–1927)

B135   Walter FAWKES to J. M. W. TURNER
Letter of *c.*1815
Trustees of the British Museum (T.B.CLIV–Y).

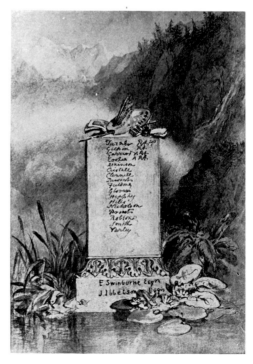

A fragment of a letter accompanying a gift of game to Turner: 'We have tormented the poor animals very much lately and now we must give them a holiday' (see No.B127).

B136 J. M. W. TURNER
Catalogue of the Fawkes Collection at 45 Grosvenor Square 1819
Nicholas Horton-Fawkes, Esq.
Fawkes' own copy, with the covers decorated in watercolour coloured by Turner. The dedication to Turner runs:
Dedication: To J. M. W. Turner, Esq. R.A. – P.P.
My Dear Sir,

The unbought and spontaneous expression of the public opinion respecting my Collection of Water Colour Drawings, decidedly points out to whom this little Catalogue should be inscribed.

To you, therefore, I dedicate it; first, as an act of duty; and, secondly, as an Offering of Friendship: for, be assured, I never can look at it without intensely feeling the delight I have experienced, during the greater part of my life, from the exercise of your talent and the pleasure of your society.

That you may year after year reap an accession of fame and fortune, is the anxious wish of
Your sincere Friend,
W. FAWKES

George O'Brian Wyndham, Third Earl of Egremont (1700–1837) was the most prodigal of Turner's patrons, purchasing some dozen oils between 1802 and 1813, when their friendship seems to have cooled, perhaps as a result of the 'Apullus' affair at the British Institution, of which Egremont was a leading official (see No.162). It was not until the late 1820s, perhaps as a result of the death of Fawkes and his reluctance to revisit Farnley, that Turner turned to Petworth for that atmosphere of easy conviviality and opportunities for working and fishing that he needed so much. In the decade up to Egremont's death he seems to have been a frequent visitor there (see Nos.325–362). The atmosphere of Turner's gouaches was vividly described by another visitor, Greville, just after Egremont's death:

[Egremont] liked to have people there who he was certain would not put him out of his way, especially those who, entering into his eccentric habits, were ready for the snatches of talk which his perpetual locomotion alone admitted of, and from whom he could gather information about passing events; but it was necessary to conform to his peculiarities, and these were utterly incompatible with conversation, or any prolonged discussion. He never remained for five minutes in the same place, and was continually oscillating between the library and his bedroom, or wandering about the enormous house in all directions: sometimes he broke off in the middle of a conversation on some subject which appeared to interest him, and disappeared, and an hour after, on a casual meeting, would resume just where had left off...

B137 Lord EGREMONT to TURNER
Letter dated 2 December 1828
E. C. and T. Griffith
Dealing with the purchase of a classical torso in Rome.

B138 **Torso Restored as Dionysius**
H.M. Treasury and the National Trust, from Petworth House (photograph)
Possibly the Torso referred to in B137, with additions by Carew (Wyndham 14).

B139 J. M. W. TURNER
The Spilt Milk *c.*1828
Watercolour, 21 × 23 (53.4 × 58.8)
The Earl of Egremont
Painted to appease Egremont's granddaughter, whose dress Turner had spoiled at breakfast.

B140 **The Deer Park, Petworth**
(Photographs)

James Holworthy (1781–1841), like Wells a founder-member of the Watercolour Society in 1804, was a close friend of Turner's between 1815 and about 1830. Some of Turner's most informal and revealing letters were written to him (see No.B89 and C. Monkhouse, 'Some Unpublished Letters by J. M. W. Turner', *Magazine of Art*, 1900, pp.400–404).

B141 James HOLWORTHY (1781–1841)
Conway Castle by Moonlight
Ink and Watercolour, 10 × 14¼ (25.4 × 36.2)
Private Collection

Charles Stokes (1785–1853) was Turner's stockbroker and a close friend in later life. He began collecting Turner's drawings in the 1820s and formed one of the most remarkable collections of *Liber Studiorum* plates and of drawings for the *Rivers of France* (see Nos.383–387). Turner appointed him an executor of his will. Stokes was an early enthusiast of lithography, an amateur geologist and an antiquary. (See L. Herrmann, *Burlington Magazine*, CXII, 1970, pp.696–9.)

B142 Mrs Dawson TURNER (1774–1850) after Sir Francis CHANTREY (1781–1842)
Charles Stokes 1821
C. W. M. Turner, Esq.
From the copy of *100 Etchings by Mrs Dawson Turner* presented by Dawson Turner to J. M. W. Turner.

B143 J. M. W. TURNER to Charles STOKES
Letter of 1 August 1851
Miss Hazel Carey
This is Turner's last recorded letter.

Turner's warmest, most brilliant and most comprehensive advocate was John Ruskin, who began his career as a critic with a long defence of Turner against Rev. John Eagles' *Blackwoods* review. Ruskin's MS was sent to Turner for approval (see Ruskin, *Works*, Library Edition, III, 635–40), but Turner dissuaded him from publishing, and the essay appeared only in 1843 as the nucleus of the first volume of *Modern Painters*. Ruskin met Turner in 1840 (*Diary*, 22 June 1840), and a warm friendship ensued. In the 1840s Turner had a conversation with a friend on Ruskin's criticism ([Mary Lloyd], *Sunny Memories*, 1880, p.34):

'Have you read *Ruskin on Me*?' I said 'No'. He replied 'but you will some day', and then he added with his own peculiar shrug, 'He sees *more* in my pictures than I ever painted!', but he seemed very much pleased

B144 Blackwood's Edinburgh Magazine, Vol.XL
October 1836
National Library of Scotland

B145 J. M. W. TURNER to John RUSKIN
Letter dated 6 October 1836
British Library (Add. MS 50119 f.101)

Joseph Gillott (1799–1873), the Birmingham pen-manufacturer, was a characteristic example of the businessman-collector-dealer who flourished in the 1840s. b) shows him buying Turner's 'Temple of Jupiter at Aegina' (Northumberland Collection) in 1843 and dealing in 'Dutch Boats', 'An avalanche' (Cat. No.87), 'Cicero's Villa' (1839, Ascott Coll.), a Van Tromp subject, 'Mercury and Argus' (1836, National Gallery of Canada), 'Shylock; the Grand Canal, Venice' (1837, The Huntington Gallery, San Marino). The story of Gillott's wooing of Turner, who was at first very reluctant to sell him anything, is given by Thornbury (2nd edition, pp.177f.). Gillott said he would barter the 'mere paper' of Birmingham Bank-notes for the 'mere canvas' of Turner, and in the event took some £5,000 worth of work away from Turner's gallery. This may be a garbled version of the trans-action documented by B.146. The appearance of the 'Mercury and Argus' in B147 suggests that another Thornbury story (pp.180ff.) about a 'Mr Dives of Liverpool' also refers to Gillott. This patron offered to buy the whole contents of Turner's Gallery for £100,000; bought the 'Mercury and Argus' and asked for a companion to be painted for it. His direct association with Turner was however short-lived, for Turner objected to his selling some pictures which had been painted on commission. Most of Gillott's acquisi-tions were through other dealers. At all events, Turner referred to Gillott in admiration as a 'Comet' in 1846, but the companion to 'Mercury' was not painted. (See *Connoisseur Year Book*, 1958, p.75.)

B146 Joseph Gillott's Cheque Book with stub for 28 January, 1845
showing a payment in cash to J. M. W. Turner of £1484.14.0
Maas Gallery

B147 Joseph Gillott's memorandum Book of Sales and Purchases of Pictures
1843–46.
Maas Gallery

DECLINING YEARS

B148 Turner's Spectacles, Watercolour Palette, Palette Knife
Visitors of the Ashmolean Museum, Oxford
These relics were collected by Ruskin. The spectacles provide evidence of Turner's failing sight (see P. D. Trevor-Roper, *The World Through Blunted Sight*, 1970, p.88).

Turner moved to Chelsea in 1846 because he wanted a studio overlooking the Thames.
The top of the house was flat, and there he would be often at daybreak watching the scenery of the river. The upper or western view he called the English view, and that down the river the Dutch view. During his last illness the weather was dull and cloudy, and he often said in a restless way, 'I should like to see the sun again'. Just before his death he was found prostrate on the floor, having tried to creep to the window, but in his feeble state had fallen in the attempt. It was pleasing to be told that at the last the sun broke through the cloudy curtain which had so long obscured its splendour, and filled the chamber of death with a glory of light' (J. W. Archer, *Once a Week*, 1 February 1862, p.166).

B149 Turner's House at Chelsea (6 Davis Place) (Photograph)
B150 James Wykeham ARCHER (1823–1904)
Turner's House at Chelsea 1852
Watercolour, 14¹¹⁄₁₆ × 10¾ (37.3 × 27.2)
Trustees of the British Museum (1874-3-14-461)
B151 J. M. W. TURNER
Sunset over Water c.1846–51
Watercolour, 10½ × 7¼ (26.8 × 18.5)
Inscr: 'Given to me by Mrs Booth August 1855. W. Bartlett 1 Bratton Terrace, Chelsea'
Sir Edmund Bacon, Bart.
A similarly inscribed drawing, in body-colour, is in the Fitzwilliam Museum, Cambridge.

B152 Turner's Will
Public Record Office, London (photograph)
Turner's estate, amounting to some £140,000, was not finally settled until 1857, and his wishes to found a single gallery of his works, and a Charitable Institu-tion, were frustrated. (See Nos.B67–8 and Finberg 1961, Ch.37.)

B153 Thomas GRIFFITH to T. T. GRIFFITH
Letter dated 5 January 1852
E. C. and T. Griffith
Turner died on 19 December 1851 and the funeral took place at St. Paul's on December 30. His dealer, Griffith (see No.B76) who was also an executor, described the scene in some detail to his son: 'You would be surprised to know the number of applications which we received from parties desirous of paying the last tribute of respect to Turner's memory . . . there was a long line of spectators five or six deep the whole way, and I believe there was not a dry eye amongst them . . .'
See also No.B75.

Chronology

1775
23 April. Joseph Mallord William Turner born at 21 Maiden Lane, Covent Garden, London, the eldest son of a barber and wig-maker.

1786
Probably went to live with his uncle at Brentford, Middlesex, in this year (see p.175).
First signed and dated drawings.

1789
Probable date of first extant sketchbook from nature made in London and the neighbourhood of his uncle's house in Sunningwell, near Oxford (the 'Oxford' sketchbook, T.B.II).
11 December. Admitted as a student of the Royal Academy Schools after a term's probation. Probably began to study with the watercolour painter of architectural subjects Thomas Malton at about the same time.

1790
First exhibit, a watercolour, at Royal Academy (No.2).

1791
September. Sketched at Bristol, Bath, Malmesbury, etc.

1792
Summer. First sketching tour in South and Central Wales.

1793
27 March. Awarded the 'Greater Silver Pallet' for landscape drawing by the Society of Arts.

1794
May. Publication of first engraving from one of his drawings.
His watercolours at the Royal Academy attract the attention of the press for the first time.
First Midland tour, largely to make drawings for engraving.
His employment in winter evenings, together with Girtin, Dayes and others, by Dr. Monro to copy drawings by J. R. Cozens and other artists, probably began in this year; it lasted for a period of three years (see Nos. B23–25).

1795
Tour in South Wales c.June–July and the Isle of Wight c.August–September, in part to execute private commissions for topographical drawings as well as for engravings.

1796
First oil painting at the Royal Academy (No.19).

1797
Exhibited two watercolours of Salisbury Cathedral, the first of nearly thirty commissions from Sir Richard Colt Hoare between now and 1805 (see No.15).
Summer. First tour in the North of England, including the Lake District.

1798
Summer. Trip to Malmesbury, Bristol and thence to North Wales.

1799
April. Recommended to Lord Elgin to make topographical drawings at Athens. Failed to agree on salary.
August–September. Stayed for three weeks with William Beckford at Fonthill (see Nos.37–9).
(?) September–October. To Lancashire and North Wales.
4 November. Elected an Associate of the Royal Academy.
November–December. Took rooms at 64 Harley Street.

1800
Some of the verses in the Royal Academy catalogue probably by Turner himself for the first time (see Nos. 43 and 48).
27 December. Turner's mother admitted to Bethlem Hospital.

1801
June–August. First tour of Scotland, returning through the Lakes.

1802
12 February. Elected a full member of the Royal Academy.
15 July–October. First visit to France and Switzerland; sketches and notes after pictures in the Louvre (see No. 91).

1804
15 April. Death of Turner's mother, probably at Bethlem Hospital.
April. Completed a gallery at 64 Harley Street for the exhibition of twenty to thirty of his own works.
Had a *pied-à-terre* on the Thames, at Sion Ferry House, Isleworth, by this year or 1805.

1806
Two oils at the first exhibition of the British Institution.
Late summer and autumn. Stayed at Knockholt, Kent, with W. F. Wells, who suggested the *Liber Studiorum* project (see p. 61).
c. October. Took a house at 6 West End, Upper Mall, Hammersmith, retaining his London home.

1807

11 June. First volume of *Liber Studiorum* published.
2 November. Elected Professor of Perspective at the Royal Academy.

1808

July (?). Stayed at Sir John Leicester's seat, Tabley Hall, Cheshire. Also sketched on the River Dee.

1809

Summer. First visit to Petworth House, the home of Lord Egremont, probably this year.

1810

Late summer. First recorded visit to Walter Fawkes of Farnley Hall, Yorkshire, repeated nearly every year till 1824.
Before 12 December. His town address changed to 47 Queen Ann Street West, round the corner from 64 Harley Street.

1811

7 January. First lecture as Professor of Painting of the Royal Academy.
July-September. Tour of Dorset, Devon, Cornwall and Somerset in connection with *The Southern Coast*, the first big series of topographical engravings to be published in book form (see No.168).
Gave up Hammersmith home, and had temporary residence at Sun Ferry House, Isleworth, while building house at Twickenham.

1812

First quotation in the Royal Academy catalogue from the 'Fallacies of Hope' (see No.88).

1813

Solus (later Sandycombe) Lodge, Twickenham, completed from his designs.
Summer. Toured Devon.

1816

July–September. Visited Farnley Hall and travelled in the north of England, in part collecting material for Whitaker's *History of Richmondshire* (see No.180).

1817

10 August–c.15 September. First visit to Belgium, the Rhine between Cologne and Mainz, and Holland. Returned September–early December via County Durham, and stayed at Farnley Hall.

1818

Commissioned to do watercolours of Italian subjects after drawings by James Hakewill for Hakewill's *Picturesque Tour in Italy* (see No.B87).
October–November. Visited Edinburgh in connection with Walter Scott's *The Provincial Antiquities of Scotland* (see No.204).

1819

March. Eight of his oils on view in Sir John Leicester's London gallery; also in subsequent years.
April–June. Sixty or more watercolours on view in Walter Fawkes' London house, and again in 1820.
August–1 February 1820. First visit to Italy: Turin Como, Venice Rome, Naples; returned from Rome via Florence, Turin and the Mont Cenis pass (see No.B90).

1820

Enlarged and transformed his Queen Ann Street house, building a new gallery 1819–21.

1821

Late summer or autumn. Visit to Paris, Rouen, Dieppe, etc.

1822

1 February–August. A number of watercolours included in exhibition organised by the publisher W. B. Cooke, and again in 1823 and 1824.
August. Visited Edinburgh for George IV's State Visit, going by sea up the east coast (see No.308).

1823

Sketched along the south-east coast.
Commissioned to paint 'The Battle of Trafalgar' for St. James' Palace; the picture was in place by May 1824.

1824

Summer and autumn. Toured east and south-east England.

1825

28 August. Set out on tour of Holland, the Rhine and Belgium.
25 October. Death of Walter Fawkes.

1826

10 August–early November. Visited the Meuse, the Moselle, Brittany and the Loire.

1827

18 June. Death of Lord de Tabley (Sir John Leicester).
Late July–September. Stayed with John Nash at East Cowes Castle, Isle of Wight, probably returning via Petworth, where he was a regular visitor until 1837.

1828

January–February. Turner's last lectures as Professor of Perspective.
August–February 1829. Second visit to Italy: Paris, Lyons, Avignon, Florence, Rome, returning via Loreto, Ancona, Bologna, Turin, Mont Cenis, Mont Tarare (see No.B91) and Lyons.

1829

Early June–18 July. About forty watercolours for the *England and Wales* engravings exhibited at the Egyptian Hall; some later shown at Birmingham.
August–early September. Visited Paris, Normandy and Brittany.
21 September. Death of Turner's father.

1830

Late August–September. Toured the Midlands.

1831

July–September. Toured Scotland, staying at Abbotsford in connection with his illustrations to Scott's poems.

1832

March. Twelve illustrations to Scott exhibited at Messrs. Moon, Boys and Graves Pall Mall; further watercolours were shown there in 1833 and 1834.

1833
August. Visited Paris; it was probably on this occasion that he went to see Delacroix.
September. Almost certainly in Venice, travelling via the Baltic, Berlin, Dresden, Prague and Vienna.

1834
Illustrations to Byron's poems exhibited at Colnaghi's.
Late July. Set off on a tour of the Meuse, Moselle and Rhine.
Winter. Four of his early oils on view at the Society of British Artists.

1836
Summer. Toured France, Switzerland and the Val d'Aosta with H. A. J. Munro of Novar.
October. Ruskin's first letter to Turner, enclosing a reply to an attack in *Blackwood's Magazine*.

1837
One oil in the British Institution 'Old Masters' Exhibition.
11 November. Death of Lord Egremont.
28 December. Resigned post of Professor of Perspective.

1840
22 June. Met Ruskin for the first time.
Early August–early October. Third visit to Venice, going via Rotterdam and the Rhine and returning through Munich and Coburg.

1841
August–October. Visited Switzerland: Lucerne, Constance and Zurich.

1842
August–October. Visited Switzerland.

1843
May. Publication of the first volume of Ruskin's *Modern Painters*, intended largely as a defence of Turner.

1844
c. August–early October. Visited Switzerland, Rheinfelden, Heidelberg and the Rhine.

1845
'Walhalla' shown at the 'Congress of European Art' at Munich.
May. Short visit to Boulogne and neighbourhood.
14 July. As eldest Academician was chosen to carry out duties of President during Shee's illness.
September–October. Visit to Dieppe and the coast of Picardy (his last trip abroad).

1846
Last firm date for a finished watercolour (see No.616).
Took a cottage on the corner of Cremorne Road and Cheyne Walk, Chelsea, at about this time.

1848
January. One painting hung in the National Gallery to represent the Vernon Gift (No.532).

1851
No works at the Royal Academy.
19 December. Died at his cottage, 119 Cheyne Walk, Chelsea. Buried at St. Paul's on 30 December.

Select Bibliography

Including Publications referred to in Abbreviated Form in the Catalogue Entries

John Ruskin, *Modern Painters*, 5 vols. 1843–60, reprinted in *Library Edition*, edited by E. T. Cook and Alexander Wedderburn, vols.III–VII, 1903–5.

John Burnet, *Turner and his Works*, with a 'Memoir' by Peter Cunningham, 1852; 2nd ed. 1859.

John Ruskin, *Notes on the Turner Gallery at Marlborough House 1856*, 1857; *Library Edition*, vol.XIII, 1904.

Walter Thornbury, *The Life of J. M. W. Turner R.A.*, 2 vols., 1862; 2nd ed. in one volume, 1876.

C. F. Bell, *A List of the Works contributed to Public Exhibitions by J. M. W. Turner, R.A.*, 1901.

Sir Walter Armstrong, *Turner*, 1902.

W. G. Rawlinson, *The Engraved Work of J. M. W. Turner, R.A.*, 2 vols., 1908 and 1913.

A. J. Finberg, *Complete Inventory of the Drawings of the Turner Bequest*, 2 vols., 1909.

A. J. Finberg, *Turner's Sketches and Drawings*, 1910; paperback reissue with an introduction by Lawrence Gowing, 1968.

A. J. Finberg, *Turner's Water-Colours at Farnley Hall*, n.d. (1912).

D. S. MacColl, *National Gallery, Millbank: Catalogue; Turner Collection*, 1920.

A. J. Finberg, *The History of Turner's Liber Studiorum with a New Catalogue Raisonné*, 1924; this retains the numbering of W. G. Rawlinson's *Turner's Liber Studiorum*, 1878.

A. J. Finberg, *In Venice with Turner*, 1930.

A. J. Finberg, *The Life of J. M. W. Turner, R.A.*, 1939; 2nd edition 1961.

Martin Davies, *National Gallery Catalogues: The British School*, 1946.

Martin Butlin, *Turner Watercolours*, 1962 and subsequent editions.

Adrian Stokes, 'The Art of Turner (1775–1851)', in *Painting and the Inner World*, 1963.

Jerrold Ziff, 'Turner and Poussin', in *Burlington Magazine*, vol.CV, 1963, pp. 215–21.

Jerrold Ziff, ' "Backgrounds, Introduction of Architecture and Landscape": a Lecture' in *Journal of the Warburg and Courtauld Institutes*, vol.XXVI, 1963, pp. 124–47.

Michael Kitson, *Turner*, 1964.

John Rothenstein and Martin Butlin, *Turner*, 1964.

John Gage, 'Turner and the Picturesque', in *Burlington Magazine*, vol.CVII, 1965, pp. 16–26, 75–81.

Lawrence Gowing, *Turner: Imagination and Reality*, 1966.

Jack Lindsay, *J. M. W. Turner, His Life and Work*, 1966.

John Gage, 'Turner's Academic Friendships: C. L. Eastlake', in *Burlington Magazine*, vol.CX, 1968, pp. 677–85.

Gerald Finley, 'Turner: an Early Experiment with Colour Theory', in *Journal of the Warburg and Courtauld Institutes*, vol.XXX, 1967, pp. 357–66.

Luke Herrmann, *Ruskin and Turner*, 1968.

John Gage, *Colour in Turner*, 1969.

Graham Reynolds, *Turner*, 1969.

Graham Reynolds, 'Turner and East Cowes Castle', in *Victoria and Albert Museum Yearbook*, vol.I, 1969, pp. 67–79.

Hardy George, 'Turner in Venice', in *Art Quarterly*, vol.LIII, 1971, pp. 84–7.

Gerald Wilkinson, *Turner's Early Sketchbooks*, 1972.

Gerald Finley, 'Turner's Colour and Optics: a "New Route" in 1822', in *Journal of the Warburg and Courtauld Institutes*, vol.XXXVI, 1973, pp.385–90.

A. G. H. Bachrach, *Turner and Rotterdam 1817, 1825, 1841*, 1974.

John Gage, 'Turner and Stourhead: The Making of a Classicist?', in *Art Quarterly*, vol.XXXVII, 1974, pp. 29–52.

Gerald Wilkinson, *The Sketches of Turner R.A., 1802–20*, 1974.

List of Lenders

Her Majesty The Queen   B70

Abbot Hall Art Gallery, Kendal   67
Aberdeen Art Gallery   13, 613
Lady Agnew   15, 127, 431
Thos. Agnew & Sons Ltd   74, 506
Artists' General Benevolent Institution   B67–8
Ashmolean Museum, Oxford   40, 185, 269, 384–7,
   552–4, 592, B10, B74–5, B148.
Lord Astor of Hever   490

Sir Edmund Bacon, Bart.   51, 265, 438–9, 589, 637, B151
Iain Bain   B98
Bembridge School, Ruskin Galleries   B79
City Museums & Art Gallery, Birmingham   179, 427,
   B90
Boston Museum of Fine Arts   518
British Library   B57–8, B72, B76, B82, B85, B87, B89,
   B96, B108–9, B111, B118, B126, B133, B145
British Museum   1, 3–9, 11–12, 14, 17–18, 22–6, 29,
   41, 43–4, 49, 50, 52–60, 62, 64, 66, 89–99, 101, 104,
   109–11, 114–26, 128–30, 168, 170, 172, 174–8, 182–3,
   187–8, 200–204, 207–35, 239–56, 259–64, 266–8,
   270–84, 287, 295–8, 300–306, 340–73, 375–82,
   388–422, 429, 432, 436, 440–65, 467–9, 498–500,
   540–50, 556–66, 575–82, 584–7, 593–600, 602, 604–6,
   609–10, 614, 617–18, 627–36, 638–9, 641–2, 644–9,
   B2–3, B13, B17–18, B33, B41, B43–4, B47–8, B54,
   B59, B81, B86, B92–3, B100–102, B104–5, B114, B131,
   B135, B150.
Bury Public Library, Art Gallery & Museum   508

Miss Hazel Carey   B143
Art Institute of Chicago   567
Alan Cole   B66
William A. Coolidge   309
Corcoran Gallery of Art, Washington   79
Courtauld Institute of Art   B31, B51
Mrs William Crabtree   113

Simon Day   181

Earl of Egremont   B139

Mrs M. D. Fergusson   293–4, 623
Brinsley Ford   B40

Gainsborough House Society, Sudbury   B29
Geological Society of London   B116
Christopher Gibbs Ltd   78
Major General E. H. Goulburn   153
E. C. and T. Griffith   B137, B153

Guildhall Library and Art Gallery   171
Fundaçao Calouste Gulbenkian, Lisbon   83, 173, 491

Earl of Harewood   27–8, 31–2
Harvard University, Houghton Library, Cambridge,
   Mass.   B107
Cecil Higgins Art Gallery, Bedford   194
Nicholas Horton-Fawkes   189–92, B127, B136
Hounslow Library Services   B7

Indianapolis Museum of Art   2, 70, 195, 206, 321

Dr F. J. G. Jefferiss   B19, B21

Mrs C. G. Keith   591

Leeds City Art Galleries   38, 193, 199, 299
Leger Galleries Ltd   69, B25
Lt Col J. L. B. Leicester-Warren   150
Levens Hall Collection   B45
Lady Lever Art Gallery, Port Sunlight   169, 205, 257,
   426, 607, 621, 626
University of Liverpool   163, 433
Musée du Louvre, Paris   620
C. L. Loyd   131, 159

Maas Gallery   B146–7
Manchester City Art Gallery   288, 292, 423–4, 588
Manning Galleries Ltd   B23
P. N. McQueen   B95
Mr & Mrs Paul Mellon   65, 184, 186, 619
Lt Col Sir George Meyrick   142
Dr H. Judith Milledge   B63
G. K. Monro   B20

National Gallery, London   75, 482
National Gallery of Scotland, Edinburgh   158
National Gallery of Victoria, Melbourne   132, 568,
   603
National Gallery of Art, Washington   310, 513, 533
National Library of Scotland, Edinburgh   B121, B144
National Maritime Museum   B34
National Museum of Wales, Cardiff   16, 197, 323–4
National Portrait Gallery   B9
National Trust   47, 72, 80, 149, 151, 331, B83
Castle Museum, Norwich   B32

Mr and Mrs Kurt F. Pantzer   430, 616
Philadelphia Museum of Art   512
Pierpont Morgan Library, New York   B80
Brian Pilkington   428, 466
Graham Pollard   B132